Diseases, Complications, and Drug Therapy in Obstetrics

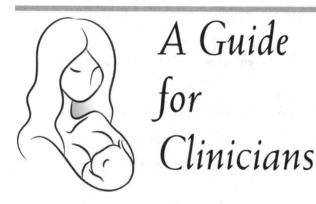

A Guide for Clinicians

Editors

Gerald G. Briggs, BPharm, FCCP
Pharmacist Clinical Specialist
MemorialCare Center for Women
Miller Children's Hospital
Long Beach Memorial Medical Center
Long Beach, California
Clinical Professor of Pharmacy
University of California, San Francisco
Adjunct Professor of Pharmacy Practice
University of Southern California, Los Angeles

Michael P. Nageotte, MD
Perinatologist
Associate Chief Medical Officer
MemorialCare Center for Women
Miller Children's Hospital
Long Beach Memorial Medical Center
Long Beach, California
Professor
Department of Obstetrics / Gynecology
University of California, Irvine

American Society of Health-System Pharmacists®
Bethesda, Maryland

Any correspondence regarding this publication should be sent to the publisher, American Society of Health-System Pharmacists, 7272 Wisconsin Avenue, Bethesda, MD 20814, attention: Special Publishing.

The information presented herein reflects the opinions of the contributors and advisors. It should not be interpreted as an official policy of ASHP or as an endorsement of any product.

Because of ongoing research and improvements in technology, the information and its applications contained in this text are constantly evolving and are subject to the professional judgment and interpretation of the practitioner due to the uniqueness of a clinical situation. The editors, contributors, and ASHP have made reasonable efforts to ensure the accuracy and appropriateness of the information presented in this document. However, any user of this information is advised that the editors, contributors, advisors, and ASHP are not responsible for the continued currency of the information, for any errors or omissions, and/or for any consequences arising from the use of the information in the document in any and all practice settings. Any reader of this document is cautioned that ASHP makes no representation, guarantee, or warranty, express or implied, as to the accuracy and appropriateness of the information contained in this document and specifically disclaims any liability to any party for the accuracy and/or completeness of the material or for any damages arising out of the use or non-use of any of the information contained in this document.

Director, Special Publishing: Jack Bruggeman
Acquisitions Editor: Rebecca Olson
Senior Editorial Project Manager: Dana Battaglia
Production Editor: Melissa Jones, Silverchair Science + Communications, Inc.
Page Design: David Wade
Cover Design: DeVall Advertising
Composition: Silverchair Science + Communications, Inc.

Library of Congress Cataloging-in-Publication Data

Diseases, complications, and drug therapy in obstetrics : a guide for clinicians / editors, Gerald G. Briggs, Michael P. Nageotte.

    p. ; cm.
 Includes bibliographical references and index.
 ISBN 978-1-58528-202-9
 1. Obstetrical pharmacology. I. Briggs, Gerald G. II. Nageotte, Michael P. III. American Society of Health-System Pharmacists.

  [DNLM: 1. Pregnancy Complications--drug therapy. 2. Embryo, Mammalian--drug effects. 3. Fetus--drug effects. 4. Lactation--drug effects. 5. Pregnancy--drug effects. WQ 240 D6116 2009]

 RG528.D57 2009
 618.3--dc22

                              2009015782

ISBN: 978-1-58528-202-9

Foreword

William E. Smith, PharmD, MPH, PhD, FASHP
Executive Associate Dean, Professor of Pharmacy
School of Pharmacy, Virginia Commonwealth University
Medical College of Virginia Campus, Richmond, Virginia

This book is the result of many years of collaboration between pharmacists, physicians, and nurses in the care of obstetric patients and drugs affecting the fetus and newborn. Pharmacists in the clinical care of pregnant obstetric patients started at a few medical centers in the late 1960s and early 1970s. Today, with the possible exception of pharmacist services in labor/delivery, the pharmacy profession still has little involvement with pregnant patients, especially in the pharmacotherapeutic care of pregnant women with chronic disease and infections. There is an unmet demand for pharmacy services in the care of these patients. Moreover, there are numerous opportunities to work with maternal-fetal medicine physicians (a subspecialty of obstetrics that cares for high-risk pregnancies) in clinical research involving the drug therapy of pregnant or breastfeeding women.

The text provides an organized compilation of subject matter that can be used in the teaching of obstetric pharmacotherapy to pharmacy students and pharmacists. Knowledge of the physiology and diseases/complications unique to pregnancy is a prerequisite to understanding why drug therapy for the pregnant patient is markedly different from that of the nonpregnant patient. The arrangement of the book provides a good first step toward that knowledge and understanding. It also raises an important question to pharmacy educators and practitioners: What services are needed to increase the protection of the pregnant patient and fetus in acute, ambulatory, and community-based pharmacy services? Hopefully, the answer to the question will catalyze the teaching of medication use in pregnant patients and newborns in the curriculums of pharmacy schools and will spur the interest of pharmacist practitioners. If this occurs, significant changes in the types and quantity of pharmacist clinical services for pregnant patients and newborns in acute and ambulatory care settings can occur.

An important feature of this text is the interprofessional relationship that has developed over the years between the editors. Gerald Briggs has been consistent and persistent in his pursuit over three decades to improve the quality of drug use in the pregnant patient to protect the fetus and newborn. He has provided clinical care to these patients, developed drug therapy guidelines, conducted research, published, and freely given his time to teach physicians, nurses, pharmacists, residents, and students.

Dr. Michael Nageotte, a superb maternal-fetal medicine physician, has assembled a highly proficient group of maternal fetal medicine physicians, labor and delivery nurses, clinical pharmacists, and other health professionals. Under his leadership, the combined efforts of this group consistently achieve extraordinary outcomes in complicated pregnancies. Their well-earned reputation has made the MemorialCare Center for Women at Long Beach Memorial Medical Center a major referral hospital for high-risk pregnancies.

The book also reflects the relationships that have developed over the years between the editors and contributors. Many of the contributors are recognized leaders in their fields. From their knowledge and clinical experience, the quality and safety of patient care have increased significantly. Their efforts to prepare and publish this textbook will benefit the care received by many more obstetric patients and newborns in the future.

Foreword

Roger K. Freeman, MD
Associate Medical Director for Women's Services
MemorialCare Center for Women
Miller Children's Hospital
Long Beach Memorial Medical Center
Long Beach, California
Clinical Professor of Obstetrics and Gynecology
University of California, Irvine

Those who participate in the obstetric care of a pregnant patient are challenged with making sure that their actions are beneficial to the mother and fetus-newborn. The use of drugs in the pregnant patient may be directed at the mother, fetus, or both. Only in pregnancy and lactation can a drug administered to one patient have a direct beneficial or detrimental effect on another being. It is for this reason that practitioners involved with pregnant and/or lactating patients must be constantly vigilant when using drugs.

Certainly there are instances in which a drug may be beneficial to both mother and fetus either directly or indirectly (eg, anti-infectives, anticonvulsants). In other circumstances a drug administered to the mother may have untoward effects on the fetus (eg, cancer chemotherapy), and drugs administered for the benefit of the fetus may have detrimental effects on the mother (eg, digoxin for treatment of fetal supraventricular tachycardia). These strategies must be undertaken with consideration for the risks. However, there are inevitably going to be instances in which there are currently unknown effects that may be detrimental to mother or fetus when treatment is directed at one or the other.

This text is aimed at educating obstetric caregivers, including physicians, pharmacists, and nurses, in the use of drugs in pregnancy. However, an equally important goal is to increase awareness of over-the-counter drugs to which patients have access. The use of such drugs is frequently unknown by the practitioner, which increases the need for obstetric caregivers to inquire about a patient's self-administered substances, both legal and illegal.

In recent years, clinical pharmacists have become increasingly pro-active in counseling patients about the drugs prescribed for them, as well as inquiring about other drugs a patient may be taking. At our hospital, clinical pharmacists are always present

v

on maternal-fetal medicine patient care rounds, and they have become much more involved in monitoring and managing the drug therapy of pregnant women with complicated conditions. This responsibility includes both hospitalized patients and ambulatory care. It is because of this increased involvement that this text is focused on pharmacists, as well as physicians and nurses who comprise the team that maximizes both safety and efficacy when drugs are used in pregnancy.

Preface

The concept for this book emerged in 2005. In our collective memories, there has always been a close working relationship between physicians and nurses and pharmacists in the MemorialCare Center for Women at Long Beach Memorial Medical Center. This professional relationship has played a major role in helping to make Women's a premier center for the care of both routine and high-risk pregnancies. Thus, it is in our best interest to assist in the training of these health care professionals for the care of obstetric patients. All nurses receive some training in obstetrics during their academic years. This has made the transition of new nurses into obstetrics an easier task.

However, such is not the case with pharmacists. For pharmacists, the absence of any training in obstetrics during their 4 years of formal postgraduate education makes such a transition a daunting journey, which can take many months to years before an acceptable level of competence is reached. It is encouraging that a number of pharmacy students come to Women's every year for an introduction to obstetrics. Their time with us is brief, but the students' feelings of accomplishment are universal in that they leave with an initial understanding and appreciation of this discipline. It is rewarding to observe these students progress from just "learning the language of Obstetrics" to becoming fledgling clinicians. Provided with the right opportunity, many of these students will become clinical pharmacists who have the ability to make outstanding contributions in the care of pregnant and lactating women. This book is one step of assistance toward making that opportunity a reality.

We are grateful for the 32 contributors who captured the essence of their topics. They covered complex subjects in a way that is easily understood, in spite of the restrictions of space and time. Each of the chapters could be expanded to many times their current size if all of the available information was included. Their ability to condense and select pertinent information and to present it in a meaningful way that promotes understanding is, in our opinion, a major accomplishment. We sincerely appreciate what they have done and thank them for their efforts.

Gerald G. Briggs, BPharm, FCCP
Pharmacist Clinical Specialist
MemorialCare Center for Women
Miller Children's Hospital
Long Beach Memorial Medical Center
Long Beach, California
Clinical Professor of Pharmacy
University of California, San Francisco
Adjunct Professor of Pharmacy Practice
University of Southern California, Los Angeles

Michael P. Nageotte, MD
Perinatologist
Associate Chief Medical Officer
MemorialCare Center for Women
Miller Children's Hospital
Long Beach Memorial Medical Center
Long Beach, California
Professor
Department of Obstetrics/Gynecology
University of California, Irvine

Contents

Section III. Treatment of Chronic Diseases in Pregnancy

Contributors

Peter J. Ambrose, PharmD, FASHP
Professor of Clinical Pharmacy
Vice Chair, Department of Clinical Pharmacy
School of Pharmacy
University of California, San Francisco

Philip O. Anderson, PharmD, FASHP
Clinical Professor of Pharmacy
Skaggs School of Pharmacy and Pharmaceutical Sciences
University of California, San Diego

Tamerou Asrat, MD
Director of Maternal Fetal Medicine
Hoag Memorial Hospital Presbyterian, Women's Pavilion
Newport Beach, California
Staff Perinatologist
MemorialCare Center for Women
Miller Children's Hospital
Long Beach Memorial Medical Center
Long Beach, California
Clinical Associate Professor
Division of Maternal Fetal Medicine
Department of Obstetrics/Gynecology
University of California, Irvine

Anjan S. Batra, MD
Assistant Professor of Pediatrics
University of California, Irvine
Director of Electrophysiology
Children's Hospital of Orange County
Orange, California

Kathleen M. Berkowitz, MD
Regional Medical Director, Sweet Success Region 6.1
Clinical Associate Professor
Division of Maternal Fetal Medicine
Department of Obstetrics/Gynecology
University of California, Irvine

Annette E. Bombrys, DO
Division of Maternal Fetal Medicine
Department of Obstetrics and Gynecology
University of Cincinnati
Cincinnati, Ohio

Gerald G. Briggs, BPharm, FCCP
Pharmacist Clinical Specialist
MemorialCare Center for Women
Miller Children's Hospital
Long Beach Memorial Medical Center
Long Beach, California
Clinical Professor of Pharmacy
University of California, San Francisco
Adjunct Professor of Pharmacy Practice
University of Southern California, Los Angeles

Eliza Chakravarty, MD, MS
Assistant Professor of Medicine
Division of Immunology and Rheumatology
Stanford University School of Medicine
Palo Alto, California

Stephanie R. Chao, PharmD, BCPS, CDE
Senior Manager of Clinical Pharmacy
Hoag Memorial Hospital Presbyterian
Newport Beach, California
Assistant Clinical Professor of Pharmacy
University of California, San Francisco

Christina Chambers, PhD, MPH
Associate Professor
Departments of Pediatrics, Family and Preventive Medicine
University of California, San Diego

John P. Elliott, MD
Director, Division of Maternal Fetal Medicine
Banner Good Samaritan Medical Center
Phoenix, Arizona
Clinical Professor
Department of Obstetrics/Gynecology
College of Medicine
University of Arizona, Tucson

Michael R. Foley, MD
Medical Director for Academic Affairs
Scottsdale Healthcare
Scottsdale, Arizona
Clinical Professor
Division of Maternal Fetal Medicine
Department of Obstetrics and Gynecology
College of Medicine
University of Arizona, Tucson

Wendy Abe Fukushima, PharmD, FCSHP
Women's Health Clinical Pharmacist
Hoag Memorial Hospital Presbyterian
Newport Beach, California

Anna M. Galyean, MD
Maternal Fetal Medicine
Magella Medical Group
Newport Beach, California

Mounira Habli, MD
Clinical Instructor
Division of Maternal Fetal Medicine
Department of Obstetrics and Gynecology
University of Cincinnati
Cincinnati, Ohio

Michael Haydon, MD
Assistant Clinical Professor
Division of Maternal Fetal Medicine
Department of Obstetrics and Gynecology
University of California, Irvine

Leslie Hendeles, PharmD
Professor
School of Pharmacy and Department of Pediatrics
University of Florida, Gainesville

Julie J. Kelsey, PharmD
Clinical Pharmacy Specialist, Women's Health
University of Virginia Health System
Department of Pharmacy Services
Charlottesville, Virginia

Carl W. Kildoo, PharmD
Director
Pharmacy Department
City of Hope
Duarte, California

Gideon Koren, MD, FRCPC, FACMT
Director, The Motherisk Program
The Hospital for Sick Children,
Professor of Pediatrics, Pharmacology, Pharmacy and Medical Genetics
The University of Toronto
Professor of Medicine, Pediatrics and Physiology/Pharmacology
    and the Ivey Chair in Molecular Toxicology
The University of Western Ontario
Toronto, Ontario, Canada

David Lagrew, Jr., MD
Medical Director, Women's Hospital
Saddleback Memorial Medical Center
Laguna Hills, California
Clinical Professor
Division of Maternal Fetal Medicine
Department of Obstetrics/Gynecology
University of California, Irvine

David F. Lewis, MD, MBA
Professor and Vice-Chair
Fellowship Program Director
Division of Maternal Fetal Medicine
Department of Obstetrics and Gynecology
University of Cincinnati
Cincinnati, Ohio

John-Charles Loo, MD
Pediatric Cardiology
Southern California Permanente Medical Group
Bellflower, California
Volunteer Clinical Faculty
University of California, Irvine

David L. Lourwood, PharmD, BCPS, FCCP
Clinical Pharmacy Specialist
Department of Pharmacy Services
Popular Bluff Regional Medical Center
Adjunct Clinical Associate Professor of Pharmacy Practice
University of Missouri-Kansas City
Adjunct Clinical Assistant Professor of Pharmacy Practice
St. Louis College of Pharmacy
University of Arkansas for Medical Sciences

Jennifer McNulty, MD
Maternal Fetal Medicine
Magella Medical Group
Long Beach, California

Michael P. Nageotte, MD
Perinatologist
Associate Chief Medical Officer
MemorialCare Center for Women
Miller Children's Hospital
Long Beach Memorial Medical Center
Long Beach, California
Professor
Department of Obstetrics/Gynecology
University of California, Irvine

Lisa O'Brien, MS, PhD(c)
Graduate Student
University of Toronto
Division of Clinical Pharmacology and Toxicology
The Hospital for Sick Children
Toronto, Ontario, Canada

Dee Quinn, MS, CGC
Director, Arizona Teratology Information Program
Executive Director, OTIS
College of Pharmacy
University of Arizona, Tucson

Michael Schatz, MD, MS
Chief, Allergy Department
Kaiser Permanente Medical Center
San Diego, California

Julie Scott, MD
Clinical Assistant
Division of Maternal Fetal Medicine
Department of Obstetrics and Gynecology
College of Medicine
University of Arizona, Tucson

Craig V. Towers, MD
Maternal Fetal Medicine
Huntington Beach, California

Kimey Ung, PharmD, BCPS
Pharmacist Clinical Specialist
MemorialCare Center for Women
Miller Children's Hospital
Long Beach Memorial Medical Center
Long Beach, California

Patricia R. Wigle, PharmD, BCPS
Assistant Professor
Clinical Pharmacy Practice
College of Pharmacy
University of Cincinnati
Cincinnati, Ohio

Elizabeth Yi, PharmD
Pharmacist Clinical Specialist
MemorialCare Center for Women
Miller Children's Hospital
Long Beach Memorial Medical Center
Long Beach, California

Reviewers

Kathryn J. Drennan, MD
Wayne State University
Detroit, Michigan

Lea S. Eiland, PharmD, BCPS
Auburn University Harrison School of Pharmacy
Huntsville, Alabama

Ruth A. Lawrence, MD, FABM, FAAP
Professor of Pediatrics and Obstetrics/Gynecology
Director of Breastfeeding and Human Lactation Study Center
University of Rochester School of Medicine
Rochester, New York

Donald R. Mattison, MD, CAPT, US Public Health Service
Senior Advisor to the Director of NICHD
Eunice Kennedy Shriver National Institute of Child Health and
    Human Development
National Institutes of Health
Bethesda, Maryland

Edward J. Quilligan, MD
Professor Emeritus of Obstetrics and Gynecology
University of California, Irvine
Director of Medical Education
Long Beach Memorial/Miller Children's Hospital
Long Beach, California

Susan Scott Ricci, ARNP, MSN, MEd
University of Central Florida Nursing faculty
Orlando, Florida

Introduction

Gerald G. Briggs and Michael P. Nageotte

In 2006, approximately 4,300,000 babies were born in the United States and slightly over 350,000 in Canada. Although the majority of the births resulted in full-term, normal, healthy newborns, a significant number were premature or involved infants with structural birth defects. Additionally, a significant number of pregnancies had major complications or ended in abortions, either spontaneous or elective. Thus, although it is easy to overlook, pregnancy is a condition that can result in both good and poor outcomes.

Regardless of the eventual outcome, drug therapy is very common in pregnancy. There are many complications that are unique to pregnancy, and nearly all are treated with drugs. Furthermore, there are many chronic diseases that predate pregnancy and require continued drug treatment during gestation. Appropriate drug therapy is usually beneficial for the mother and the developing infant, but it can adversely affect the pregnancy and the newborn, as well as the nursing infant if continued after delivery. In order to obtain optimal pregnancy outcomes, the treatment of unique complications and chronic diseases requires clinicians with specific knowledge of obstetrics. Because drugs are used so commonly during pregnancy and lactation, pharmacists providing services to women of reproductive potential also require knowledge of obstetrics. Ideally, an introduction to obstetrics should be included in the pharmacy curriculum. The purpose of this book is to help meet that goal.

This book is primarily about drug therapy in pregnancy and, to a lesser extent, during lactation. It is critical to understand that treatment of the mother in either of these conditions potentially involves exposure of at least one other unintended patient: the embryo, fetus, or nursing infant. Clinicians must have access to references to estimate the risk of the therapy to these other "patients." The various chapters in this book will assist them in meeting this obligation. However, because the pharmacologic therapy of pregnant women is undergoing continuous change, no single source, including this book, will have all of the published reports or even cover all of the drugs. Thus, in addition to this book, we recommend a reference library that contains several other sources, such as those listed below (arranged alphabetically):

Books

- Briggs GG, Freeman RK, Yaffe SJ. *Drugs in Pregnancy and Lactation. A Reference Guide to Fetal and Neonatal Risk.* 8th ed. Philadelphia: Lippincott, Williams & Wilkins, 2008.

- Hale T. *Medications and Mothers' Milk*. 13th ed. Amarillo, TX: Pharmasoft Medical Publishing, 2008.
- Koren G. *Medication Safety in Pregnancy and Breastfeeding*. New York: McGraw-Hill, 2007.
- Schaefer C, Peters P, Miller RK. *Drugs during Pregnancy and Lactation*. 2nd ed. London, UK: Academic Press, 2007.
- Schardein JL. *Chemically Induced Birth Defects*. 3rd ed. New York: Marcel Dekker, 2000.
- Shepard TH, Lemire RJ. *Catalog of Teratogenic Agents*. 12th ed. Baltimore: The Johns Hopkins University Press, 2007.

Online or Telephone

- LactMed, an online service of the National Library of Medicine. Available at: http://toxnet.nlm.nih.gov/cgi-bin/sis/htmlgen?LACT.
- Organization of Teratology Information Specialists (OTIS). Available at: http://otispregnancy.org (free counseling on exposures during pregnancy and lactation for patients and healthcare professionals; toll free 866-626-OTIS).
- REPRORISK system: A commercially-available CD-ROM that contains electronic versions of REPROTEXT, REPROTOX, Shepard's Catalog, and TERIS. The system is available from http://www.micromedex.com/products/reprorisk.

There are three sections in this book: General Considerations in Pregnancy and Lactation, Complications Unique to Pregnancy, and Treatment of Chronic Diseases in Pregnancy.

The first section covers the physiological changes that occur in every pregnancy, as well as drug-induced developmental toxicity, drug exposure during breastfeeding, pregnancy-induced changes in pharmacokinetics, over-the-counter drugs in pregnancy, and risk communication. The focus of the latter chapter is on methods of communicating risks to patients so that it is done with current information and an understanding of counseling aspects. If risk communication is done properly, it can provide a significant measure of protection from medical liability for pharmacists working with pregnant patients.

Complications unique to pregnancy are covered in the second section. Preterm labor and delivery, fetal lung immaturity, gestational hypertension, preeclampsia and eclampsia, preterm rupture of the membranes, fetal cardiac arrhythmias, labor induction, fetal cardiac arrhythmias, and complications of the placenta are examples of complications that only occur in pregnancy. Also included is a chapter on how safe and effective pain control during child birth can be achieved. This is important because for many women child birth will be the most painful experience in their life. Additionally, there is a critical need to correctly recognize and treat postpartum hemorrhage. This condition has a high potential for maternal morbidity and mortality and is a leading cause of maternal death in the period immediately after delivery.

Section III addresses the treatment of chronic diseases and other disorders in pregnancy. The diseases and disorders covered are diabetes mellitus, infections, nausea and vomiting of pregnancy, chronic hypertension, depression, asthma, epilepsy, two autoimmune disorders, thromboembolic disorders, and thyroid disease. Obviously, there are many more diseases that could have been discussed, but these are the most common in pregnancy. In each case, their treatment is complicated by the fact that at least one, and sometimes more, unintended patients are always present, the embryo(s) and/or fetus(es). Furthermore, the effects of a disease on the embryo-fetus are often much more severe than on the mother; diabetes mellitus is an excellent example. In other cases, there may be no proven benefit for the mother or the fetus from treatment, such as in mild chronic hypertension. In these situations, treatment may result only in risk. An understanding of the pregnant state, in addition to the disease pathology, is critical to achieving optimal pregnancy outcomes.

In addition to the editors, there are 32 contributors to the book. We have been very fortunate to obtain their assistance. We believe that their quick acceptance of our invitations to contribute was due to their recognition of the need for this book. All are clinicians and have special knowledge involving the treatment of pregnant women. Many are considered to be leading authorities on their subjects. In spite of their busy schedules, they have done very well in capturing the essence of their topics.

In our dual roles as editors and contributors, we hope this book will fulfill its purpose. If it does, we believe that pregnancy will be safer with improved outcomes for women everywhere.

SECTION *1*
General Considerations in Pregnancy and Lactation

Physiologic Changes in Pregnancy

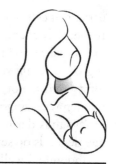

Michael P. Nageotte

LEARNING OBJECTIVES

1. Describe how the human placenta is structured as well as how it functions during fetal development.

2. State the different stages of development from fertilization to embryo formation.

3. Summarize the marked changes in maternal organ systems from the very early stages of pregnancy.

4. Describe the effects of maternal position on changes in vital signs, cardiac output, and uterine blood flow.

I. Introduction

By convention, pregnancy dating is based on the patient's last normal menstrual period. The duration of normal human pregnancy is approximately 280 days from the first day of the last normal menses. For women with regular, 28-day menstrual cycles, the expected date of delivery can be calculated using Naegele's rule. This is accomplished by adding 7 days to the date of the first day of the last menstrual period and counting back 3 months. For example, if the first day of the last menstrual period was June 6, then the expected date of delivery would be March 13. This establishes the due date or expected date of confinement. While it is biologically evident that pregnancy does not commence before ovulation (approximately 14 days after the onset of menses), gestational age remains the accepted nomenclature for clinicians and it actually includes the first 2 weeks before ovulation and conception. It is very important to maintain consistency in pregnancy dating and pharmacists should also employ Naegele's rule for dating pregnancy. Of note, certain investigators, such as embryologists, often employ fertilization ovulatory age and are consequently 2 weeks shorter in their stated pregnancy dating calculations.

Pregnancy is further divided into trimesters each of approximately 3 calendar months. The division is made by using 42 weeks, the maximum duration of a normal pregnancy, so that each trimester lasts for a total of 14 completed weeks. However, using trimesters as dating techniques is often both imprecise and inappropriate. The reader is encouraged to refer to pregnancy dating using weeks of gestation from last menstrual period rather than calculated trimester. Commonly, either to confirm dating or to establish dating accurately, ultrasound is employed. While routine use of ultrasound is not recommended in low-risk pregnancies, it is increasingly used for women receiving prenatal care. Indeed, the majority of women receive one or more ultrasounds during such care. The accuracy of ultrasound in establishing gestational age depends on several factors. These include the patient size, habitus, and presence of abdominal wall scarring. Most important, however, is the point in pregnancy at which the ultrasound is performed. When performed in the first 13 weeks of pregnancy, ultrasound is accurate for establishing dating within 7 days or fewer. This accuracy progressively decreases with advancing gestation, and re-dating of pregnancy using ultrasound later in gestation should be done with caution. The correct dating of any pregnancy is of critical importance in the counseling and management of any patient.

II. Fetal Development Terminology

With successful fertilization of the ovum by a single spermatozoa, the resulting cell is called the *zygote*. With cleavage of the zygote by mitosis, two daughter cells result and are called *blastomeres*. These cells subsequently divide and develop into a ball-like shape, which is termed a *morula* once 16 blastomeres are formed. The morula is what first enters the uterine cavity after a period of time in the fallopian tube. Shortly thereafter, the morula develops a fluid-filled cavity and is then termed a *blastocyst*. The inner cell mass of the blastocyst comprises the embryo-forming cells. With appearance of the bilaminar disc, the *embryo* is present. Eight weeks after fertilization or 10 weeks after the onset of the last menstrual period, the embryonic period ends and the further changing conceptus is termed the *fetus*. The tissues of the fetus, placenta, membranes, and other tissue, both embryonic and extra-embryonic, that result from initial zygote development are termed the *conceptus*.[1]

III. Preimplantation Conceptus

Human conception occurs in the distal fallopian tube with the presence of sperm necessarily preceding ovulation for fertilization to occur. The zygote and then morula reside in the tubal ampulla for approximately 80 hours after ovulation, then traverses the isthmic portion of the tube for 10 hours and subsequently enters the uterine cavity as the blastocyst. Over 2–3 days while floating in the endometrial cavity, the embryo develops from the blastocyst. Implantation occurs over the subsequent 2–5 days before the hormone human chorionic gonadotropin is detected in maternal serum. Implantation is thought to be a random event, although the presence of uterine scarring in the lower uterine segment as well as increased parity is associated with an increased risk for placenta previa (abnormal implanted placenta in the lower uterine segment rather than in the uterine fundus), which can place the woman at risk for hemorrhage.

IV. Placenta in Early Pregnancy

The outer cellular layers of the early embryo differentiate into the cytotrophoblasts and syncytiotrophoblasts. The syncytiotrophoblasts are the main source of placental steroid and protein hormone synthesis.[2] The syncytiotrophoblasts line the space between the placenta and the maternal inner surface of the uterus. This is called the *intervillous space* and the distal placental villi are directly exposed to maternal blood within this space. Additionally, throughout gestation there is maternal steroid and protein biosynthesis occurring in the decidualized endometrium, which lines the inner surface of the uterine cavity. Such activity is thought to be critical in the protection of the pregnancy from immunologic rejection by the host as well as critical to subsequent events unique to pregnancy, including the initiation and completion of parturition.[3] Of note, the distribution of such production of steroid and protein is not uniform throughout the uterus, with a significant degree of activity occurring within the lower uterine segment particularly with advancing gestational age.[4]

V. Placenta in Late Pregnancy

As the pregnancy enters the second and third trimesters, the placenta continues to undergo important changes. The placenta functions more as the interface for feto-maternal exchange and less that of critical hormone production and secretion. However, the hormonal production role of the placenta continues throughout pregnancy. The density of the fetal capillaries increases, cytotrophoblastic cells are fewer, and the syncytial layer becomes markedly attenuated. Such changes further facilitate transport of compounds which would not have occurred earlier in gestation, at least not to the same degree.[5] However, the fetus has dramatically changed from the first trimester and in certain ways is less at risk from exposures as organogenesis is essentially completed. Nonetheless, although structural abnormalities may not occur or not be identifiable, the potential for more subtle effects on the rapidly developing fetus should not be overlooked. Fetal organs continue to grow at different rates throughout pregnancy and well into the pediatric time period. As an example, brain growth is rapidly occurring in both the second and third trimesters, but continues to occur well after birth.

VI. Fetal Circulation

Deoxygenated fetal blood flows in the two umbilical arteries away from the fetus and toward the placenta within the umbilical cord. Once entering the placenta, these vessels repeatedly branch over the placental surface ultimately ending in fetal capillaries in the terminal villi, which are bathed by maternal blood in the above described intervillous space. Blood returns from the placenta to the fetus through the single umbilical vein within the umbilical cord with a higher level of oxygenation and nutrients after maternal exchange. This forward flow of fetal blood in the umbilical arteries is constant and maintained by the fetal heart, blood pressure, and diminished resistance to flow within the placental vasculature, normally continuing throughout both systole and diastole.[6] Such flow may be interrupted or intermittently reversed when there are changes in the vascular resistance within the placenta. In such circumstances, there is an increased risk for adverse perinatal outcome. Blood returning to the fetus is not pulsatile but essentially that of venous flow. Such flow can be interrupted by compression of the umbilical cord.

The fetus is totally dependent on the maternal circulation being maintained through the intervillous space. Maternal blood enters this space in spurts from terminal arterioles in the myometrium, driven by pulsatile maternal blood pressure. Of note, flow into and out of this intervillous space may be interrupted by maternal position, hypotension, or uterine contractions that constrict the spiral arteries feeding the space as well as the veins that drain this space as a result of the contracting myometrium temporarily obliterating blood flow in the vessels within the uterine wall.

Maternal blood actually exits these distal arterioles entering the intervillous space and directly bathes the fetal cells of the syncytiotrophoblasts lining the placental trophoblastic villi. It is important to understand that fetal blood is always contained within fetal capillaries in the placental villi and normally does not mix directly with maternal blood. Thus, the human placenta is a hemochorial placenta. Although fetal blood, DNA, and RNA are readily found in the maternal blood from early in pregnancy, when a significant transfusion of blood from the fetus into the mother occurs, sensitization of the mother may result if appropriate preventive measures are not taken. Such an event can have profound effects on subsequent pregnancies.

VII. Placental Transfer

In the hemochorioendothelial human placenta, maternal blood and solutes remain separated from fetal blood by trophoblastic tissues and the fetal endothelial cells lining the fetal capillaries. As a result, transit from the maternal intervillous space to the fetal capillary lumen occurs across a number of different cellular structures. The first step is transport across the microvillus plasma membrane of the syncytiotrophoblast. All maternal solutes first interact with the placenta at this plasma membrane. The cytotrophoblast cells are discontinuous, particularly in later gestation, and are unlikely a barrier to transit of solutes between mother and fetus. The basal lamina within the interface has a glycoprotein backbone containing anionic sites, which influence movement of large charged molecules. This is an important mechanism which essentially prevents the movement of such molecules from the maternal to the fetal circulation. The fetal capillary endothelial cells impose additional plasma membrane surfaces, which are traversed by molecules passing through cells into the lumen of fetal capillaries. From there, these molecules are carried through the umbilical vein to the fetus.

VIII. Mechanisms of Transit Across Placental Membranes

Solutes which lack specialized transport mechanisms may cross the placental barrier by extracellular or transcellular diffusional transport pathways. Permeability is determined by size, lipid solubility, ionic charge, and maternal serum protein binding. Such a mechanism is called *passive diffusion*. Up to a molecular weight of 5000 dalton, the permeability of the placenta is proportional to the free diffusion of a molecule in water. Thus, small solute transfer is controlled primarily by the maternal-fetal concentration gradient. Such transfer is further impacted by lipid solubility. Highly lipid soluble substances (termed *lipophilic*) readily diffuse across the trophoblasts while lipid insoluble (termed *hydrophilic*) substances must cross through extracellular pores between the trophoblastic cells. Such transfer is restricted by both the molecular weight of the substance and the surface area for diffusion. In fact, lipid solubility is a more important factor than molecular weight in determining solute diffusion across the uteroplacental interfaces. The functional surface area and placental blood perfusion are critical to this process as well. In addition, both active transport and facilitated diffusion occur within the placenta and utilize specific transport systems with active transport requiring energy. Thus, multiple mechanisms of transport are at work throughout gestation at the critical interface of fetal cells and maternal blood within the intervillous space and provide for the complex dynamic process of nutrient and gas exchange required for successful pregnancy. Such mechanisms are used to varying degrees at different stages of pregnancy and are dependent on a healthy, functioning placenta.

IX. Maternal Physiologic Changes of Pregnancy

A. Blood Volume

There is a marked increase in maternal blood volume during pregnancy. While the degree of change varies, the average increase at term from prepregnancy is 40%–45%.[7] It is thought that such expansion occurs due to the demands of increased uterine blood flow, to accommodate for impaired venous blood return during erect and supine positions and to compensate for the expected blood loss with delivery. This change in blood volume begins in the first trimester, increases further in the second trimester, and slowly increases again in the third trimester. There is an increase in both plasma and red blood cell volume with a relatively greater increase in plasma volume.[8] This commonly results in a decrease in the concentration of hemoglobin and a fall in hematocrit (physiologic anemia of pregnancy). Maternal iron stores will be rapidly depleted in response to fetal needs as well as from this attempted increase in red blood cell mass unless adequate iron intake is maintained. Such depletion of iron stores is more profound in pregnancies complicated by multiple gestation, bleeding, or preexisting iron deficiency. Appropriate prevention in the form of oral iron replacement is part of routine prenatal care. More aggressive replacement with intravenous iron is a most effective way of restoring adequate iron to treat anemia.

B. Cardiovascular Changes

Remarkable changes of the maternal heart and circulation occur from the very early stages of pregnancy (Table 1). By the fifth week of gestation, cardiac output is increased, resulting from a slight elevation in heart rate accompanied by a more significant decrease in systemic vascular resistance. As a consequence of these changes along with the expansion of blood volume, cardiac output is markedly elevated. This change in preload is thought to be the primary driver of the increase in cardiac output.[9] Vascular capacity increases as well, particularly on the venous side. These

Table 1. Hemodynamic Changes in Pregnancy

	Pregnancy	Intrapartum	Postpartum
Plasma volume	↑	↑	↓↓
Red blood cell mass	↑↑	↑	↓↓
Systolic blood pressure	↓	—	—
Diastolic blood pressure	↓	—	—
Systemic vascular resistance	↓	↓	↑
Heart rate	—	↑	↓
Stroke volume	↑	↑	↑
Cardiac output	↑	↑↑	↑

changes all work in concert to adjust to the significant increasing demands of the growing fetus. The fetus depends on a constant supply of maternal oxygen and nutrients by way of uterine blood flow and placental perfusion, which, in turn, will only occur with the maintenance of cardiovascular stability in the mother in the setting of all these profound hemodynamic changes. These are significant adjustments that may tax women with underlying congenital or acquired heart disease. On occasion, a patient may become symptomatic during pregnancy for the first time due to a previously undiagnosed cardiac abnormality, with the typical time for such manifestation of cardiac decompensation being in the mid- to late second trimester (20–28 weeks).

The baseline maternal pulse increases by approximately 10 beats/min. Other than a lateral movement in the cardiac electric axis due to rotation of the apex of the heart, there are no specific changes in the maternal electrocardiogram. However, benign supraventricular arrhythmias are not uncommon during pregnancy. As mentioned, cardiac output at rest increases throughout pregnancy. In the supine position, particularly in the late second and third trimesters, the cardiac output may decrease markedly and result in changes in maternal vital signs, symptoms of hypotension, and decreased uterine blood flow resulting in changes in the fetal heart rate.[10] Cardiac output can generally be maintained with the patient in the lateral recumbent position. The ability of the pregnant patient to respond to the demands of moderate or severe exercise is limited with advancing gestational age and it is important to be able to distinguish symptoms of fatigue, palpitations, light-headedness, or shortness of breath due to normal pregnancy changes from those symptoms due to underlying cardiac pathology (Table 2).

Maternal blood pressure changes during pregnancy as well, with a general decrease from prepregnancy levels. Both systolic and diastolic pressures decrease with a greater decline in the diastolic values. These changes reach their lowest levels in the second trimester and subsequently increase slightly. Blood pressure in pregnancy is most affected by maternal position and should be regularly measured with the patient sitting, having her right arm flexed and relaxed at the level of her heart. An appreciation for these dramatic changes that occur in normal pregnancy is of critical importance to be able to correctly diagnose and manage specific complaints and findings of patients. Complaints of fatigue, shortness of breath, chest pain, and irregular heart

Table 2. Central Hemodynamic Changes with Normal Term Pregnancy [Measured by Cardiac Catheterization]

	Pregnant (mean ± SD)	Postpartum (mean ± SD)	% Change	p
Cardiac output (L/min)	6.2 ± 1.0	4.3 ± 0.9	−43	.0003
Heart rate (bpm)	83 ± 1.0	71.0 ± 10.0	−17	.015
Systemic vascular resistance (dyne/cm/s^5)	1210 ± 266	1530 ± 520	−21	NS
Pulmonary vascular resistance (dyne/cm/s^5)	78 ± 22	119 ± 47	+34	.02
Colloid oncotic pressure (mmHg)	18.0 ± 1.5	20.8 ± 1.0	+14	NS
Central venous pressure (mmHg)	3.6 ± 2.5	3.7 ± 2.6	+3	NS
Pulmonary capillary wedge pressure (mmHg)	7.5 ± 1.8	6.3 ± 2.1	−19	NS
Left ventricular stroke work index (g/m/m^2)	48 ± 6	41 ± 8	−17	.04

NS = not studied, SD = standard deviation.

rhythms are classically associated with underlying cardiac pathology, but commonly occur in completely normal pregnancies.

C. Pulmonary Changes

Although there is little change in the respiratory rate in pregnancy, significant increases do occur in important respiratory functions, including tidal volume, minute ventilatory volume, and oxygen uptake.[11] As a result of elevation of the diaphragm secondary to the enlarging uterus as well as this increase in tidal volume, the functional residual capacity and residual air volume in the lungs are decreased. The partial pressure of carbon dioxide in maternal blood normally decreases also as a result of the increase in tidal volume. Dyspnea is a common complaint during pregnancy and is thought to be primarily a result of the hormone progesterone stimulating the central respiratory center. Care should be taken in correct response to respiratory complaints of pregnant patients. Women with underlying respiratory diseases, such as asthma or pneumonia, may be significantly compromised by the pregnant condition. Continued aggressive asthma care should not change during pregnancy and the appropriate choice of pneumonia antibiotic therapy is not affected by the pregnant state. Similarly, patients need not alter their asthma medications and should closely monitor their symptoms and pulmonary function throughout pregnancy.

D. Urinary Tract Changes

The kidneys change in size and function during pregnancy. Kidneys enlarge slightly while both glomerular filtration rate and renal plasma flow increase markedly. Creatinine clearance normally increases during pregnancy even in women with pre-existing renal disease. Glucosuria is not necessarily an abnormal finding while proteinuria or hematuria are not normal during pregnancy and need further evaluation.[12] Collection of urine to assess protein loss and renal function is often done in pregnancy. However, the accuracy and reproducibility of such testing may be problematic.

The specific mechanisms responsible for these alterations in renal hemodynamics during pregnancy are not completely known. The dramatic increase in renal blood flow and concordant increase in glomerular filtration rate (GFR) result primarily from reduced renal vascular resistance.[13] These changes in renal blood flow begin in very early pregnancy and to some degree precede the changes in both blood volume and cardiac output. The increase in GFR is noted as early as 6 weeks' gestation and increases by 50% over nonpregnant values by the end of the first trimester.[14] While renal plasma flow (RPF) increases more than glomerular filtration, the RPF does decline somewhat toward the end of pregnancy while the GFR remains elevated. As a result, creatinine clearance increases during pregnancy (from 110 to 150 mL/min).[15] Such vascular changes are thought to result from both prostaglandin and hormonal influences throughout gestation.

E. Gastrointestinal Tract Changes

While the intraperitoneal organs are displaced by normal pregnancy, both hormonal and mechanical factors are thought to be responsible for the delayed gastric emptying and transit times in the small and large intestines particularly during labor.[16] Constipation during pregnancy is a common complaint and is exacerbated by medications such as iron supplementation. An appreciation for changes in physical examination of the pregnant women is important in correct diagnosis of abdominal pathology. As one example, women with acute appendicitis are often misdiagnosed during pregnancy for many reasons. One is the finding that with displacement of the distal ileum secondary to the enlarging uterus, the classic physical finding of appendicitis may change or disappear. Another is the symptoms are often nonspecific and the etiology of the complaints may not be due to actual pathology. Correct diagnosis of such conditions remains a clinical challenge in spite of newer imaging and diagnostic technologies. In fact, most women with acute appendicitis during pregnancy present with typical right lower quadrant pain.[17] Careful clinical assessment and frequent monitoring along with appropriate imaging and laboratory testing is necessary in the management of abdominal pain complicating pregnancy.

Taste is often altered in pregnancy as is appetite. Gastric secretion is reduced and gastric emptying may be delayed. Heartburn, also called pyrosis, is a common complaint and likely results from the reflux of stomach acid into the esophagus. This is the consequence of the increased abdominal pressure from the enlarging uterus as well as relaxation of the gastroesophageal sphincter secondary to hormonal changes. The entire gastrointestinal tract has reduced motility, leading to the common complaint of a sensation of bloating and constipation. Nausea and vomiting are also common, affecting more than 50% of pregnant women in early gestation. For some women, nausea and vomiting continue well beyond the typical abatement at completion of the first trimester and such complaints may persist throughout the pregnancy. When severe and associated with weight loss, dehydration, and electrolyte abnormalities, a diagnosis of hyperemesis gravidarum may be made. This is a condition that requires specialized and aggressive treatment with a high likelihood of recurrence in both the current and subsequent pregnancies.[18] Various protocols for management are used in efforts to control the all too common problem of nausea and vomiting complicating pregnancy.

F. Metabolism Changes

Pregnancy is associated in every patient with changes in body shape and size. As the fetus and placenta continue to grow there are increasing demands on the maternal metabolism to adjust appropriately. Weight gain normally results from the pregnant state in women who are not otherwise morbidly obese prior to conception. It is not necessarily a problem if the obese pregnant patient gains little or no weight or actually experiences weight loss during pregnancy. This is not commonly associated with any adverse effects on fetal growth or development. Indeed, the actual correlation between specific weight gain and pregnancy outcome in a population that is not nutritionally deprived is difficult to establish.[19]

Maternal weight gain is not simply the result of the enlarging uterus and its contents. In addition, breast tissue increases as does the extracellular and intravascular volume of blood, water, and lymph throughout the body. Increases in maternal stores of cellular water occur along with fat and protein deposition. The average weight gain in pregnancy is 25–30 pounds (11.4–13.6 kilograms) with wide variations reported.[20] Although frequently a concern, absolute nutritional deficiencies are rare for pregnancies that occur in developed countries. Nonetheless, supplementation of a balanced diet with a daily multivitamin that contains folic acid, 0.4 mg, and iron is recommended for all women before as well as during pregnancy.[21] More recently, an epidemic of obesity in our population has been noted and plays a serious role in complications of pregnancy. This epidemic presents challenges at every level of care and is a serious issue in the prenatal, intrapartum, and postpartum stages of pregnancy.

G. Hepatic Changes

Some hepatic functions are affected by pregnancy. Overall serum albumin concentration declines, but albumin binding is unchanged and the total amount of albumin is normally maintained. Cholestasis is frequently documented and may cause symptoms of pruritus and findings of jaundice. Cholelithiasis is increased during pregnancy and surgical management of acute gallbladder pathology is a common consideration during pregnancy. Total alkaline phosphatase serum level essentially doubles in pregnancy but this is primarily the heat-stable isozyme produced by the placenta. Bilirubin and hepatic enzymes are slightly lower during pregnancy normally.[22] Patients with chronic hepatitis generally tolerate pregnancy well. Understanding of the potential risks for vertical transmission (ie, from mother to baby) is an important consideration for women positive for hepatitis B or hepatitis C.

H. Coagulation Changes

Levels of several coagulation factors change during normal pregnancy. Fibrinogen (factor I) levels increase markedly as do those of clotting factors VII, VIII, IX, X, and XII. Other plasma factors and platelets do not change to a great degree. Plasminogen levels increase in parallel with fibrinogen, thus maintaining an equilibrium of clotting and lysing activity. Overall fibrinolytic activity decreases during pregnancy. The concentration of certain endogenous anticoagulants falls during pregnancy. Included are both antithrombin III and factor S. Essentially, there is a shift in pregnancy toward an increased risk of venous thromboembolism from these changes, which is only further enhanced with stasis, immobilization, surgery, or other occurrences common in pregnancy and in the period of time after delivery. Thromboembolism remains one of the leading causes of maternal death in developed countries. In the United States, the relative risk of venous thromboembolism among women who are either pregnant or postpartum is 4.3 with an overall incidence of 200 cases per 100,000 woman years.[23] The risk of a first episode of venous thromboembolism is five times as high in the postpartum period compared with during pregnancy and the risk of pulmonary embolism is 15 times higher in the postpartum period compared with during pregnancy.[24]

X. Summary

Pregnancy presents dramatic change and challenge to essentially every organ system of the human body. It is of critical importance for both patient and health care provider to have an understanding of these issues so as to know what is normal and what is potentially pathologic. Further, an appreciation for these physiologic changes with consideration of the specific gestational age of the pregnancy is also of paramount importance. Pharmacists play a very important role in the provision of appropriate information, counsel, and care to women before, during, and after pregnancy. Only with an understanding of these various dynamic issues is it possible to provide the type of care these women deserve.

XI. References

1. Moore KL. *The Developing Human: Clinically Oriented Embryology*. 4th ed. Philadelphia: Saunders, 1988:8–14.
2. Bernirschke K, Kaufman P. *Pathology of the Human Placenta*. 4th ed. New York: Springer, 2000:50–76.
3. Johnson PM, Christmas SE, Vince GS. Immunological aspects of implantation and implantation failure. *Hum Reprod*. 1999;14(suppl 2):26–36.
4. MacDonald PC, Casey ML. Preterm birth. *Sci Am*. 1996;3:42–44.
5. Morriss FH Jr, Boyd RDH, Manhendren D. Placental transport. In Knobli E, Neill J, eds. *The Physiology of Reproduction*. Vol 2. New York: Raven, 1994:813–861.
6. Rudolph AM, Heymann MA. The fetal circulation. *Annu Rev Med*. 1968;19:195–202.
7. Whittaker PG, MacPhail S, Lind T. Serial hematologic changes and pregnancy outcome. *Obstet Gynecol*. 1966;88:33–39.
8. Pritchard JA. Changes in the blood volume during pregnancy and delivery. *Anesthesiology*. 1965;26:393–399.
9. Ueland K, Metcalfe J. Circulatory changes in pregnancy. *Clin Obstet Gynecol*. 1975;19:41–47.

10. Clark SL, Cotton DB, Lee W, et al. Central hemodynamic assessment of normal term pregnancy. *Am J Obstet Gynecol.* 1989;161:1439–1442.

11. Hankins GDV, Clark SL, Uckan E, et al. Maternal oxygen transport variables during the third trimester of normal pregnancy. *Am J Obstet Gynecol.* 1999;180:406–409.

12. Hytten FE, Leitch I. *The Physiology of Human Pregnancy.* 2nd ed. Philadelphia: Davis, 1971:50–54.

13. Dunlap W. Serial changes in renal hemodynamics during normal human pregnancy. *Br J Obstet Gynaecol.* 1981;88:1–8.

14. Davison JM, Dunlap W. Changes in renal hemodynamics and tubular function induced by normal human pregnancy. *Semin Nephrol.* 1984;4:198–202.

15. Kalousek G, Hlavecek C, Nedoss B. Circadian rhythms of creatinine and electrolyte excretion in healthy pregnant women. *Am J Obstet Gynecol.* 1969;103:856–861.

16. Macfie AG, Magides AP, Richmond MN, et al. Gastric emptying in pregnancy. *Br J Anaesth.* 1991;67:54–58.

17. Mourad J, Elliott JP, Erickson L, et al. Appendicitis in pregnancy: new information that contradicts long-held clinical beliefs. *Am J Obstet Gynecol.* 2000;185:1027–1029.

18. Nageotte MP, Briggs GG, Towers CV, et al. Droperidol and diphenhydramine in the management of hyperemesis gravidarum. *Am J Obstet Gynecol.* 1996;174:1801–1805.

19. Feig DS, Naylor DC. Eating for two: are guidelines for weight gain during pregnancy too liberal? *Lancet.* 1998;351:1054–1058.

20. Parker JD, Abrams B. Prenatal weight gain advice: an examination of the recent prenatal weight gain recommendations of the Institute of Medicine. *Obstet Gynecol.* 1992;79:664–667.

21. Centers for Disease Control and Prevention. Knowledge and use of folic acid by women of childbearing age—United States 1995 and 1998. *MMWR Morb Mortal Wkly Rep.* 1999;48:325–327.

22. Girling JC, Dow E, Smith JH. Liver function tests in pre-eclampsia: importance of comparison with a reference range derived for normal pregnancy. *Br J Obstet Gynaecol.* 1997;104:1215–1216.

23. Heit JA, Kobbervig CE, James AH, et al. Trends in the incidence of venous thromboembolism during pregnancy or postpartum: a 30 year study. *Ann Intern Med.* 2005;143:697–706.

24. Tapson VF. Acute pulmonary embolism. *N Engl J Med.* 2008;358;1037–1052.

QUESTIONS AND ANSWERS

1. Fertilization in the human:

   a. occurs in the distal fallopian tube only when ovulation precedes intercourse.

   b. occurs in the uterus with arrival of the egg after ovulation.

c. occurs in the distal fallopian tube only when ovulation follows intercourse.

d. commonly occurs outside the fallopian tube with transport of the embryo into the uterus subsequently.

2. Cardiac output in the pregnant woman:

a. is very resistant to various pharmacologic agents otherwise used to increase cardiac performance.

b. can be drastically changed in late pregnancy by maternal position.

c. does not measurably increase until completion of the first trimester.

d. does not increase in pregnancy in a patient with congenital heart disease.

3. During pregnancy, changes in gastrointestinal function include all of the following except:

a. delayed gastric emptying.

b. increased esophageal reflux.

c. more frequent episodes of appendicitis.

d. constipation, exacerbated by iron supplementation.

4. After fertilization in the distal fallopian tube, the correct sequence in the development of the embryo is:

a. zygote - blastocyst - morula - embryo.

b. blastocyst - morula - zygote - embryo.

c. zygote - morula - blastocyst - embryo.

d. blastocyst - zygote - morula - embryo.

5. In the placenta, the primary source of steroid and hormone production is in the:

a. cytotrophoblasts.

b. intervillous space.

c. syncytiotrophoblasts.

d. decidualized endometrium.

Answers:

1. a; 2. b; 3. c; 4. c; 5. c

Developmental Toxicity and Drugs

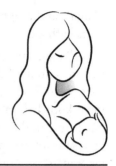

Gerald G. Briggs

LEARNING OBJECTIVES

1. State the estimated risk of congenital anomalies to a human embryo using only animal reproduction data.

2. Identify a drug known to cause developmental toxicity but needed by the mother, and outline a treatment plan that represents the lowest risk to the embryo and/or fetus.

3. Summarize the elements of developmental toxicity.

4. Describe the functions that can be employed by pharmacists to reduce the probability of developmental toxicity.

I. Introduction

Pregnancy usually results in a normal, healthy newborn but, sometimes, it is marred by the birth of an infant with a major birth defect or with other aspects of developmental toxicity. Birth defects (ie, structural anomalies) combined with deformations and chromosomal abnormalities are a leading cause of neonatal and postnatal deaths.[1] As upsetting as these outcomes can be, structural anomalies are only one aspect of abnormal development. Other aspects include growth restriction, functional-neurobehavioral deficits, and death. Collectively, these four elements are called developmental toxicity, which, in turn, is part of a larger category, reproductive toxicity.[2,3]

There are at least three misconceptions regarding the toxic effects of drugs in pregnancy. Contrary to popular belief, most birth defects are not caused by drugs. However, drug-induced and drug-deficient defects are the only birth defects that might be preventable. The latter category includes undertreatment of some diseases (eg, diabetes mellitus) and a deficiency of folic acid. A second misconception is that teratogenic drugs can cause all types of birth defects, when, in reality, defects are confined to a group of malformations that often are referred to as a syndrome (a cluster of birth defects commonly seen together).[4] The belief that drugs can only cause birth defects in the first trimester is a third misconception.[5] Drugs can cause all aspects of developmental toxicity, including birth defects, throughout gestation, from preimplantation through delivery. The only requirement is that a teratogenic exposure coincides with a critical development event.

All clinicians providing services to women of reproductive potential have a role in the prevention of drug-induced developmental toxicity. However, as a group, pharmacists are the health care professionals most accessible to the general public and the most knowledgeable about drugs. As such, the pharmacy profession should play a major role in the prevention of developmental toxicity by acting as a guardian against exposures of pregnant women to harmful drugs. Moreover, a knowledgeable pharmacist can act as a resource to provide critical information on exposures, both therapeutic and abusive, to women of reproductive age, which increases the probability of a healthy outcome. Preventing drug-induced birth defects or any type of developmental toxicity can result in a marked decrease in the significant emotional and economic cost associated with these outcomes.

Pharmacists have several critical functions in the prevention of developmental toxicity from drugs and chemicals. First, screening the therapy of women of reproductive age for drugs that are known or suspected of causing developmental toxicity is paramount. Second, pharmacists should be able to provide pregnant women or those who might become pregnant, and other health care professionals, with information for interpreting experimental animal reproduction tests, especially when there is only limited human pregnancy experience. Third, pharmacists should help ensure that women of reproductive age are taking adequate vitamins before and during pregnancy. Folic acid, 0.4 mg/d, the amount in many multivitamin preparations, taken before conception and during pregnancy is well known to prevent neural tube defects (NTDs) and other malformations.[6,7] In addition, folic acid, 4–5 mg/d, can prevent developmental toxicity from first-generation anticonvulsants. Finally, disseminating information about the dangers of exposure to potentially toxic social drugs during gestation is important. The use of any amounts of alcohol, cigarettes, cocaine, or inhaled toluene by a pregnant woman can be associated with all aspects of developmental toxicity.

To provide these services, pharmacists must have a general understanding of the principles of teratology, knowledge of the drugs known for or suspected of causing disrupted development, and access to current sources of information. This knowledge base is critical to ensure that a woman receives accurate and appropriate counseling. A pharmacist who possesses this knowledge can estimate the risk from any drug exposure in pregnancy and convey this in a confident manner to the woman or her health care provider. This knowledge transfer can markedly decrease the anxiety that women frequently experience after taking a drug during pregnancy. Additionally, pharmacists can reassure women concerned about issues of exposure for which there is no evidence of fetal harm.

II. PATIENT CASE [PART 1]

S.M. is a married 26-year-old white woman who presents with dysuria and frequency. She has never been pregnant but eventually wants to have children. Her medical history, except for two previous urinary tract infections, is negative as is her family medical history. There is no history of cigarette smoking or drug abuse, but she has an occasional glass of wine with dinner. She has no allergies, is not using any contraceptive method, and is taking no medications or vitamins. A urine culture reveals a heavy growth of *Escherichia coli* that is resistant to ampicillin but sensitive to co-trimoxazole (trimethoprim/sulfamethoxazole). Her primary care physician prescribes a 14-day course of co-trimoxazole double strength twice daily. What are the potential embryo-fetal risks of the therapy and her lifestyle if she is pregnant? How could the risks be lessened?

III. Reproductive Toxicity

Reproductive toxicity includes fertility, lactation, parturition, and developmental toxicity. Although there are many examples of drug-induced infertility (eg, some antineoplastic agents), only developmental toxicity and parturition involve the use of drugs during pregnancy.

A. Developmental Toxicity

Developmental toxicity can occur in any pregnancy, including in those cases where there are no known maternal risk factors. The toxicity relates to exposures or diseases during pregnancy that cause growth alteration, structural anomalies, functional-neurobehavioral deficits, or embryo-fetal death.

1. Growth Alteration

Mild-to-moderate growth restriction has been observed with some drugs (eg, prolonged use of corticosteroids; some β-blockers), social habits (eg, cigarette smoking), and with some diseases (eg, chronic mild hypertension). Severe growth restriction, defined as fetal weight less than the 10th percentile for gestational age, is commonly called *intrauterine growth restriction* when referring to the fetus or *small for gestational age* when referring to the infant.[8] It can be a serious complication, especially in infants whose weights are less than the 5th percentile.[8] Not only is there a decrease in weight that affects all organs, but also a significant decrease in the number of cells in the current and future brain cortex. Severe growth restriction, whether caused by drugs or other factors, is significantly associated with an increased risk of neonatal morbidity and mortality, including a markedly increased risk of cerebral palsy.[8-10]

2. Structural Anomalies

The background prevalence of structural anomalies recognized at birth is 2%–4%. The prevalence increases to approximately 5%–6% as previously hidden defects, especially of the internal organs and the brain, become evident in the months and years after birth. Structural anomalies are classified as either major or minor birth defects. Major defects are defined as those that have cosmetic or functional significance to the child (eg, a heart defect, NTD, etc.). Typically, research studies reporting birth defects refer only to major defects. Minor defects (eg, hypoplastic fingernails, strabismus, etc.) are defined as those that occur in less than 4% of the population but that have neither cosmetic nor functional significance to the child.[11] However, a small cluster of minor defects often is a signal that a major defect is present.[4,11-13]

3. Functional-Neurobehavioral Deficits

Functional-neurobehavioral deficits may not be recognized for years after birth, such as alcohol-induced mental retardation. For these reasons, the focus of drug-induced toxic effects on the embryo and fetus has shifted from considering only structural anomalies to consideration of all four aspects of developmental toxicity.[1]

4. Embryo-Fetal Death

Death in utero, either of an embryo or a fetus, is classified as a spontaneous abortion (SAB) (ie, miscarriage) if it occurs before 20 weeks' gestation and as a stillbirth at ≥20 weeks. An elective abortion, sometimes called a therapeutic abortion, is the choice of the mother and is accomplished by either drugs or surgery. Most SABs (>80%) occur in the first 12 weeks of pregnancy. The prevalence of SABs in clinically recognized pregnancies varies from 12%–26%. Chromosomal abnormalities are the main cause (50%–60%) of SABs. Other causes include uterine infections, chronic debilitating disease, hypothyroidism, poorly controlled diabetes mellitus, radiation, and drugs and chemicals. Included in the latter group are alcohol, cigarette smoking, cocaine, nonsteroidal anti-inflammatory drugs (NSAIDs), toluene inhalation, and warfarin.[6,14]

Some studies have concluded that high daily doses of caffeine (eg, ≥200 mg/d) are associated with miscarriage, but conflicting results also have been found.[6,12,14-16] The reasons probably reflect the retrospective nature of the studies, varying amounts of caffeine in beverages, concurrent cigarette smoking or alcohol intake, reporting bias (ie, caffeine consumption determined after the miscarriage), and other factors such as genetics. Moreover, nausea and vomiting is common in early pregnancy and women usually avoid coffee and other caffeinated beverages during this period. Nevertheless, moderate caffeine consumption, such as 1–2 cups of coffee per day in women who do not smoke or drink alcohol, probably is harmless.[6]

The causes of stillbirths are classified as fetal (25%–40%), placental (25%–35%), maternal (5%–10%), and unknown (25%–35%).[17] Drugs and chemicals, part of the maternal group, that cause stillbirths are the same agents that are involved in SABs.

B. Parturition

Parturition occurs at the end of pregnancy with the delivery of the fetus. Several classes of drugs are commonly used during this period. They include anti-infectives for the prophylaxis or treatment of infections, corticosteroids for fetal lung immaturity, anticonvulsants to prevent or treat seizures from eclampsia, antihypertensives for gestational hypertension and preeclampsia, tocolytics for preterm labor control, agents for cervical ripening and labor induction, and parenteral analgesics or local, regional, and general anesthesia for pain control. All of the agents used during parturition have the potential to cause fetal and/or neonatal toxicity, primarily functional-neurobehavioral deficits or death.[6,18,19] The reader should refer to the specific chapters that cover the complications and drug therapy during parturition (Chapters 7–9, 11, 15, 16, 23, and 26).

IV. Causes of Structural Anomalies

The causes of structural anomalies can be classified under five general headings: genetic, chromosome abnormalities, multifactorial inheritance, environmental (includes drugs, environmental chemicals, infections, and maternal metabolic imbalances), and unknown.[20] The percent that each of these contributes to the total is not known with certainty, but multifactorial inheritance is generally believed to be the primary cause of structural anomalies.[1]

A. Genetic

Genetic causes of structural anomalies may involve a dominant or recessive gene from either parent.[20] If the gene is dominant, there will be a family history of the defect, such as achondroplasia (ie, dwarfism). There also may be a spontaneous gene mutation that can cause any type of major birth defect. In this case there would be no family history of the malformation. A recessive gene that is carried by both parents can cause a birth defect when both are passed on to the embryo, such as infantile polycystic kidney disease. In some cases, however, disease might occur even when only one recessive gene is inherited (eg, mental retardation with phenylketonuria [PKU]). None of the defects caused by genetic factors involves drugs.[20]

B. Chromosome

Chromosome abnormalities often involve an extra normal chromosome, such as in trisomy 21 (ie, Down's syndrome), trisomy 13 (ie, Patau's syndrome), trisomy 18 (ie, Edwards' syndrome), and so forth. All of these are related to mental retardation and different malformations, and are associated with a high mortality rate. Chromosome abnormalities also may involve an extra X chromosome (47,XXX) or a missing X (eg, 45,X or Turner's syndrome). As with genetic defects, chromosome abnormalities are not caused by exposure to drugs, but may be associated with increased maternal or paternal age.[20]

C. Multifactorial

Multifactorial inheritance determines the susceptibility of the embryo and/or fetus to interact with environmental factors resulting in birth defects.[3,20] Although the actual percentage of defects that are secondary to this cause is unknown, the number appears to be growing. Examples of such defects are cleft lip with or without cleft palate, cleft palate alone, some common cardiac defects, pyloric stenosis, clubfoot, Hirschsprung's anomaly (megacolon), congenital dislocation of the hip, NTDs, and scoliosis. The cause of these defects may be an interaction between one or more embryo-fetal genes and environmental factors. Environmental factors are usually unknown, but some (and the associated birth defect) that have been identified include low socioeconomic class (NTDs), birth order (dislocation of the hip and pyloric stenosis), and drugs or chemicals, such as thalidomide, phenytoin, hydrocortisone, cigarette smoking, and alcohol.[3,21] There is evidence that susceptibility to alcohol resulting in the fetal alcohol syndrome is genetically determined by the activity of the gene producing the enzyme alcohol dehydrogenase that metabolizes ethanol to acetaldehyde.[22] One of the mechanisms involved in phenytoin-induced defects is thought to be low or absent activity of epoxide hydrolase, the enzyme responsible for metabolizing the highly reactive intermediate epoxide metabolite of phenytoin.[23]

Multifactorial inheritance is probably one of the reasons why the majority of pregnant women exposed to known teratogens have normal babies. Even potent teratogens adversely affect only a relatively few embryos or fetuses. For example, the prevalence of birth defects with thalidomide and phenytoin are about 20%–30% and less than 10%, respectively. Unfortunately, there is no method, other than family history, to determine susceptibility in the clinical setting.

Viruses known to cause human teratogenicity include cytomegalovirus, herpes simplex types 1 and 2, parvovirus B19, rubella, varicella zoster, and Venezuelan equine encephalitis virus. Two nonviruses associated with severe developmental toxicity are *Toxoplasma gondii*, a protozoan parasite that causes toxoplasmosis, and *Treponema pallidum*, a bacterium that causes syphilis. Bacterial infections involving the placenta can result in embryo-fetal death.[14,17]

Diabetes mellitus is the most common medical complication of pregnancy.[24] When poorly controlled, it is associated with all four aspects of developmental toxicity, including a high-rate of SABs, stillbirths, and structural anomalies. Although fetal growth restriction may occur if the diabetic mother has vascular disease, excessive growth (macrosomia) is a much more common result. The metabolic imbalance second only to diabetes mellitus in frequency is PKU.[25] If a fetus is homozygous for the defective gene, it will have virtually no phenylalanine hydroxylase activity and is unable to metabolize phenylalanine (an essential amino acid found in protein or from metabolism of the artificial sweetener aspartame) to tyrosine. Even fetuses that have inherited just one autosomal recessive gene, and are heterozygous and nonphenylketonuric, will have limited enzyme activity to metabolize phenylalanine. In both types, excessive amounts of phenylalanine that cross the placenta could increase to toxic concentrations in the fetus and induce mental impairment. This is a functional deficit, the magnitude of which is dependent on the amount of fetal enzyme activity and specific dietary adjustments employed during pregnancy, especially if the mother has PKU.[6,25]

D. Unknown

At the present time, the cause of a substantial number of birth defects cannot be determined. However, many of the defects that have no known cause might have been caused by multiple genes, spontaneous errors in development, multifactorial interactions, or synergistic interactions of teratogens.

V. How Is Human Developmental Toxicity Determined?

Criteria for determining if a drug causes human teratogenicity have been published.[1,4,13] These criteria also can be applied to developmental toxicity. Four of the eight published criteria are considered essential, whereas four others are helpful but not essential. The essential criteria are exposure at the critical period, a specific defect or syndrome, and either consistent findings of two or more epidemiologic studies or a rare exposure associated with a rare defect. The helpful but nonessential criteria are teratogenicity in animals, biological plausibility, proof that the agent acts in an unaltered state and not as a metabolite (important for prevention), and secular trends in which the data demonstrate an increase in the prevalence of a specific defect when a drug is available and a decrease when the drug is no longer available. Although the criteria are self-explanatory, the critical period (ie, timing) of the exposure deserves further explanation. In addition, dose also is an essential factor but is not included among the eight published criteria for the reason given below in the Dose Relationship section.

A. Critical Period

The timing of an exposure is critical because if an exposure occurs after a structure is formed, it cannot cause the defect. Organogenesis (20–55 days postconception or 34–69 days after the first day of the last menstrual period [LMP]) is the period of greatest vulnerability for birth defects because most structures are formed during this time. However, developmental toxicity can occur at any time during gestation with the only requirement being that the toxic exposure coincides with a critical development event. Some examples of critical periods (time from conception; add 14 days for time from the LMP) are neural tube defects (before 30 days), cleft lip (before 36 days), cleft palate (before 10 weeks), ventricular septal defect (before 6 weeks), and omphalocele (before 10 weeks). Exposures after these periods cannot cause these defects. Although organogenesis is usually the most vulnerable period, the central nervous system and the urogenital system are examples of systems that are very sensitive to late injury because of their ongoing development during gestation.[1,4,26]

B. Dose Relationship

There always is a dose relationship for drug exposures and developmental toxicity. The threshold dose or no-observed-effect-level (NOEL), below which there is no toxic effect, varies from drug to drug. As the dose increases above the threshold, so does the severity and frequency of developmental toxicity until, eventually, the lethal dose is reached.[1] However, this does not mean that all aspects of developmental toxicity are observed with increasing doses. One exposure might cause structural anomalies and then death, whereas another exposure might only cause death. The NOEL is frequently used with animal reproduction tests. Although it is an important value, particularly in the evaluation of animal reproduction data, the human NOEL for drugs is rarely known with certainty. Studies to determine the value would be unethical. Observational studies have identified the NOEL for some drugs, such as thalidomide and, possibly, cardioselective β-blockers (eg, atenolol, <50 mg/d)[6] and paroxetine (<25 mg/d).[6,27] However, even then the dose is an estimate because drug exposures that cause developmental toxicity are rarely quantified in terms of weight, body surface area, or plasma concentrations. Thus, this critical element for determining developmental toxicity usually cannot be assessed.[4,6]

VI. Drugs Known to Cause Developmental Toxicity

Table 1 shows drugs and substances that are known to cause human developmental toxicity, and Table 2 has additional defects that require confirmation. There are now

Table 1. Drugs and Substances Known to Cause Developmental Toxicity*

Agent	Critical Period	Developmental Toxicity
Androgens	8 wk to term	Masculinization of female fetus
ACE inhibitors Angiotensin II receptor antagonists	2nd–3rd trimesters	Fetal kidney toxicity/anuria, hypotension, oligohydramnios, pulmonary hypoplasia, hypocalvaria, limb contractures, neonatal renal failure, hypotension
Anticoagulants		
Warfarin	6th–9th wk	Fetal warfarin syndrome defects: nasal hypoplasia, stippled epiphyses, IUGR, hypoplasia of extremities, seizures, developmental delay, scoliosis, hearing loss, heart defects, death
	2nd–3rd trimester	Hemorrhage-induced brain damage, blindness, optic atrophy, microphthalmia
Anticonvulsants		
Carbamazepine	1st trimester	NTDs, craniofacial defects, nail hypoplasia, developmental delay; folic acid, 4–5 mg/d, may lower risk
	3rd trimester	Early hemorrhagic disease of the newborn
Paramethadione Trimethadione	1st trimester	Mental retardation, craniofacial and kidney/ureter defects, developmental delay
Phenobarbital Primidone	1st trimester	Mental retardation, cardiovascular and urinary tract defects; folic acid, 4–5 mg/d, may lower risk
Phenytoin	1st trimester	Fetal hydantoin syndrome: facial defects, oral clefts, VSD, IUGR, mental retardation; folic acid, 4–5 mg/d may lower risk
	3rd trimester	Early hemorrhagic disease of the newborn
Valproic acid	1st trimester	NTDs (risk 1%–2%); facial defects, IUGR, retarded psychomotor development; folic acid not protective
Antidepressants		
Lithium	1st trimester	Ebstein's anomaly (low risk)
SSRIs SNRIs	2nd–3rd trimesters	Seizures, withdrawal, serotonin syndrome, transient neurobehavioral deficits, low birth weights
Antiestrogenic		
Tamoxifen	8 wk to term	Ambiguous female genitalia
Anti-infectives		
Fluconazole	1st trimester	Craniofacial and skeletal defects, VSD, pulmonary artery hypoplasia (high dose)
Tetracyclines	2nd–3rd trimesters	Permanent discoloration of deciduous teeth
Trimethoprim	1st trimester	NTDs, cardiovascular defects (folic acid, 0.4 mg/d, reduces risk) Oral clefts (not certain if folic acid reduces risk)
Quinine (high dose)	1st trimester	Multiple defects after unsuccessful abortion attempt

(continued)

Table 1. Drugs and Substances Known to Cause Developmental Toxicity* (Continued)

Agent	Critical Period	Developmental Toxicity
Antineoplastics		
Busulfan	1st trimester	Cleft palate, pyloric stenosis, eye defects
Chlorambucil	1st trimester	Renal/ureter agenesis, cardiovascular defects
Cyclophosphamide	1st trimester	Craniofacial, eye and limb defects, genitourinary tract defects, IUGR, neurobehavioral deficits
Methotrexate	1st trimester	Craniofacial, limb defects, IUGR, neurobehavioral deficits
Antithyroids		
Methimazole	Up to 7 wk from conception	Aplasia cutis, choanal atresia, esophageal atresia with tracheoesophageal fistula, minor facial defects, hypoplastic or absent nipples, psychomotor delay, goiter
Iodine	2nd–3rd trimesters	Goiter
β-Blockers		
Atenolol	2nd–3rd trimesters	Severe IUGR of placenta and fetus (all β-blockers without intrinsic sympathomimetic activity)
Chelator		
Penicillamine	Unknown	Cutis laxa, craniofacial defects
Corticosteroids	1st trimester	Cleft lip and/or palate (risk is about 1% or less) with systemic agents
	Throughout	Mild growth restriction (300–400 g) systemic agents
Dermatologic		
Acitretin	1st trimester	Microtia, anotia, thymic aplasia, cardiovascular defects
Etretinate		
Isotretinoin		
Diagnostics		
Methylene blue (intra-amniotic)	2nd–3rd trimesters	Intestinal atresia and/or occlusion, newborn hemolytic anemia, hyperbilirubinemia, or methemoglobinemia
Diethylstilbestrol	Up to 20 wk	Multiple defects of the genital tract in female and male; vaginal-cervical clear cell adenocarcinoma in adolescents
Gastrointestinal		
Misoprostol	1st trimester	Defects secondary to attempted abortion: vascular disruption, limb defects, Möbius' syndrome (high doses)
Immunomodulators		
Thalidomide	20–36 d after conception (± 1 d)	Limb, skeletal, and craniofacial defects, brain defects, NTDs, respiratory, gastrointestinal, cardiac, and genitourinary defects

Table 1. Drugs and Substances Known to Cause Developmental Toxicity* (Continued)

Agent	Critical Period	Developmental Toxicity
Immunomosuppressives		
Mycophenolate	1st trimester	SAB; external ear defects; facial anomalies; cleft lip/palate; and defects of distal limbs, heart, esophagus, and kidneys
NSAIDs	1st trimester	Abortion, cardiac defects (ASD & VSD)
	After 32 wk	Premature closure of the ductus arteriosus
Vitamins		
Vitamin A	1st trimester	Microtia, anotia, thymic aplasia, cardiovascular defects (high doses)
Abuse drugs		
Cigarette smoking	Throughout	Risk usually <2%: defects of heart and great vessels, limbs, skull, genitourinary system, feet, abdominal wall, small bowel, and muscles High risk: abortion, stillbirths, IUGR, placenta abruption, placenta previa, preterm delivery Functional deficits: increased risk of admission to NICU; transient retinal abnormalities; SIDS; long-term effects on cognitive performance, emotional development, perceptual motor abilities, behavior, and increased childhood morbidity
Cocaine	Throughout	IUGR, vascular disruptive type defects, cerebrovascular accidents, death
Ethanol (alcohol)	Throughout	Fetal alcohol syndrome defects: craniofacial, central nervous system, heart, renogenital, cutaneous, skeletal, and muscle, IUGR, mental retardation Fetal alcohol effects: abortions, mental retardation
Toluene inhalation	Throughout	Similar to ethanol

ACE = angiotensin-converting enzyme, ASD = atrial septal defects, IUGR = intrauterine growth restriction, NICU = neonatal intensive care unit, NSAIDs = nonsteroidal anti-inflammatory drugs, NTDs = neural tube defects, RA = receptor antagonist, SAB = spontaneous abortion, SIDS = sudden infant death syndrome, SNRIs = serotonin norepinephrine reuptake inhibitors, SSRIs = selective serotonin reuptake inhibitors, VSD = ventricular septal defects.
*Adapted from Schardein,[1] Briggs et al.,[6] Shepard,[13] and Koren.[33]

21 pharmacologic classes and more than 90 individual agents that can be classified this way. Alarmingly, this list continues to expand as researchers design increasingly sophisticated studies that have adequate statistical power to detect even small risks of toxicity. This research includes multicenter case control studies, prospective cohort studies with detailed dysmorphology examinations of offspring, and the discovery that clusters of three or more minor malformations are often an indication of a hidden major defect.[11,28]

A careful examination of Tables 1 and 2 will reveal that even very toxic drugs cannot cause all types of defects or toxicity. The critical period is usually during organogenesis,

Table 2. Possible Drug-Induced Developmental Toxicity That Requires Confirmation*

Agent	Critical Period	Developmental Toxicity
ACE inhibitors	1st trimester	Cardiovascular and central nervous system defects
Anticonvulsants		
Lamotrigine	1st trimester	Cleft lip or palate
Topiramate	1st trimester	Cleft lip and palate, hypospadias[30]; growth restriction
Antidepressants		
SSRIs/SNRIs	>20 wk	Persistent pulmonary hypertension of newborn
Paroxetine	1st trimester	Cardiac (mostly ASD and VSD) but also right ventricular outflow tract obstruction, omphalocele, anencephaly, gastroschisis, abortions
Antiestrogenic		
Tamoxifen	8 wk to term	Goldenhar's syndrome
Corticosteroids (inhaled)	1st trimester	Cleft lip and/or palate
NSAIDs	1st trimester	Gastroschisis
Pseudoephedrine	1st trimester	Gastroschisis, small intestinal atresia

ACE = angiotensin-converting enzyme, ASD = atrial septal defects, NSAIDs = nonsteroidal anti-inflammatory drugs, SNRIs = serotonin norepinephrine reuptake inhibitors, SSRIs = selective serotonin reuptake inhibitors, VSD = ventricular septal defects.
*Adapted from Briggs et al.,[6] Hunt et al.,[34] and Ornoy et al.[35]

but a number of agents cause toxicity later in pregnancy. Angiotensin-converting enzyme inhibitors (ACE inhibitors), angiotensin II receptor antagonists, β-blockers without intrinsic sympathomimetic activity (ie, partial agonist), corticosteroids, tetracycline, NSAIDs, and abuse drugs can all produce various types of developmental toxicity after the first trimester.

VII. How Should the Risk of Human Developmental Toxicity Be Estimated?

A very common clinical situation occurs when a woman of reproductive age or her caregiver asks if the drug she is taking could harm a developing fetus. Ideally, the best time for the question is preconception, but more often than not it occurs during pregnancy. In the majority of cases, a definite answer is not possible. The best that can be done is to estimate the risk from the exposure. Answering the four questions below can assist in the estimation.

A. Is There Human Pregnancy Data for the Drug?

Pregnant women are exposed to drugs in one of three ways: they become pregnant while taking a drug for a current condition, they take a drug in an undiagnosed pregnancy, or they take a drug when the pregnancy is known. The first two reasons are very common because about 50% of pregnancies are unplanned. Regardless of the reason for the exposure, published human pregnancy experience is *sine qua non* for providing the best estimate of embryo-fetal risk. Unfortunately, this experience is nearly always absent for new drugs because pregnancy is an exclusion in premarketing clinical trials. Indeed, even nonpregnant women are often excluded from the trials. Even for drugs that have been on the market for 20 years, more than 90% have inadequate data to determine the risk of teratogenicity or other forms of developmental toxicity.[29] The answer to the question is typically of limited usefulness because so many drugs have little or no reported human pregnancy experience.

B. Do Other Drugs in the Same Class Cause Developmental Toxicity?

Drugs in the same pharmacologic class will usually produce similar effects in the embryo and fetus. This class effect is common. For example, all of the drugs in the following classes can produce similar toxic effects in the embryo or fetus: androgens, ACE inhibitors, corticosteroids, NSAIDs, and tetracyclines (Table 1). Drugs with similar mechanisms also may cause the same defects, such as ACE inhibitors and angiotensin II receptor antagonists, and selective serotonin reuptake inhibitors and serotonin norepinephrine reuptake inhibitors. The pharmacologic classes must not be too broad because comparisons would lead to erroneous conclusions. The following are a few examples of classes that are too broad for estimating the risk of human developmental toxicity because they include drugs that have markedly different mechanisms: antidiabetics, antidepressants, antihypertensives, antibiotics or anti-infectives, and antineoplastics. Moreover, many new drugs belong to new pharmacologic classes, such as the monoclonal antibodies used in cancer and other diseases. Thus, estimating risk by this method is frequently not possible.[6]

C. Does the Drug Reach the Embryo-Fetus?

To cause direct toxic effects, sufficient amounts of a drug must reach the maternal circulation and cross the placenta so that the threshold concentration for toxicity (ie, the NOEL) in the embryo-fetus is surpassed. Moreover, the transfer rate has to exceed the clearance rate. Unfortunately, neither of these rates is known in the clinical setting because there are no acceptable clinical methods to quantify drug concentration in the embryo or fetus, although a few drugs have been studied using in vitro placental perfusion models. However, for most drugs the best that can be done is to determine the probability of embryo-fetal exposure. The factors known to determine whether a drug crosses the placenta are maternal blood concentration, molecular weight, plasma elimination half-life, lipid solubility, ionization at physiologic pH, plasma protein binding, and placental metabolizing enzymes.[30] Maternal concentration, molecular weight, and plasma elimination half-life are the most important factors. A drug has to obtain systemic concentrations in the mother to cross the placenta, irrespective of the other factors. Some drugs, such as inhaled corticosteroids, have very low systemic bioavailability and these agents would present minimal risk of direct embryo or fetal harm. Most drugs have molecular weights less than 600 dalton, and these agents should easily cross the placenta. A long elimination half-life will place the drug at the maternal:fetal interface for an equally long time and increase the opportunity for drug transfer. Drugs that are lipid soluble cross biological membranes easier than drugs that are not. Ionization at physiologic pH and high plasma protein binding inhibit transfer across any membrane, but drugs are in equilibrium with their unionized and unbound forms, and the free forms can cross. The transfer of the free drug will be enhanced by a long elimination half-life. This concept is illustrated by warfarin sodium. It is a known human teratogen that is approximately 99% protein bound and has low lipid solubility, but the mean plasma elimination half-life is approximately 40 hours. Placental metabolism of a drug also has to be considered because the placenta is a rich source of metabolizing enzymes and can deactivate some drugs. Both betamethasone and dexamethasone are partially metabolized by the placenta, 47% and 54%, respectively, to inactive 11-ketosteroid derivatives, while prednisolone is even more significantly metabolized.[30]

D. Does the Drug Cause Developmental Toxicity in Animals?

All drugs approved in the United States by the Food and Drug Administration (FDA) must be tested in pregnant experimental animals, except for drugs that only produce effects in humans (eg, some monoclonal antibodies such as abciximab). At least one rodent, usually a rat or a mouse, and one nonrodent, usually a rabbit, are required in the testing. Testing in animals is designed to include organogenesis, other portions of pregnancy, and sometimes through weaning. The highest dose tested is the dose that produces slight maternal toxicity, such as loss of appetite or body weight, and the lowest dose corresponds to the approximate human dose. The middle dose is chosen to fit between these doses. The doses are usually reported in mg/kg/d, or other appropriate units, and are compared with the human dose based on body surface area (eg, mg/m^2) or systemic exposure. For example, the product information might state: "In rats, a daily oral dose of 100 mg/kg (four times the maximum recommended human dose based on mg/m^2) during organogenesis resulted in congenital malformations." In many cases, and depending on the toxic potency of the drug, all three doses may be a fraction of the human dose. For exposure during organogenesis, the end points include the growth restriction with reduced fetal body weights, structural defects, death as in pre- and postimplantation losses or decreased live births, and abnormal development, such as delayed skeletal ossification. Prenatal and postnatal studies extending through weaning also are conducted to determine the potential for functional deficits.[31]

Although there are no definite methods to interpret animal studies, it is important to note, as shown in Table 3, that nearly all drugs known to cause human developmental toxicity also cause developmental toxicity in at least one experimental animal species. With this understanding, a panel convened by the FDA and other groups concluded that if a drug did not cause developmental toxicity (with doses that did not cause maternal toxicity) at doses equal to or less than 10 times the human dose based on body surface area or exposure, then the drug could be considered low risk for human embryo-fetal toxicity.[2] Conversely, if a drug did cause toxicity at doses equal to or less than 10 times the human dose, then it could be classified as having risk, but the risk magnitude would be unknown. This conclusion was similar to that stated in guidelines released by the United States Environmental Protection Agency in 1991.[31] However, if the dose that caused developmental toxicity also caused maternal toxicity (eg, weight reduction), the embryo-fetal results would not be interpretable. One source has quantified the risk of developmental toxicity, based on the number of experimental animal species that had such toxicity, as moderate risk (one species), risk (two species), or high risk (three or more species).[6] These assessments were based on the animal data for all drugs known to cause human developmental toxicity (Table 3).

Table 3. Human Teratogens and Structural Defects in Animals*

Proven Human Teratogens	Animal Species				
	Mouse	Rat	Rabbit	Monkey	Other
ACE inhibitors	0	0	0		
Angiotensin II receptor antagonists	0	0	0		
Busulfan	+	+			
Carbamazepine	+	+			
Cigarette smoking					NS
Cocaine	+	+	±		
Cyclophosphamide	+	+	+	+	
Diethylstilbestrol	+	+		+	Ferret +, hamster +
Ethanol	+	+	+	+	Guinea pig +, pig +, dog +
Fluconazole (≥ 400 mg/d)		+	0		
Hydrocortisone (corticosteroids)	+	+	+		Guinea pig +, hamster +
Lithium	+	+	0		
Methimazole		±	0		
Methotrexate	+	+	+	±	Cat +
Methylene blue (intraamniotic)					NS
Misoprostol		0	+		
Mycophenolate		+	+		
Paramethadione		0		0	
Penicillamine	+	+			Hamster +
Phenobarbital/primidone	+	+	+		
Phenytoin	+	+	+	+	Cat +
Testosterone (androgens)	+	+	+	+	Hamster +
Tetracyclines	0	+	0		Guinea pig +
Thalidomide	+	+	+	+	
Toluene abuse	+	+	0		
Trimethadione	+	±		+	
Trimethoprim		+	0		
Valproic acid	+	+	+	+	Gerbil +, hamster +
Vitamin A derivatives (vitamin A [high dose], isotretinoin, etretinate, tretinoin, acitretin)	+	+	+	+	Guinea pig +, dog +, pig +, hamster +
Warfarin	0	+	0		

+ = defects observed, 0 = no defects observed, ± = conflicting studies, ACE = angiotensin-converting enzyme, NS = not studied in animals.
*Adapted from Schardein[1] and Briggs et al.[6]

VIII. FDA Risk Categories

In 1979, the FDA required the labels of all new approved drugs to contain a letter risk category for use in pregnancy. The definitions of the FDA risk categories (A, B, C, D, and X) are shown in Table 4. Although they were meant to aid health care practitioners in determining the risk of a drug if it was used in pregnancy, it soon became appar-

Table 4. U.S. Food and Drug Administration Risk Categories*

Category A: Controlled studies in women fail to demonstrate a risk to the fetus in the first trimester (and there is no evidence of a risk in later trimesters), and the possibility of fetal harm appears remote.

Category B: Either animal-reproduction studies have not demonstrated a fetal risk but there are no controlled studies in pregnant women or animal-reproduction studies have shown an adverse effect (other than a decrease in fertility) that was not confirmed in controlled studies in women in the first trimester (and there is no evidence of a risk in later trimesters).

Category C: Either studies in animals have revealed adverse effects on the fetus (teratogenic or embryocidal or other) and there are no controlled studies in women or studies in women and animals are not available. Drugs should be given only if the potential benefit justifies the potential risk to the fetus.

Category D: There is positive evidence of human fetal risk, but the benefits from use in pregnant women may be acceptable despite the risk (eg, if the drug is needed in a life-threatening situation or for a serious disease for which safer drugs cannot be used or are ineffective).

Category X: Studies in animals or human beings have demonstrated fetal abnormalities or there is evidence of fetal risk based on human experience or both, and the risk of the use of the drug in pregnant women clearly outweighs any possible benefit. The drug is contraindicated in women who are or may become pregnant.

*From Briggs et al.[6] and *Federal Register*.[36]

ent that the system resulted in over-reliance on the letters themselves.[32] In 2007, because of the concerns given below, the FDA began the process to remove the risk categories from drug labels. The primary problem with the categories is that they do not account for the physiologic changes in the fetus that occur throughout gestation. Other concerns are:

- Categories A and B cannot be equated to complete safety.
- The categories do not show a gradation of risk, where X is the highest risk and A is the lowest risk.
- Some products are labeled category X because there is no benefit to the mother (eg, oral contraceptives).
- All drugs within the same category do not share the same risk (eg, all drugs labeled as C have no human data but some have animal data suggesting risk, whereas others have no animal data; also does not take into account the human experience with other drugs in the same pharmacologic class).
- The categories do not consider exposure timing, dose, route, duration, or frequency.
- The categories do not address incidence, severity, or reversibility.[32]

IX. Information Sources

There are a number of sources that cite information about drug exposures during pregnancy. Because no single source covers all drugs, cites all published references, or arrives at the same conclusion of risk, it is helpful to have several sources available when answering questions concerning drug-induced developmental toxicity. There are also teratology information services associated with the Organization of Teratology Information Specialists (OTIS) that answer questions relating to drug exposures in a pregnant and breastfeeding woman. Listed below are suggested reference sources (listed alphabetically).

Books

(1) Briggs GG, Freeman RK, Yaffe SJ. *Drugs in Pregnancy and Lactation. A Reference Guide to Fetal and Neonatal Risk.* 8th ed. Philadelphia: Lippincott Williams & Wilkins, 2008.

(2) Koren G. *Medication Safety in Pregnancy and Breastfeeding.* New York: McGraw-Hill, 2007.

(3) Schaefer C, Peters P, Miller RK. *Drugs During Pregnancy and Lactation.* 2nd ed. London: Academic Press, 2007.

(4) Schardein JL. *Chemically Induced Birth Defects.* 3rd ed. New York: Marcel Dekker, 2000.

(5) Shepard TH, Lemire RJ. *Catalog of Teratogenic Agents.* 12th ed. Baltimore: The Johns Hopkins University Press, 2007.

Online and Telephone

(6) Organization of Teratology Information Specialists (OTIS). Available at: http://otispregnancy.org (toll free telephone 866-626-OTIS [6847])

(7) REPRORISK system; commercially available CD-ROM that contains electronic versions of REPROTEXT, REPROTOX, Shepard's Catalog, and TERIS. The system is available from Micromedex, Inc. (http://www.micromedex.com/products/reprorisk/).

X. PATIENT CASE [PART 2]

Important aspects of this case are that the patient is married, not using contraceptives, and could be in an early pregnancy. There are at least three risk factors for a poor pregnancy outcome: consumption of alcohol, not taking supplemental vitamins with folic acid, and co-trimoxazole. Alcohol, in any amount, is known to cause embryo-fetal toxicity consisting of growth restriction, structural anomalies, mental retardation, and abortion (Table 1). She should be counseled to stop all intake of alcohol. She also is at risk for NTDs and other malformations from possible inadequate dietary intake of folic acid. Moreover, trimethoprim is a dihydrofolate reductase inhibitor that has been associated with NTDs, cardiovascular defects, and cleft lip with or without cleft palate. Because folic acid, 0.4 mg/d, has been shown to reduce the risk of these birth defects, she should be immediately started on a daily multivitamin with folic acid. However, even if all of these steps are taken, she should be made aware of the fact that there is a background risk of birth defects of about 5%–6%. The pharmacist should discuss these matters with the patient and her physician before dispensing the anti-infective.

XI. Summary

There are many factors and conditions that cause developmental toxicity, but exposure to harmful drugs and chemicals, and nutritional deficiencies are the only ones that usually can be modified or eliminated. All health care professionals have an obligation to counsel women of childbearing potential how to avoid potentially toxic exposures and to correct nutritional deficiencies. This counseling also must include surveillance of prescribed or over-the-counter medications for substances known or suspected of causing embryo-fetal harm. Although preconception counseling is best, reducing or preventing these harmful factors at any time during pregnancy may markedly increase the chance of a good outcome.

Pharmacists are in a unique position to assist in the prevention of drug-induced embryo-fetal harm. They are respected health professionals who are routinely sought out by the public and other health professionals for drug information. As such, pharmacists have a professional obligation to all pregnant and potentially pregnant women to screen their medication profiles for drugs that might cause developmental toxicity and omissions in therapy, such as daily folic acid, and counsel them on the potential toxicity of social drugs and habits. Although few drugs can be implicated in causing developmental toxicity, they are the only cause that can be prevented. The effects of drugs on the embryo and fetus are complex, but understanding of this critical area should be a requirement for all pharmacists. Because of the genetic diversity of humans, every drug exposure during pregnancy has the potential to cause developmental toxicity and, combined with the lack of adequate human pregnancy experience, strongly suggests that few drugs can be called safe in pregnancy.

XII. References

1. Schardein JL. Principles of teratogenesis applicable to drug and chemical exposure. In *Chemically Induced Birth Defects*. 3rd ed. New York: Marcel Dekker, 2000:1–65.

2. Scialli AR, Buelke-Sam JL, Chambers CD, et al. Communicating risks during pregnancy: a workshop on the use of data from animal developmental toxicity studies in pregnancy labels for drugs. *Birth Defects Res A Clin Mol Teratol*. 2004;70:7–12.

3. Vorhees CV. Can prenatal exposure to a teratogenic agent have delayed long-term effects on behavior? *Teratology Primer*. Teratology Society, 2005:12–14.

4. Brent RL. Environmental causes of human congenital malformations: the pediatrician's role in dealing with these complex clinical problems caused by a multiplicity of environmental and genetic factors. *Pediatrics*. 2004;113:957–968.

5. Rodier JC. Is the fetus susceptible to adverse effects of a chemical or physical agent after the first trimester? *Teratology Primer*. Teratology Society, 2005:9–11.

6. Briggs GG, Freeman RF, Yaffe SJ. *Drugs in Pregnancy and Lactation*. 8th ed. Philadelphia: Lippincott Williams & Wilkins, 2008.

7. Goh YI, Koren G. Folic acid and congenital birth defects: a review. In Koren G. *Medication Safety in Pregnancy and Breastfeeding*. New York: McGraw-Hill, 2007:279–288.

8. American College of Obstetricians and Gynecologists. Intrauterine growth restriction. *ACOG Practice Bulletin*. Number 12, January 2000.

9. Resnik R. Intrauterine growth retardation. *Obstet Gynecol.* 2002;99:490–496.

10. Samuelsen GB, Pakkenberg B, Bogdanovic N, et al. Severe cell reduction in the future brain cortex in human growth-restricted fetuses and infants. *Am J Obstet Gynecol.* 2007;197:56.e1–7.

11. Chambers CD, Braddock SR, Briggs GG, et al. Postmarketing surveillance for human teratogenicity: a model approach. *Teratology.* 2001;64:252–261.

12. Food and Drug Administration. Office of Training and Communication, Division of Drug Information, HFD-240, Center for Drug Evaluation and Research. Reviewer Guidance: Evaluating the risks of drug exposure in human pregnancies. April 2005. Available at http://www.fda.gov/cber/gdlns/rvrpreg.htm. Accessed February 3, 2008.

13. Shepard TH. *Catalog of Teratogenic Agents.* 10th ed. Baltimore: The Johns Hopkins University Press, 2001.

14. Abortion. In Cunningham FG, Leveno KJ, Bloom SL, et al. *Williams Obstetrics.* 22nd ed. New York: McGraw-Hill, 2005:232–251.

15. Weng X, Odouli R, Li D-K. Maternal caffeine consumption during pregnancy and risk of miscarriage: a prospective cohort study. *Am J Obstet Gynecol.* 2008; 198:279.e1–8.

16. Savitz DA, Chan RL, Herring AH, et al. Caffeine and miscarriage risk. *Epidemiology.* 2008;19:55–62.

17. Fetal death. In Cunningham FG, Leveno KJ, Bloom SL, et al. *Williams Obstetrics.* 22nd ed. New York: McGraw-Hill, 2005:678–679.

18. Briggs GG, Wan SR. Drug therapy during labor and delivery. Part 1. *Am J Health Syst Pharm.* 2006;63:1038–1047.

19. Briggs GG, Wan SR. Drug therapy during labor and delivery. Part 2. *Am J Health Syst Pharm.* 2006;63:1131–1139.

20. Holmes LB. What are common birth defects in humans, and how are they diagnosed? *Teratology Primer.* Teratology Society, 2005:1–3.

21. Jelinek R. The contribution of new findings and ideas to the old principles of teratology. *Reprod Toxicol.* 2005;20:295–300.

22. Green RF, Stoler JM. Alcohol dehydrogenase 1B genotype and fetal alcohol syndrome: a HuGE minireview. *Am J Obstet Gynecol.* 2007;197:12–25.

23. Buehler BA, Delimont D, Van Waes M, et al. Prenatal prediction of risk of the fetal hydantoin syndrome. *N Engl J Med.* 1990;322:1567–1572.

24. Diabetes. In Cunningham FG, Leveno KJ, Bloom SL, et al. *Williams Obstetrics.* 22nd ed. New York: McGraw-Hill, 2005:1169–1187.

25. Sadler TW. Will alterations in maternal metabolism increase the risk of birth defects? *Teratology Primer.* Teratology Society, 2005:19–21.

26. Jones KL. Morphogenesis and dysmorphogenesis. In Jones KL. *Smith's Recognizable Patterns of Human Malformations.* 6th ed. Philadelphia: W.B. Saunders, 2006:794.

27. Berard A, Ramos E, Rey E, et al. First trimester exposure to paroxetine and risk of cardiac malformations in infants: the importance of dosage. *Birth Defects Res B Dev Reprod Toxicol.* 2007;80:18–27.

28. Chambers CD, Johnson KA, Dick LM, et al. Birth outcomes in pregnant women taking fluoxetine. *N Engl J Med*. 1996;335:1010–1015.

29. Lo WY, Friedman JM. Teratogenicity of recently introduced medications in human pregnancy. *Obstet Gynecol*. 2002;100:465–473.

30. Garland M. Pharmacology of drug transfer across the placenta. *Obstet Gynecol Clin North Am*. 1998;25:21–42.

31. Guidelines for developmental toxicity risk assessment. U.S. Environmental Protection Agency. Risk Assessment Forum, Washington, DC, EPA/600/FR-91/001, 1991. Available at http://cfpub.epa.gov/ncea/cfm/recordisplay.cfm?deid=23162. Accessed February 3, 2008.

32. Kweder SL. Drugs and biologics in pregnancy and breastfeeding: FDA in the 21st century. *Birth Defects Res A Clin Mol Teratol*. 2008;82:605–609.

33. Koren G. *Medication Safety in Pregnancy and Breastfeeding*. New York: McGraw-Hill, 2007.

34. Hunt S, Russell A, Smithson WH, et al. Topiramate in pregnancy. Preliminary experience from the UK Epilepsy and Pregnancy Register. *Neurology*. 2008;71:272–276.

35. Ornoy A, Zvi N, Arnon J, et al. The outcome of pregnancy following topiramate treatment: a study on 52 pregnancies. *Reprod Toxicol*. 2008;25:388–389.

36. *Federal Register*. 1980;44:37434–37467.

QUESTIONS AND ANSWERS

1. There is no reported human pregnancy experience for a new drug indicated for the treatment of asthma. In studies with pregnant rats and rabbits, doses that were 12 and 20 times, respectively, the maximum recommended human dose based on body surface area caused cardiac defects. Based only on these data, what is the estimated human risk for birth defects if the drug is used in pregnancy?

   a. The risk cannot be determined without human pregnancy data.

   b. There would be risk but low.

   c. There would be risk of unknown magnitude.

   d. There would be risk but only during organogenesis.

2. The elements of developmental toxicity are:

   a. growth, structural defects, neurobehavioral deficits, and death

   b. genetic, chromosomal, multifactorial, and environmental

   c. growth alteration, structural anomalies, neurobehavioral deficits, and death

   d. structural anomalies, deformations, functional deficits, and death

3. A drug known to cause a low risk of cleft lip is recommended for a woman at 7 weeks' gestation to optimize control of her non–life-threatening chronic disease. There are no other alternatives. What is the best plan to reduce the primary risk to the embryo?

   a. Try to wait for a few days before starting the drug.

   b. Try to wait until after the period of organogenesis.

   c. Start the drug now because her health is paramount.

   d. Try to wait until the first trimester is completed.

4. Some critical functions that a pharmacist can perform when advising women of reproductive age to reduce the risk of developmental toxicity from drugs are:

   a. screening drug therapy, including social drugs, for those that could cause harm

   b. estimating the human embryo-fetal risk from animal reproduction data

   c. making certain that they are taking vitamins with folic acid

   d. all of the above

Answers:

1. b; 2. c; 3. a; 4. d

Drug Use and Lactation

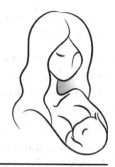

Philip O. Anderson

LEARNING OBJECTIVES

1. List five advantages of breastmilk over formula.

2. List five drug and infant factors that determine the risk of the drugs used during breastfeeding.

3. Calculate the infant's dose of a medication in breastmilk from maternal serum and milk concentration values.

4. State the infant age at which adverse reactions from drugs in breastmilk are most prevalent.

I. Introduction

Breastfeeding an infant is not only the best method of infant feeding, it is the method against which other types of infant feeding should be measured. Strong scientific evidence indicates that infants, including those in developed countries, obtain numerous benefits from breastfeeding compared to artificial feeding. These include decreases in risks of gastroenteritis, severe lower respiratory tract infections, acute otitis media, necrotizing enterocolitis, sudden infant death syndrome in the first year of life, types 1 and 2 diabetes mellitus, childhood leukemia, and obesity.[1–3] Furthermore, some studies indicate that breastfed infants might be protected against lymphoma, Hodgkin's disease, atopic dermatitis, bacteremia, bacterial meningitis, botulism, urinary tract infections, late-onset sepsis, adult hypercholesterolemia, ulcerative colitis, celiac disease, and other chronic digestive diseases.[2,3] Postneonatal (beyond 28 days of age) mortality is reduced by 21% in the United States by breastfeeding.[2] These advantages all lead to considerable cost savings for parents and the health care system.[3] For these reasons, breastfeeding is considered the "gold standard" for infant nutrition. Formula feeding falls short on all of the above factors.

The mother who nurses her infant also derives many benefits, such as more rapid uterine involution, decreased postpartum blood loss, fertility reduction (while nursing and amenorrheic), and decreased risk of breast and ovarian cancer, type 1 and 2 diabetes mellitus, and possibly osteoporosis and hip fracture later in life.[1,2] Not breastfeeding or early cessation of breastfeeding results in a higher risk of maternal postpartum depression.[1]

Exclusive breastfeeding is defined as an infant's consumption of human milk with no supplementation of any type except for medications.[4] Research currently supports the recommendation that 6 months of exclusive breastfeeding followed by continued breastfeeding plus complementary foods for up to 2 years and beyond is best for infant health and development. These recommendations have been endorsed by major national and international professional associations and agencies involved with infant health.[2,5,6] The Healthy People 2010 goals for the United States are 50% of infants exclusively breastfed at 3 months and 25% at 6 months of age.[5] Data collected by the Centers for Disease Control and Prevention for 2004 indicate that rates are far below the goals at 30.5% and 11.3%, respectively.[7]

Many factors contribute to this shortfall, one of them being the use of medications by the nursing mother.[8,9] Concern among mothers and health professionals about medications in breastmilk harming the nursing infant often leads to discontinuation of breastfeeding.[10,11] In the vast majority of cases, breastfeeding discontinuation is not necessary. Pharmacists can play an important role in maintaining breastfeeding among mothers who are taking medications if they understand and properly apply the scientific evidence.

II. In Utero Exposure

The risks of medication use during pregnancy have little to do with the drug's safety during breastfeeding. Drug exposure of the fetus is usually much greater, often by 10-fold or more, than the exposure of the infant via breastmilk. Additionally, organogenesis is completed at birth, so teratogenicity cannot occur during breastfeeding. These facts are sometimes overlooked and clinicians mistakenly try to apply pregnancy warnings or U.S. Food and Drug Administration (FDA) pregnancy categories to breastfeeding. A mother who is concerned about exposing her infant to a medication during breastfeeding is often comforted by the fact that breastmilk exposure is much lower than exposure during pregnancy.

However, medications taken by the mother during pregnancy can result in fetal exposure that has effects after birth in the breastfed infant. For example, infants of mothers who took medications during late pregnancy that can cause withdrawal symptoms when abruptly discontinued can experience neonatal withdrawal symptoms. Breastfeeding can mitigate infant withdrawal symptoms from some anticonvulsants. Several centers that encourage breastfeeding by mothers on methadone maintenance during pregnancy and postpartum have noted fewer withdrawal symptoms and shorter hospitalizations among breastfed infants.[12–15] Other drugs pass so poorly into breastmilk that infant withdrawal symptoms are not substantially mitigated by breastfeeding.

Another potential problem is administration of long-acting drugs near term and during delivery before umbilical cord clamping because they can persist in the infant's circulation after birth. Further drug ingested from breastmilk might then result in prolonged therapeutic serum concentrations, at least until the infant's drug elimination rate exceeds the rate of drug intake from milk. For example, fluoxetine and its active metabolite persist in the infant's circulation for weeks after delivery even without breastfeeding. Because fluoxetine and norfluoxetine persist in breastmilk, even without postpartum maternal intake, breastmilk can add to the infant's serum concentration.[16] Long-acting sedatives and narcotics (such as meperidine, which has a long-acting metabolite) given during delivery before cord clamping can cause newborn infants to be groggy and nurse poorly.[17,18]

III. Stages of Lactation

Just as pregnancy has several stages during its course, lactation is not a single state. A small amount of milk called *colostrum* that is rich in immunoglobulins and antioxidants is produced immediately after birth, 37–169 mL of colostrum during the first 48 hours.[3,19] In the colostral phase, large molecules such as proteins can pass readily into breastmilk from maternal serum because junctions (pores) between the mammary epithelial cells are relatively open.

By day 5 postpartum, women can produce 500–750 mL of milk daily, and by day 14 postpartum, 700–1000 mL daily. A daily value of 150 mL of milk per kilogram of infant weight is usually used to estimate milk intake of the exclusively breastfed infant once lactation is well established.[20]

These changes in nursing pattern have implications for drug therapy. During the colostral phase, the dose of drugs in breastmilk is low because of the small volume of milk. Once the milk comes in by day 5, the dose the infant receives will increase in proportion to the milk volume. Newborn infants often nurse every 2–3 hours around the clock, so trying to time medication doses with respect to nursing to reduce infant drug exposure is futile. Also, during the first 4 weeks postpartum, interference with nursing, either by medications or inappropriate advice by health professionals, can have a profound impact on milk production and breastfeeding success. After that time, lactation is usually well established and more resilient.

Returning to work is a major disruption to exclusive breastfeeding, but many workplaces now have lactation rooms. Mothers can pump milk for their infants who can be fed breastmilk by the infant's caretaker during the day and be breastfed before and after work. Although exclusive breastfeeding (or breastmilk feeding) is recommended for 6 months, many mothers begin supplementation with formula sooner. While not ideal, mixed feeding nevertheless provides health benefits over exclusive formula feeding.

Once the infant begins to take a proportion of his or her nourishment as formula or solid foods, the dose of any medication in the mother's breastmilk drops proportionately. Some infants continue to nurse once or twice a day beyond the first year, often in the morning, before naps or at bedtime. In this setting, the dose of medication that the infant receives in breastmilk is low, and timing maternal doses to occur right after nursing can minimize infant drug exposure even further.

IV. Drug Passage into Milk

A. Physiochemical Factors

Unlike pregnancy, in which drugs can pass rather directly from the mother to the infant in similar serum concentrations, a drug takes a complex route to the infant during breast-feeding.[21,22] Small water-soluble nonelectrolytes pass into breastmilk by simple diffusion through pores in the mammary epithelial membrane that separates plasma from milk. Equilibration between the two fluids is rapid, and milk levels of drugs approximate plasma levels.

For larger molecules, only the lipid-soluble, unbound, nonionized forms pass across the mammary epithelium by crossing the cell wall and diffusing across the interior of the cell to reach the milk. Most drugs pass across the mammary epithelium by passive diffusion down the concentration gradient of the nonionized, unbound drug from the high concentration in the maternal plasma into breastmilk.

Because the pH of milk is generally lower than that of plasma, milk can act as an "ion trap" for basic drugs. At equilibrium, these compounds can concentrate in milk relative to plasma. Conversely, acidic drugs are inhibited from entering milk. The pK_a of weak electrolytes is an important determinant of their equilibrium concentration in milk.

Protein binding is also an important determinant because plasma proteins bind drugs much more avidly than do milk proteins. Highly protein-bound drugs usually do not pass into milk in high concentrations.

Lipid solubility favors passage of drugs into milk, because the fat component of milk can concentrate them. However, because milk contains only a small amount fat, its capacity for concentrating drugs is limited. A few drugs are actively transported into breastmilk.[23] No single one of these factors can be applied in isolation to predict drug passage, though, because they interact with each other. For example, higher lipid solubility confers higher plasma protein binding among β-blockers, so the water-soluble β-blockers attain higher concentrations in milk than the lipid-soluble β-blockers.[24]

Numerous methods have been proposed for estimating the passage of drugs into breastmilk using the principles listed above and the physicochemical properties of the drug, but none of these methods has proven to be completely reliable.[25] Currently, the best method for determining the passage of drugs into human milk is by properly conducted clinical studies in humans. Manufacturers are not required to perform such studies, so useful information is not always available.

B. Pharmacokinetic Factors

Studies in animals and humans have found that passage of drugs into and out of breastmilk can be represented as a two-compartment pharmacokinetic model as shown in Figure 1. Because the breast is periodically emptied by the nursing infant and refilled with newly formed milk, equilibrium between plasma and milk is rarely reached. The rate of drug passage from plasma into milk is therefore important in determining the concentration of a drug in milk. Factors favoring rapid passage into milk are high lipid solubility and low molecular weight.

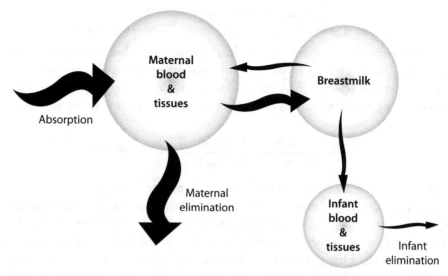

Figure 1. Pharmacokinetic Model. Originally published in reference 14, and cited in reference 21. © 1991, American Society of Health-System Pharmacists, Inc. All rights reserved. Reprinted with permission. (RO736)

As the pharmacokinetic model indicates, passage of drugs between plasma and milk occurs in both directions. When the concentration of nonionized free drug in the breastmilk is higher than it is in plasma because of maternal metabolism and excretion of the drug from the plasma, net transfer of drug from milk to plasma occurs. Thus, pumping and discarding milk does not appreciably hasten the elimination of most drugs from milk, and it does not have a marked effect on overall clearance of the drug from the mother's body because of the small fraction of the drug that is in the breastmilk.

C. Methods of Expressing the Extent of Passage

The ratio of concentrations of a drug in milk and plasma (the milk/plasma, or M/P, ratio) has often been used as a measure of a drug's passage into breastmilk.[21,22] However, the M/P ratio has shortcomings that make it meaningless as a measure of drug safety during nursing. The value is not constant as often calculated, but varies with the time after the dose and can vary with the number of doses given. It also does not take into account the potential toxicity of the drug, the extent of nursing, or the infant's age. However, if the M/P ratio is calculated using the areas-under-the-curve rather than single time-point measurements, it can be used to estimate the amount of drug in breastmilk using the following formula:

Average milk concentration (mg/mL) =
Average maternal serum concentration (mg/mL) × M/P

If the average breastmilk concentration can be determined, either by the above calculation or through data from clinical studies, the daily dosage of the drug in breastmilk can be calculated using the standard value of milk intake of 150 mL/kg/d for a fully breastfed infant and the formula:

$$\text{Average infant dosage (mg/kg/d)} =$$
$$\text{Average milk concentration (mg/mL)} \times 150 \text{ mL/kg/d}$$

To standardize the expression of drug passage into breastmilk, the currently accepted methodology is using the "weight-adjusted percentage of maternal dosage," which is sometimes referred to as the "relative infant dose." To calculate this value, the daily weight-adjusted (ie, mg/kg) dosages of the drug must be used in the calculation below:

$$\frac{\text{Daily infant dosage in breastmilk (mg/kg)}}{\text{Daily maternal dosage (mg/kg)}} \times 100$$

This value has been used to estimate the safety of medication use during breastfeeding. A weight-adjusted infant dosage less than 10% of the mother's dosage is considered acceptable for breastfeeding. Of 205 drugs in the World Health Organization's (WHO) 1996 reference book, *Drugs and Human Lactation*, 2nd ed.,[20] 87% were found to be excreted to an extent less than 10% of the weight-adjusted percentage of maternal dosage and therefore considered acceptable to use during breastfeeding. Only about 3% of the 205 drugs were excreted to an extent of greater than 25% of the weight-adjusted percentage of maternal dosage. These drugs are considered by the WHO reference to be unacceptable during breastfeeding. The likelihood that an adverse infant effect had been reported increased markedly in drugs that had an infant dosage in milk over 25% of the maternal weight-adjusted dosage.[26]

Drug clearance can also be a useful factor for identifying drugs that may accumulate in infants and thereby have a pharmacologic effect.[27] Drugs with an adult total body clearance of 0.3 L/h/kg or greater and that have no active metabolites are unlikely to cause a pharmacologic effect in a nursing infant because they are rapidly eliminated from both the mother and infant.

D. Infant Factors

The clearance of many drugs that are used primarily in adults is not known for preterm and newborn infants. However, as a general rule, these infants eliminate drugs more slowly than older infants. Therefore, preterm and newborn infants are the most susceptible to adverse effects from medications in breastmilk[28]; most reported adverse reactions from drugs in breastmilk are in infants younger than 1 month of age.[29] The two primary renal excretory mechanisms, glomerular filtration and tubular secretion, are both undeveloped in the neonate. Glomerular filtration rate (GFR) matures over 3–5 months to adult levels.[23] The preterm infant of less than 34 weeks' gestational age may have a further reduced GFR of one fourth to one half that of a full-term infant. GFR of preterm infants remains below that of full-term infants of the same postnatal age until 4 to 5 weeks after birth. Tubular secretion appears to mature over a period of several months, the rate of maturation varying somewhat depending on the drug.[30] Conversely, as infants' metabolic and excretory processes mature, the risk of adverse reactions in breastfed infants from maternal medications decreases dramatically. After 2 months of age, the risk of an adverse reaction from drugs in breastmilk is quite small.[29] Risk further decreases once complementary feeding is introduced, because drug doses from breastfeeding decrease proportionately.

Preterm and newborn infant responses to medications in breastmilk are sometimes different from those of older infants and children.[31,32] These differences may result from differences in the number or affinity of drug receptors, immaturity of the nervous system, or other factors. One of the more important and well-documented differences involves the stability of the neonatal red cell membrane, which can lead to drug-induced hemolysis during the first month of life. Because of this increased susceptibility, hemolytic drugs (ie, oxidizing agents) should be avoided by mothers breastfeeding neonates. Increased permeability of the blood–brain barrier has been reported, potentially leading to increased activity of some centrally active compounds, such as narcotics. Central nervous system (CNS) depressants are the most commonly reported causes of adverse drug reactions in breastfed newborns.[29]

Pharmacogenetics also plays a role in drug safety during breastfeeding. The only clear-cut infant death from a medication in breastmilk occurred in the infant of a mother who was a CYP2D6 "supermetabolizer" and excreted very large amounts of morphine into her milk after taking low to moderate doses of codeine for postpartum pain.[33] Another mother with this phenotype who was taking codeine reported severe drowsiness and poor feeding in her infant.[34]

Higher serum concentrations of citalopram were found in two breastfed infant twins whose mother was a poor metabolizer of citalopram because of having the CYP2C19*2/*2 mutation and resulting high maternal plasma concentrations. Five infants who were heterozygous for the CYP2C19*1/*2 genotype and whose mothers were all extensive metabolizers had average serum levels that were 3.75 times higher than five other infants with the CYP2C19*1/*1 extensive metabolizer genotype.[35] These findings indicate that both maternal and infant genotypes can influence the serum concentration in breastfed infants.

Other factors that should be considered when determining the advisability of using a particular drug in a nursing mother include the potential acute toxicity of the drug, dosage and duration of therapy, age of the infant, quantity of milk consumed, experience with the drug in infants, oral absorption of the drug by the infant, potential long-term effects, and possible interference with lactation.[21,31]

Non–dose-related adverse effects, such as allergic reactions and some hemolytic anemias, can also occur in breastfed infants; however, these reactions are relatively uncommon. The most common is gastrointestinal (GI) intolerance caused by antimicrobial agents in breastmilk, which can occur whether or not the drugs are absorbed by the infant. Antimicrobial agents are among the most commonly used maternal medications during nursing and, although serious side effects are rare, diarrhea may occur in up to 12% of infants.[36] Disruption of the infant's GI flora occasionally leads to thrush and rarely to pseudomembranous colitis, especially after repeated maternal courses of antimicrobial therapy. Severe diarrhea or blood in the infant's stool during maternal antimicrobial use is an indication to stop nursing and seek medical attention.

Although the above considerations are important, follow-up of mothers who took medications while breastfeeding their infants has shown that serious side effects are uncommon. In one study of 873 infants whose mothers were taking a medication during breastfeeding, no side effects occurred that required medical intervention.[36] An exhaustive review of the worldwide medical literature from the early 1900s up to 2002 found only 100 adverse drug reactions reported in breastfed infants, many of which were not clearly caused by maternal medication use.[29]

V. Drugs of Concern

The classes of drugs that are of most concern during breastfeeding are listed below.[29]

A. Antidepressants

Antidepressants can be separated into those that can cause problems and those that are unlikely to cause problems. Doxepin and citalopram have been associated with infant CNS depression. Fluoxetine has been associated with irritability and colic and may decrease the rate of weight gain in breastfed infants. Nortriptyline, sertraline, and paroxetine are the antidepressants of choice because they do not appear to cause such problems and amounts excreted into milk are much less than with citalopram and fluoxetine. Newer agents have not been well studied.[37,38]

B. Narcotics

Narcotics in large maternal doses have caused apnea, bradycardia, and cyanosis in breastfed infants; the highest risk period is during the first week. As noted above, the only well-documented death in a breastfed infant was caused by a narcotic. Newborn infants often become drowsy and may not nurse well or may gain weight inadequately if their mothers take high doses of codeine. One recent study found that codeine's side effects in breastfed infants were much more common if their mothers were taking a dose of 1.6 mg/kg/d than if they were taking a dose of 1 mg/kg/d.[34]

C. Long-Acting Sedatives

Phenobarbital, primidone, and diazepam have caused excessive sedation in some infants. Infants of mothers with epilepsy who received phenobarbital transplacentally during pregnancy may tolerate the drug in breastmilk better than unexposed neonates because of in utero enzyme induction. However, the net effect of these drugs is unpredictable because infants may be born with substantial amounts in their bloodstream.

D. Water-Soluble β-Blockers

Atenolol, acebutolol, and sotalol are excreted into milk in relatively large amounts. Additionally, these drugs are poorly eliminated by the undeveloped kidneys of newborns. Apnea, bradycardia, and cyanosis have been reported. Lipid-soluble, highly protein-bound drugs such as propranolol are preferred while nursing a neonate. Labetalol is also usually considered a good choice during breastfeeding in full-term infants, but sinus bradycardia and atrial premature beats occurred in a 26-week preterm infant who was given pumped breastmilk containing labetalol.[39]

E. Lithium

Lithium is excreted in large amounts (up to 25% of weight-adjusted maternal dosage) in breastmilk. Since lithium relies completely on the kidneys for elimination, its use in mothers nursing newborns is somewhat risky. However, excretion of lithium in milk is quite variable from mother to mother and lithium may be used cautiously if the baby is carefully monitored clinically and perhaps with serum lithium levels.[40]

F. Iodine-Containing Drugs

Drugs that release free iodine into the mother's bloodstream such as povidone-iodine can cause infant thyroid dysfunction. Iodine and iodides should be avoided if possible, especially applied to mucous membranes (eg, vaginal douching) or to open wounds. If used, these drugs should be used in the lowest dose for the shortest time.[41] Topical agents should be applied on the smallest area possible and in the lowest concentration possible. Nonradioactive iodinated contrast media do not release sufficient free iodine to be of concern and do not require breastfeeding interruption.[42,43]

G. Hemolytic Agents

These types of drugs should be avoided in mothers with an infant less than 1 month of age. Dapsone and long-acting sulfonamides in breastmilk have caused hemolysis in a breastfed infant.[44,45] Currently, the hemolytic agents most commonly prescribed to nursing mothers are phenazopyridine and nitrofurantoin.

VI. Drug Effects on Lactation

Several commonly used medications can interfere with lactation. Most standard references fail to mention these problems. Pharmacists can be helpful in counseling mothers to avoid these products and by recommending appropriate alternatives.

A. Drugs That Decrease Milk Supply

1. Alcohol
Alcohol's effects on lactation are complex and depend on the dose of alcohol. With four drinks or more, alcohol decreases milk production by decreasing milk letdown (via decreased oxytocin). Beer might increase maternal serum prolactin levels because of polysaccharides from barley and hops. However, nursing after one or two drinks (including beer) can decrease the infant's milk intake by 20%–23% and cause infant agitation and poor sleep patterns. The long-term effects of daily use of alcohol on the infant are unclear. Daily use of alcohol of more than two drinks may affect infants negatively and appears to decrease the length of time that mothers breastfeed their infants.[46] Nursing mothers should use alcohol moderately at most and wait 2–2.5 hours per drink before nursing.[47]

2. Anticholinergics
Smooth muscle relaxants for the GI and genitourinary tracts appear to have some negative effect on lactation. Older, more anticholinergic antihistamines can be a problem, particularly in combination with sympathomimetics (eg, in over-the-counter cold and allergy products).

3. Diuretics
Diuretics in high doses have been used therapeutically to suppress lactation. Hydrochlorothiazide in a dose of 25 mg/d or less is unlikely to cause lactation problems.

4. Dopaminergic Agents

Amantadine, antiparkinson drugs, and some agents used for restless leg syndrome should usually be avoided in nursing mothers. These are dopamine agonists that decrease serum prolactin levels via an effect on the CNS.

5. Estrogens

Estrogens, including the amounts in combination (ie, estrogen-containing) oral contraceptives suppress lactation in a dose-dependent manner. Progestin-only contraception begun at 6 weeks postpartum is the hormonal contraceptive method of choice for nursing mothers. When combined with exclusive breastfeeding, progestin-only contraceptives have an efficacy similar to combined oral contraceptives in non-nursing women. Although progestin-only contraceptives are preferred throughout the breastfeeding period, combination products containing less than 35 µg/d of ethinyl estradiol can be introduced in well-nourished women with well-established lactation for greater contraceptive efficacy after at least 6 weeks postpartum.[48] Nursing mothers should be monitored carefully for lactation adequacy if a combination product is used.

6. Cigarette Smoking

Nursing mothers who smoke usually stop breastfeeding earlier and supplement with formula sooner than nonsmokers.[49] Their infants may also have growth retardation and colic, and high levels of contaminants from smoke are found in the breastmilk. If mothers stop smoking during pregnancy, they breastfeed for longer than mothers who continue smoking.[50]

7. Sympathomimetic Vasoconstrictors

Pseudoephedrine reliably decreases milk supply because of decreased central release of prolactin and possibly oxytocin.[51] Oral phenylephrine probably has a similar effect. Nasal decongestant sprays containing oxymetazoline (eg, Afrin) are preferred decongestants for nursing mothers.

B. Galactagogues

Galactagogues are drugs or other substances that can increase milk supply. Metoclopramide, domperidone, and sulpiride are the most common clinically used drugs for this purpose. None is officially approved for this use in any country, and only metoclopramide is an FDA-approved drug. A rigorous review of studies on galactagogues found that these drugs raise baseline serum prolactin concentrations by their dopamine antagonist activity.[52] However, there is no direct correlation between baseline serum prolactin and long-term breastfeeding success in normal women or in those given a dopamine antagonist galactagogue. Furthermore, in most studies in which mothers were provided education and practice techniques that support lactation physiology, galactagogues had little or no added benefit. The safety of dopamine antagonists has not been adequately studied when used as galactagogues, but all have potential safety concerns for mothers, infants, or both.

Fenugreek is an herbal product that is frequently used as a galactagogue, although no scientific evidence exists on its use for this purpose. Its use is based primarily on historical precedent and anecdote. Although it is commonly used safely as a spice and flavoring agent, the larger amounts taken as a galactagogue can cause hypoglycemia and interact with warfarin. Allergy and asthma have also been reported from contact with fenugreek.[53,54] Milk thistle is another traditional herbal used as a galactagogue with no scientific basis.

Galactagogues should not be used as a substitute for good patient management. Pharmacists can recommend more frequent nursing as the first step in increasing milk supply. A mother with difficulties in nursing should be referred to her infant's pediatrician or a lactation consultant for further evaluation.

VII. Information Sources

Because studies on drug use during breastfeeding rarely meet the "gold standard" of being randomized and double blinded, some differences in interpretation of the available literature exist, even among experts. Differences in recommendations on the advisability of the use of drugs during breastfeeding by various information resources have been documented.[55,56]

In one study, breastfeeding information was analyzed in 10 drug information sources.[55] The *Physicians' Desk Reference*, which is based on the package insert, gave entirely negative advice about the use of 14 medications commonly used during breastfeeding and provided no documentation. The more evidence-based sources of information provided more permissive advice. The two sources rated best by the authors were Hale's *Medications and Mothers' Milk*,[56] and LactMed, a free database published by the National Library of Medicine (http://lactmed.nlm.nih.gov).

In addition to Hale's book and LactMed, which focus on drugs and breastfeeding alone, several specialty books are available that cover medication use in both pregnancy and lactation. These include Briggs GG, Freeman RK, Yaffe SJ. *Drugs in Pregnancy and Lactation. A Reference Guide to Fetal and Neonatal Risk*. 8th ed. Philadelphia: Lippincott, Williams & Wilkins, 2008; Koren G. *Medication Safety in Pregnancy and Breastfeeding*. New York: McGraw-Hill, 2007; and Schaefer C, Peters P, Miller RK. *Drugs during Pregnancy and Lactation*. 2nd ed. London: Academic Press, 2007. Other resources are the teratogen information services. Although they specialize in medication safety during pregnancy, they also provide information on drug use during breastfeeding. The nearest teratogen information service can be located through the Organization of Teratogen Information Specialists Web site at http://otispregnancy.org or at 866-626-OTIS (6847).

The FDA has recognized that the drug package insert is an unreliable and incomplete source of information on medication use during breastfeeding.[57] Consequently, in 2008, the FDA proposed major changes to drug labeling requirements with respect to lactation.[58] The proposed labeling format is shown in Figure 2.[59] The new format will initially apply to newly approved drugs. Several years will be required to revise the labeling of all marketed drugs.[60] Meanwhile, the current deficient labeling will continue to appear in the package inserts of older drugs.

Many computerized outpatient and community pharmacy systems print labels that warn against breastfeeding based on information in the package insert. These labels often cause unwarranted concern in nursing mothers about the safety of taking medications during breastfeeding, even after a knowledgeable prescriber has told them the drug is safe to

Risk Summary

For drugs that are not systemically absorbed, there is a standard statement that states that maternal use is not expected to result in infant exposure.

For drugs that are systemically absorbed, the risk summary must describe the following information or state that it is not available:

- Effects of drug on milk production
  - Presence of drug in human milk
  - If drug not detected, state limits of assay
  - If drug is detected, provide drug concentration in milk and estimated infant daily dose (actual and compared to pediatric or maternal doses)
  - Effects of the drug on the breast-fed child
- If data show that the drug does not affect the quantity and quality of breast milk and there is reasonable certainty that either the drug is not detectable in breast milk or will not adversely affect the breast-fed child, then state:
  - "The use of (name of drug) is compatible with breastfeeding."

Clinical Considerations

This section must provide, when available, information on:
- Ways to minimize exposure of the breast-fed infant to the drug
- Dosing adjustments during lactation

Data

This section must provide an overview of the data that are the basis for information in the risk summary and clinical considerations.

Figure 2. Proposed U.S. Food and Drug Administration (FDA) Lactation Labeling Format. From FDA.[59]

use. Most database suppliers are taking steps to upgrade their information based on the new FDA requirements. However, until the transition to new labeling is complete, it is incumbent on the pharmacist to be aware of the differences in labeling and to use an evidence-based source of information in judging whether to warn mothers about potential problems with medications taken during nursing using the principles described in this chapter.

VIII. PATIENT CASE

A 30-year-old woman has been taking citalopram, 40 mg/d, before and during pregnancy for chronic depression. She has responded well to this drug and has relapsed in the past when it was discontinued. The drug was withheld for 2 days prior to delivery and she gave birth to a healthy, full-term male infant with Apgar scores of 8 at 5 minutes and 9 at 10 minutes. The mother wants to breastfeed her baby, but is unsure about taking citalopram during breastfeeding.

A. Assessment

In this patient, there was an attempt to minimize the impact of citalopram on the newborn by withholding the medication before delivery. However, the half-life of citalopram is in the 30- to 40-hour hour range, so it is likely that the mother and infant both have some citalopram in their bloodstreams at delivery. Because the infant was exposed to citalopram in utero throughout gestation, there is a risk of the infant experiencing withdrawal symptoms as his serum concentrations drop. If the mother restarts citalopram, breastfeeding might mitigate the infant's withdrawal symptoms by maintaining his serum citalopram concentrations. The amount of citalopram in breastmilk is among the highest of the selective serotonin reuptake inhibitors (SSRIs) on average and occasionally causes sedation in breastfed infants, but the amount excreted in milk varies from mother to mother, so it is not possible to predict whether the infant will have withdrawal symptoms, sedation, or neither.

Usually the greatest concern is the long-term adverse effects of antidepressants in breastmilk on the infant. Although the literature is not conclusive, the studies that have been published have found no long-term effects on infants' growth and development. It is usually desirable to minimize the exposure of infants, especially newborns, to drugs in breastmilk that can affect the CNS. Many well-designed studies have demonstrated short- and long-term health benefits from breastfeeding compared to artificial feedings such as formula. The mother's needs also need to be considered. With a history of chronic depression, the likelihood that she will experience postpartum depression is high. The infants of depressed mothers have difficulties with behavior and interaction with others that can persist into the school years.

B. Plan

The many facets of this rather complex situation should be discussed with the mother to both educate her and have her participate in the final decision. Options include the following: (i) not treating the mother so she could breastfeed; (ii) treating the mother with a psychological therapy (eg, cognitive behavioral therapy, psychotherapy) instead of an antidepressant so she could breastfeed; (iii) treating the mother with an antidepressant, but not breastfeeding; (iv) treating the mother with a different antidepressant and breastfeeding; or (v) treating the mother with citalopram and monitoring the infant for side effects.

Failure to treat the mother for depression would seem to be the most undesirable option from both the mother's and infant's standpoint. Psychological therapies might be of benefit in this situation, either alone or in combination with an antidepressant, usually the same drug that was taken successfully during pregnancy. Most pharmacists would not be expected to be able to recommend psychological therapies to patients, so this decision should be made in consultation with the physician treating her depression.

Often, antidepressant therapy during pregnancy will be continued postpartum. Although the clinician should not force breastfeeding on a mother, the benefits of breast-feeding should be emphasized as should the lack of evidence of harm of small amounts of SSRI antidepressants in breastmilk. The fact that the infant will have a lower exposure to the drug via breastfeeding than during pregnancy is reassuring to most mothers. The exposure of the infant could be further reduced by switching from citalopram, 40 mg/d, to escitalopram, 10 mg/d, which are considered to be equivalent dosages. Infants will receive 40%–50% less medication in milk with this strategy. Switching to a completely different antidepressant with lower excretion into milk (eg, sertraline or paroxetine) may or may not be an option, depending on how stable she is and what her past experience is with these drugs. Again, this is a judgment to be made in consultation with her physician.

The most likely scenario is that the mother will continue with an antidepressant postpartum. Whether she breastfeeds or not, the infant should be observed carefully for withdrawal symptoms or serotonin syndrome during the first few days of life. Both conditions have similar symptoms of hyperactivity such as jitteriness, irritability, excessive crying, insomnia, tremors, and increased startle reflex. The mother can be alerted to these symptoms and told to call her pediatrician if they are seen. If she breastfeeds her infant, the mother should be alerted to the possibility of excessive drowsiness in the infant. She should also be instructed to make sure she follows up with regular pediatric appointments to ensure that her infant is growing normally. Sometimes infant sedation can lead to less breastfeeding and reduced growth. The mother should also be followed by her physician or psychiatrist to ensure that her depression is adequately treated and not worsening postpartum. Early neonatal follow-up of the infant is also important.

IX. Summary

Pharmacists can counsel nursing mothers and their health care providers about breast-feeding during medication use. Although adverse reactions are uncommon, minimizing infant drug exposure in breastmilk is often desirable. A stepwise approach to using medications in breastfeeding women can be followed in order to minimize infant exposure to medications in milk.[21] The steps outlined in Table 1 can be used to minimize exposure, starting from the strategies that are least disruptive to nursing (at the top of the list) and progressing to those that are most disruptive (at the bottom). These strategies should be used in conjunction with specific information on the drug(s) in question and information obtained from the mother and in consultation with the mother's physician. The infant's age (plus gestational age for neonates) and the drug's name are the most important pieces of information. These alone will often determine the safety of drug use. Most adverse reactions occur while breastfeeding infants younger than 2 months of age. The drug dosage and duration of therapy, the condition being treated (to recommend alternatives), maternal or infant allergies (to avoid recommending contraindicated drugs), and the quantity and pattern of nursing (to recommend dosage regimens) can all be helpful in applying the steps in Table 1.

Table 1. Stepwise Approach to Minimizing Infant Exposure to Drugs in Breastmilk

1. Withhold the drug. For the pharmacist, this often means recommending the avoidance of unnecessary over-the-counter medications or multiple-ingredient combination products when a single medication would suffice.
2. Delay therapy (until the baby is older or weaned). Some elective diagnostic procedures or therapies might be delayed if a potentially toxic drug will be used.
3. Choose an alternative drug that passes poorly into milk. Medications in the same pharmacologic class (eg, β-blockers) can pass into breastmilk in markedly different amounts.
4. Choose an alternate route of administration (eg, topical rather than systemic, inhaled rather than oral).
5. Avoid nursing at times of peak drug concentration.* This strategy is effective only for medications with short half-lives in immediate-release dosage forms.
6. Administer the drug as a single dose before the infant's longest sleep period* and/or use alternate feeding for 1–2 feedings after the dose. This strategy can help avoid postabsorption peak breastmilk concentrations, even with drugs having a long elimination half-life.
7. Temporarily withhold breastfeeding. Sometimes, mothers can pump milk before the procedure and feed their infants stored breastmilk during the period of cessation.
8. Stop breastfeeding. This is only necessary for the most toxic drugs (eg, cancer chemotherapy, some radiopharmaceuticals) and some multidrug regimens. It should be considered a "last resort" and not recommended unless absolutely necessary.

*May not be feasible while nursing a newborn.

The risks associated with discontinuing breastfeeding should be discussed with the mother. Formula exposes the infant to increased risks of infection and long-term metabolic diseases. Mothers can also be negatively affected as outlined at the beginning of this chapter.

Finally, until the new FDA lactation labeling is fully implemented and drug databases are updated accordingly, a reasonable pharmacist might consider *not* affixing some computer-generated lactation warning labels to prescription bottles when a reliable information source states that risks to the breastfed infant are minimal or nonexistent.

X. References

1. U.S. Department of Health and Human Services. Agency for Healthcare Research and Quality. Breastfeeding and maternal and infant health outcomes in developed countries. *Evidence Report/Technology Assessment Number 153. AHRQ Publication No. 07-E007.* Rockville, MD: U.S. Department of Health and Human Services. Agency for Healthcare Research and Quality. 2007.

2. Gartner LM, Morton J, Lawrence RA, et al. Breastfeeding and the use of human milk. *Pediatrics.* 2005;115:496–506.

3. Eglash A, Montgomery A, Wood J. Breastfeeding. *Dis Mon.* 2008;54:343–411.

4. Labbok M, Krasovec K. Toward consistency in breastfeeding definitions. *Stud Fam Plann.* 1990;21:226–230.

5. Anon. Healthy People 2010. 16–19. Increase the proportion of mothers who breastfeed their babies. 2000. Available at http://www.healthypeople.gov. Accessed September 10, 2008.

6. World Health Organization. Global strategy for infant and young child feeding. 2003. Geneva. Available at http://www.unicef.org/nutrition/files/Global_ Strategy_Infant_and_Young_Child_Feeding.pdf. Accessed September 10, 2008.

7. Centers for Disease Control and Prevention. Breastfeeding trends and updated national health objectives for exclusive breastfeeding—United States, birth years 2000–2004. *MMWR Morb Mortal Wkly Rep.* 2007;56:760–763.

8. Ito S, Lieu M, Chan W, et al. Continuing drug therapy while breastfeeding. Part 1. Common misconceptions of patients. *Can Fam Physician.* 1999;45:897–899.

9. Ito S, Moretti M, Liau M, et al. Initiation and duration of breast-feeding in women receiving antiepileptics. *Am J Obstet Gynecol.* 1995;172:881–886.

10. Lee A, Moretti ME, Collantes A, et al. Choice of breastfeeding and physicians' advice: a cohort study of women receiving propylthiouracil. *Pediatrics.* 2000;106:27–30.

11. Li R, Fein SB, Chen J, et al. Why mothers stop breastfeeding: mothers' self-reported reasons for stopping during the first year. *Pediatrics.* 2008;122(suppl 2):S69–S76.

12. Malpas TJ, Darlow BA. Neonatal abstinence syndrome following abrupt cessation of breastfeeding. *N Z Med J.* 1999;112:12–13.

13. Ballard JL. Treatment of neonatal abstinence syndrome with breast milk containing methadone. *J Perinat Neonat Nurs.* 2002;15:76–85.

14. Abdel-Latif ME, Pinner J, Clews S, et al. Effects of breast milk on the severity and outcome of neonatal abstinence syndrome among infants of drug-dependent mothers. *Pediatrics.* 2006;117:e1163–1169.

15. Kuhnz W, Koch S, Helge H, et al. Primidone and phenobarbital during lactation period in epileptic women: total and free drug serum levels in the nursed infants and their effects on neonatal behavior. *Dev Pharmacol Ther.* 1988;11:147–154.

16. Kim J, Riggs KW, Misri S, et al. Stereoselective disposition of fluoxetine and norfluoxetine during pregnancy and breast-feeding. *Br J Clin Pharmacol.* 2006; 61:155–163.

17. Wittels B, Glosten B, Faure EA, et al. Postcesarean analgesia with both epidural morphine and intravenous patient-controlled analgesia: neurobehavioral outcomes among nursing neonates. *Anesth Analg.* 1997;85:600–606.

18. Gaiser R. Neonatal effects of labor analgesia. *Int Anesthesiol Clin.* 2002;40:49–65.

19. Hartmann PE, Cregan MD, Ramsay DT, et al. Physiology of lactation in preterm mothers: initiation and maintenance. *Pediatr Ann.* 2003;32:351–355.

20. Bennett PN, ed. *Drugs and Human Lactation.* 2nd ed. Amsterdam: Elsevier, 1996.

21. Anderson PO. Drug use during breast-feeding. *Clin Pharm.* 1991;10:594–624.

22. Ilett KF, Kristensen JH. Drug use and breastfeeding. *Expert Opin Drug Saf.* 2005; 4:745–768.

23. Ito S, Lee A. Drug excretion into breast milk—overview. *Adv Drug Deliv Rev.* 2003;55:617–627.

24. Riant P, Urien S, Albengres E, et al. High plasma protein binding as a parameter in the selection of beta blockers for lactating women. *Biochem Pharmacol.* 1986;35:4579–4581.

25. Larsen LA, Ito S, Koren G. Prediction of milk/plasma concentration ratio of drugs. *Ann Pharmacother.* 2003;37:1299–1306.

26. Bennett PN, Notarianni LJ. Risk from drugs in breast milk: an analysis by relative dose. *Br J Clin Pharmacol.* 1996;42:P673–674. Abstract.

27. Ito S, Koren G. A novel index for expressing exposure to the infant to drugs in breast milk. *Br J Clin Pharmacol.* 1994;38:99–102.

28. McNamara PJ, Abbassi M. Neonatal exposure to drugs in breast milk. *Pharm Res.* 2004;21:555–566.

29. Anderson PO, Pochop SL, Manoguerra AS. Adverse drug reactions in breastfed infants: less than imagined. *Clin Pediatr (Phila).* 2003;42:325–340.

30. Stewart CF, Hampton EM. Effect of maturation on drug disposition in pediatric patients. *Clin Pharm.* 1987;6:548–564.

31. Anderson PO. Medication use while breast feeding a neonate. *Neonatal Pharmacol Q.* 1993;2:3–14.

32. Hale TW. Medications in breastfeeding mothers of preterm infants. *Pediatr Ann.* 2003;32:337–347.

33. Koren G, Cairns J, Chitayat D, et al. Pharmacogenetics of morphine poisoning in a breastfed neonate of a codeine-prescribed mother. *Lancet.* 2006;368:704.

34. Madadi P, Ross C, Hayden M, et al. Pharmacogenetics of neonatal opioid toxicity following maternal use of codeine during breastfeeding: a case-control study. *Clin Pharmacol Ther.* 2008 Aug 20. [Epub ahead of print].

35. Berle JO, Steen VM, Aamo TO, et al. Breastfeeding during maternal antidepressant treatment with serotonin reuptake inhibitors: infant exposure, clinical symptoms, and cytochrome P450 genotypes. *J Clin Psychiatry.* 2004;65:1228–1234.

36. Ito S, Blajchman A, Stephenson M, et al. Prospective follow-up of adverse reactions in breast-fed infants exposed to maternal medication. *Am J Obstet Gynecol.* 1993;168:1393–1399.

37. Weissman AM, Levy BT, Hartz AJ, et al. Pooled analysis of antidepressant levels in lactating mothers, breast milk, and nursing infants. *Am J Psychiatry.* 2004;161:1066–1078.

38. The Academy of Breastfeeding Medicine Protocol Committee. ABM clinical protocol #18: use of antidepressants in nursing mothers. *Breastfeed Med.* 2008;3:44–52.

39. Mirpuri J, Patel H, Rhee D, et al. What's mom on? A case of bradycardia in a premature infant on breast milk. *J Invest Med.* 2008;56:409. Abstract.

40. Moretti ME, Koren G, Verjee Z, et al. Monitoring lithium in breast milk: an individualized approach for breast-feeding mothers. *Ther Drug Monit.* 2003;25:364–366.

41. Casteels K, Punt S, Bramswig J. Transient neonatal hypothyroidism during breastfeeding after post-natal maternal topical iodine treatment. *Eur J Pediatr.* 2000;159:716–717.

42. Webb JA, Thomsen HS, Morcos SK, et al. The use of iodinated and gadolinium contrast media during pregnancy and lactation. *Eur Radiol.* 2005;15:1234–1240.

43. ACR Committee on Drugs and Contrast Media. Administration of contrast medium to breastfeeding mothers. *ACR Bull.* 2001;57:12–13.

44. Brown AK, Cevik N. Hemolysis and jaundice in the newborn following maternal treatment with sulfamethoxypyridazine (Kynex). *Pediatrics.* 1965;36:742–744.

45. Sanders SW, Zone JJ, Foltz RL, et al. Hemolytic anemia induced by dapsone transmitted through breast milk. *Ann Intern Med.* 1982;96:465–466.

46. Mennella JA. Alcohol use during lactation: effects on the mother and the breast-feeding infant. In Watson RR, Preedy VR, eds. *Nutrition and Alcohol.* Boca Raton, FL: CRC Press, 2004:377–391.

47. Ho E, Collantes A, Kapur BM, et al. Alcohol and breast feeding: calculation of time to zero level in milk. *Biol Neonate.* 2001;80:219–222.

48. Queenan JT. Contraception and breastfeeding. *Clin Obstet Gynecol.* 2004;47:734–739.

49. Horta BL, Kramer MS, Platt RW. Maternal smoking and the risk of early weaning: a meta-analysis. *Aust N Z J Psychiatry.* 2001;91:304–307.

50. Giglia R, Binns CW, Alfonso H. Maternal cigarette smoking and breastfeeding duration. *Acta Paediatr.* 2006;95:1370–1374.

51. Hale T, Ilett K, Hartmann P, et al. Pseudoephedrine effects on milk production in women and estimation of infant exposure via human milk. *Adv Exp Med Biol.* 2004;554:437–438.

52. Anderson PO, Valdes V. A critical review of pharmaceutical galactagogues. *Breastfeed Med.* 2007;2:229–242.

53. Montgomery A , Wight N. Protocol #9: Use of galactagogues in initiating or augmenting maternal milk supply. Academy of Breastfeeding Medicine. 2004. Available at http://www.bfmed.org/ace-files/protocol/prot9galactogoguesEnglish.pdf. Accessed September 10, 2008.

54. Tiran D. The use of fenugreek for breast feeding women. *Complement Ther Nurs Midwifery.* 2003;9:155–156.

55. Akus M, Bartick M. Lactation safety recommendations and reliability compared in 10 medication resources. *Ann Pharmacother.* 2007;41:1352–1360.

56. Hale T. *Medications and Mothers' Milk.* 13th ed. Amarillo, TX: Pharmasoft Medical Publishing, 2008.

57. Uhl K, Peat R, Toigo T, et al. Review of drug labeling for information regarding lactation. *Clin Pharmacol Ther.* 2003;73:P39. PII–39.

58. Department of Health and Human Services. Food and Drug Administration. Content and format of labeling for human prescription drug and biological products; requirements for pregnancy and lactation labeling. *Federal Register.* 2008;73:30831–30868.

59. U.S. Food and Drug Administration. Lactation subsection: overview. 2008. Available at http://www.fda.gov/cder/Regulatory/Pregnancy_Labeling/Example_Lactation.pdf. Accessed September 10, 2008.

60. Kweder SL. Drugs and biologics in pregnancy and breastfeeding: FDA in the 21st century. *Birth Defects Res A Clin Mol Teratol.* 2008;82:605–609.

QUESTIONS AND ANSWERS

1. List three infant diseases that are more prevalent and/or serious in formula-fed infants than in breastfed infants.

2. At what infant age does the risk of adverse reactions from drugs in breastmilk decrease markedly?

3. List three properties of medications that result in low breastmilk concentrations.

4. A study on the excretion of a new drug into breastmilk in 12 nursing mothers found that the average milk/plasma ratio of the drug was 1.5. In the package insert, you find that with a dosage of 750 mg every 12 hours, the average steady-state peak serum concentration is 2 µg/mL. If an infant's 75-kilogram mother were taking this dosage, what would be the approximate dose that an exclusively breastfed infant would receive?

   a. 750 µg/kg/d

   b. 600 µg/kg/d

   c. 450 µg/kg/d

   d. 300 µg/kg/d

5. In the case above, what is the weight-adjusted percentage of the maternal dosage for this drug?

   a. 7.5%

   b. 4.5%

   c. 3.75%

   d. 2.25%

Answers

1. Any three of the following: diarrhea, respiratory tract infections, otitis media, bacteremia, bacterial meningitis, urinary tract infections, necrotizing enterocolitis, or late-onset sepsis.

2. After 1 month of age the risk decreases substantially; after 2 months adverse reactions are rare.

3. Any three of the following: weak acid, high protein binding, very high molecular weight, poor lipid solubility, rapid drug clearance, or extent of nursing.

4. c

5. d

Clinical Pharmacokinetics in the Pregnant Patient

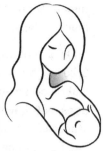

Carl W. Kildoo and Peter J. Ambrose

LEARNING OBJECTIVES

1. Identify four key physiologic changes that occur during pregnancy that affect the pharmacokinetics of drugs in general.

2. Discuss three factors that limit the ability to predict the effect of pregnancy on the pharmacokinetics and dosing needs for a given drug in a specific patient.

3. Describe the disposition of the aminoglycosides, digoxin, phenytoin, and vancomycin in the pregnant patient.

I. Introduction

Appropriate drug dosing during pregnancy is a complicated topic reflecting the dynamic physiologic and metabolic changes that occur throughout pregnancy. Additionally, there are limited data to help guide therapy. However, it is clear that there is a potential effect of pregnancy on the efficacy and safety of a given drug and this should be a consideration in drug therapy during pregnancy and in the postpartum period. Pregnancy may have significant effects on the absorption, distribution, metabolism, and excretion of many drugs.[1,2] These effects correlate with the specific physiologic changes observed in pregnancy, which include an increase in cardiac output, a decrease in serum albumin concentration, a significant increase in renal blood flow and glomerular filtration rate, and a variable effect on the metabolic pathways in the liver in which drug elimination may increase, decrease, or remain the same.[1-5]

II. PATIENT CASE [PART 1]

The patient is a 24-year-old female at 29 weeks' gestation in her first pregnancy. She is 5'7" tall and weighs 82 kilograms, resulting in a body mass index of 28. Fetal echogram does not indicate the presence of hydrops. The fetus was found to have supraventricular tachycardia on examination, with a heart rate of 220 beats per minute (bpm). The mother's blood pressure and heart rate were within normal limits (WNL).

Digoxin therapy was initiated with a loading dose of 1.0 mg IV; given as 0.5 mg, 0.25 mg, and 0.25 mg, with 6 hours between each dose. A serum digoxin concentration obtained 6 hours after the last dose was 0.7 ng/mL. The assay employed does not have significant interference from digoxinlike immunoreactive substances (DLIS) in serum from patients who are pregnant or have liver dysfunction, and from neonates, as reported by the package insert in the manufacturer's assay kit. The mother's heart rate and blood pressure remained WNL, while the fetal heart rate essentially did not change. At that time, a maintenance dose of 0.5 mg IV every 12 hours was initiated. On the next day, the serum digoxin concentration was 1.3 ng/mL, 6 hours after the previous dose. The fetal heart rate decreased to 110 bpm, while the mother's heart rate and blood pressure remained WNL. The maintenance dose was continued and achieved an eventual steady-state concentration of 1.6 ng/mL, with a fetal heart rate of 80–100 bpm; mother's heart rate and blood pressure remained WNL.

The above case reflects some of the pharmacokinetic changes that are observed in pregnancy and demonstrates the importance for clinicians to be aware of assay-interfering substances for serum digoxin concentrations in pregnant patients. Questions to consider, which are highlighted in this chapter, include:

- Is the high dose consistent with expected changes in renal and metabolic elimination?
- What effect would a decrease in serum albumin have on the plasma protein binding of digoxin in pregnant patients?
- Does digoxin significantly cross the placenta to exert an effect on the fetus?
- What is the potential problem with the assay-interfering substances regarding digoxin in the pregnant patient?

Additionally, there is a general discussion of the physiologic and metabolic changes occurring in pregnancy, and the resulting change on the pharmacokinetic profile of various drugs. (See also Chapter 1, Physiologic Changes in Pregnancy.)

III. Physiologic and Metabolic Changes

There is an increase in cardiac output during pregnancy that may be as much as a 60% increase at its maximal effect. This process begins in early pregnancy and appears to reach its peak effect in the second trimester.[1,5,6] During the third trimester there appears to be a significant amount of interpatient variability in cardiac output.[6] The increase in cardiac output in pregnancy is accompanied by a decrease in peripheral resistance. Despite a compensatory increase in blood volume, there is an overall decrease in blood pressure of approximately 10%. These effects result in an increase in blood flow to the kidneys, liver, uterus, and placenta.[1,5,6] In addition to the increase in intravascular volume, there is a significant increase in total body water.[7]

A. Physiologic Changes in Kidney Function

A number of changes in renal physiology and hemodynamics occur during pregnancy that regulate the dynamic fluid and electrolyte needs during gestation. These changes can also influence the renal elimination of drugs to a significant degree. Studies have demonstrated that renal plasma flow and glomerular filtration rate (GFR) increase during normal pregnancy, with a sustained increase in GFR of 40%–80% above prepregnant or postpartum values.[8–12] Further, the kidney increases in size, likely due to the increase in renal blood flow and renal vascular volume.[13] As a result of this increase in GFR, concentrations of blood urea nitrogen and serum creatinine decline. The rise in GFR has been observed in pregnant women with diabetes and with gestational hypertension, as well.[8] One study measured serial 24-hour creatinine clearances at weekly intervals in healthy pregnant women and found an average increase of 25% above baseline during the fourth week of pregnancy, which continued to rise to a 45% increase during the ninth week.[14] It has also been shown that creatinine clearance remains elevated during the second trimester of pregnancy, and then declines during the last 6 weeks of pregnancy, and essentially returns to baseline over the last 6 weeks before delivery.[15,16] Measured creatinine clearances were found to increase soon after delivery, and were back to baseline 6 days after delivery. It should be kept in mind that creatinine clearance may not necessarily predict GFR to the same degree as in nonpregnant subjects, since renal tubular handling of creatinine may be significantly different.

No reliable formula has been developed to estimate creatinine clearance in normal pregnancy based on serum creatinine concentrations and other patient characteristics. Use of the popular Cockcroft-Gault equation to estimate creatinine clearance in adults would not necessarily be appropriate, as the formula was not developed or validated in this patient population.[17] Further, the production rate of creatinine is likely different in this population, in addition to differences in renal tubular secretion and reabsorption. In a recent study comparing GFR measured by inulin clearance with that estimated by the modification of diet in renal disease (MDRD) formula, modified for various stages of pregnancy, the formula underestimated GFR by approximately 42 mL/min (27%) on average.[18]

Studies have demonstrated that the increase in GFR observed in normal pregnancy is not observed in preeclampsia.[8,19,20] The GFR in preeclamptic women, at least in late pregnancy, tends to remain unchanged in comparison to prepregnancy or postpartum values. This appears to be due to structural changes in the kidney associated with preeclampsia that result in impaired intrinsic glomerular ultrafiltration.[19] In a study comparing measured 24-hour creatinine clearance values to those estimated by the Cockcroft-Gault, MDRD, and the modified MDRD equations in pregnant patients (≥24 weeks' gestation) diagnosed with preeclampsia, on average the Cockcroft-Gault equation overestimated the measured creatinine clearance by 30%, whereas the MDRD and modified MDRD equations underestimated by averages of 14% and 9%, respectively.[21] A new formula was derived from the data in this study, but it has not been validated in studies with other subjects.

B. Physiologic and Metabolic Changes in the Liver

1. Physiologic Changes in the Liver

The primary changes that may alter the metabolic function of the liver and the pharmacokinetic profile of many drugs during pregnancy are an increase in liver blood flow, changes in the metabolic activity of liver enzymes, and a decrease in concentration of albumin that can result in a change in protein binding. Liver blood flow increases as a result of the increase in cardiac output that occurs. An increase of up to 160% in liver blood flow during the third trimester has been reported.[22] The metabolism of high-extraction drugs, such as morphine and propranolol, would be expected to be cleared from the body more rapidly with such a significant increase in liver blood flow. However, reports for these drugs have not confirmed such an increase, but are more variable.[23,24] Additional study is needed to determine if the increase in liver blood flow has a consistent effect on drug elimination, realizing that other metabolic changes may attenuate or potentiate the overall effect.

The concentration of serum albumin decreases in pregnancy. No data are available to document that this is related to a decrease in production as some have theorized. Rather, the decrease in concentration appears to be connected to a dilutional effect related to the increase in plasma volume, and may also reflect some increase in urinary excretion of albumin in the later stages of pregnancy.[1,2,25,26] This decrease in serum albumin concentration affects the binding of drugs that are highly bound to albumin, such as phenytoin. However, this decrease in protein binding does not result in a change in therapeutic efficacy, as the free drug concentration, which is the active moiety, remains unchanged unless pregnancy also affects the metabolism of the free drug. The total (bound and unbound) drug concentration is reduced because there is less bound drug in the plasma. Therefore, in a pregnant patient, it should be requested that the laboratory determine the free drug serum concentration for drugs that are highly bound to plasma proteins such as phenytoin.[27] If such testing is not available for a particular drug, the effect of decreased plasma protein binding on total drug concentration needs to be considered when interpreting serum drug concentrations and in adjusting therapy. With regard to the case history, digoxin is also bound to serum albumin; however, a change in serum albumin concentration would not have a significant on the unbound concentration of digoxin, as it is 70%–80% unbound already.

2. Metabolic Changes in the Liver

Changes may be seen during pregnancy in various metabolic enzyme systems, including the cytochrome P-450 (CYP) and uridine 5'-diphosphate glucuronosyltransferases (UGT) enzyme systems. CYP enzymes are a superfamily of hemoproteins. Of most interest are the three major families (CYP1, CYP2, and CYP3). The specific isoenzymes that are primarily involved in metabolism of drugs commonly used in pregnant patients are CYP1A2, CYP2A6, CYP2C9, CYP2C19, CYP2D6, and CYP3A4.[1,2] This nomenclature is a genetically based description of the isoenzyme. For CYP1A2, in addition to "CYP" referring to the cytochrome P-450 system, "1" indicates the genetic family, "A" is the genetic subfamily, and "2" is the specific gene.

The effect of pregnancy on the CYP enzymes appears to vary depending on the isoenzyme and the stage of pregnancy. For some isoenzymes, data are not available for all stages of pregnancy or the effect is only known for a limited number of drugs metabolized by the pathway. Table 1 summarizes the effect of pregnancy on key isoenzymes and drugs potentially affected.

Table 1. Changes in Drug Metabolism Activity in Pregnancy*

Enzyme Pathway	Change in Activity	Drugs of Interest	Comments
CYP1A2	Decreased	Theophylline, clozapine, olanzapine, ondansetron, propranolol, cyclobenzaprine	Caffeine half-life also prolonged
CYP2A6	Increased	Nicotine, cotinine	Cotinine is active metabolite nicotine; may have decreased effect of nicotine gum
CYP2C9	Increased	Phenytoin, glyburide	Monitoring of phenytoin concentrations indicated
CYP2C19	Decreased	Lansoprazole, omeprazole, pantoprazole	Potential for increased efficacy of proton pump inhibitors
CYP2D6	Increased	Many β-blockers, including metoprolol; many tricyclic antidepressants and SSRIs (including citalopram, duloxetine, fluoxetine, paroxetine); codeine	Decreased concentration of SSRI documented and may be associated with recurring symptoms of depression
CYP3A4	Increased	Most calcium channel blockers, including nifedipine; most benzodiazepines; most HIV protease inhibitors; most nonsedating antihistamines; methadone	May have withdrawal symptoms in patients on methadone maintenance
UGT1A1	Increased	Acetaminophen	Unknown clinical consequence
UGT1A4	Increased	Lamotrigine	Significant decrease in serum lamotrigine concentrations; increase in seizure activity unless monitoring and dose adjustment occurs
UGT2B7	Increased	Lorazepam	Unknown clinical consequence

*From Hodge et al.,[1] Anderson,[2] and U.S. Food and Drug Administration.[81]

There are additional details of interest to understand the functioning of the CYP system and the potential effect of pregnancy. The activity of some isoenzymes such as CYP2C9, CYP2C19, and CYP2D6 are genetically controlled with genetic polymorphism associated with differing effect on drugs. For example, for CYP2D6, there are different phenotypic expressions depending on the genetic variation with resulting activity of CYP2D6 in a given patient described as "poor," "intermediate," "extensive," or "ultrarapid" metabolizers. Other pathways, including of particular interest CYP3A4, can have their activity induced or inhibited by interfering substrates.

Predicting the effect of pregnancy for a given drug can be further complicated by three factors. This includes interpatient variability in enzymatic activity, in which a patient who is a "poor metabolizer" for the isoenzyme may not have the same effect from pregnancy as a patient who has "intermediate," "extensive," or "ultra-rapid" metabolic activity for the pathway. Also, some drugs are metabolized by more than one isoenzyme or eliminated by more than one pathway and, therefore, pregnancy may have differing effects on the activity of the different pathways.[1,2] Hence, specific clinical information is needed for each individual drug. Additionally, patients may be on other medications that may induce or inhibit the activity of the isoenzyme, thus modifying the effect of pregnancy.

An example of these complicating factors can be seen in pregnant patients receiving methadone therapy. The primary enzyme responsible for metabolizing methadone is CYP3A4. However, there is evidence that other CYP isoenzymes are involved in its metabolism including 2D6, 1A2, 2C9, 2C19, and 2B6. Therefore, generalities for the effect of pregnancy on CYP3A4 cannot be directly applied, and specific studies for methadone are needed. For methadone, data are available to help guide therapy to some extent. Mean methadone clearance in nine pregnant women increased from 0.17 L/h/kg in the first trimester to 0.21 L/h/kg representing a 24% increase. This resulted in a decrease in the mean trough plasma methadone concentration from 0.12 mg/L in the first trimester to 0.07 mg/L in the third trimester. However, there was wide interpatient variability, with not all patients having an increase in clearance.[28] Clinically, if a patient experiences withdrawal symptoms while on methadone therapy during pregnancy, it has been suggested that the daily dose be increased by 5–10 mg or a divided dose regimen be used.[1] Again, for many drugs metabolized by multiple isoenzymes or eliminated by different mechanisms (eg, both metabolism and renal excretion), the drug-specific information needed on the effect of pregnancy is not available.[2]

Uridine 5'-diphosphate glucuronosyltransferases are enzymes that metabolize drugs by glucuronidation. The activity of UGT1A1, UGT1A4, and UGT2B7 increases in pregnancy. The clinical effect of this increased activity is currently only known for UGT1A4, which metabolizes lamotrigine. There is a significant decrease in serum lamotrigine concentrations during pregnancy due to this increased enzymatic activity. Without appropriate dosage adjustment, there is a loss of seizure control.[1,29] In a report of 12 pregnancies in nine women receiving lamotrigine as monotherapy, increased seizure activity was noted in nine of the 12 pregnancies.[30] The increase in seizure activity was noted between 12 and 28 weeks' gestation in eight pregnancies and at week 40 in the ninth. Dosage adjustment was made in seven women to regain seizure control. Subsequently, three of the seven women with previous increases in dosage had side effects (dizziness, diplopia, or ataxia) between 3 and 10 days after delivery. The serum lamotrigine concentrations were in the high-normal range (12–14 mg/L) in these patients, and their symptoms resolved with a decrease in dose. Table 1 includes summary information for the UGT pathways and drugs metabolized via these enzymes.

IV. Placental-Fetal Compartment

The existence of the placental-fetal compartment in the pregnant patient also contributes to changes in drug disposition. The placenta acts as a permeable barrier between the maternal and fetal blood circulations and is perfused by both systems. It functions to transport oxygen and nutrients from the mother to the growing fetus, while also providing a mechanism for metabolic waste exchange from the fetus to the mother for elimination. Thus, whether intentional or not, the fetus is exposed to xenobiotics ingested by the mother.

Drugs cross the placenta to varying degrees, resulting in a wide range of fetal-maternal drug concentration ratios. A number of factors and processes determine the rate and extent to which drugs cross the placental barrier. Passive diffusion is the principal mechanism involved in drug transport across the placenta from the maternal to the fetal circulation, according to the maternal-fetal concentration gradient. Factors that affect the ability of a compound to cross the placenta to the fetal circulation include placental blood flow and the physicochemical properties of the specific compound, such as pK_a, lipid solubility, and molecular size.[31–33]

Differences in the maternal and fetal plasma protein concentrations and their respective affinities for drugs are also determinants of the amount of drug that passes through the placenta.[31] In general, drugs with low maternal plasma protein binding are more readily available for diffusion. Further, the pH of the blood in the fetal circulation is very slightly more acidic than in the maternal blood. Some weak bases are then likely to be nonionized in the maternal blood and more permeable through the placenta and into the fetal circulation. In the fetal circulation with the slightly lower pH, these weak bases then become ionized and are less permeable for diffusion back to the maternal circulation, a process that has been termed "ion trapping."[31]

There are a number of enzymes expressed in the placenta that can metabolize xenobiotics during transplacental passage. However, the degree of drug metabolism via this mechanism is relatively insignificant, except for certain steroid substrates that the placenta regulates. Similarly, although the maturing liver in the fetus can progressively perform more and more complex phase I and phase II metabolic reactions, the fetal liver is still quite immature, and biotransformation of drugs is relatively minor in comparison to the metabolic capacity of the maternal liver. Hence, both placental and fetal metabolism of drugs are insignificant when applying clinical pharmacokinetics to drug therapy in terms of the total clearance of a drug.

The placenta also highly expresses transporter proteins that are thought to protect the fetus by facilitating the efflux of xenobiotics from the fetal circulation back to the maternal circulation. These proteins are termed the adenosine triphosphate–binding cassette transporters, consisting of P-glycoprotein, multidrug resistance–associated proteins, and the breast cancer resistance protein.[34,35] For example, glyburide is actively secreted from the fetal circulation against the maternal-fetal blood concentration gradient via transport by some of these proteins.[34]

Drugs that are renally cleared are also cleared by the maturing fetal kidney, and those drugs are excreted into the amniotic fluid. As with metabolic clearance, the small amount of renal clearance by the fetus is essentially insignificant; however, drugs can concentrate in the amniotic fluid with chronic administration.

V. Physiologic Changes in the Gastrointestinal Tract

The composition of gastrointestinal secretions has been reported to be altered during pregnancy, with conflicting reports of an overall decrease in gastric acid secretion.[36] The gallbladder increases in size, motility is decreased, and the composition of bile tends to change and be more dilute during pregnancy. Such effects could potentially alter drug stability and solubility and affect the rate of oral absorption. Gastrointestinal motility has been reported to be diminished in pregnancy, likely due to the actions and changes in concentration of motilin, somatostatin, estradiol, and progesterone.[37–40] Some investigators have observed a decrease in gastric emptying, whereas others have not.[36,41] Intestinal motility has also been reported to be reduced, resulting in a prolonged transit time.[39,42]

VI. Alterations in Pharmacokinetic Parameters

A. Absorption

There are numerous factors that determine the rate and extent of absorption of drugs after oral administration. Many of these factors relate to the physicochemical properties of the drug and the pharmaceutics of the specific product (eg, dosage form, excipients). Further, bioavailability is also a function of patient-specific physiologic factors, such as gastric secretions, gastrointestinal motility, metabolism via first pass through the liver, and metabolism by gut flora.

A slower rate in gastric emptying would delay the delivery of drug to the small intestine, and could potentially delay the onset of action and reduce the rate of absorption of a drug. A decrease in intestinal motility would increase the amount of time that a drug takes to pass through the intestine, and can potentially increase the extent of absorption, particularly for sustained-release products. The absorption process is quite complex and the exact net effect of these factors must be studied for individual drugs. However, data are only available for a very limited number of drugs.

In a study comparing the pharmacokinetics of ampicillin during and after pregnancy, no difference in the oral bioavailability was found, although significant changes in other pharmacokinetic parameters were observed.[43] In a similar study, the oral bioavailability of cephradine in healthy pregnant patients was observed to be 24% higher during pregnancy in comparison to postpartum values; however, the difference was not statistically significant.[44] In a small study of patients at different stages of pregnancy, the mean oral bioavailability of phenytoin was approximately 90%, which is comparable to nonpregnant values.[45]

B. Volume of Distribution

The volume of distribution of drugs may increase in pregnancy depending on the characteristics of a given drug. This is primarily related to an increase in extracellular fluid and total body water, and a decrease in plasma protein binding. Consequently, a decrease in peak blood concentrations after a dose of the drug can occur.[2] This change in volume of distribution is of most clinical significance for the aminoglycoside antibiotics, which are water-soluble drugs that distribute into extracellular fluid, and for which the peak serum concentration is directly related to the efficacy of the drug.

C. Clearance

1. Renal Elimination
The renal elimination of drugs is a function of GFR, as well as active tubular secretion and reabsorption. The latter two processes are dependent on saturable membrane

transport, and although these mechanisms have been shown to be remarkably different for endogenous substances during pregnancy, it is not possible to translate them to the disposition of drugs in general.[16] However, it is prudent to suspect that renal tubular secretion and reabsorption may be altered in pregnancy for drugs that undergo these routes, although the exact effects must be studied for individual drugs. Furthermore, the extent of any change in renal clearance will depend on the term during pregnancy that the drug is studied or used. Table 2 summarizes various studies on the effect of pregnancy on the renal elimination of multiple drugs.[2]

2. Metabolism
CYP1A2

The majority of the data regarding the effect of pregnancy on CYP1A2 is from studies using caffeine as the substrate, with some data available regarding the effect on theophylline clearance.[1,2] For other drugs that can be used in pregnancy and are metabolized by CYP1A2, no data are currently available.[1]

Pregnancy decreases the activity of CYP1A2, with the effect being greatest in the later stages. There is wide interpatient variability, which suggests that genetics may be involved in the activity of CYP1A2.[1,2,46] Based on caffeine metabolism, it was reported that CYP1A2 activity was reduced in comparison with postpartum activity by 32.8% ± 22.8% in the first trimester, 48.1% ± 27% in the second trimester, and 65.2% ± 15.3% in the third trimester.[46] The clearance of theophylline has been reported to decrease during the third trimester with an increase in the mean theophylline half-life to 13 hours compared with a postpartum value of 9.5 hours.[47] Hence, the dose of theophylline may need to be reduced in later stages of pregnancy to prevent adverse effects.[1] However, two other studies found only a nonsignificant trend toward an increase in clearance. This may be related to two other isoenzymes (CYP2E1 and CYP3A4), which are minor pathways for the elimination of theophylline but could potentially offset the full effect of decreased activity of CYP1A2. The activity of CYP3A4 appears to increase in pregnancy, whereas the effect on CYP2E1 is unknown.[2] This is another example of the difficulty of predicting the effect of pregnancy on a specific drug when it is eliminated by multiple pathways. If used during pregnancy, monitoring of serum theophylline concentrations is warranted, particularly in the third trimester.

CYP2A6

CYP2A6 is responsible for the metabolism of nicotine and its metabolite cotinine. Based on studies performed during the second and third trimesters, pregnancy increases the activity of this enzyme.[1-3] While the effect of hormonal changes in pregnancy on this increased activity has not been directly evaluated, patients using oral contraceptives have an increased metabolism of both nicotine and cotinine.[48] The effect of this increased CYP2A6 activity on nicotine replacement therapies has provided conflicting data. Lower serum concentration of nicotine has been reported with nicotine gum during pregnancy, whereas no effect was noted in women using the nicotine patch.[1,49,50]

CYP2C9

The activity of CYP2C9 increases during pregnancy. Phenytoin, which is metabolized primarily by 2C9 and also by the 2C19 pathway, is the primary drug of interest. The clear-

Table 2. Effect of Pregnancy on Drugs Eliminated Unchanged by the Kidneys

Study	Drug (Route of Administration)	Study Design	Results during Pregnancy Compared with Postpartum or Nonpregnant Controls
Chamber-lain et al.[82]	Ampicillin (IV)	Third trimester and 6 wk postpartum (n = 22)	CL ↑ 22% and $t_{1/2\beta}$ ↓ 20% (NS)
Philipson[43]	Ampicillin (IV/PO)	9–33 gw and 3–12 mo postpartum (n = 26)	CL and CL_R ↑ 50%[†]; $t_{1/2\beta}$ ↓ 12%[†]
Assael et al.[83]	Ampicillin (IM)	21–40 gw (n = 14) and healthy controls (n = 6)	CL ↑ 79%[††]
Philipson and Stiern-stedt[84]	Cefuroxime (IV)	11–35 gw, at delivery, and postpartum after termi-nation of breastfeed-ing and resumption of normal menses (n = 7)	CL ↑ 42%, CL_R ↑ 37%,[†] and $t_{1/2\beta}$ ↓ 24%
Nathorst-Boos et al.[85]	Ceftazidime (IV)	First and third trimesters, and postpartum after termination of breast-feeding (n = 12)	CL ↑ 38% and 65%, respectively
Philipson et al.[44]	Cephradine (PO/IV)	Second trimester and postpartum after termi-nation of breastfeeding and resumption of nor-mal menses (n = 12)	CL ↑ 39%[†] and $t_{1/2\beta}$ ↓ 26%[†]
Philipson et al.[44]	Cefazolin (IV)	Second trimester and postpartum after termi-nation of breastfeed-ing and resumption of normal menses (n = 6)	CL ↑ 31%[†] and $t_{1/2\beta}$ ↓ 35%[†]
Heikkila and Erkkola[86]	Piperacillin (IV)	At delivery (n = 8) and healthy controls (n = 5)	CL ↑ 184%[††] and no differ-ence in $t_{1/2\beta}$
Heikkila et al.[87]	Mecillinam (IV)	First trimester (n = 10) compared with at term (n = 10), and healthy subjects (12)	No difference in CL; $t_{1/2\beta}$ ↑ 77% and 42%, respec-tively
Heikkila et al.[87]	Pivmecillinam (PO)	10–32 gw (n = 6) com-pared with healthy con-trols (n = 6)	No difference in CL or $t_{1/2\beta}$
Hurst et al.[88]	Atenolol (PO)	Third trimester and 6 wk postpartum (n = 10)	No difference in CL
Thorley et al.[89]	Atenolol (PO)	22–38 gw (n = 11) com-pared with historical controls	No difference in $t_{1/2\beta}$
Hebert et al.[90]	Atenolol (PO)	Second and third trimes-ters and 3 mo postpar-tum (n = 17)	CL_R ↑ 38% and 36%[†]; $t_{1/2\beta}$ ↓ 12% and 11%,[†] respectively; no differ-ence in CL

(continued)

Table 2. Effect of Pregnancy on Drugs Eliminated Unchanged by the Kidneys [Continued]

Study	Drug (Route of Administration)	Study Design	Results during Pregnancy Compared with Postpartum or Nonpregnant Controls
O'Hare et al.[91]	Sotalol (PO/IV)	Third trimester and 6 wk postpartum (n = 6)	CL ↑ 60%[†] and $t_{1/2\beta}$ ↓ 29% after IV administration; no effect on $t_{1/2\beta}$ after PO administration
Luxford and Kellaway[92]	Digoxin (PO)	Third trimester and 6–12 wk postpartum (n = 15)	CL_R ↑ 21%[†]
Schou et al.[93]	Lithium (PO)	Third trimester and 6–7 wk postpartum (n = 4)	CL ↑ 100%
Ensom and Stephenson[94]	Dalteparin sodium (SC)	Prepregnancy, and first, second, and third trimesters (n = 9)	CL ↑ 100% in first, second, and third trimesters[†††]
Blomback et al.[95]	Dalteparin sodium (SC)	32–35 gw (n = 15) compared with historical controls (n = 12)	CL ↑ 64%
Casele et al.[96]	Enoxaparin sodium (SC)	First and third trimesters, and 6–8 wk postpartum (n = 13)	CL ↑ 46% and 17%, respectively[†]

CL = clearance, CL_R = renal clearance, gw = gestational weeks, IM = intramuscular, IV = intravenous, NS = statistically nonsignificant, PO = oral, SC = subcutaneous, $t_{1/2\beta}$ = terminal elimination half-life, ↓ = decrease, ↑ = increase, † = $p < .05$ vs postpartum, †† = $p < .05$ vs nonpregnant controls, ††† = $p < .05$ vs prepregnancy.
Reprinted from Anderson[2] with permission.

ance of phenytoin increases during pregnancy.[27] Because phenytoin is highly bound to albumin, the clearance of total drug is potentially misleading and it is the clearance of free phenytoin that is clinically relevant. There is at least a 20% increase in free phenytoin clearance with a reported corresponding decrease in free concentration of 18%–31%.

CYP2C19

The activity of CYP2C19 appears to decrease during pregnancy. This is based on data with the antimalarial drug proguanil and the protease inhibitor nelfinavir. Neither of these drugs is currently used in the United States in pregnant patients. Data are lacking for other drugs used during pregnancy such as omeprazole. However, the area under the plasma concentration vs time curve for omeprazole was 38% higher in nonpregnant subjects taking estrogen-containing oral contraceptives.[1] It appears that pregnancy may decrease the activity of CYP2C19 through increased estrogen levels. While a dosage adjustment may be considered for omeprazole, lansoprazole, and pantoprazole due to this effect of pregnancy, in view of the wide dosage range for these drugs and the goal of therapy, a dosage adjustment is not indicated.

CYP2D6

Generally, it has been thought that it was not possible to induce the enzymatic activity of CYP2D6 because it is primarily under genetic control. However, there are studies that indicate an increase in CYP2D6 activity in pregnant women. Drugs tested include metoprolol, dextromethorphan, citalopram, and fluoxetine.[1,51,52] In addition to these specific drugs, CYP2D6 metabolizes several other commonly used drugs, including various antidepressants, neuroleptic agents, and β-adrenergic receptor blockers.[1,2,53] For antidepressants, the clinical impact of the effect of pregnancy is not clear at this time. In relatively small studies, the trough serum concentrations of citalopram and fluoxetine were significantly lower in pregnant patients than in nonpregnant patients.[1,51,53] Few patients needed an adjustment in their dose for symptoms of depression. Contrary to this, it has been reported that two thirds of 34 pregnant women receiving fluoxetine, sertraline, or paroxetine required an increase in dose to maintain efficacy of the antidepressant.[1,51] Based on available information, if symptoms of depression recur in a pregnant patient receiving an antidepressant metabolized by 2D6, a dosage increase should be considered.

CYP3A4

A majority of drugs are metabolized to some extent by CYP3A4, including many drugs used during pregnancy. Studies of nifedipine, methadone, and indinavir indicate that the activity of CYP3A4 is increased during pregnancy.[1,2] The available information is limited to small studies in patients with significant interindividual variability. Additionally, the time course of the effect has not been determined. Currently, no generalizations can be made on the timing or size of dosage adjustments. Many drugs that are metabolized by CYP3A4 are also substrates of the drug transporter P-glycoprotein. Therefore, the overall effect of pregnancy on the elimination of these drugs is difficult to predict as the effect of pregnancy on P-glycoprotein is not known.[2]

Uridine 5'-Diphosphate Glucuronosyltransferases

The activity of the UGT system, which is involved in the glucuronidation of drugs, appears to be increased in pregnancy. The specific UGT pathways of primary interest are 1A1, 1A4, 1A6, and 2B7. Data from oral contraceptive studies indicate that the estrogen component promotes an increase in UGT activity. Therefore, the effect of pregnancy on these pathways may be hormonally related.[1]

The clinical significance of this increased activity has only been established for the anticonvulsant lamotrigine. Approximately 90% of its metabolism is via N-glucuronidation by UGT1A4. Studies have documented significant increases in lamotrigine clearance that can result in a loss of seizure control unless the serum concentrations are monitored and the dose is adjusted accordingly.[1,27]

The clearance of acetaminophen and lorazepam is increased during pregnancy due to higher activity of the UGT1A1 and 1A6 pathways for acetaminophen and UGT2B7 pathway for lorazepam.[1] However, the clinical need to adjust dosage during pregnancy has not been established at this time.

VII. Drugs of High Interest in Pregnancy

A. Antiepileptic Agents

Maintaining therapeutic serum concentrations of antiepileptic agents throughout pregnancy is essential to minimizing the risk of seizure activity, which can adversely affect both the mother and fetus. For older antiepileptic agents (eg, phenytoin, carbamazepine, valproic acid, phenobarbital), it is important to not only understand the significance and timing of the effect of pregnancy on the metabolism of these drugs, but also the changes in plasma protein binding that occur in pregnancy because these drugs are highly bound. CYP pathways are primarily involved in the elimination of these drugs, except valproic acid, of which only approximately 10% is eliminated by CYP pathways; glucuronidation accounts for approximately 50% of valproic acid's elimination. For second-generation antiepileptic agents (eg, lamotrigine, topiramate, gabapentin, levetiracetam, oxcarbazepine), much of the drug elimination occurs by non-CYP routes. Lamotrigine and mono-hydroxycarbazepine, the active metabolite of the prodrug oxcarbazepine, are primarily metabolized by glucuronidation via UGT enzymes, whereas topiramate, gabapentin, and levetiracetam are primarily excreted in the urine as unchanged drug.[1-3,27,30]

In general, pregnancy results in either a decrease in serum concentration of antiepileptic drugs with the potential for increased seizure activity, or it has a minimal effect. The pattern and significance of change is difficult to predict for a given patient. Therefore, serum concentration monitoring is recommended throughout pregnancy and in the postpartum period.[1,13,25] It is generally recommended that serum concentration monitoring be performed at least in each trimester and then postpartum, whereas more frequent monitoring (eg, monthly) has been recommended by some authors. Frequent monitoring during pregnancy and postpartum should be performed for antiepileptic drugs in which significant changes in drug elimination have been reported and significant dosage adjustment is anticipated.[27,30]

Phenytoin clearance increases during pregnancy and then decreases postpartum. However, as previously discussed in Alterations in Pharmacokinetic Parameters, CYP2C9, to evaluate the significance of this effect, it is important to take into account the high affinity of phenytoin for albumin and the decrease in serum albumin that occurs during pregnancy. The result of these factors is a relative decrease in bound phenytoin and an increase in the free fraction of active, unbound phenytoin. If the relatively large reported decrease in total serum phenytoin (bound and unbound drug) concentrations (55%–61%) is used without consideration of changes in plasma protein binding, a much larger effect on phenytoin clearance is concluded. However, when properly using the free (unbound) concentration data, a more modest increase in clearance is determined. The reported decrease in free phenytoin concentrations during pregnancy is 18%–31%. The increase in phenytoin metabolism during pregnancy is related primarily to the increased activity for the CYP2C9 pathway. Due to the changes in protein binding that occur during pregnancy, it is important to measure the free phenytoin serum concentration.[1,27]

Carbamazepine is primarily metabolized by CYP3A4 and is highly bound to plasma albumin. As discussed above for phenytoin, because of this high protein binding it is important to use the free concentration in interpreting data and determining therapy. While pregnancy generally increases the activity of CYP3A4, the data reported for carbamazepine indicate a wide variety of effects, with reported decreases in free carbamazepine serum concentrations of 0%–28%.[27] When a decrease in serum concentration was noted, it was primarily in the third trimester.

Phenobarbital is primarily metabolized by CYP2C9, along with CYP2C19. The general pattern reported is an increase in the phenobarbital clearance throughout pregnancy, which is most significant in late pregnancy. This effect decreases during the postpartum period.[27]

Valproic acid (VPA) is metabolized by several pathways, with glucuronidation representing about 50% of its metabolism. VPA is highly bound to plasma albumin and, as noted for the other older antiepileptic agents, this protein binding decreases during pregnancy. The metabolism of VPA has been reported to increase throughout pregnancy, reaching its greatest activity during the third trimester.[27]

As previously noted, the newer antiepileptic agents are primarily eliminated by non-CYP pathways and have low or negligible protein binding. While topiramate, gabapentin, and levetiracetam are primarily excreted in the urine as unchanged drug, both topiramate and levetiracetam have some elimination via metabolic pathways. It has been reported that the clearance of topiramate increases with CYP inducers. Enzymatic hydrolysis is responsible for approximately 30% of the elimination of levetiracetam.[1,27,29,30,54] Only lamotrigine has been well studied. A significant increase in clearance has been reported for lamotrigine during pregnancy, with a peak increase of >300%.[27] In view of the significant effect that pregnancy has on the clearance of lamotrigine and the resulting potential loss of seizure control, it is recommended that monitoring of serum lamotrigine concentrations be as frequent as monthly. Additionally, the serum concentration needs to be monitored postpartum to guide a dosage decrease to prevent potential adverse effects.

B. Antibiotics

1. Aminoglycosides

Dosages of the aminoglycoside antibiotics (amikacin, gentamicin, and tobramycin) are based on a pharmacokinetic approach, and therapeutic drug monitoring is commonly employed when indicated. In general, the apparent volume of distribution is correlated to the extracellular fluid compartment, and the clearance is essentially equal to creatinine clearance. When administered to pregnant patients, the aminoglycosides rapidly pass through the placenta and enter the fetal blood circulation and the amniotic fluid.[55] Multiple studies have demonstrated that lower serum concentrations of the aminoglycosides are achieved in nonpreeclamptic pregnant patients in comparison to nonpregnant women, and that higher doses are necessary.[56,57] This can be attributed to both an increase in the apparent volume of distribution and a more rapid clearance in pregnant subjects. Further, although an increase in apparent volume of distribution would prolong the elimination half-life, studies have demonstrated that the half-life of the aminoglycosides is actually quite short (approximately 1.5 hours on average) and may be significantly shorter than in nonpregnant subjects.[58–60] This is consistent with the considerable increase in creatinine clearance, resulting in a more rapid aminoglycoside clearance. The degree of these changes likely depends on the stage of pregnancy, as changes in body fluids and creatinine clearance are dynamic throughout gestation and during postpartum. Studies of the aminoglycosides in normal pregnancy demonstrate wide interpatient variability in the pharmacokinetic parameters and in the peak serum levels achieved.[58–60] Mean values reported for the volume of distribution generally range from 0.2 to 0.3 L/

kg; however, it is not always clear from these studies what weight was actually used to determine this value (ie, ideal body weight, actual body weight, some "adjusted" body weight). Mean values observed for clearance range from approximately 120 mL/min to 150 mL/min or higher. In one study comparing the pharmacokinetic parameters of tobramycin in separate groups of pregnant women during the second and third trimesters of pregnancy, the mean half-life was significantly longer during the third trimester (1.60 vs 2.39 hours, respectively), the mean clearance was decreased (2.00 vs 1.58 mL/min/kg, respectively), while the mean volume of distribution was not significantly different (0.24 vs 0.27 L/kg, respectively).[61] This is consistent with studies demonstrating a decline in the creatinine clearance during the later stages of pregnancy.[15,16]

In preeclamptic pregnant patients, the very rapid clearance and very short half-life may not be observed because GFR does not increase significantly as it does in normal pregnancy. More detailed studies are necessary to adequately characterize the disposition of the aminoglycosides in normal and preeclamptic pregnant patients, particularly in using population parameters to estimate the volume of distribution and clearance during various stages of gestation. Further, monitoring serum aminoglycoside levels, particularly for serious infections, would be advisable.

In postpartum patients, the mean apparent volume of distribution has been reported to be approximately 0.35–0.38 L/kg (ideal body weight), with creatinine clearance values of 120–140 mL/min/1.73 m^2 and corresponding half-lives of 2.0–2.5 hours.[62–64] In postpartum patients with severe preeclampsia, the mean clearance was reported to be reduced by 33% compared to normotensive patients, and the mean half-life increased by about the same proportion, with no change in apparent volume of distribution.[65]

2. Vancomycin

Vancomycin is predominantly eliminated unchanged in the urine and its clearance is essentially equal to creatinine clearance.[66] It distributes to a wide range of tissues and fluids, and it crosses the placenta.[55,67,68]

Studies of the pharmacokinetics of vancomycin in the pregnant patient are lacking. In a case report of a 33-year-old woman in her 26th week of gestation, both the clearance (251 mL/min) and apparent volume of distribution (1.48 L/kg) of vancomycin were increased in comparison to average pharmacokinetic values.[68] The elimination half-life was 4.6 hours, which is within the usual range for relatively young patients. In a more recent report, four women at term who were scheduled to undergo cesarean delivery received 1 gram of vancomycin infused over 1 hour and had peak serum vancomycin concentrations that ranged between 9.6 and 19.6 µg/mL, measured between 26 and 76 minutes after the infusion ended.[68] Based on the limited information available on vancomycin for this patient population, monitoring serum vancomycin concentrations is advisable. Increases in the clearance and apparent volume of distribution of vancomycin during pregnancy would be expected to coincide with pregnancy-related changes in renal function and hemodynamics.

C. Digoxin

Digoxin is eliminated via metabolism and renal excretion; in young healthy adults, the renal route is the predominant mechanism for elimination.[2] The apparent volume of distribution of digoxin is relatively large (approximately 5–7 L/kg), indicating that the drug significantly distributes into the tissue compartment. In addition to treating cardiac conditions in the mother, digoxin crosses the placenta and has been administered to pregnant women to treat fetal supraventricular tachycardia and congestive heart failure in utero, which was successful in the above case history.[69–71]

Early studies of digoxin pharmacokinetics in pregnancy are difficult to interpret and compare due to the subsequent finding of a previously unknown assay-interfering endogenous substance(s) in the plasma of pregnant patients, which spuriously elevated measured serum digoxin concentrations. These interfering substances have been termed digoxinlike immunoreactive substances (DLIS).[72–75] The actual concentration of DLIS has been shown to fluctuate during gestation, likely due to changes in the rate of production.[76] Further, different commercially available digoxin assays have variable cross-reactivity and yield significantly different results.[77,78] In our case history, a digoxin assay was employed where DLIS was known not to be a significant factor.

In one of the earliest studies of digoxin pharmacokinetics in pregnancy, the serum digoxin concentration in five pregnant patients taking daily doses of 0.25 mg of digoxin orally, the average serum digoxin concentration at delivery was 0.6 ng/mL.[79] Subsequently, the average serum digoxin concentration in these five women was 1.1 ng/mL on the same dose 1 month postpartum. This could be attributed to an increase in digoxin clearance, a decrease in bioavailability, or a combination of both during pregnancy. In a more recent prospective study, the average plasma clearance of digoxin in five pregnant women (excluding a sixth patient who received indomethacin) receiving 0.5–1.0 mg every 12 hours was 314 mL/min; the average volume of distribution was 6.1 L/kg, and the mean elimination half-life was 20.4 hours.[80] This is consistent with the increase in GFR previously discussed, and a rapid clearance is indeed observed in the case history.

Our experience has been that young, healthy, pregnant patients require doses in the range of 0.25–1 mg daily (given in divided doses) to achieve serum digoxin concentrations in the mid- to upper therapeutic range and to control fetal supraventricular tachycardia. Doses are typically titrated from a starting dose of 0.25–0.5 mg every 12 hours, until the desired effect is obtained or until the risk of toxicity to mother or baby becomes a concern. When monitoring serum digoxin concentrations in the pregnant patient, it is imperative that the drug assay used has negligible interference from DLIS. In addition, pregnant patients and the fetus should be monitored closely for clinical signs and symptoms of toxicity.

VIII. Summary

The vast and complex physiologic changes that occur during pregnancy have significant effects on drug disposition. Understanding these changes can generally guide the clinician to tailor dosages for patients at various stages of pregnancy. Nevertheless, there is wide interpatient and intrapatient variability, and adequate monitoring of serum drug levels should be used when indicated.

IX. References

1. Hodge LS, Tracy TS. Alterations in drug disposition during pregnancy: implications for drug therapy. *Exper Opin Metab Toxicol.* 2007;3:357–371.

2. Anderson GD. Pregnancy-induced changes in pharmacokinetics—a mechanistic-based approach. *Clin Pharmacokinet.* 2005;44:989–1008.

3. Loebstein R, Lalkin A, Koren G. Pharmacokinetic changes during pregnancy and their clinical relevance. *Clin Pharmacokinet.* 1997;33:329–343.

4. Krauer B, Krauer F. Drug kinetics in pregnancy. *Clin Pharmacokinet.* 1977;2:167–181.

5. Duvekot JJ, Cheriex EC, Pleters FA, et al. Early pregnancy changes in hemodynamics and volume homeostasis are consecutive adjustments triggered by a primary fall in systemic vascular tone. *Am J Obstet Gynecol.* 1993;169:1382–1392.

6. Van Oppen AC, Stigter RH, Bruinse HW. Cardiac output in normal pregnancy: a critical review. *Obstet Gynecol.* 1996;87:310–318.

7. Krauer B, Krauer F, Hytten FE. Drug disposition and pharmacokinetics in the maternal-placental-fetal unit. *Pharmac Ther.* 1980;10:301–328.

8. Krutzen E, Olofsson P, Back SE, et al. Glomerular filtration rate in pregnancy: a study in normal subjects and patients with hypertension, preeclampsia and diabetes. *Scan J Clin Lab Invest.* 1992;52:387–392.

9. Duvekot JJ, Cheriex EC, Pieters AA, et al. Early pregnancy changes in hemodynamics and volume homeostasis are consecutive adjustments triggered by a primary fall in systemic vascular tone. *Am J Obstet Gynecol.* 1993;169:1382–1392.

10. Varga I, Rigo J, Somos P, et al. Analysis of maternal circulation and renal function in physiologic pregnancies; parallel examinations of the changes in cardiac output and the glomerular filtration rate. *J Mater Fetal Med.* 2000;9:97–104.

11. Moran P, Baylis PH, Lindheimer MD, et al. Glomerular ultrafiltration in normal and preeclamptic pregnancy. *J Am Soc Nephrol.* 2003;14:648–652.

12. Jeyabalan A, Conrad KP. Renal function during normal pregnancy and preeclampsia. *Front Biosci.* 2007;12:2425–2437.

13. Beydoun SN. Morphologic changes in the renal tract in pregnancy. *Clin Obstet Gynecol.* 1985;28:249–256.

14. Davison JM, Noble MCB. Serial changes in 24 hour creatinine clearance during normal menstrual cycles and the first trimester of pregnancy. *Br J Obstet Gynaecol.* 1981;88:10–17.

15. Davison JM, Dunlop W, Ezimokhai M. 24-hour creatinine clearance during the third trimester of normal pregnancy. *Brit J Obstet Gynaecol.* 1980;87:106–109.

16. Davison JM. The physiology of the renal tract in pregnancy. *Clin Obstet Gynecol.* 1985;28:257–265.

17. Cockcroft DW, Gault MH. Prediction of creatinine clearance from serum creatinine. *Nephron.* 1976;16:31–41.

18. Smith MC, Moran P, Ward MK, et al. Assessment of glomerular filtration rate during pregnancy using the MDRD formula. *BJOG.* 2008;115:109–112.

19. Lafayette RA, Druzin M, Sibley R, et al. Nature of glomerular dysfunction in pre-eclampsia. *Kidney Int.* 1998;54:1240–1249.

20. Moran P, Baylis PH, Lindheimer MD, et al. Glomerular ultrafiltration in normal and preeclamptic pregnancy. *J Am Soc Nephrol.* 2003;14:648–652.

21. Alper AB, Yi Y, Webber LS, et al. Estimation of glomerular filtration rate in pre-eclamptic patients. *Am J Perinatol.* 2007;24:569–574.

22. Nakai A, Sekiya I, Oya A, et al. Assessment of the hepatic arterial and portal venous blood flows during pregnancy with Doppler ultrasonography. *Arch Gynecol Obstet.* 2002;266:25–29.

23. Smith MT, Livingstone I, Eadie MJ, et al. Chronic propranolol administration during pregnancy. Maternal pharmacokinetics. *Eur J Clin Pharmacol.* 2007;25:481–490.

24. Gerdin E, Salmonson T, Lindberg B. Maternal kinetics of morphine during labour. *J Perinatal Med.* 1990;18:479–487.

25. Cheung CK, Lao T, Swaminathan R. Urinary excretion of some proteins and enzymes during normal pregnancy. *Clin Chem.* 1989;35:1978–1980.

26. Erman A, Neri A, Sharoni R, et al. Enhanced urinary albumin excretion after 35 weeks of gestation and during labour in normal pregnancy. *Scand J Clin Lab Invest.* 1992:52:409–413.

27. Pennell PB. Antiepileptic drug pharmacokinetics during pregnancy and lactation. *Neurology.* 2003;61(suppl 2):S35–S42.

28. Wolff K, Boys A, Rostami–Hodjegan A, et al. Changes to methadone clearance during pregnancy. *Eur J Clin Pharmacol.* 2005;61:763–768.

29. Tomson T, Battino D. Pharmacokinetics and therapeutic drug monitoring of newer antiepileptic drugs during pregnancy and the puerperium. *Clin Pharmacokinet.* 2007;46:209–219.

30. De Haan G-J, Edelbroek P, Segers J, et al. Gestation-induced changes in lamotrigine pharmacokinetics: a monotherapy study. *Neurology.* 2004;63:571–573.

31. Koren G. Changes in drug disposition in pregnancy and their clinical implications. In Koren G, ed. *Maternal-Fetal Toxicology.* 2nd ed. New York: Marcel Dekker, Inc., 1994:3–13.

32. Loebstein R, Lalkin A, Koren G. Pharmacokinetic changes during pregnancy and their clinical relevance. *Clin Pharmacokinet.* 1997;33:328–343.

33. Syme MR, Paxton JW, Keelan JA. Drug transfer and metabolism by the human placenta. *Clin Pharmacokinet.* 2004;43:487–514.

34. Gedeon C, Behravan J, Koren G, et al. Transport of glyburide by placental ABC transporters: implications in fetal drug exposure. *Placenta.* 2009;27:1096–1102.

35. Behravan J, Piquette-Miller M. Drug transport across the placenta, role of the ABC drug efflux transporters. *Expert Opin Drug Metab Toxicol.* 2007;3:819–830.

36. Myers SA, Gleicher N. Physiologic changes in normal pregnancy. In Gleicher N, ed. *Principles and Practice of Medical Therapy in Pregnancy.* 2nd ed. East Norwalk, CT: Appleton & Lange, 1992:35–52.

37. Davison JS, Davison MC, Hay DM. Gastric emptying time in late pregnancy and labour. *J Obstet Gynaecol Brit Commonw.* 1970;77:37–41.

38. Christofides ND, Ghatei MA, Bloom SR, et al. Decreased plasma motilin concentrations in pregnancy. *Br Med J.* 1982;285:1453–1454.

39. Wald A, Van Thiel DH, Hoechstetter L, et al. Effect of pregnancy on gastrointestinal transit. *Dig Dis Sci.* 1982;27:1015–1018.

40. Holst N, Jenssen TG, Burhol PG. Plasma concentrations of motilin and somatostatin are increased in late pregnancy and postpartum. *Br J Obstet Gynaecol.* 1992;99:338–341.

41. Macfie AG, Magides AD, Richmond MN, et al. Gastric emptying in pregnancy. *Br J Anaesth.* 1991;67:54–57.

42. Parry E, Shields R, Turnbull AC. Transit time in the small intestine in pregnancy. *J Obstet Gynaecol Br Commonw.* 1970;77:900–901.

43. Philipson A. Pharmacokinetics of ampicillin during pregnancy. *J Infect Dis.* 1977;136:370–376.

44. Philipson A, Stiernstedt G, Ehrnebo M. Comparison of the pharmacokinetics of cephradine and cefazolin in pregnant and non-pregnant women. *Clin Pharmacokinet.* 1987;12:136–144.

45. Lander CM, Smith MT, Chalk JB, et al. Bioavailability and pharmacokinetics of phenytoin during pregnancy. *Eur J Clin Pharmacol.* 1984;27:105–110.

46. Tracy TS, Venkataramanan R, Glover DD, et al. Temporal changes in drug metabolism (CYP1A2, CYP2D6 and CYP3A activity) during pregnancy. *Am J Obstet Gynecol.* 2005;192:633–639.

47. Gardner MJ, Schatz M, Cousins I, et al. Longitudinal effects of pregnancy on the pharmacokinetics of theophylline. *Eur J Clin Pharmacol.* 1987;32:289–295.

48. Benowitz NL, Lessov-Schlaggar CN, Swan GE, et al. Female sex and oral contraceptive use accelerate nicotine metabolism. *Clin Pharmacol Ther.* 2006;79:480–488.

49. Oncken CA, Hatsukami DK, Lupo VR, et al. Effects of short-term use of nicotine gum in pregnant smokers. *Clin Pharmacol Ther.* 1996;59:654–661.

50. Ogburn PL, Hurt RD, Croghan IT, et al. Nicotine patch use in pregnant smokers: nicotine and cotinine levels and fetal effects. *Am J Obstet Gynecol.* 1999;181:736–743.

51. Heikkinen T, Ekblad U, Palo P, et al. Pharmacokinetics of fluoxetine and norfluoxetine in pregnancy and lactation. *Clin Pharmacol Ther.* 2003;73:330–337.

52. Wadelius M, Darj E, Frenne G, et al. Induction of CYP2D6 in pregnancy. *Clin Pharmacol Ther.* 1997;62:400–407.

53. Heikkinen T, Ekblad U, Kero P, et al. Citalopram in pregnancy and lactation. *Clin Pharmacol Ther.* 2002;72:184–191.

54. Tomson T, Palm R, Källén K, et al. Pharmacokinetics of levetiracetam during pregnancy, delivery, in the neonatal period, and lactation. *Epilepsia.* 2007;48:1111–1116.

55. Briggs GG, Freeman RK, Yaffe SJ. *Drugs in Pregnancy and Lactation.* 8th ed. Philadelphia: Lippincott Williams & Wilkins, 2008.

56. Weinstein AJ, Gibbs RS, Gallagher M. Placental transfer of clindamycin and gentamicin in term pregnancy. *Am J Obstet Gynecol.* 1976;124:688–691.

57. Graham JM, Blanco JD, Oshiro BT, et al. Gentamicin levels in pregnant women with pyelonephritis. *Am J Perinatol.* 1994;11:40–41.

58. Zaske DE, Cipolle RJ, Strate RG, et al. Rapid gentamicin elimination in obstetric patients. *Obstet Gynecol.* 1980;56:559–564.

59. Lazebnik N, Noy S, Lazebnik R, et al. Gentamicin serum half-life: a comparison between pregnant and non-pregnant women. *Postgrad Med J.* 1985;61:979–981.

60. Locksmith GJ, Chin A, Vu T, et al. High compared with standard gentamicin dosing for chorioamnionitis: a comparison of maternal and fetal serum drug levels. *Obstet Gynecol.* 2005;105:473–479.

61. Bourget P, Fernandez H, Delouis C, et al. Pharmacokinetics of tobramycin in pregnant women: safety and efficacy of a once-daily dose regimen. *J Clin Pharm Ther.* 1991;16:167–176.

62. Briggs GG, Ambrose P, Nageotte MP. Gentamicin dosing in postpartum women with endometritis. *Am J Obstet Gynecol.* 1989;160:309–313.

63. Munar MY, Lawson LA, Samuels P, et al. Gentamicin pharmacokinetics in postpartum women with endomyometritis. *DICP.* 1991;25:1306–1309.

64. Cropp CD, Davis GA, Enson MH. Evaluation of aminoglycoside pharmacokinetics in postpartum patients using Bayesian forecasting. *Ther Drug Monit.* 1998;20:68–72.

65. McNeeley SG, Beitel R, Lee M, et al. Delayed gentamicin elimination in patients with severe preeclampsia. *Am J Obstet Gynecol.* 1985;153:793–796.

66. Rushing TA, Ambrose PJ. Clinical application and evaluation of vancomycin dosing in adults. *J Pharm Technol.* 2001;17:33–38.

67. Bourget P, Fernandez H, Delouis C, et al. Transplacental passage of vancomycin during the second trimester of pregnancy. *Obstet Gynecol.* 1991;78:908–911.

68. Laiprasert J, Klein K, Mueller BA, et al. Transplacental passage of vancomycin in noninfected term pregnant women. *Obstet Gynecol.* 2007;109:1105–1110.

69. King CR, Mattioli L, Goertz KK, et al. Successful treatment of fetal supraventricular tachycardia with maternal digoxin therapy. *Chest.* 1984;85:573–575.

70. Van Engelen AD, Weijtens O, Brenner JI, et al. Management outcome and follow-up of fetal tachycardia. *J Am Coll Cardiol.* 1994;24:1371–1375.

71. Simpson JM, Sharland GK. Fetal tachycardias: management and outcome of 127 consecutive cases. *Heart.* 1998;79:576–581.

72. Pudek MR, Seccombe DW, Whitfield MF. Digoxin-like immunoreactivity in premature and full-term infants not receiving digoxin therapy. *N Engl J Med.* 1983;308:904–905.

73. Graves SW, Valdes R Jr, Brown BA, et al. Endogenous digoxin-immunoreactive substance in human pregnancies. *J Clin Endocrinol Metab.* 1984;58:748–751.

74. Koren G, Farine D, Maresky D, et al. Significance of the endogenous digoxin-like substance in infants and mothers. *Clin Pharmacol Ther.* 1984;36:759–764.

75. Scherrmann JM, Sandouk P, Guedeney X. Digitalis-like factors and digoxin pharmacokinetics. *Chest.* 1986;89:468–469.

76. Seccombe DW, Pudek MR, Whitfield MF, et al. Perinatal changes in a digoxin-like immunoreactive substance. *Pediatr Res.* 1984;18:1097–1099.

77. Ng PK, LeGatt D, Coates J, et al. Measuring endogenous digoxin-like substance and exogenous digoxin in the serum of low-birth-weight infants. *Am J Hosp Pharm.* 1985;42:1977–1979.

78. Cook JD, Koch TR, Cook MS, et al. Inaccuracies in digoxin measurement. *Clin Biochem.* 1988;21:353–357.

79. Rogers MC, Willerson JT, Goldblatt A, et al. Serum digoxin concentrations in the human fetus, neonate and infant. *N Engl J Med.* 1972;287:1010–1013.

80. Azancot-Benisty A, Jacqz-Aigrain E, Guirgis NM, et al. Clinical and pharmacologic study of fetal supraventricular tachyarrhythmias. *J Pediatr.* 1992;121:608–613.

81. U.S. Food and Drug Administration. Pharmacogenomics from the Ground Up, Session 1: Concepts and Tools in Pharmacogenomics. Available at http://www.fda.gov/cder/genomics/Concepts_Pharmacogenomics.PDF. Accessed April 26, 2008.

82. Chamberlain A, White S, Bawdon R, et al. Pharmacokinetics of ampicillin and sulbactam in pregnancy. *Am J Obstet Gynecol.* 1993;168:667–673.

83. Assael BM, Como ML, Miraglia M, et al. Ampicillin kinetics in pregnancy. *Br J Clin Pharmacol.* 1979;8:286–288.

84. Philipson A, Stiernstedt G. Pharmacokinetics of cefuroxime in pregnancy. *Am J Obstet Gynecol.* 1982;142:823–828.

85. Nathorst-Boos J, Philipson A, Hedman A, et al. Renal elimination of ceftazidime during pregnancy. *Am J Obstet Gynecol.* 1995;172:163–166.

86. Heikkila A, Erkkola R. Pharmacokinetics of piperacillin during pregnancy. *J Antimicrob Chemother.* 1991;28:419–423.

87. Heikkila A, Pyykko K, Erkkola R, et al. The pharmacokinetics of mecillinam and pivmecillinam in pregnant and non-pregnant women. *Br J Clin Pharmacol.* 1992;33:629–633.

88. Hurst AK, Shotan A, Hoffman K, et al. Pharmacokinetic and pharmacodynamic evaluation of atenolol during and after pregnancy. *Pharmacotherapy.* 1998;18:840–846.

89. Thorley KJ, McAinsh J, Cruickshank JM. Atenolol in the treatment of pregnancy-induced hypertension. *Br J Clin Pharmacol.* 1981;12:725–730.

90. Hebert MF, Carr DB, Anderson GD, et al. Pharmacokinetics and pharmacodynamics of atenolol during pregnancy and postpartum. *J Clin Pharmacol.* 2005;45:25–33.

91. O'Hare MF, Leahey W, Murnaghan GA, et al. Pharmacokinetics of sotalol during pregnancy. *Eur J Clin Pharmacol.* 1983;24:521–524.

92. Luxford AM, Kellaway GS. Pharmacokinetics of digoxin in pregnancy. *Eur J Clin Pharmacol.* 1983;25:117–121.

93. Schou M, Amdisen A, Steenstrup OR. Lithium and pregnancy: II. Hazards to women given lithium during pregnancy and delivery. *BMJ.* 1973;2:137–138.

94. Ensom MH, Stephenson MD. Pharmacokinetics of low molecular weight heparin and unfractionated heparin in pregnancy. *J Soc Gynecol Investig.* 2004;11:377–383.

95. Blomback M, Bremme K, Hellgren M, et al. A pharmacokinetic study of dalteparin (Fragmin) during late pregnancy. *Blood Coagul Fibrinolysis.* 1998;9:343–350.

96. Casele HL, Laifer SA, Woelkers DA, et al. Changes in the pharmacokinetics of the low-molecular-weight heparin enoxaparin sodium during pregnancy. *Am J Obstet Gynecol.* 1999;181:1113–1117.

QUESTIONS AND ANSWERS

1. In pregnancy, the serum albumin concentration:

   a. remains essentially the same throughout gestation.

   b. is decreased, most likely due to a dilutional effect.

   c. is more concentrated than in nonpregnant women.

   d. changes unpredictably during gestation.

2. Changes in renal function during pregnancy include:

   a. an initial decline in GFR due to an increase in fluid requirements.

   b. a significant and sustained increase in GFR.

   c. a progressive decrease in renal blood flow due to compression by the expanding fetus.

   d. a progressive decline in GFR.

3. With respect to drugs that are metabolized by the liver:

   a. the rate of metabolism is predictably lower for drugs with high extraction ratios.

   b. the metabolic clearance is significantly higher in the third trimester due to the added metabolism by the fetal liver.

   c. the magnitude of any change in metabolic clearance is clinically insignificant.

   d. the overall effect is difficult to predict due to the complex changes in the various metabolic pathways.

4. With respect to the pharmacokinetics of phenytoin in pregnancy:

   a. monitoring free (unbound) serum concentrations is preferred to monitoring total (bound and unbound) serum phenytoin concentrations.

   b. the volume of distribution is decreased as a result of a decrease in plasma protein binding.

    c. the metabolic clearance is slightly decreased in the second trimester.

    d. the free fraction (percent unbound in the plasma) decreases as a result of a decrease in plasma albumin concentration.

5. With regard to digoxin:

    a. it can yield a false-positive pregnancy test.

    b. it does not significantly affect the fetus due to placental transport proteins that secrete digoxin against the maternal-fetal blood concentration gradient.

    c. high doses are often required due to a very rapid rate of elimination in pregnant women.

    d. lower does are often necessary in pregnant women due to changes in cardiovascular physiology and response.

Answers:

1. b; 2. b; 3. d; 4. a; 5. c

Use of Over-the-Counter Medications in Pregnancy

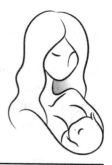

Craig V. Towers

LEARNING OBJECTIVES

1. Describe the seven different ways in which medications can affect a pregnancy.

2. Explain the reasoning behind why certain over-the-counter analgesic medications may produce undesirable effects in a pregnancy.

3. Discuss and analyze the physiology behind why certain over-the-counter cold and respiratory medications may produce adverse reactions in a pregnancy.

4. List and differentiate the over-the-counter drugs that should be avoided or used with caution in pregnancy.

I. Introduction

More than 100,000 over-the-counter drug products are available for purchase by the general public in the United States alone. There are several key factors regarding over-the-counter drug ingredients that must be realized when addressing this topic. First, all of the over-the-counter products basically consist of several hundred active ingredients that are used alone or in combination with other ingredients. Second, pharmaceutical companies use brand names or trade names when marketing these medications. As time progresses, the active ingredients may change within a given over-the-counter medication; however, the brand or trade name will remain the same because the public has become familiar and comfortable with the product and considers it safe and effective. Therefore, the best approach when reviewing this topic is to primarily focus on the active ingredients.

An important issue to remember when evaluating over-the-counter medications is that these agents can be purchased without a prescription.[1] Many individuals have a belief that if a drug can be purchased without a prescription then it must be safe. When dealing with pregnant women, there is also a concept (held by many) that these drugs cannot affect the baby. Essentially, every drug has the potential of affecting a pregnancy both positively or negatively. Thus, no one can claim that a drug, especially an over-the-counter product, is 100% safe. Based on these factors, it might be easy to adopt the belief that all pregnant women should just avoid over-the-counter medicines. On the surface, this approach may seem reasonable; however, some of these medications may actually help a pregnancy and lead to a better overall outcome. An example of this would be a pregnant woman who is on bedrest and has a pregnancy complication that requires minimal straining. If she were to develop constipation, significant straining would be needed to have a bowel movement; therefore, the use of stool softeners in this case would be prudent. Likewise, "stress" is an unknown commodity in pregnancy and is handled differently from person to person. Stress is difficult to study but has been implicated in producing contractions and can also affect vital signs. Thus, minimizing stress by treating certain bothersome symptoms may decrease anxiety and help the pregnancy.

Finally, there are several different ways in which a drug can affect a pregnancy, including (i) producing birth defects (teratogenic effects), (ii) damaging or affecting one of the unborn baby's organs, (iii) producing problems that appear later in life, (iv) interfering with the function of the placenta, (v) interfering with labor, (vi) interfering with how the baby adapts after birth, and (vii) adversely affecting the mother, which may indirectly affect the baby or pregnancy. Regarding these seven issues, none of the over-the-counter medications on the market today (when taken at prescribed dosages) has been proven to be teratogenic, nor is there any evidence that they may produce an effect that appears later in life (as was seen with diethylstilbestrol). However, over-the-counter medicines may have an affect in the other five areas, and these will be discussed as each category of drug is covered. As may be expected, many of the drugs that are available over-the-counter have not been studied in pregnant women.[2] Therefore, in certain cases, the drug's actions will be covered and how those may impact a pregnancy.

II. PATIENT CASE (PART 1)

A 32-year-old pregnant woman was having twice weekly antenatal testing (fetal monitoring) performed due to a history of an unexplained stillbirth. The normal fetal heart rate ranges between 110–160 beats per minute (bpm). On one particular visit at 34 weeks' gestation she was placed on the monitors and a fetal tachycardia of about 180 bpm was noted. Her only complaint was that she had developed a cold about 2 days before the visit. With this information, what questions and evaluation should the physician ask and obtain from the patient to explain the findings of the fetal tachycardia?

III. Analgesic Medications

A. Aspirin

Aspirin or acetylsalicylic acid is one of the most common over-the-counter drugs, if not the most common, used in pregnancy.[3] Many studies have examined this drug in pregnancy and there is no conclusive evidence that it causes birth defects.[4-7] In addition, if a single dosage of aspirin were used to treat a one-time pain (such as a tension headache), the likelihood for problems would be very small. However, more frequent aspirin usage or chronic use is not harmless.

Because this drug inhibits the action of the enzyme prostaglandin synthetase,[8] it may result in prolonging a gestation or cause labor to be dysfunctional if used near term. Prostaglandins play a major role in parturition and the inhibition of this enzyme can affect the production of these mediators. In addition, aspirin is also an irreversible inhibitor of the enzyme platelet cyclooxygenase,[8] and thus, it can prolong the bleeding time. Platelets that are affected by aspirin become irreversibly nonfunctional and the bleeding time will not return to normal until enough new platelets are made by the body to replace the affected ones (for most individuals, this will occur within 4–5 days). Therefore, if a pregnant woman were to suffer antenatal hemorrhage from a placenta previa or placental abruption, the hemorrhage could become worse if aspirin were recently ingested. Furthermore, all women will bleed in the process of giving birth and the amount of bleeding can also increase after the intake of aspirin. It is important to remember that most women do not know when labor will occur. Aspirin also crosses the placenta, with higher concentrations found in the neonate's blood at delivery when compared to the mother's. Therefore, this risk of bleeding can also extend to the newborn.[9] Because of the potential risks of prolonging the gestation, dysfunctional labor, antenatal hemorrhage, postpartum hemorrhage, and newborn hemorrhage, aspirin is not generally recommended for use in the latter half of pregnancy.

B. Nonsteroidal Anti-Inflammatory Drugs

Several nonsteroidal anti-inflammatory drugs (NSAIDs) are available over-the-counter, including ibuprofen, naproxen, and ketoprofen. As time progresses, it is likely that other prescription NSAIDs will also move to an over-the-counter status. NSAIDs are similar to aspirin in their effects and concerns when dealing with pregnancy. Although these drugs have not been evaluated as extensively as aspirin, there are no conclusive reports that NSAIDs are teratogenic.[3-7] Likewise, a single dosage used to treat a one-time pain is unlikely to lead to any significant problems.

The primary action of NSAIDs is through the inhibition of prostaglandin production. However, their action (different from aspirin) is reversible or not permanent.[8] These medications, if used frequently or chronically, can prolong gestation or cause labor to be dysfunctional. In fact, some NSAIDs have been used in treating premature labor (discussed in Chapter 7). NSAIDs can also affect platelet function and prolong the bleeding time and if used in close proximity to a bleeding episode (such as labor, scheduled cesarean section, or bleeding from a placenta previa or placental abruption) can result in further or greater hemorrhage. This risk of bleeding, though real, is less evident when compared to aspirin due to the reversible nature of their mechanism of action.[8]

Two other areas of concern exist with NSAIDs, especially when chronically used in the latter part of pregnancy. One of these is the potential for the development of oligohydramnios and the second is the potential in utero effects that may occur in the fetus and/or newborn after delivery.[10,11] As part of their mechanism of action, NSAIDs can also inhibit prostaglandin-mediated renal function.[8] This effect is not usually seen in normal healthy adults, but it appears that in some cases, it can occur in utero with the fetus. The fetal kidneys produce the amniotic fluid and if kidney function decreases, a low amount of amniotic fluid will develop. An abnormally low amount of amniotic fluid is called oligohydramnios. Because this category of medication has been used to treat premature labor, there have been reports of the development of oligohydramnios in some gestations.[11] Patients who are being treated for preterm labor with NSAIDs are often followed by sonography for this occurrence. However, if a pregnant woman is frequently using these drugs to treat other symptoms (such as chronic aches and pains), oligohydramnios, if it developed, might go undiagnosed leading to potential damage and even death of the fetus.

Like aspirin, NSAIDs cross the placenta. In utero, the oxygenated blood that is returning to the fetus from the placenta enters the right heart and then is shunted to the left side by way of the foramen ovale and the ductus arteriosus. The ductus arteriosus in the fetus is a large vessel that connects the pulmonary artery to the descending aorta. The patency of the ductus arteriosus is maintained in utero by prostaglandins, and this vessel normally closes after delivery because of metabolic changes that occur in the newborn shortly after birth. Because NSAIDs are potent inhibitors of prostaglandin synthesis and these medications cross the placenta, there have been reports of premature constriction of the ductus arteriosus in utero leading to primary pulmonary hypertension in the newborn.[10] Similarly, a risk of bleeding in the newborn has been reported when this medication was frequently used in close proximity to delivery. Thus, because of the potential risks of prolonging the gestation, dysfunctional labor, antenatal hemorrhage, postpartum hemorrhage, oligohydramnios, newborn hemorrhage, and premature constriction of the ductus arteriosus, NSAIDs are generally not recommended for use in the latter half of pregnancy.

C. Acetaminophen

Acetaminophen is an over-the-counter analgesic medication, but it does not have the anti-inflammatory action of aspirin or NSAIDs. Several studies have looked at first trimester use of acetaminophen in pregnancy and this drug does not appear to be teratogenic.[3-7] This medication differs from aspirin and NSAIDs because it is a very weak inhibitor of prostaglandin synthesis and cyclooxygenase.[8] Thus, it does not affect the bleeding time nor does it have any effect on uterine contractions. It freely crosses the placenta but again does not have any apparent interactions with the fetus. The primary concern with acetaminophen is overdosage. An acetaminophen overdose can be fatal by producing liver necrosis and there have been reports of this occurring during pregnancy that have led to fetal damage as well. However, barring an overdosage or any allergic issues a patient may have, acetaminophen is the primary analgesic of choice during pregnancy.

D. Methyl Salicylate

Methyl salicylate is one of the main ingredients in over-the-counter creams that can be applied for muscle aches and pains. These creams also contain menthol and camphor. Methyl salicylate is similar to aspirin in its pharmacokinetics and mechanism of action.[8] This drug has not been studied in pregnancy so any teratogenic effect is unknown; however, it would probably be similar to that of aspirin. The primary issue for this over-the-counter medication is that it is not for oral intake. This means that most people, including pregnant women, believe that these creams are completely safe because they are topically applied. Nevertheless, methyl salicylate is absorbed into the bloodstream when applied topically, although the amount is small when used as directed. If used chronically over large areas, the amount will increase, leading to a prolonged bleeding time and the risks of hemorrhage, as seen with aspirin. Furthermore, there have been reports of salicylate overdosage and even death when these creams were applied to extensive body areas for prolonged periods of time.[12] Because of the enlarging uterus, pregnancy can often result in general body "aches and pains" because of rapid changes in body dynamics involving weight gain, weight distribution, and center of gravity. Therefore, some pregnant women may want to use these topical creams for treatment of their muscle aches and pains. However, because methyl salicylate is absorbed into the bloodstream, creams that contain this agent should probably be avoided near delivery and should not be applied to extensive areas on the body during pregnancy.

IV. Cold Medications/Respiratory Medications

A. Decongestants

Decongestants are a group of drugs that are used to clear nasal passages and "unstuff" a stuffy nose. They perform this task by constricting blood vessels. Decongestants are sympathomimetic drugs that have either α-adrenergic activity or both α-adrenergic and β-adrenergic activity.[8] α-Adrenergic activity is found within numerous organs, and these agents also interact with smooth muscle fibers found in blood vessels and the uterus. Alpha activity will increase heart rate, constrict blood vessels (thereby increasing blood pressure), decrease insulin release from the pancreas and promote glycogenolysis within the liver (in order to elevate blood glucose), and cause uterine muscle fibers to contract. β-Adrenergic activity is divided into β_1 action and β_2 action. β_1 action is mainly seen in the heart and will increase the heart rate. β_2 action will also cause glycogenolysis (thereby increasing blood glucose levels) but will relax blood vessels, relax uterine muscle fibers, and relax the muscles in the lungs. β_2 drugs are used in treating asthma and are also used as a form of tocolytic agent (discussed in Chapter 18).

Decongestants can be taken orally and are also found in direct nasal products that include sprays, drops, or jellies. The direct nasal medications consist of oxymetazoline, xylometazoline, naphazoline, propylhexedrine, levmetamfetamine, and phenylephrine. Although none of these drugs has been extensively evaluated, the studies that do exist have not identified any as being teratogenic.[4–7] All of these medications are primarily potent α-adrenergic drugs. In addition, even though they are placed locally within the nasal passages, some of the drug is absorbed into the bloodstream. If nasal decongestant medications were to be used sparingly and intermittently, it is unlikely that they would lead to any complications in pregnancy. However, nasal congestion unrelated to a cold or flu is common in pregnancy and can last for several weeks and even months. The reason for this may be that blood vessels are more dilated during pregnancy. Therefore, if nasal spray usage were more frequent or chronic, this could lead to larger amounts of the drug entering the bloodstream, which could affect blood pressure, blood glucose, and promote uterine contractions.[13] Another important issue to understand regarding nasal decongestant usage is the phenomenon of "rebound congestion." Rebound congestion is a disorder that occurs with decongestant nasal products after use over a period of several days whereby the nasal congestion becomes worse after the drug wears off. This can lead to more frequent use, resulting in higher blood concentrations of the drug.

Decongestants also come in oral form consisting primarily of phenylephrine and pseudoephedrine. Phenylephrine is primarily a potent α-adrenergic drug as discussed above; however, pseudoephedrine has both α-adrenergic and β-adrenergic effects. Pseudoephedrine has probably been analyzed the most in pregnancy, and studies have not identified this drug as being teratogenic.[4–7] All of the decongestant drugs can elevate blood pressure, and therefore, should probably be avoided or used with caution in patients with hypertension or preeclampsia. In addition, they can all elevate blood glucose and this could affect patients with diabetes. None of the decongestant drugs has been studied in relation to uterine contractions; however, α-adrenergic action will promote contractions, so decongestants should be used with caution in patients with or who are at risk for premature labor.[13] This factor should also be considered by patients with preterm premature rupture of the membranes and those with incompetent cervix where minimizing contractions is of paramount importance. Pseudoephedrine is the one decongestant that may have a different effect on the uterus in that its α-adrenergic action would promote contractions, whereas its β-adrenergic action would decrease contractions. This issue, however, has not been studied in any detail.

Levmetamfetamine is an amphetamine drug but it has no central nervous system stimulating effects as seen with other amphetamines. All three-dimensional objects have mirror images and the same is true for chemicals and drugs. These mirror images in chemistry are labeled levo for left and dextro for right, and in some cases the pharmacokinetics and mechanism of action will differ between a drug's levo and dextro configurations. Levmetamfetamine is the levo-oriented drug of dextro-methamphetamine; however, it has no central nervous system euphoric effects, only the α-adrenergic effects.[8] Thus, it is available as an over-the-counter decongestant.

In summary, decongestant medications, if used in pregnancy, should be taken sparingly and avoided or used with caution in patients with or who are at risk for hypertension, preeclampsia, diabetes, premature labor, preterm premature rupture of the membranes, and incompetent cervix.

B. Antihistamines

The antihistamines are a group of drugs that are primarily used to treat rhinorrhea, sneezing, and itchy watery eyes. Many antihistamine medications are found over-the-counter and include first-generation drugs of diphenhydramine, doxylamine, clemastine, chlorpheniramine, dexchlorpheniramine, brompheniramine, dexbrompheniramine, pheniramine, triprolidine, pyrilamine, chlorcyclizine, phenindamine, and thonzylamine, along with second-generation drugs of loratadine and cetirizine.[14] In general, these drugs are used to counter the effects of histamine, which is often released in response to an allergic reaction, such as hay fever, or in response to an infection with a cold or flu virus. Once histamine is released, it attaches to cell receptors that are either H_1 receptors or H_2 receptors.[8] The H_2 receptors are primarily found within the intestinal tract and will be discussed under the section regarding gastrointestinal medications. H_1 receptors are highly concentrated in the nasal passages, lungs, and skin, and when histamine attaches to these receptors, local irritation and inflammation can develop. The mechanism of action for antihistamine drugs is that they block the histamine receptors, which results in minimizing the overall effect of the histamine release.[8] However, this action is only temporary.

As with most over-the-counter drugs, none of the antihistamines has been extensively evaluated in pregnancy, but from the studies that have been reported, as a group they do not appear to be teratogenic.[3–7,14] Antihistamines do not have any direct action on the heart or affect blood glucose, nor do they interact with the uterus or uterine vasculature.[8] The primary issue with antihistamine agents is their side effect of drowsiness, and a few of these are also found in over-the-counter nighttime sleep aids. This effect is primarily due to the anticholinergic action found with antihistamines, especially the first-generation medications. Some first-generation antihistamine drugs are marketed as being less sedating when compared to others. However, in general, all first-generation antihistamine medicines can produce drowsiness. Because of their anticholinergic action, the first-generation antihistamine drugs should be used with caution in patients with narrow-angle glaucoma and in people who have difficulties with urination. The second-generation antihistamines of loratadine and cetirizine have minimal anticholinergic action and, therefore, are less sedating than the others.

C. Expectorants

Expectorants are medications that are used to thin out mucus or phlegm so that it can be coughed up more easily. Essentially, only one expectorant is approved by the U.S. Food and Drug Administration (FDA) for use in over-the-counter medications and that is guaifenesin. Guaifenesin has minimal actions within the body and by itself does not appear to have many side effects. It has been analyzed in early pregnancy by several studies and it does not appear to be teratogenic.[3–7]

Potassium iodide and iodinated glycerol, at one time, were available as expectorants in over-the-counter medications; however, the FDA no longer approves their use because they are considered noneffective. These two drugs are mentioned because they may be found in natural products that are available over-the-counter. Iodide drugs are not recommended for use in pregnancy because they can cross the placenta and potentially inhibit the thyroid function of the fetus, leading to hypothyroidism and goiter.[3]

D. Cough Suppressants

Cough suppressants are antitussives, a group of drugs that are used to relieve or slow down coughing. The primary ingredient in most preparations is dextromethorphan. Four others can be found listed as treatments for coughing: diphenhydramine, chlophedianol, camphor, and menthol. Narcotic medications were the initial class of drugs found to possess antitussive properties. Narcotic drugs, however, are habit-forming and can lead to dependence and addiction. Dextromethorphan is the mirror image drug of a potent narcotic, levorphanol, but it does not have any analgesic effects, nor is it addicting like the narcotics.[8] It does, however, have antitussive properties. A few studies have analyzed the use of this drug in pregnancy, and it does not appear to be teratogenic.[4–7,15] In recent years, dextromethorphan has been consumed in larger amounts in order to produce a euphoric effect. No information exists as to what consequence might occur in a pregnancy after the use of larger quantities. In recommended dosages, dextromethorphan appears to be safe for use in pregnancy.

Diphenhydramine is an antihistamine that has occasionally been listed as a cough suppressant. This drug was discussed above under antihistamines and its antitussive effect is reported to be centrally active; however, some studies have questioned its effectiveness in this regard. Chlophedianol is FDA-approved, but few, if any, over-the-counter products contain this drug. It appears to be similar to diphenhydramine and is stated to be centrally active,[8] but there are no studies regarding its use in pregnancy.

Camphor and menthol are topical antitussive medications. Camphor is found in topical rubs and nasal mists. Menthol is also found in topical rubs and nasal mists as well as in throat lozenges, sprays, and cough drops. The exact mechanism of action for these two drugs is not fully known, but it is believed that they have mild local anesthetic action.[8] No studies have been reported to suggest that either of these is teratogenic. In addition, millions of cough drops are consumed annually in the United States alone and no untoward effects have been described.

E. Throat Lozenge Medications

Throat lozenges, cough drops, and throat sprays are most often used in soothing a sore throat. Several drugs can be found within these products including dyclonine, benzocaine, camphor, menthol, phenol (carbolic acid), resorcinol, boric acid, and cetylpyridinium. Menthol and camphor were just discussed under cough suppressants. Regarding the others, again, little or no information exists concerning their use in pregnancy. Dyclonine and benzocaine are local anesthetics of the ester type and the mechanism of action for these drugs is that they produce numbness in the applied area.[8] Benzocaine has been reported to cause methemoglobinemia, which is a disorder that alters normal hemoglobin so that it is unable to carry oxygen.[16] Most of these reports have occurred in infants and young children following the use of excessive amounts; however, a few cases have occurred after the use of recommended doses. If this were to occur in pregnancy, the decreased oxygen levels could affect the pregnancy. It is uncertain whether benzocaine crosses the placenta. Therefore, benzocaine should be used with caution during pregnancy.

Phenol (carbolic acid) is similar to camphor in that it appears to have local anesthetic properties, but the drug is not an anesthetic.[8] This medication is actually an antiseptic and disinfectant and may also produce some of its effect by preventing an overgrowth of bacteria in the applied location. Resorcinol, boric acid, and cetylpyridinium are also listed as topical antiseptics and disinfectants.[8] Therefore, the mechanism of action for these medications may be somewhat similar to that of phenol. In summary, all of the drugs contained in throat medications are readily absorbed into the bloodstream but very little is known regarding their effect on pregnancy and whether or not these agents cross the placenta. As previously stated, millions of these products are used annually in the United States and no major untoward events have been reported.

F. Asthma and Allergy Medications

Until recently, there were three over-the-counter preparations that could be purchased for use in asthma: theophylline, ephedrine, and epinephrine. The FDA removed the first two, leaving only epinephrine. Epinephrine is only available as a product that has to be inhaled. It is not available in pill form. Its mechanism of action for treating asthma is bronchodilation by way of its β_2-adrenergic effect. However, as briefly discussed under the section regarding decongestants, epinephrine has very strong α-adrenergic action and can elevate heart rate, constrict blood vessels, and increase blood glucose levels.[8] Therefore, this drug should be used with caution in patients with hypertension, pre-eclampsia, and diabetes. Health care providers should follow pregnant women with asthma closely because asthma may affect other aspects of the pregnancy and other related prescription medications may be preferred over epinephrine for use during the gestation (discussed in Chapter 18). Health care providers need to be aware of the medicines that are used in treating asthma and how frequently they are needed as the pregnancy progresses. Therefore, it is not recommended that pregnant women with asthma self-medicate without the knowledge of their health care providers. The effect of epinephrine on the uterus has not been fully studied. Its α-adrenergic action would promote uterine contractions, whereas its β-adrenergic action would do the opposite.

Cromolyn sodium is used in preventing respiratory allergies. This drug is only available as an inhaled product. Its mechanism of action differs from that of antihistamines in that it works by preventing the release of histamine from certain cells found within the body rather than blocking the effect once histamine has been released.[8] Few studies have evaluated the use of this drug in pregnancy.[3,17] From the reports that do exist, this medication does not appear to be teratogenic. It is poorly absorbed into the bloodstream, has very few side effects, and it is uncertain whether it crosses the placenta. Based on this information and barring any allergy to the drug itself, there does not appear to be any contraindication to the use of cromolyn sodium in pregnancy.

V. Gastrointestinal Medications

A. Antacids and Antiflatulents

Antacids are available over-the-counter in three basic forms: direct-acting medications, histamine-2 (H_2) receptor antagonists, and proton pump inhibitors. The direct-acting medications include calcium carbonate, magnesium hydroxide, and aluminum hydroxide. These products are bases in nature that when mixed with the acid in the stomach result in a neutralizing effect.[8] None of these products has been found to be teratogenic.[3] Magnesium tends to increase intestinal motility while aluminum decreases it, which is why these two drugs are often found together in the same over-the-counter product.[8] The absorption of aluminum, calcium, and magnesium is variable; however, because they alter the gastric pH, they can affect the absorption of other medications, such as antibiotics. Thus, pregnant women who are prescribed other medications by their health care providers need to be asked about antacid use because heartburn is a disorder commonly experienced by pregnant women. One direct-acting medication that should be avoided during pregnancy is sodium bicarbonate. This drug is readily absorbed and if used extensively, can lead to alkalosis.

The H_2 receptor antagonists include cimetidine, ranitidine, famotidine, and nizatidine. Histamine is released into the stomach by several different mechanisms that include paracrine stimulation, nerve impulses from the vagus nerve, or by way of released gastrin.[8] The released histamine then in turn activates gastric parietal cell H_2 receptors leading to the release of stomach acid. The H_2 receptor antagonists are the antihistamines of the intestinal tract and work by blocking these H_2 histamine receptors, thereby decreasing the amount of acid that is released.[8] Numerous studies have evaluated these drugs in pregnancy and to date they have not been found to be teratogenic; however, these agents do cross the placenta.[3] Because the direct-acting medications are minimally absorbed and short acting, they are considered as first-line treatment choices in pregnancy. The H_2 receptor antagonists are only recommended in pregnant women in whom the direct-acting medications fail and whose symptoms cannot be controlled with lifestyle changes.[18]

Recently, omeprazole was made available over-the-counter, and this antacid is a proton pump inhibitor. It is likely that other proton pump inhibitors will be made available over-the-counter in the future. This drug differs from the others in that it directly inhibits gastric acid secretion from the parietal cell.[8] Few studies have analyzed the effect of this drug in pregnancy, but what has been reported to date does not suggest that it is teratogenic.[19] Because it also crosses the placenta, it is not recommended as a first-line drug for usage in pregnancy similar to the H_2 receptor antagonist agents. Furthermore, this drug is long acting in that it is an irreversible inhibitor on the enzyme H^+,K^+-ATPase; therefore, its action persists after the drug disappears from the bloodstream.[8]

Simethicone is an antiflatulent that helps decrease the development of gas. Few studies have analyzed this drug in pregnancy, but it does not appear to have any untoward effects.[3] This is probably because it is not readily absorbed, and there is no data to suggest that it would cross the placenta.

B. Antiemetics

A few antiemetics are available over-the-counter and these primarily consist of dimenhydrinate, meclizine, cyclizine, and doxylamine. All of these are H_1 receptor antagonist antihistamines similar to the antihistamines used for treating allergy, cold, or flu symptoms. These drugs, however, appear to have stronger anticholinergic properties that result in the ability to somewhat treat motion sickness.[8] This effect on treating motion sickness (of which nausea is a common symptom) has led some to use these products in hopes that they will minimize nausea that may be caused by other etiologies, such as nausea and vomiting of pregnancy. Their effectiveness in this regard is uncertain.

Doxylamine was part of a commonly prescribed medication called Bendectin that was used by millions of pregnant women in treating nausea and vomiting of pregnancy from the 1950s through the 1970s. The manufacturer ceased production over litigation issues in the early 1980s, although this drug has never been proven to be teratogenic (see Chapter 24).[20] A few studies have analyzed the use of dimenhydrinate, meclizine, and cyclizine in pregnancy and these also do not appear to be teratogenic. As with the other antihistamines, the main concern with the use of these medications is drowsiness.

C. Antidiarrheal Medications

The available over-the-counter antidiarrheal medications vary somewhat in their makeup and mechanism of action. The primary ones are kaolin and pectin, bismuth subsalicylate, loperamide, and diphenoxylate/atropine. Kaolin and pectin are often considered the first-line treatments in pregnancy because these substances are not absorbed and it also does not appear that they would cross the placenta.[2] Thus, they would be considered safe for use in pregnancy. Bismuth subsalicylate is hydrolyzed in the gastrointestinal tract into bismuth salts and sodium salicylate.[8] Bismuth is not well absorbed into the bloodstream; however, salicylate is, and this substance could have similar effects to those that are seen with aspirin usage. Because of the potential risks of prolonging the gestation, dysfunctional labor, antenatal hemorrhage, postpartum hemorrhage, and newborn hemorrhage, salicylates are not generally recommended for use, especially in the latter half of pregnancy.

Loperamide and diphenoxylate are both piperidine opioid drugs. It has long been established that the opioid class of drugs works well in treating diarrhea. An obvious concern, however, is their addictive nature. The two over-the-counter opioid medications of loperamide and diphenoxylate have become the drugs of choice for treating diarrhea because they poorly penetrate the central nervous system. A few studies have evaluated these products in pregnancy, and it does not appear that either is teratogenic.[3] Diphenoxylate is structurally similar to meperidine, and it is usually combined with atropine to minimize any abuse or overdose potential. Atropine is well absorbed after oral intake and readily crosses the placenta. This drug can affect the appearance of a fetal heart monitor tracing by increasing the heart rate and decreasing the variability.[21] Therefore, diphenoxylate/atropine is not recommended or should be used with caution in pregnancy (especially the latter half of gestation). Loperamide is not combined with atropine and is considered the second-line drug of choice in pregnancy if kaolin and pectin are ineffective.

D. Stool Softeners and Laxatives

Stool softeners and laxatives can be organized into four basic categories: bulk-forming agents, surfactants, osmotic, and stimulant. Most constipation can be resolved by increasing the water and fiber content of the diet along with exercise.[22] Bulk-forming agents include bran, agar, psyllium, methylcellulose, and calcium polycarbophil. These products add bulk to the stool, which then retains more water, leading to a softening and a decrease in transit time.[8] Because these substances are poorly absorbed they are considered safe to use in pregnancy. The primary surfactant product that is available over-the-counter is docusate sodium. The mechanism of action for this drug is that it alters the permeability of the intestine, leading to an increase in water content and thus a softening.[8] A few studies have analyzed this medication in pregnancy and in summary it is considered safe for use during pregnancy.[4–7] When taken in normal dosages, it is mild in action.

The other two categories overlap somewhat and have stronger actions. The osmotic laxatives include magnesium hydroxide, magnesium sulfate, and magnesium citrate. In smaller dosages, some of these medications are used as antacids (as previously covered). However, in larger amounts, they have a cathartic effect due to direct stimulation from magnesium along with the fact that they are poorly absorbed, pulling more water into the intestinal tract.[8] Stimulants include bisacodyl, senna, and cascara. Bisacodyl is a diphenylmethane and is the mildest of these three and the few studies that have occurred in pregnancy have not found it to be teratogenic. Only approximately 5%–10% of the drug is absorbed and it is uncertain how readily it can cross the placenta. Its stimulant effect is on the colon itself, so its action will not usually occur until several hours after the dose is taken. Senna and cascara are anthraquinones[8] that also directly stimulate the colon and thus their action is also delayed somewhat after intake. These two products, however, are much stronger in their stimulation when compared to bisacodyl. The few studies that have evaluated these drugs in pregnancy have not found them to be teratogenic.[3]

Two other available laxatives are castor oil and mineral oil. Mineral oil is a mixture of aliphatic hydrocarbons obtained from petroleum, and these are ingestible. Its mechanism of action is that it softens the stool and interferes with water reabsorption in the colon, which in turn increases the water content. Minimal studies exist regarding its use in pregnancy. The main concern with this drug is that it can decrease the absorption of fat-soluble vitamins[8] and, therefore, should be used with caution in pregnancy. Castor oil is a surfactant laxative (and also a stimulant), however, it is much stronger than docusate sodium. In the small intestine, castor oil is converted into glycerol and ricinoleic acid.[8] Ricinoleic acid reduces the net absorption of water, but it also stimulates intestinal peristalsis. Few studies have evaluated this medication in pregnancy, but it does not appear to be teratogenic. Regarding pregnancy, it is not recommended that the stronger cathartic laxatives (cascara, senna, castor oil, and the magnesium products at laxative dosages) be used without the knowledge of or the direction of the patient's health care provider.[22]

VI. Miscellaneous Medication Categories

A. Vaginal Preparations

The over-the-counter vaginal preparations on the market today primarily involve the antifungal agents of butoconazole, clotrimazole, miconazole, and tioconazole. Numerous studies have examined these medications in pregnancy and none of the reports has identified these as being teratogenic.[3-7,23,24] At the present time, the over-the-counter products are all topical in the form of creams or suppositories. The Centers for Disease Control and Prevention recommends using only topical vaginal anti-fungal agents in pregnancy; therefore, the over-the-counter products are considered the drugs of choice.

No consensus statement from any national association has been released regarding douching in pregnancy. Many obstetric health care professionals usually recommend against douching while pregnant because a woman never really knows if her cervix has dilated somewhat. In addition, bacteria that normally reside in the lower vagina (such as group B streptococcus) may be pushed higher into the canal, increasing the risk of infection. If douching is performed, one type that should be avoided is betadine because this product is a form of iodine that can be absorbed into the bloodstream and affect the fetal thyroid function, as discussed with potassium iodide.[3]

Spermicides primarily contain nonoxynol-9 and octoxynol-9. Although unlikely to be used once a woman realizes that she is already pregnant, these products are not 100% effective in preventing pregnancy. Similarly, it usually takes several weeks to even a couple of months before many women realize they are pregnant and these products may have been used in that time period. Therefore, women may be concerned once they discover this fact and may have questions. Numerous studies have evaluated the use of spermicides in the first trimester of pregnancy and in summary it does not appear that they are teratogenic.[3] In fact, the FDA submitted a statement regarding this fact.[25]

B. Caffeine

Caffeine is naturally occurring in coffee as well as teas and is found in other food products, such as certain carbonated beverages. The amount of caffeine in these food substances varies widely from approximately 40 mg to more than 200 mg in an 8-ounce glass. Caffeine can also be found in some over-the-counter products used as central nervous system stimulants or as part of cold preparations to boost energy. The amount of caffeine in these products is similar to the levels found in the food items. Numerous evaluations of this drug have not found it to be teratogenic.[3,26] Caffeine readily crosses the placenta with fetal levels that are in equilibrium with maternal levels.[3] Caffeine can elevate an individual's heart rate and fetal tachycardia has been reported following its use in pregnancy. This substance is not contraindicated for use in pregnancy; however, taking extra caffeine in tablet form beyond what might be obtained from a person's diet is not recommended.

C. Smoking Cessation Drugs

Smoking cessation products primarily contain nicotine and the use of this drug by itself has not been sufficiently studied in pregnancy, leading to controversy. Smoking in pregnancy has been associated with numerous complications including low birth weight, intrauterine growth restriction, premature membrane rupture with preterm delivery, and elevated carboxyhemoglobin levels.[27] It is believed that many of these disorders are related to nicotine, but could be caused by other substances found in cigarette smoke. It does not appear that nicotine is teratogenic.[3,27] The American College of Obstetricians and Gynecologists has submitted a Committee Opinion on this topic and strongly urges that health care providers help patients achieve smoking cessation by way of education and counseling.[27] Nicotine products should only be considered when nonpharmacologic methods fail. If used, it is also recommended that the amount be minimized as much as possible by using the intermittent agents (gums, sprays, and inhalers) instead of the continuous-release products (patches).

D. Vitamins and Homeopathic Preparations

All vitamins are considered safe for use in pregnancy at the recommended dosages.[3] The primary concern with excess vitamin intake is the fat-soluble vitamins of A, D, E, and K. Vitamin A is one vitamin that can be teratogenic in high dosages.[28] It is recommended that all women of reproductive age take a folic acid supplement of 0.4 mg per day to minimize the potential risk of spina bifida. If a woman has delivered a child with a neural tube defect, then it is recommended that she take 4 mg daily beginning before conception.[28] To obtain this amount of folic acid, the woman should not use a megavitamin that may have excess vitamin A. Regarding the three other fat-soluble vitamins (D, E, and K), no adverse reports for use in pregnancy have been published.

Thousands of homeopathic preparations are available over-the-counter, and this topic is too large to adequately cover in a few paragraphs. What is important to understand is that a substance that may be listed as "homeopathic" or "natural" can often bring a false sense of security to consumers, including pregnant women. In its entirety, very little research has been performed on over-the-counter products in pregnancy and even less has occurred with "natural" products or even herbal medications. Therefore, it is not recommended that pregnant women use these products, especially if little is known about the contents. One example to discuss is an over-the-counter product that is available for treating leg cramps. Leg cramps or leg discomfort is common in pregnancy. This homeopathic product contains quinine, which in the past was used as an abortifacient drug.[29] The amount of quinine in this product is probably small; however, the use of quinine is not recommended in pregnancy.

E. Nighttime Sleep Aids

The nighttime sleep aids primarily consist of two antihistamines (doxylamine and diphenhydramine) that were previously discussed above. The dosage levels are similar, and neither of these was contraindicated for use in pregnancy.

F. Scabicides and Pediculicides

Over-the-counter scabicide and pediculicide products primarily contain one of two drugs, which are pyrethrins with piperonyl butoxide and permethrin. Pyrethrins are extracts from the chrysanthemum flower and topical absorption is poor.[8] Therefore, this product is often the first-line drug of choice when treating head lice in pregnancy. Pyrethrins with piperonyl butoxide do not kill unhatched nits and thus a second treatment is recommended in 7–10 days. This drug combination is also not effective in treating scabies.[8]

Permethrin is similar to pyrethrins, but is effective against all forms of lice (head, body, and pubic), as well as scabies. Very little knowledge is available on the use of this drug in pregnancy.[30] Again, because it is topical there is a question as to how much is actually absorbed into the bloodstream. Permethrin does not kill unhatched eggs, so a second treatment is indicated in 7–10 days.

G. Inactive Ingredients

The last topic to cover is the inactive ingredients. Just because they are listed under the inactive category does not mean that they have no effect. The inactive ingredients can include sugar, sugar substitutes, alcohol, caffeine, preservatives, and numerous other chemicals. The amount of these substances is usually small, but patients, including pregnant women, may not think of over-the-counter drugs as "food" and the sugar content, if present, could affect the results of a fasting blood glucose test if taken before the blood draw. Likewise, patients with phenylketonuria are to avoid the amino acid phenylalanine, which can be found in the sugar substitute aspartame.

VII. PATIENT CASE (PART 2)

The patient evaluation revealed that her uterus was nontender, she was afebrile with a normal blood pressure, but she was tachycardic with a maternal heart rate of 110 bpm. In questioning the patient, she had no medical disorders, was on no prescribed medications, and she noted good fetal movement. In further talking with the patient, it was discovered that she was using an over-the-counter cold remedy and she divulged that the normal dosage and scheduling had not helped with her symptoms, so she had "doubled up." To obtain an effect, she was taking double the dosage, twice as often. The differential diagnosis for fetal tachycardia includes fetal issues of compromise (hypoxia, anemia, heart failure, or sepsis) or a fetal tachyarrhythmia. Fetal issues usually result in decreased or absent fetal movement. The maternal causes include fever, drug usage, an intrauterine infection, or hyperthyroidism. Because she had good fetal movement, no signs of infection, a negative past medical history, and was afebrile, the most likely cause was the excessive usage of the over-the-counter cold remedy medication. In addition, this was probably the cause of the maternal tachycardia. She was told to discontinue the medication and return in a few hours for repeat monitoring. On return, her heart rate was now normal at 82 bpm and the fetal monitor tracing had also returned to normal with a baseline of 150 bpm. Examples of the fetal monitor strips are seen in Figure 1.

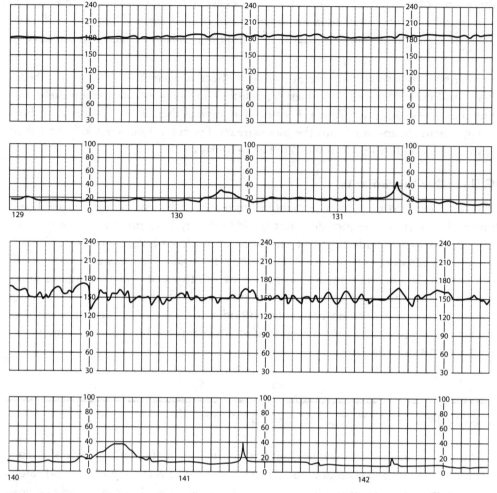

Figure 1. The top tracing depicts the fetal tachycardia in the 180 beats per minute (bpm) range. The lower tracing shows the fetal heart strip when it returned to normal with a baseline of 150 bpm.

VIII. Summary

Because over-the-counter medications can be purchased without a prescription, many people (including pregnant women) do not consider these agents to be the same as a prescribed drug. This means that patients need to be specifically asked if they are using any medicines, prescribed and over-the-counter, when obtaining a history. As depicted in the case history along with the information supplied in this chapter, it is apparent that over-the-counter drugs can affect both the mother and the baby. However, it is prudent to also be aware that some of these medications can be helpful in certain pregnancies based on the clinical situation. Table 1 is a summary of those active ingredients that should be used with caution or avoided during pregnancy.

Table 1. Over-the-Counter Drugs to Avoid or to Use with Caution in Pregnancy

Over-the-Counter Medication	Potential Adverse Reaction or Reason for Using with Caution
Antihistamines (first-generation)	Should be used with caution in patients with narrow-angle glaucoma and in people who have difficulties with urination
Aspirin	May prolong the gestation, produce dysfunctional labor, increase hemorrhage (antenatal and/or postpartum), produce oligohydramnios, lead to newborn hemorrhage or premature constriction of the ductus arteriosus (primarily chronic usage in the latter half of gestation or when used near delivery)
	Should be avoided for several days before scheduled surgery (ie, planned cesarean section)
Benzocaine	Could cause methemoglobinemia
Bismuth subsalicylate	Potential adverse reactions similar to aspirin
Decongestants	Should be avoided or used with caution in patients with or who are at risk for hypertension, preeclampsia, diabetes, premature labor, preterm premature rupture of the membranes, or incompetent cervix
Diphenoxylate/ atropine	May affect the appearance of a fetal heart monitor tracing by increasing the heart rate and decreasing the variability—use with caution (especially the latter half of gestation)
Epinephrine	Should be avoided or used with caution in patients with or who are at risk for hypertension, preeclampsia, diabetes, premature labor, preterm premature rupture of the membranes, or incompetent cervix
Iodides and betadine	May adversely affect fetal thyroid gland function (primarily the second and third trimesters)
Methyl salicylate	Potential reactions similar to aspirin
Mineral oil	May decrease the absorption of fat-soluble vitamins
Nonsteroidal anti-inflammatory drugs	May prolong the gestation, produce dysfunctional labor, increase hemorrhage (antenatal and/or postpartum), produce oligohydramnios, lead to newborn hemorrhage or premature constriction of the ductus arteriosus (primarily chronic usage in the latter half of gestation or when used near delivery)
	Should be avoided for 24 hours before scheduled surgery (ie, planned cesarean section)
Quinine	Can adversely affect fetal viability
Sodium bicarbonate	Could produce alkalosis
Vitamin A (in excess)	May be teratogenic (first trimester use)

IX. References

1. Werler MM, Mitchell AA, Hernandez-Diaz S, et al. Use of over-the-counter medication during pregnancy. *Am J Obstet Gynecol*. 2005;193:771–777.

2. Black RA, Hill DA. Over-the-counter medications in pregnancy. *Am Fam Physician*. 2003;67:2517–2524.

3. Briggs GG, Freeman RK, Yaffe SJ. *Drugs in Pregnancy and Lactation*. 8th ed. Philadelphia: Lippincott Williams & Wilkins, 2008.

4. Rosa F, Baum C. *Medicaid Surveillance of Drugs in Pregnancy and Birth Defects*. Rockville, MD: U.S. Food and Drug Administration, Freedom of Information, 1995.

5. Jick H, Holmes LB, Hunter JR, et al. First-trimester drug use and congenital disorders. *JAMA*. 1981;246:343–346.

6. Aselton P, Jick H, Milunsky A, et al. First-trimester drug use and congenital disorders. *Obstet Gynecol.* 1985;65:451–455.

7. Heinonen Op, Slone D, Shapiro S. *Birth Defects and Drugs in Pregnancy.* Littleton, MA: Publishing Sciences Group, 1977.

8. Brunton LL, Lazo JS, Parker KL, eds. *Goodman & Gilman's The Pharmacologic Basis of Therapeutics.* 11th ed. New York: McGraw-Hill, 2005.

9. James AH, Brancazio LR, Price T. Aspirin and reproductive outcomes. *Obstet Gynecol Surv.* 2008;63:49–57.

10. Koren G, Florescu A, Costei AM, et al. Nonsteroidal anti-inflammatory drugs during pregnancy during the third trimester and the risk of premature closure of the ductus arteriosus: a meta-analysis. *Ann Pharmacother.* 2006;40:824–829.

11. Savage AH, Anderson BL, Simhan HN. The safety of prolonged indomethacin therapy. *Am J Perinatol.* 2007;24:207–213.

12. Azer M, Bailey H. Toxicity, salicylate. November 2007. Available at http://www.emedicine.com/MED/topic2057.htm. Accessed April 11, 2008.

13. Rayburn WF, Anderson JC, Smith CV, et al. Uterine and fetal Doppler flow changes from a single dose of a long-acting intranasal decongestant. *Obstet Gynecol.* 1990;76:180–182.

14. Gilbert C, Mazzotta P, Loebstein R, et al. Fetal safety of drugs used in the treatment of allergic rhinitis: a critical review. *Drug Saf.* 2005;28:707–719.

15. Einarson A, Lyszkiewicz D, Koren G. The safety of dextromethorphan in pregnancy: results of a controlled study. *Chest.* 2001;119:466–469.

16. Kane GC, Hoehn SM, Behrenbeck TR, et al. Benzocaine-induced methemoglobinemia based on the Mayo Clinic experience from 28 478 transesophageal echocardiograms: incidence, outcomes, and predisposing factors. *Arch Intern Med.* 2007;167:1977–1982.

17. Gluck JC, Gluck PA. Asthma controller therapy during pregnancy. *Am J Obstet Gynecol.* 2005;192:369–380.

18. Katz PO, Castell DO. Gastroesophageal reflux disease during pregnancy. *Gastroenterol Clin North Am.* 1998;27:153–167.

19. Diav-Citrin O, Arnon J, Shechtman S, et al. The safety of proton pump inhibitors in pregnancy: a multicenter prospective controlled study. *Aliment Pharmacol Ther.* 2005;21:269–275.

20. Brent RR. Editorial. The Bendectin saga: another American tragedy. *Teratology.* 1983;27:283–286.

21. Schifferli P, Caldeyro-Barcia R. Effects of atropine and beta-adrenergic drugs on the heart rate of the human fetus. In Boreus L, ed. *Fetal Pharmacology.* New York: Raven Press, 1973:259–279.

22. Prather CM. Pregnancy-related constipation. *Curr Gastroenterol Rep.* 2004;6:402–404.

23. Czeizel AE, Toth M, Rockenbauer M. No teratogenic effect after clotrimazole therapy during pregnancy. *Epidemiology.* 1999;10:437–440.

24. Mastroiacovo P, Mazzone T, Botto LD, et al. Prospective assessment of pregnancy outcomes after first-trimester exposure to fluconazole. *Am J Obstet Gynecol.* 1996;175:1645–1650.

25. Anonymous. Data do not support association between spermicides, birth defects. *FDA Drug Bull.* 1986;16:21.

26. Browne ML. Maternal exposure to caffeine and risk of congenital anomalies: a systematic review. *Epidemiology.* 2006;17:324–331.

27. The American College of Obstetrics and Gynecology. *Smoking Cessation During Pregnancy.* Committee Opinion No. 316. Washington, DC: ACOG, October 2005.

28. The American College of Obstetrics and Gynecology. *Neural Tube Defects.* ACOG Practice Bulletin No. 44. Washington, DC: ACOG, July 2003.

29. Smith JP. Risky choices; the dangers of teens using self-induced abortion attempts. *J Pediatr Health Care.* 1998;12:147–151.

30. Kennedy D, Hurst V, Konradsdottir E, et al. Pregnancy outcome following exposure to permethrin and use of teratogen information. *Am J Perinatol.* 2005;22:87–90.

QUESTIONS AND ANSWERS

1. All of the following drugs, if used excessively or chronically, could lead to a prolonged bleeding time **except**:

   a. methyl salicylate

   b. acetaminophen

   c. ketoprofen

   d. aspirin

   e. bismuth subsalicylate

2. Of the following over-the-counter decongestant drugs, which one has both α-adrenergic activity as well as β-adrenergic action?

   a. phenylephrine

   b. oxymetazoline

   c. propylhexedrine

   d. pseudoephedrine

   e. naphazoline

3. The direct-acting oral antacid that should probably be avoided in pregnancy because of the risk of developing alkalosis is:

   a. aluminum hydroxide

    b. calcium carbonate

    c. magnesium hydroxide

    d. calcium polycarbophil

    e. sodium bicarbonate

4. The laxative whose mechanism of action is brought about after it is converted into ricinoleic acid in the small intestine is:

    a. cascara

    b. senna

    c. castor oil

    d. bisacodyl

    e. mineral oil

5. The one vitamin that could be teratogenic if large amounts were ingested is:

    a. vitamin a

    b. vitamin b

    c. vitamin d

    d. vitamin e

    e. vitamin k

Answers:

1. b; 2. d; 3. e; 4. c; 5. a

Teratology Risk Assessment and Counseling

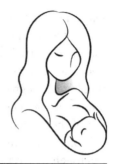

Dee Quinn

LEARNING OBJECTIVES

1. Describe the frequency and circumstances of medication use in pregnant and preconceptional women.

2. Identify strengths and weaknesses of animal and human reproductive data.

3. Compare the current and proposed U.S. Food and Drug Administration use in pregnancy labeling.

4. Outline the information needed from the client to provide a teratology risk assessment.

5. Summarize key sources of teratology information.

I. Introduction

Birth defects are known to occur in 3%–5% of all newborns. They are the leading cause of infant mortality in the United States and account for more than 20% of all infant deaths.[1] Heart defects make up about one third to one fourth of all birth defects and are present in approximately 1 in every 100–200 babies.[2] Other common birth defects include neural tube defects (spina bifida and anencephaly) and oral clefts, both of which occur in approximately 1 in 1000 pregnancies.[2]

Although significant progress has been made in identifying etiologic causes of some birth defects, approximately 65% have no known or identifiable cause. Of this number, it is estimated that 10% of all birth defects are caused by a prenatal exposure or teratogen.[1] These exposures include, but are not limited to, medication or drug exposures, maternal infections and diseases, and environmental and occupational exposures. An additional factor that must be considered is the high background rate of spontaneous abortions, occurring in approximately 15%–20% of *recognized* pregnancies.[3]

In the middle of the 20th century, the use of thalidomide and the recognition of congenital rubella syndrome brought to the forefront the issues of exposures during pregnancy.[4] Since that time, significant progress has been made, such that reproductive exposures are now considered an important aspect of women's health. In recent years, pregnant women have been identified as a special population in the drug development and approval process with particular attention to the ethical concerns regarding their participation in this process.[5] Questions about prenatal exposures with uncertain effects are increasingly common due to factors such as an increase in the number of pregnant women with chronic medical conditions, use of novel treatments, and a general increase in the use of medications. Empowered by a clearer understanding of the reproductive effects of a specific exposure and the integration of this information into a meaningful "answer" for an individual or family, clients can avoid teratogenic exposures when possible, manage medical conditions with the safest known treatment, and make informed reproductive choices.

II. PATIENT CASE (PART 1)

Ms. K is a 37-year-old, gravida 3, para 1, spontaneous abortion 1 woman who has been treated for depression and anxiety for the past 3 years with sertraline, 100 mg/d. She just did a home pregnancy test, which was positive. Her last normal menstrual period (LMP) was 6 weeks ago and she is concerned about the effects of sertraline on the developing baby. Although this was an unintended pregnancy, she says she would like to continue "unless there are really serious problems for the baby." She heard from a friend that antidepressants aren't safe in pregnancy. She has one healthy, 2-year-old daughter, no other medical problems, and there is no history of inherited disorders or birth defects in her or her partner's family. She is employed as an accountant. She is followed by a therapist monthly, while the sertraline is prescribed by her primary care provider. Her first obstetric visit is in 2 weeks.

III. Prevalence of Medication Use in Reproductive-Age Women

Prescription drug use among pregnant women is frequent, with estimates of 50%–66% exposed to at least one medication during gestation.[6,7] Other studies have shown that women in the United States fill an average of three nonvitamin prescriptions during pregnancy.[8] One retrospective study using an automated HMO database of medication use between 1996 and 2000, found that 59% of pregnant women had been prescribed a medication other than a vitamin or mineral supplement and almost half received medications in U.S. Food and Drug Administration (FDA) category C, D, or X.[9] Use of over-the-counter (OTC) products during pregnancy is also significant, with many women using analgesics and allergy and cold medications.[10] OTC products may be viewed by the public as safe to use during pregnancy due to their availability without prescription.[10] The use of dietary supplements during pregnancy has been estimated at 13%.[11] Animal reproductive studies are not performed on dietary supplements or herbal products.[12] As these products are generally considered to be safe and natural, pregnant women may opt to use these products in lieu of prescription medications. Patients are often unaware that these products are not regulated by the FDA, may have significant pharmacologic activity, and are very poorly studied in pregnant women.

It is important to recognize that half of pregnancies in the United States are unplanned.[13] For this reason, women of reproductive age should receive information concerning potential teratogenicity for all medications. Recent patterns of medication use in the adult U.S. population indicate that 82% of reproductive-age women took a medication (prescription or OTC drug, vitamin/mineral, or herbal/supplement) in the previously studied week.[14] The National Ambulatory Medical Care Survey documented that use of a pregnancy class D or X medication by reproductive-age women occurred in 1 out of every 13 ambulatory visits. In addition, contraceptive counseling was provided in fewer than 20% of these visits.[15] Recommendations for improvement in preconception care have been outlined,[16,17] and include an increase in consumer awareness, preventative visits, interventions for identified risk, and enhancement of health care coverage and public health programs. A current recommendation for preconception care that has been shown to decrease the incidence of spina bifida is the use of 0.4 mg of folic acid in all women of reproductive age.[18]

Despite scientific advances in clinical teratology and the small number of known teratogens, exposures before and during pregnancy still cause great anxiety and misunderstanding among both the public and health care professionals. In fact, perception of teratogenic risk may adversely affect the ability of the clinician to treat medically dangerous conditions during pregnancy. Bendectin, an antinauseant containing vitamin B_6 and doxylamine, was introduced in the United States in 1956. Allegations of associations with limb defects led the manufacturer to voluntarily remove the drug from the market amid increasing legal and insurance costs, as well as negative publicity. Numerous studies with significant sample sizes and statistical power have not found an association with limb defects or other adverse pregnancy outcomes.[19] As Bendectin was the only medication approved to treat nausea and vomiting of pregnancy, clinicians were and are still left with alternatives for which there are fewer reproductive data. While Diclectin is approved in Canada to treat nausea and vomiting of pregnancy, there is no approved drug therapy in the United States.[20] However, some clinicians suggest that women combine Unisom (doxylamine) and vitamin B_6 that are available OTC to treat this condition.

Several studies have shown that women and their health care providers perceive teratogenic risk as substantially greater than that obtained from a careful analysis of the literature.[21,22] However, health care providers are more likely to assign greater safety to medications than are patients.[23] Several studies have shown that perception of risk by women is often guided by their previous experiences and knowledge.[23,24] In addition, clients provided with information on reproductive health do not always act on the basis of "actual" risk but more on their perception of the risk.[25] This inflated assessment of risk can result not only in inadequate medical management but also in termination of an otherwise wanted pregnancy. Use of an evidence-based information and counseling service, such as that provided by Teratology Information Services (TIS), has been shown to substantially decrease the use of termination of pregnancy.[26,27] Teratology Information Services, such as those organized under OTIS

(Organization of Teratology Information Specialists), have also been shown to prevent congenital malformations, support appropriate medical management and nutritional supplementation, correct misperceptions of risk, and facilitate knowledge transfer and translation.[28–30]

There are numerous reasons for this inflated perception of risk, including the scarcity of evidence-based data, particularly concerning common exposures. Clinicians often find original reproductive studies time-consuming and difficult to interpret. Resources, when available, may be unknown or difficult to access for providers. Additionally, the complexity of this information precludes the development of a simple but accurate "list" of known teratogens. Lists of medications considered to be "safe" or "unsafe" for use in pregnancy have serious limitations and can result in mismanagement of pregnancies.[31] Improvements in knowledge transfer of teratology-related research are essential for health care providers, consumers, and public officials to practice evidence-based medicine.[32]

The media plays an increasing role in patient education. Medical information is available to the public via the Internet, newspapers, television, and print media. Some of these sources may be unregulated, incomplete, and sensational.[20,33] A study of popular magazines found that 55% of the pregnancy exposure information provided was misleading or inaccurate.[34] In another recent example cited by the Motherisk program, all 43 women who responded to an FDA advisory concerning third trimester use of antidepressants in pregnancy described an increase in anxiety following the report, with three discontinuing antidepressant use abruptly and six others considering discontinuation without medical consultation. Numerous examples of misunderstanding of the advisory were found.[33] In addition, the public is poorly educated about reproductive health, particularly in complex areas such as reproduction and embryonic development.

Although risk assessment and counseling may result in the decision to stop a medication, it is important to recognize that continued pharmacologic treatment for conditions such as hypertension, diabetes, asthma, and mental illness may be necessary to protect the health of both the woman and her fetus. Clinicians must not only make risk assessments after inadvertent exposures, but also determine treatment regimens in recognized pregnancies. Given the lack of up-to-date information and often conflicting scientific data, health care providers and clients must make decisions with the best available information. Decisions about the use of medications during pregnancy should be made with the following in mind: the severity and course of the maternal illness, efficacy of the medication, and known reproductive data. Examples of risk assessments for specific exposures are covered in Chapter 2, Developmental Toxicity and Drugs. Reference texts and additional resources are also listed at the end of this chapter.

Pharmacists are in a unique position to answer questions concerning exposures for pregnant and preconceptional women. Their expertise in pharmacology is recognized by the public, and they are often consulted with questions concerning reproductive toxicity. However, they may feel unprepared to do so. Several studies have demonstrated that pharmacists worldwide are inadequately prepared to provide evidence-based risk assessments to pregnant women and their health care providers[35,36] and that they do so infrequently.[37]

IV. Availability of Reproductive Data

Overall, there is a general lack of adequately powered and well-designed studies needed to ascertain the safe use of medications in pregnancy. There is little information on the use of medications during pregnancy before a drug is marketed and when available, may be difficult for health care providers to access. Given that pregnant women are generally excluded from clinical trials for ethical reasons and premarketing animal data do not necessarily reflect the risks to human pregnancy, little information concerning teratogenicity of a newly marketed drug is available. In addition to the lack of premarketing human reproductive data, there is no standard requirement for postmarketing surveillance of potential reproductive toxicants after FDA approval.[38] The length of time to identify drugs associated with reproductive toxicity has been identified as a significant concern. One recent study demonstrated insufficient human pregnancy safety data available for >80% of 468 new drugs marketed over a recent 20-year study period in the United States.[39] In addition, there were significant differences between risks assigned by the two systems studied (FDA and TERIS).[39]

Many clinicians use the FDA pregnancy categories as the basis for teratology risk assessment, although they were not intended for this purpose.[39] The current FDA pregnancy labeling system using categories A, B, C, D, and X was implemented in 1979 as a five-letter classification system for drug use in pregnancy.[40] It was meant to provide a guideline for assessment of teratogenic risk; however, many clinicians use this risk classification system as their main or only source of information concerning medication use in pregnancy. The FDA pregnancy categories are determined primarily based on animal reproductive and developmental toxicity studies, as few human data are available at the time of approval. Although the simplicity makes use of this system appealing, the current system has been criticized as being inconsistent, ambiguous, incomplete, and difficult for clinicians to interpret and use.[12,41,42] Many clinicians incorrectly use the five-letter system to estimate risk for individual patients.[39,43] Also of concern is that worldwide classification systems vary significantly. In a comparison of similar classification systems used by Australia, Sweden, and the FDA, there was only 26% concordance in the risk category for more than 200 commonly used drugs.[44] Although differences in the use of categories accounted for some of the lack of concordance, varying interpretations of the available scientific literature were also noted to be significant.[45]

Between 1994 and 2007, the Teratology Society developed specific recommendations for improving pregnancy labeling.[12,42] Beginning in 1997, additional efforts were conducted by the FDA Labeling Task Force.[45,46] These efforts have led the FDA to announce plans to revamp prescription drug labeling for use during pregnancy and breastfeeding.[47] Issued in May 2008, the proposed rule removes the letter categories, which are replaced by a narrative containing the following sections:

- Fetal Risk Summary—would describe what is known about the effects of the drug on the fetus, and if there is a risk, whether this risk is based on information from animals or humans. The proposal calls for a risk conclusion based on the available data and provides a number of examples depending on the quality and quantity of that data. This would be followed by a summary of the most important data on the drug's effects.

- Clinical Considerations—would include information about the effects of the pre-conception use of the drug. This section also would feature discussions about the risks of the disease to the mother and the baby, dosing information, and tell how to address complications.

- Data—would describe in more detail the available data regarding use of the drug in humans and from animal studies that were used to develop the Fetal Risk Summary.

The pregnancy section would also include information about whether there is a pregnancy exposure registry for the drug. A similar summary will be provided for lactation. Newly approved drugs will use this format, whereas labeling for previously approved drugs will be phased in gradually. Implementation of this proposal is anticipated to begin in 2010.[47]

Currently, the FDA requires manufacturers to submit voluntary drug experience reports; however, there is no standard requirement to conduct postmarketing surveillance. This system of identification of adverse reproductive effects is inefficient and often misleading.[39] In recent years, the use of pregnancy registries and population-based surveillance studies has provided an additional method of data collection.[48–51] Pregnancy registries collect postmarketing data on outcomes of pregnancies exposed to specific agents. The current system of passive collection of adverse pregnancy outcomes provides important but limited data.[50] Suggestions for a well-designed pregnancy registry include recruitment of an adequate number of exposed pregnancies, aggressive follow-up, and careful assessment of pregnancy outcomes.[50,52] The FDA maintains a current list of pregnancy exposure registries,[53] accessible to providers and consumers. An additional method of data collection has been described. This multicenter, prospective cohort design, used by OTIS, allows for evaluation of a spectrum of adverse pregnancy outcomes ranging from spontaneous abortion to functional deficits.[54] The European Network of Teratology Information Services uses a similar system to collect outcomes of exposed pregnancies.[55] All of the above systems currently operate without overarching guidance, support, or direction and as such, are not the comprehensive surveillance system needed to ensure the early and effective detection of birth defects related to prenatal exposures.[56] To address these concerns, a public health system that includes a central source of up-to-date information, development and coordination of research activities, and the availability of counseling services with standard communication messages are essential.[57]

Marketing of a known human teratogen, such as isotretinoin, poses additional difficulties.[8] Following documentation of continued pregnancy exposures to isotretinoin under voluntary pregnancy prevention programs,[58] the FDA now requires its manufacturers to adhere to a mandatory system with registration of the prescriber, pharmacist, and client. Information concerning the current pregnancy prevention program, IPLEDGE, is available on the web.[59] At present, there are significant variations in labeling for pregnancy category X drugs, which address risk management strategies for minimizing pregnancy occurrence.[43] A need for consistency of product labeling for category X drugs has been noted.[43]

V. Developing a Risk Assessment

Risk assessment and counseling in teratology demand knowledge of several principles. Close attention must be paid to details of timing and dose of the exposure; family, medical, and pregnancy history; and literature review. Communication and counseling skills are equally important, as this information must be correctly transmitted and understood by the client and/or her health care provider. Development of a risk assessment should include the topics below.

A. Timing

By convention, human gestational age is calculated by using the first day of the patient's LMP, although conception does not occur until 2 weeks later. This 2-week difference should be clarified when providing exposure information in early pregnancy. Also, keep in mind that animal reproductive data generally use weeks postconception, while human reproductive data use LMP.

Following conception in humans, there is approximately a 2-week period during which the fertilized egg moves through the fallopian tube and becomes implanted in the wall of the uterus. During this preimplantation or "all-or-nothing" period, if one cell is damaged, another can replace it and normal development will continue. However, if too many cells are damaged, the pregnancy will miscarry.[60] In addition, blood supply between the mother and the embryo is just being established and it is likely that any exposure (with the rare exception of an agent that has a very long half-life) will have limited access to the developing fetus. This preimplantation period corresponds to the time from conception to the first missed period, a time when many women become aware of the pregnancy. In general, exposures during this time do not increase the risk for birth defects in that pregnancy.

After implantation, the organogenesis period (5–10 weeks post-LMP) is characterized by rapid development of fetal structures. This is the period most sensitive to teratogenic effects, particularly those that cause structural anomalies. Knowledge of embryologic development is critical to providing risk assessments for first trimester exposures. An agent that can cause an increase in neural tube defects, such as spina bifida, can only do so during its development. For example, while valproic acid is associated with a 1%–2% incidence of neural tube defects,[61] to cause a defect, this exposure must occur before neural tube closure at 28 days postconception.[62] Exposures after this time do not disrupt an already formed structure. The fetal period, corresponding with 11–40 weeks is characterized by rapid growth and development, particularly of the central nervous system. Exposures with adverse effects will generally lead to growth retardation and/or intellectual impairment, although effects such as renal dysfunction in babies exposed in the second and third trimesters to angiotensin-converting enzyme inhibitors can be seen.[63]

B. Dose

The frequency, duration, and route of an exposure are also important considerations. It has been suggested that any exposure, in a high enough dose, can disrupt fetal development. In contrast, teratogenic effects occur only when the dose of an agent exceeds a specific threshold.[1] Although threshold doses are not well documented for most human teratogenic agents, some exposures are clearly insufficient to cause malformations. For example, exposure to high levels of mercury leading to severe central nervous system damage are well described after two episodes of mercury contamination in Japan and Iraq. However, humans are exposed to mercury in everyday life, in part through fish consumption. The benefits of eating fish containing omega fatty acids during pregnancy have been described.[64] Due to concerns about overexposure to mercury, the FDA currently recommends that pregnant women not eat specific fish (shark, swordfish, tile fish, and mackerel) and limiting other fish intake to 12 oz. per week.[65] The route of exposure should also be considered. The significant differences in the amount of access to the fetus should be taken into account for dermal, inhalation, oral, and parenteral exposures.

Pharmacogenetics, the study of the relationship between genetically determined metabolic pathways and individual responses to medications, holds promise for our ability to provide individualized risk assessments. It is well documented that no teratogen causes anomalies in 100% of exposed pregnancies.[1] The potential teratogenicity of an exposure is clearly influenced by maternal and fetal genotypes, which can result in differences in cell sensitivity, placental transport, metabolism, receptor binding, or drug distribution.[66] Current research is under way to look at individual genetic susceptibility that may predict specific outcomes.

C. Family, Medical, and Pregnancy History

Questions about family, medical, and pregnancy history are also essential to the development of a risk assessment. It is important to understand the current medical condition being treated, as well as any others that may co-exist. Exposure to other agents should also be explored. Be aware that most patients do not consider alternative therapies, including herbal preparations, as medications and are unlikely to discuss these exposures unless specifically asked.

D. Literature Review

Animal data are essential for the development of a risk assessment. Given the ease of controlling experimental conditions and their short gestational period, this is an important mechanism for the development of reproductive toxicity data and potential mechanisms of adverse effects. Animal studies may not predict the effects in humans due to differences in metabolism and physiology, marked interspecies variation, higher and more chronically administered doses, and maternal toxicity. To date, no one species has been predictive of human response.

Studies examining exposure to medications should include attention to the maternal disease states, in addition to the use of comparison groups that are selected with this confounder in mind. The range of outcomes should ideally include not only structural birth defects but also adverse neonatal effects and neurodevelopmental outcomes. Studies evaluating neurodevelopment in exposed children are particularly difficult, as they require long follow-up, as well as attention to additional factors, such as socioeconomics and parental cognitive assessment. Recent suggestions that prenatal exposures may play a role in adult disorders will require evaluation throughout the life span. Due to the rarity of both congenital anomalies and exposures to specific medical therapies, studies with large numbers of subjects are scarce. Although prospective, controlled studies provide the best data, these types of studies may be limited by ethical concerns of including pregnant women. Increasing efforts to collect postmarketing surveillance data are essential to improving the data available on exposures during pregnancy.

For the development of a risk assessment, information concerning exposures during pregnancy should be collected from multiple sources. No single methodology can delineate the spectrum of adverse outcomes from a potentially teratogenic exposure. Although teratogenic agents have been described by astute practitioners through case reports, such reports can be misleading. Thalidomide was recognized to cause limb reduction defects within 4 years of its use,[54] in large part due to the rarity of that birth defect. In contrast, adverse fetal outcomes with more subtle patterns of malformation or neurobehavioral effects are unlikely to be detected early.

Case reports and series are most useful when they describe a characteristic set of birth defects in the context of well-defined exposures. While case reports provide important red flags, they cannot be used to predict the range of fetal outcomes or the magnitude of the human risk. They are most useful for generating hypotheses which can be addressed in subsequent studies.

Epidemiologic studies are the only means to assess statistical power and, therefore, the range and magnitude of risk to human pregnancies. The two types of epidemiologic studies generally used in teratology are cohort and case-control studies. In cohort studies, the frequency of adverse outcomes in exposed women is compared to either the general population or an unexposed group. Thus, cohort studies allow for the study of multiple outcomes and can be prospective or retrospective. Prospective cohort studies provide the most useful information concerning reproductive toxicity as exposure data are collected before knowing the outcome and confounders can be ascertained. This ability to control recall bias is a major strength of cohort studies. However, cohort studies looking at rare reproductive outcomes can be difficult to conduct. Case-control studies allow for the study of multiple exposures. The frequency of maternal exposure to an agent is compared between children with and those without birth defects. Case-control studies have the advantage of assessing the relationship between maternal exposures and rare fetal outcomes without the need for large numbers of women. Given that they are by nature retrospective, they may suffer from bias.

Other types of studies provide additional information. Survey data have been collected from providers and clients; however, conclusions may be inconclusive due to poor response rates. Birth defects surveillance studies can determine the incidence of birth defects in the general population, as well as evaluate those related to pregnancy exposures. Examples include the National Birth Defects Prevention Study[67] and The

National Children's Study.[68] Meta-analyses can also be useful in teratology. They allow for the estimation of risk by combining the findings of multiple, often smaller, studies. However, consideration must be given to methodologic study differences.

Several assessments of the magnitude of the risk are used in these studies. The absolute risk is defined as the incidence of disease within a given population. A measure of excess risk in the population is the attributable risk (AR). For example, if an exposed group showed 10% malformations compared to a 5% incidence in the nonexposed group, the AR is 5%. This is the risk, over and above the baseline population risk, that can be attributed to the exposure. Keep in mind that confounding factors may account for part of the difference in risk, occasionally leading to an overestimation of risk. Relative risk (RR), generally used in cohort studies, compares the risk of disease (ie, birth defects) in exposed versus control groups. Odds ratio (OR) measures the incidence of exposure, not of disease. Therefore, OR does not consider prevalence of the disease. This is generally calculated in case-control studies.

Evidence from all sources, such as animal reproductive data, human case reports, pregnancy registries, and epidemiologic studies, should be evaluated to determine the strength of a purported association. The following criteria are helpful in assessing these associations.[69]

Strength of the Association
- What is the statistical likelihood that the association did not occur by chance alone?
- The larger the magnitude of association, the more likely it is to be causal.
- Most known human teratogens have very large RRs.

Consistency of the Association
- Is the same association seen in several studies with different populations?

Specificity of the Association
- Are unique patterns of malformations noted?
- How often does the drug exposure occur without causing the effect, and how often does the effect occur without exposure?

Appropriate Timing
- Did the exposure occur at the critical developmental period?

Dose-Response Relationship
- Does the occurrence and magnitude of outcomes increase with the dose of the exposure?

Biological Plausibility
- Does the association make biological sense?
- Are there alternative explanations for the association?

VI. Provision of Risk Assessment and Counseling

Provision of a teratology risk assessment involves not only the estimation of risk, but also the ability to communicate that risk to the client in a meaningful way. Communication is the skillful and understandable use of language. While each client interaction will differ, several basic principles of communication should be observed. A confidential location is essential to promote client trust and provision of information in a setting in which it can be integrated. Sensitivity to cultural and educational backgrounds is essential. Use clear and simple terms, avoiding medical jargon when possible. Listening to understand and promoting opportunities for the client to elaborate are useful techniques in obtaining relevant information.[70] Information that should be elicited from the client includes medical, family and previous pregnancy history; timing, route and dose of the exposure; reason for the exposure; and any other exposures that have occurred during the pregnancy.

The primary question is not whether a medication is "safe" to use during pregnancy but what is the risk/benefit analysis in a particular pregnancy. All assessments should be framed in the context of whether the exposure places the pregnancy at an *increased risk* above the 3%–5% background risk found in all pregnancies. Improved communication, through the use of a risk/benefit analysis, will result in better pregnancy management and reduce litigation.[71]

Any discussion of risk should be framed with the likelihood of a positive outcome balanced by the likelihood of a negative outcome. Framing the risk by presenting the positive information first has been shown to correlate with a more accurate risk assessment[72] and was shown to mitigate falsely elevated perceptions of teratogenic risk.[73] Be aware that descriptors, such as positive/negative or normal/abnormal, and words such as often, rarely, never, high, and low may have "meaning" to the client that may differ from that of the communicator.

Keep in mind that individuals have varying degrees of comfort with numerical risks. You can ask directly if they "feel comfortable with numbers" or use questions such as "when reading, do you skip over the numbers?" Presentation of specific risk figures may require several approaches. For example, if drug X causes congenital heart defects in 2% of prenatally exposed babies, the alternative event of 98% who do not have heart defects should also be presented. For clients who are not comfortable with percentages, the risk for malformation can be framed as 2/100, with the alternative risk of 98/100. A useful tool to enhance client understanding is visualization: ask the client to imagine a room of 100 people; 98 would not have a child with the birth defect while 2 would. Comparisons to the background risk for birth defects of 3%–5% should be included in these discussions. In the above example, the 2% risk should be compared not only to the overall background risk in all pregnancies, but also to that of the 0.5%–1% background risk for congenital heart defects.[2] Discussion of the background risk for birth defects allows the client to understand that an exposure and an adverse outcome may not be causally related. This is also an opportunity to educate the client about fetal development. In addition, an appreciation that all pregnancies begin with a risk, even in those with no prenatal exposures, can be reassuring to the client.

Clients may perceive risk as binary, that is, either the outcome will or won't happen. Also, if an adverse outcome has already happened, they may view their risk as 100%. It is important to explore the meaning of specific risks to the client. It may be valuable for the client to explore the negative outcomes of an exposure, including the long-term implications. Referrals to perinatal or genetic counseling services may be necessary. The client should be encouraged to view the management decision in terms of what is correct in her situation, rather than a correct versus incorrect decision.

The information must be balanced and tailored to the client. Asking the occupation of the client can assist in evaluating her education level and health literacy. Discussions of birth defects and developmental disabilities should be done with sensitivity to the client. For example, although the medical profession may use descriptors such as "a Down's child," the preferred description should be "person first," such as a child with Down's syndrome. For questions concerning the prognosis of specific birth defects, consider referrals to a perinatologist, genetic counselor, or pediatrician.

Risk analysis can be viewed within the context of heuristic principles, defined as those serving as an aid to learning or problem-solving by experimental and trial-and-error methods. The word heuristic originates from "eureka," meaning to find. They are often described as a mental shortcut or a "rule of thumb," and while helpful, can also lead to biases. One example of a heuristic principle is that of anchoring. Here a prior belief serves as a frame of reference. To elicit client knowledge, it is important to ask what information she has heard and where she heard it. Be aware that the use of anchoring may limit the extent of learning new information. Another heuristic principle that is applied in teratology counseling is availability, that is, how easily a potential outcome can be brought to mind. In general, greater availability results in a higher assessment of risk. It may be important to discuss the client's familiarity with birth defects and disabilities, pharmacology, human physiology, and scientific methods. The heuristic principle of representativeness may influence individuals to use a small sample to predict outcome in a larger group, or generalize a situation. Questions, such as "Tell me more about the person you know with xyz," may be helpful. These principles have a direct bearing on the client's perception of the potential impact of the consequences.

The scarcity of well-controlled, prospective data contributes to considerable ambiguity in teratology counseling. Clients can be made comfortable with less than "black and white" answers by providing the available evidence-based data along with an understanding of the difficulties in collecting these data. Given the amount of uncertainty in these situations, the provider should recognize that clients may need time and space to incorporate this information. Anticipatory guidance may include a discussion that a decision made today may not be the same one made in the future. The health care provider should be available for additional questions and review.

During the development of a risk/benefit analysis, the client may ask, "What would you recommend to your wife, sister, etc.?" Since these decisions need to be made in the context of conflicting and somewhat uncertain scientific data, balanced against the need for medical treatment, information must be integrated into the client's values and life experiences in a way that is meaningful to her. The focus of this question should be how to make the decision. One useful tool is to frame the risk/benefit analysis into scenarios. For example, presentation of a scenario such as "I once knew a family who chose this response," allows the client to "try on" concepts. A review of the best and worst potential outcomes may also help solidify a client's thinking. A brief discussion of her support system, including various medical professionals who may be involved her in care, may be helpful. After provision of a risk assessment and risk/benefit analysis, the counselor can ask the client to restate the information. Additional questions such as "Is this what you thought you would hear?" or "Has this information changed your thinking?" are useful in assessing client understanding.

VII. PATIENT CASE [PART 2]

This case presents many of the issues common to questions concerning exposures during pregnancy. The client and clinician must take into account both the potential fetal risks from exposures and the impact of untreated maternal disease on both the mother and the fetus. The risk of mental illness may be significantly greater than any potential risks to the fetus from psychotropic medications.[74] Maternal depression has been associated with increased rates of prematurity and low infant birth weight.[75] One study described the risk of relapse of major depression in women who discontinued use of antidepressant medication compared to those who continued pharmacologic therapy. Of the 201 women in the sample, 43% experienced a relapse, half of those in the first trimester. Relapses were seen in 26% of those who continued therapy versus 68% of women who discontinued.[74] In addition, women who discontinued medication relapsed significantly more frequently over the course of their pregnancy. Risk from first trimester use of selective serotonin reuptake inhibitors (SSRIs) has generally not been shown to be elevated.[76] Additional concerns about the use of SSRIs in the latter half of pregnancy have been described and include a 20%–30% incidence of poor neonatal adaption[77] and an approximately 1% incidence of persistent pulmonary hypertension of the newborn (PPHN).[78] Perception of risk may be so significant that women abruptly stop their medications "for the baby" but neglect to include a risk/benefit analysis of the harms of mental illness in pregnancy.[79]

For this case, a discussion of the above risks and benefits specific to her situation is imperative. It would be important to determine what information she has already received. Multiple medical consultations may be necessary for the client to develop a risk assessment and management decisions. Medical management options may include gradual withdrawal of sertraline, continued use with potential discontinuation in later pregnancy, or continued throughout pregnancy. However, changes in medical management should be anticipated. While the risk for structural birth defects in this case is not increased above the background, a discussion of the effects of poor neonatal adaptation and PPHN should be provided to the client. A summary of the information should be provided and client understanding verified. Referrals to appropriate resources are essential.

VIII. Summary

In summary, provision of risk assessments to women and their health care providers with questions concerning exposures during pregnancy can be challenging. This chapter has provided an outline for the collection and interpretation of available reproductive data, which are essential to providing well-researched, up-to-date information on exposures during pregnancy. These data should be provided in conjunction with the patients' medical condition and are best presented as a risk/benefit analysis. All risks should be compared to the 3%–5% background risk for birth defects which is present in all pregnancies. Risk communication strategies have been outlined that should assist the provider in translating this complicated medical information into meaningful answers for pregnant clients. The following checklist may be helpful for individualized risk assessments:

- Collection of teratology data on a specific agent
- Interpretation of data based on client information
- Elicit client's knowledge and source
- Summarize the information in clearly understandable terms
- Discuss 3%–5% background risk and any other risk that applies
- Review risk verus benefit
- Identify relevant resources

> "A good decision is based on knowledge and not on numbers."
>
> —Plato

IX. Resources

A. Online and Telephone

(1) Organization of Teratology Information Specialists (OTIS)—provides toll-free telephone consultation for health care providers and patients concerning the reproductive risks of prenatal exposures. Also participates in multicenter research projects and prepares educational fact sheets for providers and clients.

  Telephone: 866-626-6847

  Web site: http://www.otispregnancy.org

(2) REPROTOX®—database for scientists, health care providers, and government agencies containing summaries on the effects of exposures on human pregnancy, reproduction, and development.

  Web site: http://www.reprotox.org

(3) The Teratogen Information System (TERIS)—database of summaries of individual agents designed to assist health care providers in assessing the risk of exposures in pregnant women.

  Web site: http://depts.washington.edu/terisweb/teris

(4) Office of Women's Health, U.S. Food and Drug Administration—lists existing postmarketing pregnancy registries that monitor exposure to specific medications during pregnancy.

>Web site: http://www.fda.gov/womens /registries

(5) NIEHS Center for the Evaluation of Risks to Human Reproduction (CERHR)—provides scientifically based assessments of potential for environmental agents to cause adverse reproductive outcomes.

>Web site: http://cerhr.niehs.nih.gov

(6) March of Dimes—a Web site designed for the public that provides general information on having a healthy pregnancy.

>Web site: http://www.marchofdimes.com

(7) National Birth Defects Prevention Network—provides information and links to birth defects surveillance programs in the United States.

>Web site: http://www.nbdpn.org

B. Texts

(1) Briggs GG, Freeman RK, Yaffe SJ. *Drugs in Pregnancy and Lactation: A Reference Guide to Fetal and Neonatal Risk.* 8th ed. Baltimore: Lippincott, Williams & Wilkins, 2008.

(2) Koren G. *Medication Safety in Pregnancy and Breastfeeding.* New York: McGraw-Hill, 2007.

(3) Schardein JL. *Chemically Induced Birth Defects.* 3rd ed. New York: Marcel Dekker, 2000.

(4) Shepard TH, Lemire RJ. *Catalog of Teratogenic Agents.* 12th ed. Baltimore: The Johns Hopkins University Press, 2007.

X. References

1.   Brent RL. Environmental causes of human congenital malformations: the pediatrician's role in dealing with these complex clinical problems caused by a multiplicity of environmental and genetic factors. *Pediatrics.* 2004;113(suppl 4):957–968.

2.   Centers for Disease Control and Prevention, National Center on Birth Defects and Developmental Disabilities. Available at http://www.cdc.gov/ncbddd/bd/faq1.htm#Whatisabirthdefect. Accessed June 19, 2008.

3.   Fisher B, Rose NC, Carey JC. Principles and practice of teratology for the obstetrician. *Clin Obstet Gynecol.* 2008;1:106–118.

4.   Leen-Mitchell M, Martinez L, Gallegos S, et al. Mini-review: history of organized teratology information services in North America. *Teratology.* 2000;61:314–317.

5.   Chambers CD, Zuhre NT, Johnson D, et al. Human pregnancy safety for agents used to treat rheumatoid arthritis: adequacy of available information and strategies for developing post-marketing data. *Arthritis Res Ther.* 2006;8:215–225.

6.   King C. Genetic counseling for teratogen exposure. *Obstet Gynecol.* 1986;67:843.

7. Buitendjik S. Medication in early pregnancy; prevalence of use and relationship to maternal characteristics. *Am J Obstet Gynecol*. 1991;165:33–40.

8. Honein MA, Moore CA, Erickson JD. Can we ensure the safe use of known human teratogens? *Drug Safety*. 2004;27:1069–1080.

9. Andrade SE, Gurwits JH, Davis RL, et al. Prescription drug use in pregnancy. *Am J Obstet Gynecol*. 2004;191:398–407.

10. Werler M, Mitchell A, Hernandez-Diaz S, et al. Use of over-the-counter medications during pregnancy. *Am J Obstet Gynecol*. 2005;193;771–777.

11. Tsui B, Dennehy CE, Tsourounis C. A survey of dietary supplement use during pregnancy at an academic medical center. *Am J Obstet Gynecol*. 2001;185:433–437.

12. Scialli AR, Buelke-Sam JL, Chambers CD, et al. Communicating risks during pregnancy: a workshop on the use of data from animal developmental toxicity studies in pregnancy labels for drugs. *Birth Defects Res A Clin Mol Teratol*. 2004;70;7–12.

13. Henshaw SK. Unintended pregnancy in the United States. *Fam Plann Perspect*. 1998;30:24–46.

14. Kaufman DW, Kelly JP, Rosenberg L, et al. Recent patterns of medication use in the ambulatory adult population of the United States: the Sloane survey. *JAMA*. 2002;287:337–344.

15. Schwarz EB, Maselli J, Norton M, et al. Prescription of teratogenic medications in United States ambulatory practices. *Am J Med*. 2005;118:1240–1249.

16. Centers for Disease Control and Prevention. Recommendations to improve pre-conception health and health care—United States. *MMWR Morb Mortal Wkly Rep*. 2006;55(RR06):1–23.

17. Cragan JD, Friedman JM, Holmes LB, et al. Ensuring the safe and effective use of medications during pregnancy: planning and prevention through preconception care. *Matern Child Health J*. 2006;10:S129–S135.

18. Centers for Disease Control and Prevention. Recommendations for the use of folic acid to reduce the number of cases of spina bifida and other neural tube defects. *MMWR Morb Mortal Wkly Rep*. 1992;41(RR-14):1–7.

19. Brent R. Bendectin and birth defects: hopefully, the final chapter. *Birth Defects Res A Clin Mol Teratol*. 2003.67:79–87.

20. Ornstein M, Einarson A, Koren G. Bendectin/Diclectin for morning sickness: a Canadian follow-up of an American disaster. *Reprod Toxicol*. 1995;9:1–6.

21. Koren G, Bologa M, Long D, et al. Perception of teratogenic risk by pregnant women exposed to drugs and chemicals during the first trimester. *Am J Obstet Gynecol*. 1989;160:1190–1204.

22. Sanz E, Gomez-Lopez T, Martinez-Quintas MJ. Perception of teratogenic risk of common medications. *Eur J Obstet Gynecol Reprod Biol*. 2001;95:127–131.

23. Pole M, Einarson A, Pairaudeau N, et al. Drug labeling and risk perceptions of teratogenicity: a survey of pregnant women and their health professionals. *J Clin Pharmacol*. 2000;40;573–577.

24. Bonari L, Koren G, Einarson TR, et al. Use of antidepressants by pregnant women: evaluation of perception of risk, efficacy of evidence based counseling and determinants of decision making. *Arch Womens Ment Health.* 2005;8:214–220.

25. O'Doherty K, Suthers GK. Risky communication: pitfalls in counseling about risk, and how to avoid them. *J Genet Couns.* 2007;16;409–417.

26. Koren G, Pastuszak A. Prevention of unnecessary pregnancy terminations by counseling women on drug, chemical, and radiation exposure during the first trimester. *Teratology.* 1990;41;657–661.

27. DeSantis M, Straface G, Cavaliere A, et al. Teratological risk evaluation and prevention of voluntary abortion. *Minerva Ginecol.* 2006;58:91–99.

28. Hancock R, Koren G, Einarson A, et al. The effectiveness of Teratology Information Services (TIS). *Reprod Toxicol.* 2007;23:125–132.

29. Hancock R, Ungar W, Einarson A, et al. Providing information regarding exposures in pregnancy: a survey of North American Teratology Information Services. *Repro Toxicol.* 2008;25:381–387.

30. Clementi M, DiGuanantonio E, Ornoy A. Teratology Information Services in Europe and their contribution to the prevention of congenital anomalies. *Commun Genet.* 2002;5:8–12.

31. Scialli AR. Identifying teratogens: the tyranny of lists. *Reprod Toxicol.* 1997; 11:555–559.

32. Einarson A, Lockett D. Do we have a knowledge transfer and translation plan at Teratology Information Services? *Reprod Toxicol.* 2006;22:542–545.

33. Einarson A, Schachtschneider A, Halil R, et al. SSRIs and other antidepressant use during pregnancy and potential neonatal effects: impact of a public health advisory and subsequent reports in the news media. *BMC Pregnancy Childbirth.* 2005;20;11.

34. Gunderson-Warner S, Martinez LP, Martinez IP, et al. Critical review of articles regarding pregnancy exposures in popular magazines. *Teratology.* 1990;42:469–472.

35. Lyszkiewicz DA, Gerichhausen S, Björnsdóttir I, et al. Evidence based information on drug use during pregnancy: a survey of community pharmacists in three countries. *Pharm WorldSci.* 2001;23:76–81.

36. Damase-Michel C, Vié C, Lacroix I, et al. Drug counseling in pregnancy: an opinion survey of French community pharmacists. *Pharmacoepidemiol Drug Saf.* 2004; 13:711–715.

37. Merlob P, Stahl B, Kaplan B. Drug use in pregnancy and breast feeding: the role of the pharmacist. *Int J Risk Saf Med.* 1998;11:45–47.

38. U.S. Food and Drug Administration. Reviewer guidance: evaluating the risks of drug exposure in human pregnancies. Available at http://www.fda.gov/cder/guidance/6777fnl.pdf. Accessed June 22, 2008.

39. Lo WY, Friedman JM. Teratogenicity of recently introduced medications in human pregnancy. *Obstet Gynecol.* 2002;100:465–473.

40. Federal Register. Washington, DC: Office of the Federal Register, National Archives and Records Administration. *Federal Register.* 1979;44:37434–37467.

41. Doering P, Boothby L, Cheok M. Review of pregnancy labeling of prescription drugs: is the current system adequate to inform of risks? *Am J Obstet Gynecol.* 2002;187;333–339.

42. Public Affairs Committee of the Teratology Society. Teratology Public Affairs Committee position paper: pregnancy labeling for prescription drugs: ten years later. *Birth Defects Res A Clin Mol. Teratol.* 2007;79:627–630.

43. Uhl K, Kennedy DL, Kweder SL. Risk management strategies in the Physician's Desk Reference product labels for pregnancy category X drugs. *Drug Saf.* 2002;25:885–892.

44. Addis A, Sharabi S, Bonati M. Risk classification systems for drug use during pregnancy. Are they a reliable source of information? *Drug Saf.* 2000;23:245–253.

45. U.S. Food and Drug Administration. 2001a. Concept paper on pregnancy labeling. Summary of comments from a public hearing and model pregnancy labeling based on recommendations. Available at http://www.fda.gov/ohrms/dockets/ac/99/transcpt/3516r1.doc. Accessed June 22, 2008.

46. U.S. Food and Drug Administration, Center for Drug Evaluation and Research, Center for Biologics Evaluation and Research. *Reviewer Guidance: Evaluating the Risks of Drug Exposure in Human Pregnancies.* Rockville, MD: Food and Drug Administration, April 2005.

47. U.S. Food and Drug Administration. Available at http://www.fda.gov/bbs/topics/NEWS/2008/NEW01841.html. Accessed June 21, 2008.

48. Reiff-Eldridge R, Heffner CR, Ephross SA, et al. Monitoring pregnancy outcomes after prenatal drug exposure through prospective pregnancy exposure registries: a pharmaceutical company commitment. *Am J Obstet Gynecol.* 2000; 182:159–163.

49. Shields KE, Wilholm BE, Hostelley LS, et al. Monitoring outcomes of pregnancy following drug exposure: a company-based pregnancy registry program. *Drug Safety.* 2004;27:353–367.

50. Kennedy DL, Uhl K, Kweder SL. Pregnancy exposure registries. *Drug Safety.* 2004;27:215–228.

51. Holmes LB, Wyszynski DF, Lieberman E. The AED (antiepileptic drug) pregnancy registry: a 6-year experience. *Arch Neurol.* 2004;61:673–678.

53. Honein MA, Paulozzi LJ, Cragan JD, et al. Evaluation of selected characteristics of pregnancy drug registries. *Teratology.* 1999;60:356–364.

54. U.S. Food and Drug Administration. General Information about Pregnancy Exposure Registries. Available at http://www.fda.gov/womens/registries/default.htm. Accessed June 21, 2008.

55. Chambers CD, Braddock SR, Briggs GG, et al. Postmarketing surveillance for human teratogenicity: a model approach. *Teratology.* 2001;64;252–261.

56. Schaefer C, Hannemann D, Meister R. Post-marketing surveillance system for drugs in pregnancy—15 years experience of ENTIS. *Reprod Toxicol.* 2005;20:331–343.

56. Mitchell AA. Systematic identification of drugs that cause birth defects: a new opportunity. *N Engl J Med.* 2003;349:2556–2559.

57. Lagoy CT, Cragan JD, Rasmussen SJ. Medication use during pregnancy and lactation: an urgent call for public health action. *J Women's Health.* 2005;14:104–109.

58. Robertson J, Polifka JE, Avner M, et al. A survey of pregnant women using isotretinoin. *Birth Defects Res A Clin Mol Teratol.* 2005;73:881–887.

59. IPLEDGE. Available at http://www.ipledgeprogram.com/Default.aspx. Accessed June 21, 2008.

60. Rutledge JC. Developmental toxicity induced during the early stages of mammalian embryogenesis. *Mutat Res.* 1997;396:113–127.

61. Lammer EJ, Sever LE, Oakley G. Teratogen update: valproic acid. *Teratology.* 1987;45:465–473.

62. Sadler TW. Central nervous system. In Sadler TW. *Langman's Medical Embryology.* 9th ed. Philadelphia: Lippincott Williams & Wilkins, 2004.

63. Brent RL, Beckman D. Angiotensin-converting enzyme inhibitors, an embryopathic class of drugs with unique properties: information for clinical teratology counselors. *Teratology.* 1991;43:543–546.

64. McGregor J, Allen J, Harria M, et al. The omega-3 story: nutritional prevention of preterm birth and other adverse pregnancy outcomes. *Obstet Gynecol Surv.* 2001;56:S1–S13.

65. U.S. Food and Drug Administration. Backgrounder for the 2004 FDA/EPA Consumer Advisory: What You Need to Know About Mercury in Fish and Shellfish. Available at http://www.fda.gov/oc/opacom/hottopics/mercury/backgrounder.html. Accessed June 22, 2008.

66. Polifka JE, Friedman JM. Clinical teratology: identifying teratogenic risks in humans. *Clin Genet.* 1999;56:409–420.

67. Centers for Disease Control and Prevention. Profiles of the centers for birth defects research and prevention. Available at www.cdc.gov/ncbddd/bd/centers.htm. Accessed January 31, 2009.

68. U.S. Department of Health and Human Services. The National Children's Study. Available at http://www.nationalchildrensstudy.gov. Accessed June 22, 2008.

69. Scialli AR. *A Clinical Guide to Reproductive and Developmental Toxicology.* Boca Raton, FL: CRC Press, 1992.

70. Ormond K, Haun J, Duquette D, et al. Recommendations for telephone counseling. *J Genet Couns.* 2000;9;63–71.

71. Polifka J, Faustman E, Neil N. Weighing the risks and the benefits: a call for the empirical assessment of perceived teratogenic risk. *Reprod Toxicol.* 1997;11;633–640.

72. Zikmund-Fisher BJ, Fagerlin A, Keeton K, et al. Does labeling prenatal screening test results as negative or positive affect a woman's responses? *Am J Obstet Gynecol.* 2007;197;528.e1–528.e6.

73. Jasper JD, Goel R, Einarson A, et al. Effects of framing on teratogenic risk perception in pregnant women. *Lancet.* 2001;358;1237–1238.

74. Cohen LS, Altshuler LL, Harlow BL, et al. Relapse of major depression during pregnancy in women who maintain or discontinue antidepressant treatment. *JAMA*. 2006;295:499–507.

75. Bonari L, Pinto N, Ahn E, et al. Perinatal risks of untreated depression during pregnancy. *Can J Psychiatry*. 2004;49:726–735.

76. Alwan S, Reefhuis J, Rasmussen S, et al. Use of selective serotonin-reuptake inhibitors in pregnancy and the risk of birth defects. *N Engl J Med*. 2007;356:2684–2692.

77. Oberlander TF, Warburton W, Misri S, et al. Neonatal outcomes after prenatal exposure to selective serotonin reuptake inhibitor antidepressants and maternal depression using population-based linked health data. *Arch Gen Psychiatry*. 2006; 63:898–906.

78. Chambers C, Hernandez-Diaz S, Van Marter L, et al. Selective serotonin-reuptake inhibitors and risk of persistent pulmonary hypertension of the newborn. *N Engl J Med*. 2006;354:579–587.

79. Einarson A, Shelby P, Koren G. Abrupt discontinuation of psychotropic drugs during pregnancy: fear of teratogenic risk and impact of counseling. *J Psychiatry Neurosci*. 2001;26:44–48.

QUESTIONS AND ANSWERS

1. The percentage of women who use at least one medication during pregnancy is estimated at:

   a. 10%

   b. 50%

   c. 90%

   d. 3%

2. List the three categories of reproductive data in the newly proposed FDA pregnancy label.

3. List three resources for teratology data.

4. List the three areas of information needed from the client to provide a teratology risk assessment.

5. The type of study that provides the most useful data for pregnancy risk assessment is:

   a. case-control studies

      b. case reports

      c. meta-analyses

      d. prospective cohort studies

Answers:

1. b; 2. fetal risk summary, clinical considerations, data; 3. TIS, TERIS, REPROTOX, Briggs, etc; 4. timing of exposure, dose frequency and duration, and family, medical, and pregnancy history; 5. d

SECTION 2
Complications Unique to Pregnancy

Preterm Labor and Delivery

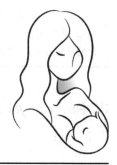

Annette E. Bombrys and
David F. Lewis

LEARNING OBJECTIVES

1. Describe the scope of the problem of preterm delivery.

2. Analyze the causes of preterm labor.

3. Compare and contrast the drugs used to arrest preterm labor and their side effects.

I. Introduction

Preterm birth is defined as a birth before the completion of 37 weeks of gestation. The lower threshold of gestational age at which preterm delivery is defined is variable but generally accepted to be at viability (23–24 weeks' gestation) and/or estimated fetal weight of ≥500 grams. Preterm delivery can be indicated, when a maternal or fetal complication warrants delivery, or spontaneous, as a consequence of preterm labor (PTL) or preterm premature rupture of membranes before the onset of labor.[1]

Preterm deliveries account for 12% of all births in the United States. The rates of preterm deliveries are rising in developed countries with the advances in assisted reproductive technologies and increased rates of multifetal gestations.[1] In 2001, $5.8 billion were spent on hospital care costs for preterm or low-birth-weight infants.[2] Despite advanced knowledge regarding the mechanisms and risk factors for PTL, the rate of preterm deliveries continues to rise.

II. PATIENT CASE (PART 1)

A 24-year-old white female gravida 1 at 25 weeks' gestation presents with complaints of contractions that began 4 hours ago and are getting stronger in strength and occurring more frequently. She was recently treated for a sexually transmitted disease but lost the prescription. The rest of her medical and surgical history is negative. She has had an uncomplicated prenatal course. She is examined and found to be 3 centimeters dilated, 100% cervical effacement, and has a bulging bag of water at +1 station. Assessment of her contractions reveals she is contracting every 3 minutes, and they palpate quite strong.

III. Pathophysiology

PTL can be viewed as a disease process with a multifactorial pattern. Risk factors for spontaneous PTL include genital tract infection, nonwhite race, multiple gestation, age <18 years, cigarette smoking, uterine anomalies, bleeding in the second trimester, low prepregnancy weight, and a history of previous preterm birth.[3] A history of a previous preterm delivery is the most predictive risk factor. In general, PTL before 32 weeks' gestation is often associated with clinical or subclinical evidence of infection, nonwhite race, long-term neonatal morbidities, and greater risk of recurrence in subsequent pregnancies. Conversely, PTL and delivery after 32 weeks' gestation is associated with increased uterine activity and volume (hydramnios), or multifetal gestation. Also, neonatal morbidity is less and the risk of recurrence is lower.

Preterm delivery is the leading cause of perinatal morbidity and mortality. Preterm fetuses are at significant risk for disease specific to prematurity, including respiratory distress syndrome (RDS), intraventricular hemorrhage (IVH), bronchopulmonary dysplasia, patent ductus arteriosus, necrotizing enterocolitis (NEC), sepsis, apnea, and retinopathy. Neonatal morbidities associated with long-term consequences include chronic lung disease, IVH grades III and IV, NEC, and hearing and vision impairment.[4]

IV. Detection, Screening, and Diagnosis of Preterm Labor

PTL is defined as regular uterine contractions with dilation and/or effacement of the cervix resulting in delivery of a preterm infant. Traditionally, dilation ≥2 centimeters with effacement ≥80% and regular uterine contractions have been used to diagnose PTL. Signs and symptoms of PTL include increased vaginal discharge, pelvic pressure, back pain, menstrual-like cramps, and uterine contractions. Assessment by digital examination has the drawback of being a subjective test and significant interobserver variability exists. When digital examinations of the cervix and contraction frequency are used independently, the ability to diagnose PTL is low. When combined, the accuracy increases. To improve the diagnostic accuracy for PTL, cervical length and fetal fibronectin can be incorporated in the PTL evaluation.[5,6] Ultrasonographic evaluation of cervical length is inversely related to the risk of preterm birth in both singleton and multifetal gestations.[7-10] Cervical length is more positively associated with history of spontaneous preterm birth than are digital cervical examinations. Cervical length measurement of ≥30 millimeters indicates that PTL is unlikely to occur in women with symptomatic contractions.[7-10]

Fetal fibronectin is a protein of the choriodecidual junction. The presence or absence of fetal fibronectin from vaginal swab is used to predict the risk of preterm delivery. A positive test has a sensitivity of 90%. The negative predictive value of a fetal fibronectin test is 97% of delivery within 2 weeks in patients with cervical dilation of ≤3 centimeters with uterine contractions. The predictive accuracy of the fetal fibronectin decreases significantly when the length of the cervix exceeds 3 centimeters.[11,12]

V. Prevention of Preterm Labor

Progesterone is a naturally occurring steroid hormone that acts through its receptor ligand–activated nuclear transcription regulators to establish and maintain a pregnancy. Multiple trials have evaluated the use of various progesterone preparations for the prophylaxis of recurrent preterm birth.[13] 17α-hydroxyprogesterone caproate (17 OHP) has been studied the most recently for the prevention of preterm birth.

Indications: The American College of Obstetrics and Gynecology recommends that if progesterone is to be given for the prevention of preterm birth, it is only indicated in women with a history of spontaneous preterm birth at <37 weeks' gestation.[14]

Mechanism of Action: The mechanism by which progesterone given to high-risk women is able to maintain uterine quiescence and prevent preterm birth is unknown. There is increasing evidence that the withdrawal of progesterone is associated with normal parturition and progesterone maintains this at the level of the uterus.[13]

Pharmacokinetics: Progesterone is rapidly absorbed from IM injection. Progesterone is almost exclusively bound to plasma proteins, especially albumin. Progesterone is metabolized to its metabolites by the liver and excreted renally. It takes approximately 8 hours following injection to reach peak serum levels.[15]

Dosage and Administration: 17 OHP is given as an IM injection prepared as 50 mg/mL in oil.[16]

Side Effects: Side effects include skin site reactions, fever, insomnia, nausea, cerebral edema, cerebral thrombosis, edema, depression, somnolence, changes in cervical secretions, and cholestatic jaundice.[16]

Contraindications: Hypersensitivity to progesterone or any of its by-products, current history of venous or arterial thrombosis, carcinoma of the breast or genital tract, or active thrombophlebitis.[16]

Evidence-Based Review of Efficacy: There have been 17 trials that have specifically focused on 17 OHP and prevention of preterm birth.[16] The most recent trial, by Meis et al. and the Maternal Fetal Medicine Unit Network, reported, in a randomized double-blinded placebo-controlled trial, a substantial reduction in the rate of preterm delivery in high-risk women with a documented history of preterm delivery.[17] The rate of preterm delivery was 6.3% in the 17 OHP group and 54.9% in the placebo (*p* <.001). Of note, the study also reported a significant reduction in the rate of NEC, need for supplemental oxygen, and IVH in the neonate.[17]

VI. Treatment of Preterm Labor

The goal of treatment of PTL is, at minimum, pregnancy prolongation while corticosteroids are administered to enhance fetal lung maturity. At best, the goal is pregnancy prolongation to term or until a significant gain in gestational age or fetal weight is obtained.[18]

A. Nonpharmacologic Therapy

The patient thought to be in or at risk for PTL should be placed on modified bed rest. PTL is frequently associated with urinary tract infections, and a urinalysis should be performed.[19] Uterine irritability and contractions are associated with dehydration, and adequate hydration, either orally or parenterally, is frequently initiated. Although bed rest and hydration are standard interventions employed by most obstetricians, there is no proven benefit of these modalities in the treatment of uterine contractions.[20–22]

B. Pharmacologic Therapy

Tocolytics are agents used to inhibit myometrial smooth muscle contractions (Tables 1 and 2). Pharmacologic therapy is initiated in patients with a diagnosis of PTL between 24 and 34 weeks' gestation. Absolute contraindication to tocolytics include severe pre-eclampsia, severe abruptio placentae, severe bleeding from any causes, chorioamnionitis, fetal death, fetal anomaly incompatible with life, and severe fetal growth restriction. Relative contraindications include mild chronic hypertension, mild abruptio placentae, stable placenta previa, maternal cardiac disease, hyperthyroidism, uncontrolled diabetes mellitus, fetal distress, fetal anomalies, fetal growth restriction, and advanced cervical dilation. The current tocolytics used in the United States include magnesium sulfate, β-adrenergic receptor agonists, calcium channel blockers, cyclooxygenase inhibitors, and nitroglycerine. Oxytocin receptor agonists are used in Europe, but not in the United States because they have not been approved by the FDA.

All patients with PTL are given antibiotic prophylaxis for group B streptococcus and corticosteroids for fetal lung maturation unless a contraindication exists. Corticosteroids and antibiotic therapy will be discussed in Chapter 8, Preterm Premature Rupture of Membranes.

1. Magnesium Sulfate

Magnesium sulfate has been studied extensively and is considered a first-line clinical agent. There have been recent suggestions that magnesium sulfate should be abandoned as a first-line tocolytic agent due to neonatal effects and unclear clinical benefit.[23–26]

Mechanism of Action: Pharmacologic doses that inhibit myometrial contractions are achieved at levels of 5–8 mg/dL.[23,27–29] The exact mechanism by which magnesium sulfate acts is unknown. It is proposed that magnesium sulfate inhibits myometrial contractions by antagonizing calcium at the cellular level and in the extracellular space, reducing intracellular levels of calcium and preventing activation of the actin and myosin complexes in smooth muscle. Magnesium may also act directly on calcium channels by competing for binding sites.[30]

Pharmacokinetics: After IV bolus of 4 or 6 grams, mean serum concentrations were 5.56 ± 0.30 mg/dL and 2.57 ± 0.17 mg/dL, respectively. The volume of distribution for magnesium is 32.3 L, with most of the magnesium collecting in bone, skeletal muscle, and blood cells. Following a 4-gram bolus, the half-life is 610 ± 137 minutes.[30] Magnesium is renally excreted. In studies on preeclamptic women, 75% of the infused dose of magnesium is excreted during the infusion and ≥90% is excreted within 24 hours.[31] Magnesium readily crosses the placenta with serum levels in the fetus correlating with the mother.[15] Maternal toxicity appears at levels ≥9 mg/dL. Patellar reflexes become absent between 9 and 13 mg/

Table 1. Mechanism of Action, Dose, Side Effects, and U.S. Food and Drug Administration Label of Current Tocolytics

Tocolytic Drug	Mechanism of Action	Dosing	Side Effects
Magnesium sulfate	Decreases levels of intracellular calcium, preventing activation of actin and myosin complexes	4- to 6-gram bolus followed by 1–4 grams per hour	Maternal: warmth, flushing, headache, nausea, blurred vision, maternal toxicity appears at levels ≥9 mg/dL; absent patellar reflexes between 9 and 13 mg/dL; respiratory distress ≥14 mg/dL Fetal: changes in heart rate variability, postnatally—respiratory and motor depression
β-Adrenergic-receptor agonist	Binding to the β_2-adrenergic receptors → increases levels of intracellular cyclic AMP → activation of protein kinase → inactivation of myosin light-chain kinases → diminished myometrial contractility	Terbutaline: 250 µg SQ every 20 min for up to 3 doses Ritodrine: IV infusion rate of 50 µg/min Salbutamol: bolus injection of 184 µg	Maternal: tachycardia, nausea, shortness of breath, chest pain, cardiac dysrhythmias, hypotension, pulmonary edema, and tachyphylaxis Fetal: increase in fetal heart rate
Calcium channel blockers	Block transmembrane flow of calcium through slowly activating voltage-gated L-type channels	Nifedipine: initial dose is 10–20 mg PO, repeat every 3–6 h as needed, followed by 30–60 mg of the long-acting formulation every 8–12 h or 10 mg PO every 10 min (40 mg in 1 h) followed by 20-mg long-acting tablet orally at 90 min Nicardipine: 60 mg PO every 6 h or IV infusion of 2–4 mg per hour	Maternal: hypotension, tachycardia, flushing, dizziness, and nausea Fetal: none
Cyclooxygenase inhibitors	Block the conversion of arachidonic acid to prostaglandins	Loading dose of 50–100 mg PO followed by 25–50 mg every 6 h for 48 h	Maternal: gastritis, proctitis, hematochezia, renal toxicity, and prolonged bleeding times Fetal: oligohydramnios and closure of the ductus arteriosus

(continued)

Table 1. Mechanism of Action, Dose, Side Effects, and U.S. Food and Drug Administration Label of Current Tocolytics [Continued]

Tocolytic Drug	Mechanism of Action	Dosing	Side Effects
Nitric oxide donors	Increase cyclic guanosine monophosphate → inactivate myosin light-chain kinases → smooth muscle relaxation	50-mg patch and repeat in 1 h if needed; remove and replace patch every 12 h	Maternal: headache, hypotension, flushing, dizziness, lightheadedness, and peripheral edema Fetal: none
Oxytocin-receptor antagonist	Competes with oxytocin for binding on myometrial membrane → inhibition of second messenger → decrease intracellular calcium → smooth muscle relaxation	IV infusion 300 µg/min ± 6.75 µg bolus	Maternal: none Fetal: fetal and neonatal death at <28 wk

AMP = adenosine monophosphate

Table 2. Pharmacokinetics of Current Tocolytic Agents

Tocolytic Drug	Serum Concentrations	Half-Life (min)	Volume of Distribution	Metabolism/ Excretion	Placental Passage
Magnesium sulfate	4-gram bolus: 5.56 ± 0.30 (mean); 6-gram bolus: 2.57 ± 0.17 (mean)	610 ± 137	32.3 L	Renal	Yes
β-Adrenergic-receptor agonist	28 ± 11 µg/L	5.9 ± 6.0 min initially and 156 ± 51 min following initial fall-off	6.95 ± 3.54 L/kg	NA	Yes
Calcium channel blockers	Peak: 38.6 ± 18 µg/L	81	NA	Liver/renal	Yes
Cyclooxygenase inhibitors	Peak: 442 ± 73 µg/L	15–16	18.3 ± 6.8 L	Liver	Yes
Nitric oxide donors	NA	2–8	NA	Liver/renal	NA
Oxytocin-receptor antagonist	Peak: 442 ± 73 µg/L	16.2 ± 2.4	18.3 ± 6.8 L	NA	Minimal

NA = not available

dL and respiratory distress occurs at levels >14 mg/dL.[30] Clinical utility of magnesium levels for dosing, adverse effects, and efficacy is controversial.

Dosage and Administration: Magnesium can be given as a 4- or 6-gram bolus IV over 20 minutes initially and maintenance of 1–4 grams per hour. Magnesium is titrated based on clinical response and maternal toxicity.

Side Effects: Maternal side effects include warmth, headache, nausea, vomiting, lethargy, dry mouth, blurred vision or diplopia, hypocalcemia, respiratory arrest, ileus, and hypoxia secondary to pulmonary edema.[32] Fetal and neonatal side effects include alterations in heart rate variability, respiratory and motor depression, drowsiness, transient lethargy, hypocalcemia, and hypotonia. Bone mineralization abnormalities have been associated with prolonged use.[32] There are reports of increased risk of fetal and neonatal death in infants exposed to magnesium sulfate.[26,33]

Contraindications: Magnesium sulfate is contraindicated in patients with hypersensitivity to any component of its formulation or cardiac/myometrial damage. Magnesium sulfate should be used with caution in patients with renal disease and impaired creatinine clearance.[15]

Evidence-Based Review of Efficacy: The largest randomized placebo-controlled trial did not show any benefit of magnesium sulfate for pregnancy prolongation over placebo.[34,35] A recent meta-analysis reported that magnesium was effective in extending births to term compared with placebo or no tocolytic treatment.[18] There is still obvious controversy regarding the efficacy of magnesium sulfate for preterm birth.

Recently, the association of magnesium sulfate and neuroprotective effects of the fetus has been revisited, and there appear to be long-term neurologic protective effects for preterm fetuses treated with magnesium sulfate.[36]

2. β-Adrenergic Receptor Agonists

β-Adrenergic receptor agonists have been studied extensively and are considered a first-line clinical agent. Terbutaline is currently the only parenteral β-adrenergic receptor agonist available in the United States.

Names: Several β-adrenergic receptor agonists exist. Terbutaline (Brethine®) is the most commonly used β-agonist used in the United States. In addition to terbutaline, other β-agonists used outside the United States include ritodrine, isoxsuprine, hexoprenaline, fenoterol, metaproterenol (orciprenaline), and salbutamol.

Mechanism of Action: The mechanism by which β-adrenergic receptor agonists cause myometrial relaxation is by binding to the $β_2$-adrenergic receptors and increasing the levels of intracellular cyclic adenosine monophosphate (AMP). Cyclic AMP activates protein kinase, which inactivates myosin light-chain kinase, which diminishes myometrial contractility (Figure 1).[26] It also lowers levels of intracellular calcium, leading to smooth muscle relaxation.[30]

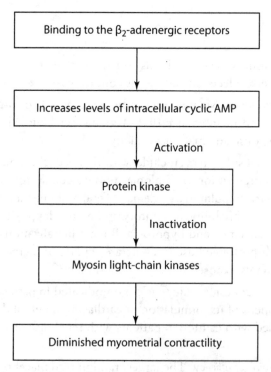

Figure 1. Mechanism of Action of $β_2$-Adrenergic Receptor Agonists. AMP = adenosine monophosphate.

Pharmacokinetics: After therapeutic SQ administration, terbutaline is rapidly absorbed with a half-life of 7 minutes. Mean plasma clearance is 30% higher compared to the nonpregnant state. There is no change in the volume of distribution. Peak serum concentrations are 0.7 µg/L. Mean steady-state plasma concentrations are 30% lower during pregnancy.[30]

Ritodrine, given IV, has steady-state concentrations of 28 ± 11 µg/L and volume of distribution of 6.95 ± 3.54 L/kg. Ritodrine is extensively bound to extravascular tissue. Half-life is 5.9 ± 6.0 minutes initially and 156 ± 51 minutes after the initial rapid fall-off.[30]

There are limited data regarding the pharmacokinetics of salbutamol in pregnancy. What is known is that mean peak concentrations are 8.33 ± 1.9 µg/L and total clearance of 501 ± 185 mL/min.[30]

Terbutaline and ritodrine cross the placenta with a fetomaternal ratio of 0.30.

Dosage and Administration: Usual dosing for terbutaline is 250 µg SQ every 20 minutes for up to 3 doses. Ritodrine is given by IV infusion rate of 50 µg/min. Salbutamol is given as a bolus injection of 184 µg.[30]

Side Effects: Maternal side effects include tachycardia, nausea, shortness of breath, chest pain, cardiac dysrhythmias, hypotension, and pulmonary edema. Rapidly decreasing response to the medication, called *tachyphylaxis*, can develop.[30] Fetal effects include increase in fetal heart rate after administration.[30]

Contraindications: Hypersensitivity to any component of the drug, cardiac arrhythmias associated with tachycardia, and tachycardia from digitalis toxicity.[15]

Evidence-Based Review of Efficacy: β-agonists are effective in stopping PTL and delaying pregnancy for 48 hours compared to placebo.[23] A meta-analysis has confirmed these findings of the effectiveness of β-adrenergic receptor agonists in delaying delivery and reducing the frequency of preterm birth and low birth weight when compared to placebo.[37]

3. Calcium Channel Blockers

Calcium channel blockers were introduced as a tocolytic agent in 1980.[38] They have been studied extensively and are considered a first-line clinical agent.

Names: Currently used calcium channel blockers for tocolysis include nifedipine (Procardia®, Procardia XL®, Adalat®) and nicardipine (Cardene®). Nifedipine is the most commonly used agent in the United States.

Mechanism of Action: Calcium channel blockers exert their effect on the myometrium by blocking transmembrane flow of calcium through slowly activating voltage-gated L-type channels. Calcium channel blockers are not specific to the myometrium; therefore, effects are seen in the vascular and nonvascular (bronchial, gastrointestinal, and genitourinary) smooth muscle, non-contractile tissues, and cardiac tissue (negative inotropic effect). There are two types of calcium channels: type 1 and type 2. Type 2 channels have less effect on cardiac tissue than type 1. Nifedipine acts on the type 2 channels.[30]

Pharmacokinetics: After oral administration, nifedipine is rapidly absorbed from the gastrointestinal tract. Nifedipine is metabolized through the liver leaving approximately 60% of the drug in active form following first-pass metabolism. The metabolites are excreted in the urine and feces.[30] Due to the physiologic changes of pregnancy, the peak serum concentrations (38.6 ± 18 µg/L at 40 minutes) and half-life (81 minutes after sublingual administration) are decreased and the clearance rate is increased. The duration of action is limited to 6 hours because of these physiologic changes.[39] Nifedipine crosses the placenta with a fetomaternal ratio of 0.77–0.93.[40,41]

Nicardipine is also absorbed through the gastrointestinal tract after oral administration. Nicardipine is a more potent smooth muscle vasodilator than nicardipine. Serum concentrations of the drug decline quickly after 2 hours. Nicardipine does cross the placenta with a fetomaternal ratio of 0.2–0.5, with levels being lower after IV infusion.[42]

Dosage and Administration: The initial dose of nifedipine is 10 or 20 mg PO and may be repeated every 3–6 hours until desired response is achieved, followed by 30–60 mg of the long-acting formulation every 8–12 hours until a course of antenatal corticosteroids is complete.[42] Nifedipine can also be given 10 mg PO every 10 minutes (40 mg in 1 hour) followed by a 20-mg long-acting tablet PO at 90 minutes.[43]

The initial dose of nicardipine is 60 mg PO every 6 hours. IV infusion can be initiated at a rate of 2–4 mg per hour.[30] Nicardipine is also metabolized by the liver.

Side Effects: Common side effects of calcium channel blockers include mild to moderate decrease in blood pressure with increase in pulse (exaggerated in patients with dehydration), headache, cutaneous flushing, dizziness, and nausea. There are no fetal effects of the medications.[32]

Contraindications: Contraindications to calcium channel blockers include hypersensitivity to any component of the drug and advanced aortic stenosis.[15]

Evidence-Based Review of Efficacy: Meta-analysis of available literature reported that calcium channel blockers, when compared with other tocolytics, appear to be more effective in reducing the number of preterm births within 7 days and before 34 weeks. Calcium channel blockers appear to reduce the frequency of RDS, NEC, IVH, and neonatal jaundice. In this meta-analysis, calcium channel blockers were mainly compared with β-adrenergic receptor agonists.[26]

Three randomized controlled trials report the same efficacy of calcium channel blockers and magnesium sulfate in various birth outcomes and pregnancy prolongation.[23, 44–46]

A recent cost-effective analysis of tocolytic medications showed nifedipine and indomethacin to be superior to magnesium or β-adrenergic receptor agonists.[47]

4. Cyclooxygenase Inhibitors
Cyclooxygenase (COX) inhibitors are also referred to as nonsteroidal anti-inflammatory drugs and were first introduced as a tocolytic agent by Zuckerman in 1974. COX inhibitors have been studied extensively and are considered a first-line clinical agent.

Names: The most common and extensively studied COX inhibitor used in pregnancy is indomethacin (Indocin®). Other medications include ibuprofen, naproxen, and sulindac.

Mechanism of Action: Indomethacin is a nonspecific COX inhibitor that blocks the conversion of arachidonic acid to prostaglandins. By blocking the action of prostaglandins, there is a decrease in the formation of myometrial gap junctions with a subsequent decrease in available intracellular calcium, leading to uterine quiescence.[26]

Pharmacokinetics: Indomethacin, after oral administration, has peak serum concentrations in 1–2 hours (serum concentration of 442 ± 73 µg/L). The half-life is 15–16 minutes. Indomethacin is tightly bound to plasma proteins.[30] Indomethacin is primarily metabolized by the liver. The volume of distribution is 18.3 ± 6.8 L with a plasma clearance of 41.8 ± 8.2 L/h.[30] Indomethacin crosses the placenta with umbilical cord values equivalent to maternal levels within 5 hours. Serum concentrations are detectable in the neonate. Fetomaternal ratio approaches 100%.[30]

Dosage and Administration: Indomethacin can be given both PO and rectally with PTL <32 weeks. The rectal form is no longer available in the United States. Indomethacin is usually given as a loading dose of 50 mg PO (range 50–100 mg) followed by 25 mg PO (range 25–50 mg) every 6 hours for 48 hours. Amniotic fluid volume levels are evaluated before initiation of therapy and at 48–72 hours. Treatment beyond 48 hours requires fetal ductal flow evaluation with Doppler echocardiography (see Side Effects and Contraindications).[30]

Side Effects: The most common maternal side effect is gastritis. Other maternal side effects include proctitis, hematochezia, renal toxicity with oliguria and electrolyte imbalances, and prolonged bleeding times.[32]

The main fetal complications associated with indomethacin therapy include oligohydramnios and closure of the ductus arteriosus. This ductal constriction has been found to be reversible. In animal studies, oligohydramnios is caused by decreased renal vasodilation from prostaglandins leading to diminished renal blood flow and urinary output. Doppler studies have failed to show this association in humans but several case reports have questioned the possibility of fetal renal toxicity. Oligohydramnios is usually associated with prolonged therapy beyond 48–72 hours. Premature constriction of the ductus arteriosus can lead to cardiac ischemia, failure, and hydrops fetalis. Like oligohydramnios, premature closure of the ductus arteriosus is usually associated with prolonged therapy beyond 48–72 hours and the likelihood increases as gestation age advances, especially beyond 32 weeks. Savage et al. reviewed retrospectively 124 cases of prolonged indomethacin therapy. Median gestational age at onset of therapy was 23 3/7 weeks, with median duration of therapy of 30 days. They demonstrated a 6.5% rate of ductal constriction and 7.3% rate of oligohydramnios. Overall composite neonatal morbidity was 29%. The rates of complications were independent of gestational age at onset, duration, and dosing of indomethacin therapy.[48]

Other possible complications include NEC, IVH, and primary pulmonary hypertension in the neonate.[32] Meta-analysis of indomethacin and adverse neonatal outcomes reported an association between indomethacin use and increased risk of periventricular leukomalacia and NEC.[49]

Contraindications: Contraindications to indomethacin include hypersensitivity to the drug, gestational age ≥32 weeks, and fetal conditions including growth restriction, renal anomalies, ductal-dependent cardiac defects, twin-twin transfusion syndrome, and oligohydramnios.

Evidence-Based Review of Efficacy: There have been two small trials regarding the efficacy of indomethacin as a tocolytic agent. One study showed a benefit in prolonging labor >48 hours from treatment and the other showed a pregnancy prolongation of >1 week. Neither study was able to prove a benefit on neonatal outcome. Meta-analysis by King et al. reported a significant reduction in women delivering at <37 weeks, increase in gestational age at delivery, and increase in birth weight compared to placebo, but failed to show a difference in other neonatal outcomes.[50]

A recent cost-effective analysis of tocolytic medications showed indomethacin and nifedipine to be superior to magnesium or β-adrenergic receptor agonists.[47]

5. Nitric Oxide Donors

Nitric oxide (NO) donors were first introduced as tocolytic agents in 1994. These agents are not used as first-line tocolytic agents. They are most commonly used in pregnancy for hypertensive crisis and as a rapid tocolytic agent for breech delivery.

The only NO donor used and studied in pregnancy is nitroglycerin (also known as *glyceryl trinitrate*).

Mechanism of Action: NO is a vasodilator. It is a potent smooth muscle relaxant generated from the oxidation of L-arginine by NO synthase. NO increases cyclic guanosine monophosphate levels, leading to the inactivation of the myosin light-chain kinases, causing smooth muscle relaxation (Figure 2).[15]

Pharmacokinetics: Nitroglycerin is given IV or transdermal for acute tocolysis because the oral availability is poor (10%–20%). Nitroglycerin is metabolized by the liver and excreted by the kidneys. The half-life is 2–8 minutes with the total duration of effect of 15–30 minutes. Pharmacokinetic effects specific to pregnancy have not been studied in detail.

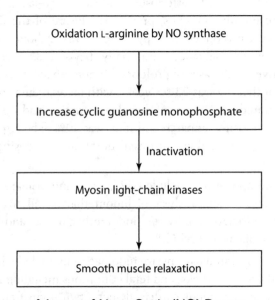

Figure 2. Mechanism of Action of Nitric Oxide (NO) Donors.

Dosage and Administration: A 50-mg nitroglycerin transdermal patch is placed initially, and a second patch may be placed in 1 hour if contractions have not ceased. Patch or patches are removed and replaced every 12 hours.[51]

Nitroglycerin is given IV as a 100-µg bolus and then a continuous infusion at a rate of 1–10 µg/kg/min.[52]

Side Effects: The most common side effect is headache, occurring in approximately 40% of patients. Other common side effects include profound hypotension, flushing, dizziness, lightheadedness, and peripheral edema.[15]

Contraindications: Contraindications to NO donors include hypersensitivity to organic nitrates or any by-products, close-angle glaucoma, concurrent use with phosphodiesterase-5 inhibitors, head trauma or cerebral hemorrhage, and severe anemia.[15]

Evidence-Based Review of Efficacy: The use of IV nitroglycerin for tocolysis does not appear to be an effective treatment in prolonging gestation.[26] Given transdermally, nitroglycerin appears to be as effective as β-adrenergic receptor agonists in prolonging gestation and superior to placebo in composite neonatal outcomes.[26]

6. Oxytocin-Receptor Antagonist

Atrosiban, an oxytocin-receptor antagonist, is widely used in Europe. It has not been approved for use in the United States.

Names: The only oxytocin-receptor antagonist available is atosiban.

Mechanism of Action: Atosiban is a peptidic oxytocin receptor antagonist that competes with oxytocin for its binding site on the myometrial plasma membrane. Binding of atosiban inhibits the second messenger process that, under normal circumstances, leads to an increase in intracellular free calcium and contractions (Figure 3).[30]

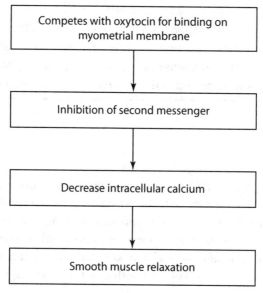

Figure 3. Mechanism of Action of Oxytocin-Receptor Antagonist.

Pharmacokinetics: After IV administration, the half-life of atosiban is 16.2 ± 2.4 minutes with peak serum concentrations of 442 ± 73 µg/L. Peak concentrations appear 2–8 minutes after infusion. Volume of distribution is 18.3 ± 6.8 L. Plasma clearance is 41.8 ± 8.2 L/h. Atosiban has 97% bioavailability. There is minimal transplacental passage of the drug.[30]

Dosage and Administration: Atosiban can be given as a continuous IV infusion of 300 µg/min or as a bolus of 6.75 mg followed by 300 µg/min continuous infusion.[30,53]

Side Effects: At this time, there do not appear to be any significant maternal side effects. Atosiban was not approved by the FDA because of concerns surrounding the excess fetal and infant deaths with the administration of atosiban at <28 weeks.[26]

Contraindications: Not currently approved for use in the United States.

Evidence-Based Review of Efficacy: A recent meta-analysis did not show a difference in neonatal outcomes or pregnancy prolongation compared to placebo. Several studies have shown an association with lower birth weights when atosiban was compared to placebo and β-adrenergic receptor agonists.[26]

VII. PATIENT CASE (PART 2)

On physical examination, the patient's vital signs are stable and she is afebrile. Speculum examination is negative and fetal fibronectin and cultures are taken. Her cervical examination reveals her to be 3 centimeters dilated, 100% cervical effacement, and has a bulging bag of water at +1 station. She is contracting every 3 minutes and they palpate quite strong. Fetal heart rate tracing is reassuring. Transvaginal cervical length is 2.0 centimeters with funneling. Fetal fibronectin results return positive. The patient is given magnesium sulfate, 6-gram bolus IV, followed by a continuous infusion of 2 grams per hour. She also received betamethasone, 12 mg IM, immediately and repeated again in 24 hours. Two hours later, contractions have subsided and her cervix remains unchanged.

VIII. Summary

In spite of efforts to prevent PTL and delivery, the rates of preterm birth continue to rise. As a group, tocolytics appear to be beneficial in prolonging labor long enough for the positive effect of corticosteroids on fetal lung maturity. However, while prolonging pregnancy, there has been no improvement in neonatal outcomes. Of all the presently used tocolytics, calcium channel blockers have the safest drug profile, lowest cost, and similar efficacy when compared with other tocolytic agents.

IX. References

1. ACOG Committee Opinion. Use of progesterone to reduce preterm birth. *Obstet Gynecol.* 2003;102(Pt 1):1115–1116.

2. Russell RB, Green NS, Steiner CA, et al. Cost of hospitalization for preterm and low birth weight infants in the United States. *Pediatrics.* 2007;120:e1–9.

3. ACOG Practice Bulletin. Assessment of risk factors for preterm birth. Clinical management guidelines for obstetrician-gynecologists. Number 31, October 2001. (Replaces Technical Bulletin number 206, June 1995; Committee Opinion number 172, May 1996; Committee Opinion number 187, September 1997; Committee Opinion number 198, February 1998; and Committee Opinion number 251, January 2001). *Obstet Gynecol.* 2001;98:709–716.

4. Villar J, Abalos E, Carroli G, et al. Heterogeneity of perinatal outcomes in the preterm delivery syndrome. *Obstet Gynecol.* 2004;104:78–87.

5. Leitich H, Brunbauer M, Kaider A, et al. Cervical length and dilatation of the internal cervical os detected by vaginal ultrasonography as markers for preterm delivery: a systematic review. *Am J Obstet Gynecol.* 1999;181:1465–1472.

6. Leitich H, Egarter C, Kaider A, et al. Cervicovaginal fetal fibronectin as a marker for preterm delivery: a meta-analysis. *Am J Obstet Gynecol.* 1999;180:1169–1176.

7. Andersen HF, Nugent CE, Wanty SD, et al. Prediction of risk for preterm delivery by ultrasonographic measurement of cervical length. *Am J Obstet Gynecol.* 1990;163:859–867.

8. Goldenberg RL, Iams JD, Miodovnik M, et al. The preterm prediction study: risk factors in twin gestations. National Institute of Child Health and Human Development Maternal-Fetal Medicine Units Network. *Am J Obstet Gynecol.* 1996; 175(Pt 1):1047–1053.

9. Iams JD, Goldenberg RL, Meis PJ, et al. The length of the cervix and the risk of spontaneous premature delivery. National Institute of Child Health and Human Development Maternal Fetal Medicine Unit Network. *N Engl J Med.* 1996; 334:567–572.

10. Imseis HM, Albert TA, Iams JD. Identifying twin gestations at low risk for preterm birth with a transvaginal ultrasonographic cervical measurement at 24 to 26 weeks' gestation. *Am J Obstet Gynecol.* 1997;177:1149–1155.

11. Smith V, Devane D, Begley CM, et al. A systematic review and quality assessment of systematic reviews of fetal fibronectin and transvaginal length for predicting preterm birth. *Eur J Obstet Gynecol Reprod Biol.* 2007;133:134–142.

12. Mateus J, Pereira L, Baxter J, et al. Effectiveness of fetal fibronectin testing compared with digital cervical assessment of women with preterm contractions. *Am J Perinatol.* 2007;24:381–385.

13. Sfakianaki AK, Norwitz ER. Mechanisms of progesterone action in inhibiting prematurity. *J Matern Fetal Neonatal Med.* 2006;19:763–772.

14. ACOG Practice Bulletin. Management of preterm labor. Number 43, May 2003. *Int J Gynaecol Obstet.* 2003;82:127–135.

15. Goletiani NV, Keith DR, Gorsky SJ. Progesterone: review of safety for clinical studies. *Exp Clin Psychopharmacol.* 2007;15:427–444.

16. Meis PJ, Aleman A. Progesterone treatment to prevent preterm birth. *Drugs.* 2004;64:2463–2474.

17. Meis PJ, Klebanoff M, Thom E, et al. Prevention of recurrent preterm delivery by 17 alpha-hydroxyprogesterone caproate. *N Engl J Med.* 2003;348:2379–2385.

18. Berkman ND, Thorp JM Jr, Lohr KN, et al. Tocolytic treatment for the management of preterm labor: a review of the evidence. *Am J Obstet Gynecol.* 2003;188:1648–1659.

19. Mercer BM, Goldenberg RL, Moawad AH, et al. The preterm prediction study: effect of gestational age and cause of preterm birth on subsequent obstetric outcome. National Institute of Child Health and Human Development Maternal-Fetal Medicine Units Network. *Am J Obstet Gynecol.* 1999;181(Pt 1):1216–1221.

20. Goldenberg RL, Cliver SP, Bronstein J, et al. Bed rest in pregnancy. *Obstet Gynecol.* 1994;84:131–136.

21. Guinn DA, Goepfert AR, Owen J, et al. Management options in women with preterm uterine contractions: a randomized clinical trial. *Am J Obstet Gynecol.* 1997;177:814–818.

22. Maxwell CV, Amankwah KS. Alternative approaches to preterm labor. *Semin Perinatol.* 2001;25:310–315.

23. Treatment of preterm labor with the beta-adrenergic agonist ritodrine. The Canadian Preterm Labor Investigators Group. *N Engl J Med.* 1992;327:308–312.

24. Mittendorf R, Dambrosia J, Pryde PG, et al. Association between the use of antenatal magnesium sulfate in preterm labor and adverse health outcomes in infants. *Am J Obstet Gynecol.* 2002;186:1111–1118.

25. Scudiero R, Khoshnood B, Pryde PG, et al. Perinatal death and tocolytic magnesium sulfate. *Obstet Gynecol.* 2000;96:178–182.

26. Simhan HN, Caritis SN. Prevention of preterm delivery. *N Engl J Med.* 2007;357:477–487.

27. Gordon MC, Iams JD. Magnesium sulfate. *Clin Obstet Gynecol.* 1995;38:706–712.

28. Harbert GM Jr, Cornell GW, Thornton WN Jr. Effect of toxemia therapy on uterine dynamics. *Am J Obstet Gynecol.* 1969;105:94–104.

29. Petrie RH. Preterm parturition. Tocolysis using magnesium sulfate. *Semin Perinatol.* 1981;5:266–273.

30. Tsatsaris V, Cabrol D, Carbonne B. Pharmacokinetics of tocolytic agents. *Clin Pharmacokinet.* 2004;43:833–844.

31. Idama TO, Lindow SW. Magnesium sulphate: a review of clinical pharmacology applied to obstetrics. *Br J Obstet Gynaecol.* 1998;105:260–268.

32. Pryde PG, Besinger RE, Gianopoulos JG, et al. Adverse and beneficial effects of tocolytic therapy. *Semin Perinatol.* 2001;25:316–340.

33. Grimes DA, Nanda K. Magnesium sulfate tocolysis: time to quit. *Obstet Gynecol.* 2006;108:986–989.

34. Cox SM, Sherman ML, Leveno KJ. Randomized investigation of magnesium sulfate for prevention of preterm birth. *Am J Obstet Gynecol.* 1990;163:767–772.

35. Crowther CA, Hiller JE, Doyle LW. Magnesium sulphate for preventing preterm birth in threatened preterm labour. *Cochrane Database Syst Rev.* 2002: CD001060.

36. Crowther CA, Hiller JE, Doyle LW, et al. Effect of magnesium sulfate given for neuroprotection before preterm birth: a randomized controlled trial. *JAMA.* 2003;290:2669–2676.

37. Anotayanonth S, Subhedar NV, Garner P, et al. Betamimetics for inhibiting preterm labour. *Cochrane Database Syst Rev.* 2004:CD004352.

38. Ulmsten U, Andersson KE, Wingerup L. Treatment of premature labor with the calcium antagonist nifedipine. *Arch Gynecol.* 1980;229:1–5.

39. Prevost RR, Akl SA, Whybrew WD, et al. Oral nifedipine pharmacokinetics in pregnancy-induced hypertension. *Pharmacotherapy.* 1992;12:174–177.

40. Silberschmidt AL, Kuhn-Velten WN, Juon AM, et al. Nifedipine concentration in maternal and umbilical cord blood after nifedipine gastrointestinal therapeutic system for tocolysis. *BJOG.* 2008;115:480-485.

41. Smith P, Anthony J, Johanson R. Nifedipine in pregnancy. *BJOG.* 2000;107:299–307.

42. Carbonne B, Jannet D, Touboul C, et al. Nicardipine treatment of hypertension during pregnancy. *Obstet Gynecol.* 1993;81:908–914.

43. Papatsonis DN, Bos JM, van Geijn HP, et al. Nifedipine pharmacokinetics and plasma levels in the management of preterm labor. *Am J Ther.* 2007;14:346–350.

44. Floyd RC, McLaughlin BN, Perry KGJ, et al. Magnesium sulfate or nifedipine hydrochloride for acute tocolysis of preterm labor: efficacy and side effects. *J Maternal-Fetal Invest.* 1995;5:25–29.

45. Glock JL, Morales WJ. Efficacy and safety of nifedipine versus magnesium sulfate in the management of preterm labor: a randomized study. *Am J Obstet Gynecol.* 1993;169:960–964.

46. Lyell DJ, Pullen K, Campbell L, et al. Magnesium sulfate compared with nifedipine for acute tocolysis of preterm labor: a randomized controlled trial. *Obstet Gynecol.* 2007;110:61–67.

47. Hayes E, Moroz L, Pizzi L, et al. A cost decision analysis of 4 tocolytic drugs. *Am J Obstet Gynecol.* 2007;197:383.e1–6.

48. Savage AH, Anderson BL, Simhan HN. The safety of prolonged indomethacin therapy. *Am J Perinatol.* 2007;24:207–213.

49. Amin SB, Sinkin RA, Glantz JC. Metaanalysis of the effect of antenatal indomethacin on neonatal outcomes. *Am J Obstet Gynecol.* 2007;197:486.e1–10.

50. King J, Flenady V, Cole S, et al. Cyclo-oxygenase (COX) inhibitors for treating preterm labour. *Cochrane Database Syst Rev.* 2005(2):CD001992.

51. Bisits A, Madsen G, Knox M, et al. The Randomized Nitric Oxide Tocolysis Trial (RNOTT) for the treatment of preterm labor. *Am J Obstet Gynecol.* 2004;191:683–690.

52. El-Sayed YY, Riley ET, Holbrook RH Jr, et al. Randomized comparison of intravenous nitroglycerin and magnesium sulfate for treatment of preterm labor. *Obstet Gynecol.* 1999;93:79–83.

53. Atosiban Investigators Group. Treatment of preterm labor with the oxytocin antagonist atosiban: a double-blind, randomized, controlled comparison with salbutamol. *Eur J Obstet Gynecol Reprod Biol.* 2001;98:177–185.

QUESTIONS AND ANSWERS

1. Preterm birth is defined as:

   a. birth before 36 completed weeks of gestation.

   b. birth before 37 completed weeks of gestation.

   c. birth before 38 completed weeks of gestation.

   d. birth before 39 completed weeks of gestation.

2. The most predictive risk factor for spontaneous preterm labor is:

   a. multiple gestation

   b. history of previous preterm birth

   c. age <18 years

   d. uterine anomalies

   e. all of the above

3. Which of the following is used to prevent preterm birth?

   a. cervical length measurement

   b. fetal fibronectin

   c. 17α-hydroxyprogesterone caproate

   d. none of the above

4. All of the following are used as first-line tocolytics except:

   a. magnesium sulfate

   b. β-adrenergic receptor agonist

   c. calcium channel blockers

   d. COX inhibitors

   e. nitric oxide donors

5. Oxytocin receptor antagonists are not approved for use in the United States because:

    a. maternal side effects are significant.

    b. fetal side effects are minimal.

    c. of excessive fetal and infant deaths at <28 weeks.

    d. not enough evidence supports or refutes its use.

6. All of the following are TRUE except:

    a. The rate of preterm birth continues to rise.

    b. Tocolysis appears beneficial in prolonging labor for the administration of corticosteroids.

    c. Tocolytic therapy is associated with improved neonatal outcomes.

    d. Calcium channel blockers appear to be the safest tocolytic currently used.

Answers:

1. b; 2. b; 3. c; 4. e; 5. c; 6. c

Preterm Premature Rupture of Membranes

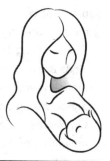

Mounira Habli and David F. Lewis

CHAPTER
8

LEARNING OBJECTIVES

1. Explain the etiology of preterm premature rupture of membranes.

2. Describe the clinical presentation of preterm premature rupture of membranes.

3. Outline the treatment goals in the management of this condition.

4. Identify the classes of drugs and their purposes.

I. Introduction

Premature rupture of membranes (PROM) is defined as spontaneous rupture of amniotic membranes before the onset of labor. Preterm premature rupture of membranes (PPROM) is when membrane rupture occurs before 37 weeks of gestation. Prolonged PPROM refers to PPROM without delivery for an interval greater than 24 hours.

PPROM occurs in 3%–5% of all pregnancies. It accounts for 25%–40% of all preterm births, complicating 140,000 pregnancies annually in the United States.[1] PPROM is a primary contributor to perinatal morbidity and mortality, accounting for nearly 50% of long-term morbidity and 60% of perinatal mortality.[2] PROM at any gestational age is generally associated with a *latency period*, defined as the interval from time of rupture to onset of labor. Latency is inversely proportional to gestational age. The mean interval between rupture and delivery (latency period) between 20 and 26 weeks is 12 days as compared to the 32–34 weeks' latency period being 4 days. Between 20 and 36 weeks, 60%–70% of patients with PPROM deliver within 48 hours versus 80% when PPROM occurs between 33 and 36 weeks.[3] The ultimate goal of managing patients with PPROM is to safely acquire as much time in utero as possible while being mindful of the risks to the mother and fetus.

II. PATIENT CASE [PART 1]

Mrs. M.S., an 18-year-old primigravida at 25 weeks' gestation, presents with a chief complaint of a gush of fluid from her vagina. She reports an uncomplicated prenatal course and denies any urinary symptoms or fever. She has a negative medical and surgical history. She denies use of illicit drugs, tobacco, and alcohol. She is taking prenatal vitamins and no other medications. On evaluation, her vital signs are stable and her oral temperature is 36.9°C (98.4°F). Her abdominal examination reveals a nontender uterus. Upon sterile speculum examination, her cervix appears long and closed with a copious amount of fluid coming through the cervix. On microscopic examination of a dried specimen, a typical fern pattern is seen, indicative of amniotic fluid. A Nitrazine paper test of the fluid creates the classic blue color response indicative of amniotic fluid and rupture of membranes. An ultrasound reveals a singleton fetus in a vertex presentation with an estimated fetal weight of 990 grams and no amniotic fluid present. Fetal and uterine assessment by external electronic monitoring reveals a fetal heart rate pattern that is reassuring without evidence of uterine contractions. The diagnosis of PPROM at 25 weeks' gestation without labor or evidence of infection is established. The patient is admitted to labor and delivery.

III. Pathophysiology

The etiology of PPROM, while multifactorial and an interplay of genetic and environmental conditions, is unknown in more than 50% of cases. Many mechanisms have been proposed, including local inflammation, local infection of the membranes (chorioamnionitis), intra-amniotic infection, decreased membrane collagen content, localized membrane defects, and excessive membrane stretch (uterine overdistention).[1] The fetal membranes are made of two layers, the amnion and the chorion. The two layers are connected by collagen-rich connective tissue.[3] Changes in collagen content and type and cellular apoptosis with advancing gestational age weaken the membranes, leading to rupture of membranes.[4,5] These changes are secondary to either physical stresses or enzymatic imbalance effects, such as increased collagenase and protease activity.[6,7]

There is evidence that links PPROM to several infectious processes involving the urogenital tract. Genital tract pathogens that have been associated with PPROM include *Neisseria gonorrhoeae*, *Chlamydia trachomatis*, and *Trichomonas vaginalis*.[8] Bacterial vaginosis has been linked to PPROM, but it is not clear if it is the inciting pathogen or if it facilitates membrane rupture through direct action on fetal membranes.[8] Preliminary studies have suggested an association between maternal genotype for inflammatory proteins and the risk of spontaneous preterm birth due to preterm labor or PROM.[9]

IV. Prediction and Prevention of Premature Rupture of the Fetal Membranes

Prediction and prevention of PPROM relies on an understanding of pathophysiology and clinical markers for subsequent membrane rupture. Identification of risk factors for PPROM is critical to identifying women with the highest risk for PPROM and then intervening when appropriate. Examples of specific risk factors whose treatment might reduce the risk of PPROM in certain individuals include cigarette smoking, urinary tract and sexually transmitted infections, and severe polyhydramnios. However, while there are many trials that have addressed the prediction and prevention of preterm birth (PTB), there are few that have focused on prediction and prevention of PPROM specifically. One of these trials was conducted by the National Institute of Child Health & Human Development-Maternal Fetal Medicine Units (NICHD-MFMU).[10] This trial prospectively evaluated factors in a current pregnancy that might predict PPROM. They reported that nulliparous women have an increased risk of PPROM in the presence of a short cervical length, medical complications, working during pregnancy, and low body mass index (BMI <19.8). In multiparous women, a prior episode of PPROM and preterm labor, positive fetal fibronectin, and short cervix increase the risk of PPROM. Women with two or three risk factors had a dramatically increased risk for PTB from PPROM. Despite efforts to identify factors that might increase the risk of PPROM, there is still not a definitive protocol addressing how to predict and/or prevent PPROM in women with high risk factors.

V. Risk Factors

Fifty percent of PPROM cases have no risk factors. A number of clinical risk factors have been identified, including connective tissue disorders (eg, Ehlers-Danlos syndrome), urogenital tract infection, abnormal genital tract bacterial colonization, chorioamnionitis, recent coitus, low socioeconomic status, uterine over-distention, second- and third-trimester bleeding, low BMI (<19.8 kg/m^2), nutritional deficiencies of copper and ascorbic acid, antepartum bleeding in one or more trimesters, maternal cigarette smoking, cervical conization or cerclage, pulmonary disease in pregnancy, and preterm labor or symptomatic contractions in the current gestation or prior PTB linked to the occurrence of PPROM.[1-4] In addition, there are several conditions, such as amniocentesis, cervical cerclage, and loop electrosurgical excision procedure, that are linked to the occurrence of PPROM (Table 1).

VI. Diagnosis

The diagnosis of ruptured membranes depends on history, physical examination, and laboratory findings. More than 80% of patients will give a history that suggests the diagnosis. Most patients present with several complaints such as a gush of fluid, leakage of fluid, continuous perineal dripping, wet pants, increase in vaginal discharge, light vaginal bleeding, and/or labor pains. The diagnosis of PPROM is established by performing a sterile speculum examination in addition to the history. Sterile speculum examination will provide confirmatory evidence of ruptured membranes if the following are present:

- Pooling of amniotic fluid in the posterior fornix of the vagina with evidence of fluid emanating from the cervical canal either spontaneously or through valsalva maneuver.
- Positive fern test: The fern test is a microscopic examination of vaginal pool fluid swabbed on a slide and air-dried. The fluid is obtained with a sterile swab from fluid

Table 1. Risk Factors for Preterm Premature Rupture of Membranes

Stress
Single women
Low socioeconomic status
Anxiety
Depression
Life events (divorce, separation, death)
Abdominal surgery during pregnancy
Multiple gestation
Polyhydramnios
Uterine anomaly or fibroids
Diethylstilbestrol
Cervical factors
History of second trimester abortion
History of cervical surgery
Infection
Placental pathology

pooled in the posterior vaginal fornix or free flowing from the cervical os. Under the microscope, the smear shows arborized crystals ("ferning") due to the interaction of amniotic fluid proteins and salts. False positive results can occur due to cervical mucus. However, the results of the tests are not affected by presence of contaminants like meconium or change in pH.

- Positive Nitrazine paper test: Amniotic fluid has an alkaline pH value. Nitrazine paper turns blue in the presence of alkaline pH. False positive results can occur from substances such as blood, semen, alkaline urine, soap, or antiseptic solutions.

A combination of two or more of the above tests (ferning or Nitrazine or patient history) provides an accuracy of 93.1%. However, in some patients it is difficult to diagnose despite an extensive history and physical examination.

Sterile speculum examination also can provide the opportunity to visually assess cervical dilatation and effacement, check for cervicitis, the presence of small fetal parts or cord, and to obtain appropriate cultures (eg, endocervical *Neisseria gonorrhoeae*, *Chlamydia trachomatis*, and anovaginal *Streptococcus agalactiae*) and vaginal smears or swabs to check for other vaginal infections, such as bacterial vaginosis, *Trichomonas*, or yeast infection. Group B streptococcus (GBS) cultures from the lower third of the vagina and perineum should also be obtained after confirmation of PPROM. Digital exam should be avoided unless imminent delivery is suspected. Another test that can be considered when the history, fern test, and Nitrazine are equivocal is fetal fibronectin (FFN). FFN is one of the most commonly used tests in preterm labor patients. FFN is an extracellular glycoprotein that attaches the fetal membranes and uterine decidua. The amniotic fluid contains more than 50,000 ng/mL of FFN. FFN is normally absent between 22 and 37 weeks. The test is done between 24 and 34 weeks if there has been no cervical exam or sexual intercourse in the previous 24 hours. Other suggested laboratory tests include complete blood count with differential, platelets, fibrinogen (if the patient is bleeding), urine for analysis, culture, sensitivities, and toxicology screen.

Fetal assessment should include a nonstress test (NST) and ultrasound examination. The NST is used to assess fetal well-being and for uterine tocodynamometry for uterine contractions. Ultrasound is done to assess the gestational age, fetal presentation, estimated fetal weight, and amniotic fluid volume, to rule out obvious fetal anomalies, and to determine placenta location. Many patients with PPROM will have a low amniotic fluid volume (<5 centimeters) that can aid in diagnosis. Other tests such as amniocentesis under ultrasound guidance may be indicated if intrauterine infection is suspected. Laboratory tests that can be performed on the fluid to help identify infection include gram stain, white cell count, and glucose level. The "gold standard" for the diagnosis of infection is isolation of the microorganisms on culture. However, a positive culture rate with fluid from amniocentesis is 25%–40%.

VII. PATIENT CASE [PART 2]

The patient was admitted to the birthing suite and placed on a fetal monitor to access fetal well-being (fetal heart rate pattern) and contractions. The fetus appeared in good health by fetal heart rate monitoring; however, the mother was found to be actively contracting. She was started on IV antibiotics: ampicillin and erythromycin. The mother was also given IM betamethasone to promote fetal lung maturation. Because of the presence of contractions, it was decided to attempt tocolysis with IV magnesium sulfate. The patient was kept in labor and delivery for 48 hours on the above drugs to complete the corticosteroid course. During this time she was observed closely for evidence of infection. At the end of 48 hours, the magnesium sulfate was discontinued and she was sent to the antenatal unit for a daily NST and was closely monitored for infection. The patient went into labor on hospital day 24 and delivered vaginally a 1445-gram neonate who was transferred to the neonatal intensive care unit. The additional 24 days in utero increased survival by more than 50% and markedly decreased short- and long-term morbidity in the infant.

VIII. Treatment

A. General Measures

Management of PPROM is based primarily on an individual assessment of the estimated risk for maternal, fetal, and neonatal complications (Figure 1). Whether conservative management or expeditious delivery will be pursued, the ultimate goal is to minimize maternal and fetal morbidity and mortality. The challenges of management of PPROM are multiple and often conflicting. If the mother exhibits signs of infection, then regardless of the gestational age, delivery is indicated. If there is no evidence of infection or fetal compromise then it is believed that leaving the fetus in utero improves outcome. Each day in utero increases the survival rate, decreases the number of days in the neonatal intensive care unit, and decreases morbidity in these neonates.

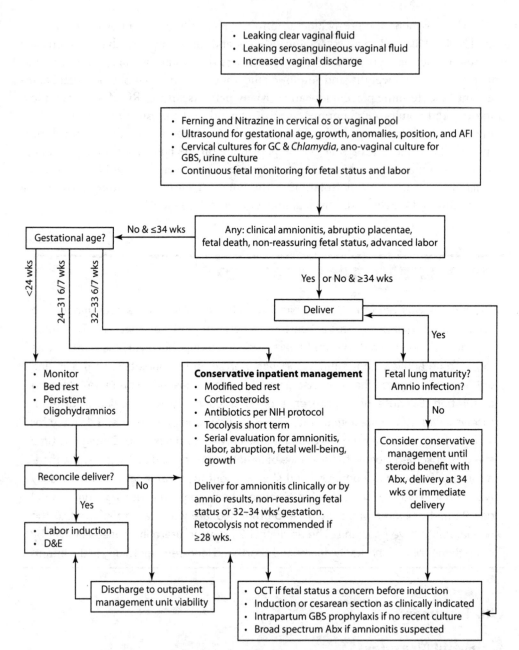

Figure 1. Algorithm for Management of Preterm Premature Rupture of Membranes. Abx = antibiotics, AFI = amniotic fluid index, D&E = dilation and evacuation, GBS = group B streptococcus, GC = gonococcus, NIH = National Institutes of Health, OCT = oxytocin challenge test.

1. Initial Assessment

On admission, each patient should be evaluated to confirm the diagnosis of PPROM, including sterile speculum examination and cultures. Fetal assessment should include NST, contraction monitoring, and ultrasound for gestational age evaluation and fluid measurement. All of these results should be made available to the pediatrician to help in maternal counseling and neonatal management. The goal of treatment of PPROM is primarily to increase the latency period to permit interventions that have been shown to reduce neonatal morbidity and mortality. These interventions include maternal transfer to a tertiary center, administration of corticosteroids to reduce risk of respiratory distress syndrome and intraventricular hemorrhage, and antibiotic prophylaxis to increase the latency period. Delivery is generally planned to take place at 34 weeks (although some institutions now advocate delivery at 32–33 weeks with confirmed PPROM) or regardless of gestational age if there is clinical evidence of intrauterine infection, nonreassuring fetal status, active labor, or fetal death. Otherwise management is based on gestational age (see Figure 1).

Gestational Age <23 Weeks

At these very early gestational ages PPROM has a dismal prognosis. The amniotic fluid is vital to lung development. With anhydramnios from 16–23 weeks, the risk of pulmonary hypoplasia is high. Infants who survive without pulmonary hypoplasia are at risk of death and long-term severe neurologic morbidity due to extreme prematurity. Women at <23 weeks are usually offered induction of labor and delivery of a nonviable pregnancy.

Gestational Age 23–31 6/7 Weeks

Patients are admitted for hospitalization after the diagnosis is confirmed. The fetus should be evaluated with ultrasound and NST as outlined in the Diagnosis section above. Tocolysis (see Chapter 7, Preterm Labor and Delivery) is initiated and continued for 48 hours for steroid administration and antibiotic therapy. During the hospital stay, serial maternal evaluation includes daily assessment for any evidence of intrauterine infection or placental abruption and serial evaluation for fetal well-being (daily NST and fetal growth evaluation every 3 weeks). Delivery indications are clinical or amniocentesis evidence of intrauterine infection, nonreassuring fetal status, active labor, or evidence of abruption or cord prolapse. Elective delivery is generally performed once the fetus is 32–34 weeks' gestation.

Gestational Age >34 Weeks

Patients with PPROM after 34 0/7 weeks are generally delivered after transfer to an institution that can care for the neonate. At these gestational ages, the risk to the mother and the neonate of expectant management are greater than the risks of delivery.

B. Protocol for Expectant Management of Preterm Premature Rupture of Membranes

1. Corticosteroids

There are two corticosteroids from which to choose: betamethasone, 12 mg IM q24h for 2 doses, or dexamethasone, 6 mg IM q12h for 4 doses. Of all the interventions done in preterm gestations, administration of corticosteroids is the most beneficial. Antenatal corticosteroids reduce the risks of respiratory distress syndrome (20% vs 35.4%), intraventricular hemorrhage (7.5% vs 15.9%), and necrotizing enterocolitis (0.8% vs 4.6%), without increasing the risks of maternal (9.2% vs 5.1%) or neonatal (7.0% vs 6.6%) infection. Corticosteroids should be administered from viability until 34 weeks unless infection is diagnosed or fetal lung maturity is established. These agents are not recommended after 34 0/7 weeks' gestation.[12–14] Corticosteroids act on the type II pneumocytes of the lung to increase the production of surfactant (see also Chapter 9, Fetal Lung Maturity).

2. Antibiotics

The goal of antibiotic therapy during conservative management of PPROM is to increase the latency period (duration from rupture of membranes to delivery). The premise is that antibiotic therapy treats subclinical infections (the major etiology of PPROM is thought to be subclinical infection) and/or prevents ascending infection (bacteria passing through the cervix into the uterus from the vagina), thus prolonging pregnancy. Antibiotic therapy in the setting of expectant management of PPROM has been shown to reduce intrauterine infection, postpartum endometritis, neonatal sepsis, respiratory distress syndrome, necrotizing enterocolitis, pneumonia, and intraventricular hemorrhage as compared to expectant management with no antibiotic therapy.[15,16]

The NICHD-MFMU Research Network reported results of a clinical trial involving women with PPROM from 24–32 0/7 weeks' gestation treated with ampicillin (2 grams IV q6h) and erythromycin (250 mg IV q6h) for 48 hours, followed by limited duration oral therapy (5 days) with amoxicillin (250 mg PO q8h) and enteric-coated erythromycin-base (333 mg PO q8h). These agents were chosen because they provide broad-spectrum antimicrobial coverage and have demonstrated safety when used in pregnancy. The study compared antibiotics to placebo and demonstrated a marked improvement in the outcome in the group that received the antibiotics. Protocols such as this one have become the standard of care in the management of PPROM.[17]

3. Between 32 and 34 Weeks

Delivery is recommended at ≥34 weeks, or if fetal lung maturity is demonstrated, or if there is evidence of infection, or if a nonreassuring fetal status evolves. At this gestational period, fetal pulmonary maturity can be assessed from either vaginal pool or amniocentesis specimens (see Chapter 9, Fetal Lung Maturity).

4. Intrapartum Management

Vaginal delivery is preferred and recommended unless cesarean delivery is indicated for specific maternal or fetal reasons. Patients can receive pain medications during labor, including epidural analgesic (see Chapter 16, Pain Control in Labor). Continuous electronic fetal monitoring is used during labor. GBS prophylaxis is given if indicated. Patients with PPROM have a significantly higher rate of cesarean delivery due to nonreassuring fetal heart rate patterns. This probably is due to the high incidence of subclinical infection.

IX. Group B Streptococcus Prophylaxis Guidelines

The Centers for Disease Control and Prevention recommendation for universal prenatal GBS prophylaxis is as follows[18]:

- Screening for vaginal and rectal GBS colonization of all pregnant women at 35–37 weeks' gestation.
- Penicillin remains the first-line agent for intrapartum antibiotic prophylaxis, with ampicillin an acceptable alternative.
- Penicillin G, 5 million units IV as the initial dose, then 2.5 million units IV q4h until delivery; alternatively, ampicillin, 2 grams IV as the initial dose, then 1 gram IV q4h until delivery.

- For penicillin-allergic women, their history of penicillin allergy should be assessed during prenatal care; women not at high risk for anaphylaxis should be given cefazolin, 2 grams IV as the initial dose, and then 1 gram IV q8h until delivery.

- For women at high risk for anaphylaxis, clindamycin and erythromycin susceptibility testing, if available, should be performed on isolates obtained during GBS prenatal carriage screening.

- Women with clindamycin- and erythromycin-susceptible isolates should be given either clindamycin, 900 mg IV q8h until delivery, *or* erythromycin, 500 mg IV q6h until delivery. If susceptibility testing is not possible, susceptibility results are not known, or isolates are resistant to erythromycin or clindamycin, the following regimen can be used for women with immediate penicillin hypersensitivity: vancomycin, 1 gram IV q12h until delivery.

- Women whose culture results are unknown at the time of delivery should be managed according to the risk-based approach: the obstetric risk factors (ie, delivery at <37 weeks' gestation, duration of membrane rupture ≥18 hours, or temperature ≥38.0°C [≥100.4°F]).

- Women with negative vaginal and rectal GBS screening cultures within 5 weeks of delivery do not require intrapartum antimicrobial prophylaxis for GBS even if obstetric risk factors develop (ie, same as above).

- Women with GBS bacteriuria in any concentration during their current pregnancy or who previously gave birth to an infant with GBS disease should receive intrapartum antimicrobial prophylaxis.

- In the absence of GBS urinary tract infection, antimicrobial agents should not be used before the intrapartum period to treat asymptomatic GBS colonization.

- Routine intrapartum antibiotic prophylaxis for GBS-colonized women undergoing elective cesarean delivery without labor or rupture of membranes is not recommended.

X. Special Therapy

Amnioinfusion has been suggested as a therapeutic option. There are no adequate controlled trials to support neonatal benefits, although one study did show an increase in cord pH in pregnancies with PPROM that had an amnioinfusion.[19]

XI. Summary

- PPROM occurs in 3%–5% of all pregnancies, accounting for 25%–40% of all preterm deliveries.

- PPROM is a significant cause of infectious perinatal morbidity and mortality.

- Latency period is defined as the interval from time of rupture to onset of labor. Latency is inversely proportional to gestational age.

- Some causes of preterm PROM are potentially preventable, including cigarette smoking, urogenital tract infections, and poor maternal nutrition.

- Expectant management of the pregnancy complicated by PPROM is recommended between 23 and 24 weeks unless evidence of intrauterine infection or maternal and fetal indications for delivery.
- Antenatal corticosteroid administration and broad-spectrum antibiotic administration have been shown to reduce neonatal morbidities.

XII. References

1. Robertson PA, Sniderman SH, Laros Jr RK, et al. Neonatal morbidity according to gestational age and birth weight from five tertiary care centers in the United States, 1983 through 1986. *Am J Obstet Gynecol*. 1992;166:1629–1645.

2. Ventura SJ, Martin JA, Taffel SM, et al. Advance report of final natality statistics, 1993. Monthly vital statistics report from the Centers for Disease Control and Prevention. *Monthly Vital Statistics Report CDC*. 1995;44:1–88.

3. Gabbe SG, Niebyl JR, Simpson JL. Obstetrics: normal and abnormal pregnancies. In Mercer B. *Preterm Premature Rupture of Membranes*. 4th ed. Philadelphia: Churchill Livingstone. 2002:755–827

4. Kitzmiller J. Preterm premature rupture of the membranes. In Fuchs F, Stubblefield PG, eds. *Preterm Birth Causes, Prevention and Management*. New York: Macmillan. 1984:298–346.

5. Lei H, Kalluri R, Furth EE, et al. Rat amnion type IV collagen composition and metabolism: implications for membrane breakdown. *Biol Reprod*. 1999;60:176–182.

6. McLaren J, Taylor DJ, Bell SC. Increased concentration of pro-matrix metalloproteinase 9 in term fetal membranes overlying the cervix before labor: implications for membrane remodeling and rupture. *Am J Obstet Gynecol*. 2000;182:409–416.

7. Lavery JP, Miller CE, Knight RD. The effect of labor on the rheologic response of chorioamniotic membranes. *Obstet Gynecol*. 1982;60:87–92.

8. Romero R, Mazor M, Wu YK, et al. Infection in the pathogenesis of preterm labor. *Semin Perinatol*. 1988;12:262–279.

9. Macones GA, Parry S, Elkousy M, et al. A polymorphism in the promoter region of TNF and bacterial vaginosis: preliminary evidence of gene-environment interaction in the etiology of spontaneous preterm birth. *Am J Obstet Gynecol*. 2004; 190:1504–1508.

10. Mercer BM, Goldenberg RL, Meis PJ, and the NICHD-MFMU Network, et al. The preterm prediction study: prediction of preterm premature rupture of the membranes using clinical findings and ancillary testing. *Am J Obstet Gynecol*. 2000;183:738–745.

11. Mercer BM, Goldenberg RL, Moawad RL, et al. The preterm prediction study: effect of gestational age and cause of preterm birth on subsequent obstetrical outcome. *Am J Obstet Gynecol*. 1999;181:1216–1221.

12. Harding JE, Pang J, Knight DB, et al. Do antenatal corticosteroids help in the setting of preterm rupture of membranes? *Am J Obstet Gynecol*. 2001;184:131–139.

13. Lewis DF, Brody K, Edwards MS, et al. Preterm premature ruptured membranes: a randomized trial of steroids after treatment with antibiotics. *Obstet Gynecol.* 1996;88:801–805.

14. Vermillion ST, Soper DE, Chasedunn-Roark J. Neonatal sepsis after betamethasone administration to patients with preterm premature rupture of membranes. *Am J Obstet Gynecol.* 1999;181:320–327.

15. Egarter C, Leitich H, Karas H, et al. Antibiotic treatment in premature rupture of membranes and neonatal morbidity: a meta-analysis. *Am J Obstet Gynecol.* 1996;174:589–597.

16. Kenyon S, Boulvain M, Neilson J. Antibiotics for preterm rupture of membranes. *Cochrane Database Syst Rev.* 2003;CD001058.

17. Mercer BM, Miodovnik M, Thurnau GR, et al. Antibiotic therapy for reduction of infant morbidity after preterm premature rupture of the membranes. A randomized controlled trial. National Institute of Child Health and Human Development Maternal-Fetal Medicine Units Network. *JAMA.* 1997;278:989–995.

18. Schrag S, Gorwitz R, Fultz-Butts K, et al. Prevention of perinatal group B streptococcal disease. Revised guidelines from CDC. *MMWR Morb Mortal Wkly Rep.* 2002;51(RR-11):1–22.

19. Nageotte MP, Bertucci L, Towers CV, et al. Prophylactic amnioinfusion in pregnancies complicated by oligohydramnios: a prospective study. *Obstet Gynecol.* 1991;77:677–680.

QUESTIONS AND ANSWERS

1. How is PPROM diagnosed?

2. What is the clinical reason for not delivering patients with PPROM immediately?

3. What increases the latency period of patients with PPROM?

4. What drugs improve outcomes in PPROM?

5. What is thought to be the major cause of PPROM?

Answers:

1. Several clinical and historical evaluations have shown to be helpful: (a) most patients give a history of a large gush of fluid per vagina; an exam is required to make sure this is not just the patient urinating due to the excess pressure of the fetus on the maternal bladder; (b) sterile speculum exams are performed to

look for pooling of amniotic fluid in the vagina; (c) Nitrazine paper is used to check the pH of amniotic fluid, which is alkaline and will turn the paper a dark blue color; and (d) a fern test is a microscopic evaluation of dried fluid from the vagina; the proteins in the amniotic fluid crystallize to a classic "ferning" pattern, meaning it has the appearance of the leaf of the fern plant.

2. The longer the fetus stays in utero, the lower the neonatal morbidity and mortality. This is especially beneficial in the very preterm fetus (<28 weeks' gestation) where a few days can markedly improve the chance of survival.

3. Antibiotics have been shown to lengthen the period from rupture of membranes to delivery in patients with PPROM.

4. Corticosteroids decrease morbidity and mortality if administered to any preterm fetus before delivery; antibiotics decrease both maternal and neonatal infectious morbidity and prolong latency, which can play a major role in improving outcome in these neonates; and tocolytics (eg, magnesium sulfate) can prolong the pregnancy at least long enough for administration of corticosteroids.

5. Subclinical infection is the major etiology of PPROM. Bacteria ascend through the cervix into the lower uterine segment to cause a subclinical infection. Neutrophils and macrophages are mobilized to eliminate the infection. The neutrophils lyse and release proteolytic enzymes that not only help kill the bacteria but also damage and weaken the fetal membranes, making them susceptible to rupture.

Fetal Lung Maturity

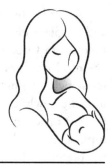

Kathleen M. Berkowitz

CHAPTER

9

LEARNING OBJECTIVES

1. Describe the phases of fetal lung development and the effect of medications on each stage.

2. Outline the physiologic changes in lung function and compliance occurring at birth.

3. State the effect of various maternal and fetal conditions on the development of fully functional fetal lungs.

4. State the indications for and tests available to determine if fetal lung maturity is present.

I. Introduction

For a newborn baby to breathe effectively, its lungs must have completed physical and biochemical processes of maturation. Respiratory transition from intrauterine to extra-uterine function proceeds rapidly through a series of tightly choreographed changes and depends on simultaneous cardiac adaptations. Retained fluid must be cleared, circulation to the pulmonary bed established, and the lungs must be compliant enough to maintain inflation once breathing has begun.

There are four phases of physical lung maturation in fetal life. During the first or embryonic phase at 4–6 weeks' gestation, fetal lung buds and the diaphragm develop. The second phase is the pseudoglandular phase lasting approximately 6–16 weeks' gestation. The general architecture of the lungs is laid out during this time. Mucous glands and cilia develop and fetal breathing motions can be noted in the early second trimester. The third phase of fetal lung development is the canalicular phase, lasting until approximately 26 weeks' gestation. The distal airways form during this time and type II alveolar cells start to develop. The final phase of fetal lung development is marked by both biochemical and physical changes. Cellular apoptosis occurs. Type I cells flatten and thin, creating a permeable basement layer of cells. Type II pneumocytes predominate and produce lipids to decrease the frictional work of breathing. This is one of the final phases of fetal maturation and often does not complete until about 37 weeks' gestation.

At birth, the first breath is triggered by physical and chemical stimulants. Touch and temperature changes initiate the first breath, which requires about −40 to −70 centimeters H_2O pressure. The functional reserve capacity is set at this time, and the chemical changes induced by increasing PaO_2 act to decrease pulmonary vascular resistance. The pressure changes induce the foramen ovale to close, redirecting blood into the newly compliant pulmonary capillary bed. Because the pulmonary system is the last major organ system to achieve competency for the transition to extrauterine survival, it was the first hurdle faced by neonatologists trying to ensure the survival of the preterm infant. The legacy of that struggle remains. At times, it seems almost as if preterm fetuses are considered no more than the sum of their lung capacity. Efforts to determine fetal fitness for birth still revolve around documentation of fetal lung maturity. The occurrences of other near term complications, such as jaundice, feeding difficulties, apneic/bradycardic events and susceptibility to infection, become distant second thoughts once fetal lung maturity has been confirmed. Even in the presence of biochemical evidence of lung maturity, other factors, such as infection and retained lung fluid, can still cause respiratory insufficiency. The practitioner should be aware that significant neonatal morbidity may still be present despite biochemical evidence of lung maturation. The complications associated with relative immaturity of other major organ systems must not be discounted.[1] In a study of patients with ruptured membranes at 32–34 weeks' gestation, the presence of indices of fetal lung maturity was not associated with decreased incidence of major neonatal morbidity.[2]

II. CLINICAL PRESENTATION—PATIENT CASE (PART 1)

J.M. is a 39-year-old gravida 4, para 2-0-1-2, white woman with diabetes and hypertension. Her last child was born approximately 10 years ago and she recently remarried. As her new husband has no children, the couple decided to attempt pregnancy. After three cycles of in vitro fertilizations, they are finally pregnant. She is approximately 12 weeks pregnant and has just been released from the care of her reproductive infertility specialist. She presents to your office for her first prenatal visit, thrilled to inform you that she is carrying twins.

Objective Information: J.M. has good glycemic control and has well-controlled mild to moderate essential hypertension. Her medications include a three times per day insulin regimen, use of an extended release calcium channel blocker, and prenatal vitamins. She has had a recent EKG and checkup with her primary care doctor. She has no evidence of diabetic retinopathy or nephropathy. She has a home blood pressure cuff and logs her blood pressure daily. Blood pressure range is 130–140 mmHg systolic pressure and 80–90 mmHg diastolic pressure. She has minimal proteinuria, recently estimated at 180 mg per day.

III. Pathophysiology

The reader should be unsurprised to see that this case is tailor-made to discuss the varying influences of maternal comorbidities on the expression of fetal lung maturation. Competent function of the lung after birth requires completion of anatomic and biochemical processes. Maternal medical conditions and exposure to medications can regulate these processes, which are very dependent upon the interplay between vasodilatory and vasoconstrictive forces. Vasodilatory forces stimulate angiogenesis, promote alveolar development, and are important in establishing endothelial permeability.[3] Vasoconstrictive forces impair or disrupt alveolar development and expression of lipids by type II pneumocytes.[4]

Anatomic and biochemical maturational processes are summarized in Table 1.[5] Anatomic maturation of the lung is relatively resistant to the influences of hypoxia, fetal homeostasis, and medical therapies. Biochemical pathways are sensitive to these influences, as is most apparent during the third trimester. Cortisol, thyroxine, and

Table 1. Anatomic and Biochemical Processes of Fetal Lung Development: How the Fetal Lung Attains Physiologic Preparedness for Extrauterine Function

Gestational Age	Anatomic Process	Biochemical Process	Physiologic Expression
5–17 wk: Pseudoglandular phase	Lung bud formation; formation of primary, secondary, and tertiary bronchioles	Columnar cells fill with glycoproteins	Formation of bronchopulmonary segments; no gas exchange possible
16–25 wk: Canalicular phase	Enlargement of bronchiolar lumina, vascularization of lung tissue; formation of respiratory bronchioles (terminal sacs)	Expression of lamellar inclusion bodies in some type 2 cells; methylation of lecithin (this process is easily affected by fetal homeostatic changes)	Increased vascularization and formation of respiratory bronchioles permit limited gas exchange after 24 wk
25 wk–birth: Terminal sac period	Epithelial lining of terminal sacs thins; mesenchyme thins and lymphatics develop; capillary invasion of lung tissue accelerates	Type I and type II pneumocytes can secrete lamellar bodies, lecithin and phospholipids	Adequate gas exchange; poor lung compliance
Late third trimester to age 8: Alveolar period	Increasing numbers of alveoli and continued thinning of alveolo-capillary membrane	After wk 36, production of phosphatidylcholine and surfactant	Good gas exchange; good lung compliance

estrogen stimulate the production of surfactant by the type II pneumocytes. The degree of lung compliance is influenced by the concentrations of three main phospholipids—phosphatidylcholine or lecithin, phosphatidylinositol, and phosphatidylglycerol (surfactant or PG). All three lipids are synthesized from the same substrate, phosphatidic acid. Lecithin and phosphatidylinositol appear first, followed by PG. The presence of PG is the best predictor that the lung has attained maximal compliance. Maternal medical conditions that favor the production of PG are thought to enhance fetal lung maturity, whereas those that favor production of phosphatidylcholine and phosphatidylinositol are thought to delay fetal lung maturation.

Hypertension is thought to produce an oxidative stress on the fetus, raising cortisol levels and thus stimulating the production of surfactant. This hypothesis grew from observational studies in the 1970s and '80s that showed that the incidence of respiratory distress syndrome was lower in neonates born to mothers with hypertension.[6,7] Biochemical studies from that era also showed differences in the concentrations of various phospholipids.[8–10] More recently, it has been shown that this effect may be expressed only in small for gestational age babies.[11] Normally grown preterm fetuses of women with hypertensive disease actually have lower lecithin-sphingomyelin (L/S) ratios than preterm fetuses of women without hypertensive disease.[12] Likewise, early observations in diabetic pregnancies suggested delays in fetal lung maturation. The biochemical pathways that supported those observations showed a preponderance of phosphatidylcholine and phosphatidylinositol and a relative lack of PG.[13] There have been significant improvements in management of diabetes in pregnancy; patients with good glycemic control are not thought to have delayed fetal lung maturity in the current era. Current research has focused on the role of pro-angiogenic factors and anti-angiogenic factors on the expression of a "mature" lipid profile by the fetal lung. One pro-angiogenic factor is vascular endothelial growth factor (VEGF), which stimulates the growth of capillary beds. In the human lung, VEGF is expressed in the amniotic fluid in the second trimester and can be found in the alveolar basement membranes and placenta at term. It acts as a potent vasodilator in the neonate, inducing a decrease in pulmonary vascular resistance and enhancing pulmonary membrane permeability. Hypoxic conditions upregulate VEGF gene activity. Amniotic fluid VEGF levels have been found to be lower in diabetic patients and higher in amniotic fluid specimens from women with preeclampsia.[14] Infection causes direct lung injury to the epithelium and increases interstitial fluid production. Finally, genetic polymorphisms are postulated to modulate the fetal response to these stresses.

IV. CLINICAL PRESENTATION—PATIENT CASE (PART 2)

J.M.'s pregnancy proceeds to 33 weeks' gestation before trouble ensues. She has continued to have mild to moderate hypertension and her glucose control has been good. Her twins have grown appropriately, and there has been no evidence of urinary tract infection. She presents to the office with complaints of increased dependent edema. She is found to have significant dependent edema, a blood pressure of 160/100, and a significant increase in proteinuria. A diagnosis of pre-eclampsia is made and she is hospitalized. A set of laboratory values is obtained and shows no evidence of HELLP (*h*emolysis, *e*levated *l*iver enzyme levels and *l*ow *p*latelets) syndrome or severe preeclampsia. Fetal heart rate patterns are reassuring. J.M.'s blood pressure ranges from 130–150 mmHg systolic and 90–94 mmHg diastolic over the next 6 hours.

V. Diagnosis of Fetal Lung Maturity

For this patient, the first decision to make concerns the degree of maternal and fetal risk associated with continuation of the pregnancy. If her condition will allow continued observation and evaluation, it may be acceptable to attempt to prolong the pregnancy. Such attempts should be made only if there is reasonable certainty that pharmacologic therapy can improve the outcomes for the fetuses, the mother, or both. In this situation, the burden of fetal prematurity is still fairly high. If fetal lung maturity can be ascertained, then there is less fetal benefit to be gained by waiting, and more maternal risk is incurred. Older studies of twin pregnancies have reported that twins achieve fetal lung maturation sooner than expected for singleton pregnancies.[15,16] Approximately half of twin pairs achieved biochemical parameters consistent with fetal lung maturity by 32 weeks' gestation. There was up to 25% discordance in indices of maturity noted between twin sacs, however. Discordant fetal size, gender, and zygosity were not found to have consistent effects upon biochemical indices of fetal lung maturation. More recent studies of twin pregnancies have not shown acceleration in indices of fetal lung maturity when twins are compared to singleton pregnancies.[17]

In this situation, it would be preferable not to incur additional fetal or maternal risk should fetal lung maturity be present. Given that neither the patient nor the fetuses are in extremis, an amniocentesis is indicated to obtain fluid for evaluation of biochemical indices of fetal lung maturity. It is preferable to tap both fetal amniotic sacs because of the discrepancies that can be present between twin pairs. However, some practitioners are willing to forego tapping one twin sac and rely on historical data showing that discordance between twins is usually less than 25%. They simply adjust the cut-off value for maturity upward by 25% and assume that even if the unsampled twin has lower biochemical indices, it will still be sufficient for expression of fetal lung maturity.

There are many tests available for estimation of fetal lung maturity. The first test described a mature lung profile as one in which measurable amounts of PG were detected by thin layer chromatography. However, PG is usually the last phospholipid expressed and does not usually become present until 36–37 weeks' gestation. This limits the clinical utility of the test. It was also noted that as phosphatidylinositol levels fell, fetal lung compliance improved. The proportion of some phospholipids was difficult to assay, however. Dr. Gluck and his colleagues developed a method of two-way thin layer chromatography, in which the ratio of phosphatidylcholine (lecithin) to sphingomyelin was measured. This could then be used to predict the presence of fetal lung compliance.[18] A thin layer chromatography plate is prepared and a sample of amniotic fluid applied. The plate is then dipped in an eluting solution and allowed to migrate upon the surface of the plate. After a defined time, the plate is rotated ("two-way") 90 degrees and the eluting solution again forces the lipids to separate. Due to the different speeds at which lecithin and sphingomyelin migrate upon the plate, the lipids are widely separated. A comparison is then made of the relative sizes of the lipid blots. An L/S ratio of greater than 2.0 indicates fetal lung maturity. If the plate is only allowed to elute in one direction, the lecithin blot will contain other phospholipids and be larger than that seen using two-way chromatography. Laboratories using "one-way" chromatography will report an L/S ratio of 2.4 as indicative of fetal lung maturity. The cut-off value of 2.0 or 2.4 was established as the level at which very few infants would develop respiratory distress syndrome. The cut-off value was originally chosen to maximize the negative predictive value (the absence of respiratory distress syndrome) because of the difficulties in dealing with even mild respiratory distress syndrome in the 1960s and 1970s.

Many fetuses with an "immature" fetal lung profile will not develop respiratory distress syndrome. Only 25% of infants with an L/S ratio of 1.0 to 1.5 developed respiratory distress in a 1973 study.[19] It should be noted that contaminants of amniotic fluid will also influence the L/S ratio. Blood has an L/S ratio of approximately 1.8–1.9.[20] Very immature samples of amniotic fluid will thus appear more "mature" and very mature samples will appear less "mature" when contaminated with blood. Meconium contamination renders a sample useless for evaluation of the L/S ratio, as the L/S ratio of meconium varies from 1.1 to 3.6. PG is not present in blood or meconium, so a contaminated sample can still be assayed for PG. Thin layer chromatography tests are difficult to perform and time consuming. If the plate cracks, the testing must be repeated. These limitations led to investigation of other methods for ascertainment of fetal lung maturity.

PG can be assayed by rapid immunologic agglutination tests, which can be performed in about 15 minutes. Amniostat-FLM is a commercially available test that has been available since the early 1980s. The "shake" test and its variant, the foam stability index, are rapid tests that use the principle of surface tension stabilization to determine fetal lung maturity. If significant concentrations of lipids with surface tension stabilizing properties are present, a ring of foam will form around the edge of a container when the fluid is shaken. In the "shake" test, amniotic fluid is mixed in a 50:50 concentration with ethanol and placed in a test tube. It is shaken vigorously for 15 seconds and then placed upright in a rack for 15 minutes. If the ring of foam persists for 15 minutes, fetal lung maturity is inferred to be present. In the foam stability index test, varying concentrations of amniotic fluid and ethanol are mixed. The relative concentration at which the ring of foam is noted to be stable indicates the degree of pulmonary maturity. A cut-off value of 47% correlates well with the presence of an L/S ratio greater than 2.0. The fluorescent polarization test measures the microviscosity of the amniotic fluid. The higher the lipid aggregation, the more intensely it binds a fluorescent dye. The fluorescence is measured by an automatic analyzer. The TDx-FLMII test has been commercially available for several years. A value of 55 mg per gram is considered to reflect the presence of fetal lung maturity. Results for this test are also influenced by contamination of the specimen with blood. Lamellar bodies are packets of lipid extruded by type II pneumocytes. They are approximately the size of platelets and can be counted on an automatic hemoanalyzer. Actual counts are affected by centrifugation, freezing, and the type of autoanalyzer used. In general, counts of about 50,000 indicate pulmonary maturity.

A practical clinical approach is to perform a cascade of tests. Rapid, simple tests are performed first and utilize cut-off values with high negative predictive values. If the rapid, simple tests fail to demonstrate lung maturity, the more complex and expensive tests are added. This approach minimizes the time needed to obtain results and decreases the laboratory costs associated with the more elaborate tests.[21] As with all tests, the prevalence of the disease affects the predictive value of the test result. If a disease is in high prevalence, then the chance of obtaining a "false positive" result is low. As the disease becomes more uncommon, the chance that a "positive" result will be a false positive increases. This should be kept in mind in relation to the gestational age at which the amniotic fluid is obtained, as respiratory distress syndrome is very rare after 37 completed weeks' gestation.

VI. CLINICAL PRESENTATION—PATIENT CASE (PART 3)

J.M. undergoes amniocentesis of each twin sac. There are no complications to the procedure and two uncontaminated specimens are obtained. The samples are sent for cascade analysis. After about 18 hours, the L/S ratios are obtained for both fetuses. Twin A has an L/S ratio of 1.8 and Twin B has an L/S ratio of 1.6. Maternal condition is re-assessed and found to be stable. Both fetuses have reassuring fetal heart rate tracings after amniocentesis.

VII. Pharmacologic Agents to Induce Fetal Lung Maturity

The most important assessment is that concerning the stability of mother and fetuses. Significant decompensation in either should prompt consideration for delivery. As the condition for all three patients appears stable, it is appropriate to turn to pharmacologic agents to assist in inducing fetal lung maturity. As indicated earlier, cortisol, estrogen, and thyroxine stimulate the type II pneumocytes to produce mature lipid profiles. Studies using estrogen, thyroxine, and prolactin failed to produce clinical results.[22–24] However, Dr. Liggins and his colleagues published a landmark trial of corticosteroid administration for induction of fetal lung maturity in 1972.[25] It is one of the best studies ever published and remains clinically relevant today. This trial showed that infants born at less than 32 weeks' gestation who had received betamethasone for at least 24 hours before delivery had significantly decreased rates of respiratory distress syndrome and mortality. Corticosteroids act on the type II pneumocytes to induce the synthesis of precursors for surfactant and increase the production of phosphatidylcholine. They also act on the fetal intestinal tract to induce digestive enzyme production, keratinize fetal skin, and stabilize the fetal germinal matrix to reduce the risk for intracranial hemorrhage. The effects upon the pulmonary system are most marked after 27–28 weeks' gestation, but some benefits can be found as early as 24 weeks' gestation. Below that gestational age, the alveolar stage of lung development has not begun and there are no anatomic structures upon which corticosteroids could act. Beyond 34 weeks' gestation, the incidence of respiratory distress syndrome drops so that any beneficial effects of steroid administration can no longer be detected. Treatment with corticosteroids is effective in multiple gestation, patients with ruptured membranes, and those with maternal medical complications.[26,27] Care must be taken in administering these agents, as patients with metabolic complications such as diabetes or infections can decompensate when treated with corticosteroids. Fetal response to steroid administration is maximal within 48 hours of the first dose, and the clinical effects of the steroid course can be seen for 1–2 weeks. Because of the possible effects of repeated courses of steroids on fetal growth and metabolic parameters, only a single course of therapy is recommended at this time (Table 2). Recommended drug regimens are outlined in Table 3. It should be noted that there is a potential anatomic

Table 2. Guidelines for Use of Antenatal Corticosteroids for Fetal Maturation*

NIH 2000 Consensus Statement	ACOG Committee Opinion 402
• Benefits of antenatal administration of corticosteroids to fetuses at risk of preterm delivery outweigh the risks. • All fetuses at 24–34 weeks' gestation at risk of preterm delivery should be considered candidates for treatment. • Decision to use steroids should not be altered by fetal race, gender, or availability of surfactant replacement therapy. • Patients eligible for therapy with tocolytics are eligible for treatment. • Because treatment for less than 24 hours is associated with significant reductions in mortality, RDS, and IVH, antenatal corticosteroids should be given unless immediate delivery is anticipated. • For PPROM at less than 30–32 weeks' gestation in the absence of clinical chorioamnionitis, antenatal corticosteroid use is recommended because of the high risk of IVH at these early gestational ages. • In complicated pregnancies in which delivery before 34 weeks' gestation is likely, antenatal corticosteroid use is recommended unless there is evidence that corticosteroids will have an adverse effect on the mother or delivery is imminent.	• A single course of corticosteroids is recommended for all pregnant women at 24–34 weeks of gestation at risk of preterm delivery within 7 days • A single course of antenatal corticosteroids should be administered to women with PROM before 32 weeks of gestation. The efficacy of corticosteroid use at 32–33 completed weeks of gestation for PPROM is unclear based on available evidence, but may be beneficial. • There are no data regarding the efficacy of corticosteroid use before viability, and it is not recommended at this time. • Because of insufficient scientific evidence, repeat corticosteroid courses are not recommended.

IVH = intraventricular hemorrhage, PPROM = preterm premature rupture of membranes, PROM = premature rupture of membranes, RDS = respiratory distress syndrome.
*From National Institutes of Health,[26] and American College of Obstetricians and Gynecologists.[27]

Table 3. Comparison of Treatment Regimens: Optimal Benefit Begins 24 Hours after Initiation of Therapy and Lasts 7 Days

Medication	Regimen	Comments
Betamethasone	2 doses of 12 mg of betamethasone given IM 24 h apart	Longer half-life, better bioavailability Significant reduction in mortality May protect against some forms of periventricular leukomalacia
Dexamethasone	4 doses of 6 mg of dexamethasone given IM 12 h apart	Has not been shown to decrease overall mortality May be more available for administration than betamethasone

cost to the antenatal administration of corticosteroids. In vitro studies of the effect of dexamethasone on the morphologic development of human lung have shown that higher concentrations of dexamethasone cause marked reductions in alveolar lumen size and reduced the volume density of type II pneumocytes.[28] This highlights the importance of following the recommended dosing schedule. Some practitioners, when faced with a patient whom they feel may deliver precipitously, will modify the dosing schedule so that all of the recommended doses are received in a shortened time interval. If this were to result in higher concentrations of medication within the fetal compartment, there might be a reversal of the beneficial effects of dexamethasone, which are seen at the lower concentrations in in vitro studies.

VIII. CLINICAL PRESENTATION—PATIENT CASE (PART 4)

J.M. receives two 12-mg doses of betamethasone 24 hours apart. She is noted to have a decompensation in glucose levels on the second day after administration of corticosteroids, which is treated with an insulin drip. The effect of corticosteroid administration wanes over the next week and she returns to her normal subcutaneous doses of insulin. She spontaneously ruptures her membranes at $33\frac{1}{2}$ weeks' gestation, giving birth without incident. After a 2-week stay in the neonatal intensive care unit, the family is taught how to use the apnea monitor and demonstrates competency in basic lifesaving techniques. The babies are then discharged home; further evaluation of neonatal complications will occur for the next 2 years of life.

IX. Summary

Fetal lung maturation is the sum of anatomic and biochemical processes that allow for adequate gas exchange. The transition from intrauterine to extrauterine function must be accomplished quickly. Maternal medical conditions can affect this maturation process via dysregulation of vasoactive and vasoconstrictive enzyme pathways. For a patient at risk to deliver prematurely, amniocentesis can be performed to determine if fetal lung maturity is present. There are several reliable tests commercially available. If a fetus is at risk for preterm delivery, corticosteroids should be administered to mitigate the risks of preterm birth. Corticosteroids induce fetal lung maturation mainly by action on biochemical pathways, although there may be some undesirable morphologic changes in the lung associated with their use. The benefits of corticosteroid therapy far outweigh the risks. Care should be taken when administering corticosteroids to a woman with diabetes or infection, as corticosteroids could make her susceptible to an intensification of those conditions. A single course of therapy is recommended. It should be noted that even in cases when fetal lung maturity has been proved, other morbidities may occur. The patient and her family should be counseled extensively concerning these risks and the risks of delivery without the use of corticosteroids.

X. References

1. Ghidini A, Hicks C, Lapinski RH, et al. Morbidity in the preterm infant with mature lung indices. *Am J Perinatol.* 1997;14:75–78.

2. Refuerzo JS, Blackwell SC, Wolfe HM, et al. Relationship between fetal pulmonary maturity assessment and neonatal outcome in premature rupture of the membranes at 32–34 weeks gestation. *Am J Perinatol.* 2001;18:451–458.

3. Lassus P, Ristimaki A, Olavi Y, et al. Vascular endothelial growth factor in human preterm lung. *Am J Respir Crit Care Med.* 1999;159:1429–1433.

4. Levy M, Muarey C, Chailley-Heu B, et al. Developmental changes in endothelial vasoactive and angiogenic growth factors in the human perinatal lung. *Ped Res.* 2005;57:248–253.

5. Katz M, Meizner I, Insler V. Development and maturation of the fetal lung. In *Fetal Well Being: Physiological Basis and Methods of Clinical Assessment.* Boca Raton, FL: CRC Press, 1990.

6. Yoon JJ, Kohl S, Harper RG. The relationship between maternal hypertensive disease of pregnancy and the incidence of idiopathic respiratory distress syndrome. *Pediatrics.* 1980;65:735–739.

7. Chiswick ML. Prolonged rupture of membranes, pre-eclamptic toxaemia, and respiratory distress syndrome. *Arch Dis Child.* 1976;51:674–679.

8. Whitsett JA, Stahlman MT. Impact of advances in physiology, biochemistry and molecular biology on pulmonary disease in neonates. *Am J Respir Crit Car Med.* 1998;157:S67–S71.

9. Bustos R, Kulovich MV, Gluck L, et al. Significance of phosphatidylglycerol in amniotic fluid in complicated pregnancies. *Am J Obstet Gynecol.* 1979;133:899–903.

10. Kulovich MV, Gluck L. The lung profile. II Complicated pregnancy. *Am J Obstet Gynecol.* 1979;135:64–70.

11. Varner MW, Dildy GA, Hunter C, et al. Amniotic fluid epidermal growth factor levels in normal and abnormal pregnancies. *J Soc Gynecol Invest.* 1996;3:17–19.

12. Winn HN, Klosterman A, Amon E, et al. Does preeclampsia influence fetal lung maturity? *J Perinat Med.* 2000;28:210–213.

13. Quirk JH, Bleasdale JE. Fetal lung maturation in the pregnancy complicated by diabetes mellitus. In DiRenzo GC, Hawkins PF, eds. *Perinatal Medicine: Updates and Controversies.* London: Wiley, 1984.

14. Vourela P, Helske CH, Alitalo K, et al. Amniotic fluid soluble vascular endothelial growth factor receptor-1 in pre-eclampsia. *Obstet Gynecol.* 2000;95:353–357.

15. Leveno KJ, Quirk PJ, Whalley PJ, et al. Fetal lung maturation in twin gestation. *Am J Obstet Gynecol.* 1984;148:405–411.

16. Whitworth NS, Magann EF, Morrison JC. Evaluation of fetal lung maturity in diamniotic twins. *Am J Obstet Gynecol* 1999;180(Pt 1):1438–1441.

17. Winn HN, Romero R, Roberts A, et al. Comparison of fetal lung maturation in preterm singleton and twin pregnancies. *Am J Perinatol.* 1992;9:326–328.

18. Gluck L, Kulovich MV, Borer RC. The interpretation and significance of the lecithin-sphingomyelin ratio in amniotic fluid. *Am J Obstet Gynecol.* 1974;120:142–148.

19. Gluck L, Kulovich MV, Borer RC, et al. Diagnosis of the respiratory distress syndrome by amniocentesis. *Am J Obstet Gynecol.* 1973;115:541–550.

20. Cotton DB, Spillman T, Bretaudiere JP. Effect of blood contamination on lecithin to sphingomyelin ratio in amniotic fluid by different detection methods. *Am J Obstet Gynecol.* 1975;121:321–323.

21. Garite TJ, Freeman RK, Nageotte MP. Fetal maturity cascade: a rapid and cost-effective method for fetal lung maturity testing. *Obstet Gynecol.* 1986;67:619–622.

22. Ballard PL, Gluckman PD, Brehier A, et al. Failure to detect an effect of prolactin on pulmonary surfactant and adrenal steroids in fetal sheep and rabbits. *J Clin Invest.* 1978;62:879–883.

23. Australian collaborative trial of antenatal thyrotropin-releasing hormone (ACTOBAT) for prevention of neonatal respiratory distress syndrome. *Lancet.* 1995;345:877–880.

24. Ballard RA, Ballard PL, Cnaan A, et al. Antenatal thyrotropin-releasing hormone for prevention of lung disease in preterm infants. *N Engl J Med.* 1998;338:493–498.

25. Liggins GC, Howie RN. A controlled trial of antepartum glucocorticoid treatment for prevention of the respiratory distress syndrome in premature infants. *Pediatrics.* 1972;50:515–522.

26. National Institutes of Health. Antenatal corticosteroids revisited: repeat courses. *NIH Consensus Statement* 2000;17:1–18.

27. American College of Obstetricians and Gynecologists. Antenatal corticosteroid therapy for fetal maturation. ACOG Committee Opinion. Number 402. March 2008. *Obstet Gynecol* 2008;111:805–808.

28. Odom MJ, Snyder JM, Boggaram V, et al. Glucocorticoid regulation of the major surfactant associated protein (SP-A) and its messenger ribonucleic acid and of morphological development of human fetal lung in vitro. *Endocrinol.* 1988;123:1712–1720.

QUESTIONS AND ANSWERS

1. Corticosteroids should be administered

    a. weekly, once risk for preterm birth is identified

    b. only in patients with ruptured membranes

    c. to patients at 23 weeks' gestation

    d. to patients with intact membranes at 30 weeks with preterm labor

2. Betamethasone is preferred over the administration of dexamethasone because

    a. of cost and availability

    b. it requires fewer injections

    c. it has been associated with better mortality rates than dexamethasone

    d. it has shorter half life

3. Which of the following patients should be considered for amniocentesis?

    a. 27 weeks' gestation with hypertension

    b. 33 weeks' gestation with twins, preterm labor

    c. 38 weeks' gestation, severe preeclampsia

    d. 31 weeks' gestation, preterm labor with diabetes

4. Alveolar phase of lung development continues until age 8.

    True or False

Answers:

1. d; 2. c; 3. b; 4. T

Multifetal Gestation

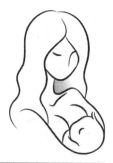

John P. Elliott

LEARNING OBJECTIVES

1. Identify at least three major physiologic changes that significantly affect multifetal gestations.

2. Recognize that each additional fetus in the uterus will reduce the average gestational age at delivery by 3.5 weeks.

3. List six circumstances that increase the risk of pulmonary edema when tocolytic drugs are used in pregnancy.

4. Name a class of drugs that causes an increase in contractions when given in multifetal gestations.

I. Introduction

Multifetal gestations are those with more than one fetus developing in the uterus. In the past, these pregnancies were relatively infrequent, with twins representing just over 1% of all births (approximately 1:90). Monozygotic twins (one embryo splitting into two identical fetuses) occur at a constant rate (3.5/1000) in all populations, while dizygotic twinning (two eggs ovulated, fertilized, and implanted in the same cycle) varies by age, race, and within families. Approximately two-thirds of twins are dizygotic and one-third are monozygotic, and of the monozygotic twins, two-thirds are monochorionic (one placenta) and one-third are dichorionic (two separate placentas). For twins, 99% are diamniotic (have their own sac), but 1% will share both the placenta and one single amnion (sac).[1]

The number of multifetal births in a population can be estimated by applying Hellin's rule,[2] which states that if the rate of twins in a population is known (1/N), then the rate of spontaneous triplets will be $1/N^2$, and quadruplets will be $1/N^3$, etc. Using this estimate in the United States, spontaneous twin births occur in 1 in 90 births, so triplets would occur 1 in 8100, quads 1 in 729,000, and quintuplets 1 in 64 million.

Multifetal gestations are far more common than those statistics would suggest. By far the most important factor in the increasing incidence of multiple gestations is the advances that have occurred in infertility therapy. Twins now represent approximately 3.4% of all births[3] and triplets may occur in 1 in 500 births. This dramatic increase has a fallout in terms of influence on mortality and morbidity for these babies, most of which is related to prematurity.[4]

II. PATIENT CASE [PART 1]

Let me introduce you to J.M. She is a 32-year-old woman who wanted to start her family. She required infertility assistance and underwent ovarian stimulation and intrauterine insemination with her husband's sperm. In a life-changing accident, six eggs were released, fertilized, and began to grow in her uterus. At 19 weeks' gestation, she was admitted to the hospital for treatment of severe iron deficiency anemia with IV iron and epoetin alfa (Epogen) to stimulate red blood cell (RBC) production by her bone marrow. During the admission, she developed preterm contractions, which were treated with a subcutaneous (SC) terbutaline pump. Additional tocolysis became necessary as the pregnancy progressed. At 27 weeks, the patient was stable and betamethasone was administered (12 mg IM q24h ×2) to benefit the six fetuses after delivery. The steroids triggered preterm labor (PTL) with cervical change.[5] Magnesium sulfate ($MgSO_4$) was initiated and at one point was being administered at 5.5 g/h. Her PTL was arrested and she was maintained on $MgSO_4$, SC terbutaline, and ibuprofen. The patient was physically and psychologically exhausted and wanted delivery. We were able to extend the pregnancy to 31 4/7 weeks, when a cesarean section was performed for delivery. The patient received several uterotonic drugs including oxytocin (Pitocin); miso-prostol (Cytotec), 1000 mg/rectum; and methylergonovine (Methergine), 0.2 mg IM. The uterus contracted strongly and estimated blood loss was only 800 mL. Postoperatively, the patient developed tachycardia, dyspnea, and tachypnea and had blood pressure of 150/105 mmHg. A diagnosis of cardiomyopathy[6] was made and treatment with dobutamine, furosemide, nitroglycerine, and felodipine supported her poor cardiac output (4.8 L/min) and ejection fraction of 15%. She recovered rapidly from the cardiomyopathy and was discharged on postpartum day 9. The six babies all were discharged without known serious morbidity at 36.5 weeks of age.

III. Pathophysiology

Pregnancy has a profound impact on maternal anatomy and physiology, which is further exaggerated by the addition of extra fetuses. Maternal blood volume (which is increased by 40% in singleton pregnancy)[7] is increased by about 70%[8] in twins and more in high-order multiples (HOM). There is a dilutional anemia due to greater expansion of plasma volume compared to RBC increase.[9] Additionally, a significant increase in the glomerular filtration capacity of the kidneys results in more rapid elimination of medications that are cleared by the kidney. There is an alteration in clotting factors, making pregnant women more likely to suffer venous thromboembolism. Multifetal gestations are placed at greater risk for almost every complication of pregnancy.

There are no published figures regarding maternal mortality in a multiple gestation. The best estimate is about 1:3000 high-order pregnancies compared with about 1:10,000 for singleton pregnancies.[10] Hemorrhage, pulmonary embolus, and hypertensive complications are the common causes of death, while morbidity in the mother is increased by many factors. The increased iron and folate depletion by multiple fetuses creates iron deficiency anemia in approximately 20% of twins[11] and 30%–40% of HOM. Megaloblastic anemia is uncommon.[12] Preeclampsia is increased in twins to approximately 20%–25%[13] and in HOM gestation it occurs in up to 60%–70%.[14] This is probably related to more paternal antigens in multiple placentas. Placental hormones including human placental lactogen affect the action of insulin, increasing the incidence of gestational diabetes.[15] The overexpansion of the uterus at the time of delivery increases the risk of uterine atony and excessive blood loss.[16] Peripartum cardiomyopathy is increased in older women and multiple gestations.[17] Pulmonary edema is a risk in pregnancy. Factors predisposing to pulmonary edema include fluid overload, infection, multiple gestation, anemia, and hypertension.[18]

The fetuses are also at risk for greater mortality and morbidity than singleton gestations. Intrauterine demise of one fetus in a twin pregnancy is reported to occur during the second or third trimester in 2%–5% of pregnancies.[19] Monochorionic twins are at greater risk for mortality and morbidity due to the vascular connections that occur between the circulations of the fetuses. Fetal death can occur due to unequal sharing of blood in what is called twin-twin transfusion syndrome (TTTS). TTTS occurs in 5%–30% of monochorionic twins. Placental insufficiency is also more common in multifetal gestation, leading to an increase in stillbirth and small for gestational age (<3rd percentile) or intrauterine growth restricted (<10th percentile) babies. Neonatal death rates are increased for multifetal gestations, mostly due to the increased preterm delivery rate of these pregnancies.

The morbidity of multifetal fetuses is increased considerably over singleton pregnancies. Congenital malformations, which occur in 3%–4% of singleton pregnancies, occur in 7%–8% of twins, with the most common defects being cardiac malformations, neural tube defects, facial clefting, gastrointestinal anomalies, and abdominal wall defects.[20] The morbidity from prematurity is substantial. As a general rule, each additional fetus in the uterus takes approximately 3.5 weeks off the mean gestational age at delivery. The mean gestational age for delivery of twins is 36.5 weeks, triplets 33 weeks, quadruplets 29.5 weeks, and quintuplets 28 weeks. This places multiple babies at risk for gestational age–related morbidity.[21] Premature delivery is due to PTL, preeclampsia, preterm premature rupture of membranes, severe growth restriction, fetal jeopardy in utero, and, with HOM gestations, iatrogenic prematurity.[22] Multiple gestations are also at greater risk for cerebral palsy (CP). The largest known risks for CP are prematurity, low birth weight (<2500 grams), and very low birth weight (<1500 grams).[23] Multifetal pregnancies result in more babies that fit into those risk categories.

IV. Detection

Multifetal gestation should be suspected in all patients who have infertility therapy. Additionally, patients with a history of twins in the mother's family, those with a uterine size larger than dates, and patients with an abnormal elevated maternal serum alpha fetoprotein screening test are at increased risk of twinning. These patients should have a screening ultrasound (US) examination. In the early 1970s, about half of multifetal gestations were not diagnosed until childbirth, but now, in patients receiving prenatal care, it would be quite unusual to find a surprise at birth.

Real-time US examination revolutionized obstetric care in the late 1970s. This provided a safe methodology for assessing the fetus, placenta, amniotic fluid, and maternal structures, including the uterus, cervix, and adnexa. US is particularly useful in multifetal gestations. After establishing that there is more than one embryo, the most important determination is the chorionicity of the placenta. This is most easily determined in the first trimester by transvaginal US.[24,25] At 4–5 weeks, the number of chorionic sacs can be counted. At week 6, the yolk sac and fetal poles can be visualized and fetal cardiac activity should be visualized. Two chorionic sacs with two yolk sacs will determine dichorionic/diamniotic twins. One chorionic sac with two yolk sacs would define a monochorionic pregnancy. The amniotic membrane may be difficult to visualize until week 8 of gestation. At 10 weeks and beyond, chorionicity can be determined by assessing the amniotic membrane. In pregnancies with a fused placental mass, there will be a wedge-shaped extension of placenta between the layers of amnion.[26] The membrane will also appear "thick," which identifies separate chorions or placentas. A thin, wispy membrane that is frequently difficult to visualize will indicate a monochorionic placenta. Early US in the first trimester is 100% accurate in determining chorionicity. US performed in the second or third trimester is less accurate in determining chorionicity (approximately 90%).[27] Factors to assess include fetal gender, the presence of two separate placental masses, and assessment of the amniotic membrane. An important point for the clinician in management is that if the chorionicity can not be determined accurately, the twins should be assumed to have monochorionic placentation and managed as if they are at risk for TTTS. Monozygotic twins will have dichorionic/diamniotic (Di/Di) placentation 66% of the time, monochorionic/diamniotic (Mo/Di) placentation 33%, and monochorionic/monoamniotic (Mo/Mo) 1%. Monoamniotic twins are at risk for sudden mortality from umbilical cord occlusion due to cord entanglement.[28]

V. Treatment

The goal of management of multiple gestation pregnancies is to deliver the patient at the "best" gestational age, which would balance prematurity with the potential harmful effects of placental aging. Studies have confirmed that the lowest fetal mortality for twins occurs at 36–38 weeks. For triplets, the ideal delivery is between 35 and 36 weeks and with quadruplets it is between 33 and 34 weeks' gestation. In our practice, we recommend the following:

		Delivery age
Twins	Di/Di	37–38 wk
	Mo/Di	36–37 wk
	Mo/Mo	32–34 wk
Triplets		35 wk
Quads		34 wk
Quints		34 wk
Sextuplets		33 wk

Individual cases may be carried further with normally growing fetuses each having its own placenta. Earlier delivery may be necessary for intrauterine growth restriction, oligohydramnios, or abnormal fetal assessment.

A. Nonpharmacologic Therapy

Diet in a multifetal gestation is extremely important. Total weight gain for twin pregnancies is targeted at 40–45 pounds with 24 pounds by 24 weeks. For triplets the ideal weight gain is 50–75 pounds, and for quadruplets it is 75–100 pounds.[29] Luke and Eberlein recommend a 3500- to 4000-calorie diet that is rich in red meat protein.[29] Other recommendations include one prenatal vitamin in the first trimester and two a day in the second and third trimesters. Supplemental iron should be given in the second and third trimesters and calcium (3 g/d), magnesium (1.2 g/d), and zinc (45 mg/d) added in the second trimester as well. Because PTL is so prevalent in multifetal pregnancies, there are some interventions that can reduce the incidence of contractions. These are not treatments for PTL, but merely reduce background contractions.[30] The first is decreased physical activity. Touching the uterus generally stimulates a contraction, so the theory is to minimize uterine stimulation by decreasing activity (bed rest with bathroom privileges). The second intervention is decreased psychological stress, which can be accomplished by patient education and confidence in the plan of management. Biofeedback techniques may also be helpful.

As mentioned previously, monochorionic placentation creates a risk for TTTS. The risk results from vascular anastomoses (particularly arteriovenous) that are unbalanced and create volume overload of one fetus (recipient) and volume depletion of the other (donor). This leads to amniotic fluid differences in the sac of the donor (oligohydramnios) and the recipient (polyhydramnios). Size discordance frequently occurs with the recipient growing normally, and the donor grows smaller (≥1.5-week difference). Treatment has been with therapeutic amniocentesis[31] in the past, and many cases are now treated by selective laser coagulation of these anastomoses.[32,33] Despite therapy, there is a high rate of mortality and morbidity, including CP from hypovolemia in the donor (even if there is survival of both babies), and morbidity and mortality related to prematurity.[21]

B. Pharmacologic Therapy

As is true for any pregnancy, multifetal gestations cause multiple changes in the anatomy and physiology of the mother. The intravascular volume is increased by 20%–

80% and cardiac output and stroke volume are enhanced. Blood flow to all organs is increased, including the kidneys, which results in an increase in the creatine clearance. This results in more rapid elimination of medications that are excreted by the kidney. The peak dose of drugs after administration is lower and the half-life is shorter. This tends to result in requiring a larger dose of a given drug or administering it more frequently to achieve therapeutic results.

Tocolytic drugs are administered in pregnancy to treat PTL. PTL complicates about 40% of twin gestations and up to 90% of quadruplet gestations.[12] The most commonly prescribed drug for acute tocolysis is $MgSO_4$. This therapy has been criticized as being ineffective[34]; however, close examination of studies of $MgSO_4$ as a tocolytic in singleton gestations reflect that there is increasing success with increasing dosage of the drug when the outcome is delay of delivery for 48 hours.[35] In HOM gestations it was clearly demonstrated that higher doses of $MgSO_4$ were required to achieve therapeutic serum levels of the drug,[36] which is what determines the success of a tocolytic medication.

One of the most important therapeutic advances in the effort to improve the outcome of premature infants is the beneficial effects that have been demonstrated in premature babies whose mothers had been treated with betamethasone before delivery.[37] The benefits include decreased mortality, decreased incidence and severity of respiratory distress syndrome, decreased incidence of intraventricular hemorrhage, and lower incidence of patent ductus arteriosus. An unexpected side effect of betamethasone administration in HOM gestations was the demonstration that steroids caused PTL and even preterm delivery after routine administration.[5] This property of causing an increase in contractions is also reflected in the daily diurnal variation in cortisol in the body, in which cortisol release is increased between 4 PM and 3 AM, with an increase in contractions observed.

Pulmonary edema is a complication of tocolytic therapy. It is associated with $MgSO_4$ tocolysis, but the magnesium administration plays a small permissive role in patients who develop this complication. In our experience, pulmonary edema will occur only in the presence of one or more risk factors for cardiac stress. These would include underlying cardiac disease, fluid overload, hypertension, anemia, multifetal gestation, or infection. $MgSO_4$ does lower the colloid oncotic pressure slightly,[37] which would slightly alter the balance of forces favoring fluid to leave the intravascular space into the tissues, including the lungs. To minimize pulmonary edema in the treatment of PTL in multifetal gestations, careful attention must be given to balancing the input and output.[38]

C. Monitoring and Follow-Up

Multifetal pregnancies should be carefully followed every 1–2 weeks. Cervical length US should be performed between 18 and 24 weeks to assess risk for preterm delivery. In monochorionic pregnancies, fluid assessment should also be done every 1–2 wks from 16 to 24 weeks. Growth US is also recommended every 3–4 weeks. Assessment of the cervix by digital exam should be done every 2 weeks. Home contraction monitoring and fetal fibronectin testing may be used by clinicians to assess the ongoing status of the pregnancy.[30]

VI. PATIENT CASE [PART 2]

J.M. gave birth at 31 4/7 weeks. The delivery time was a compromise between the significant discomfort and maternal risk of a sextuplet pregnancy balanced against the risks of prematurity for her six babies. At delivery the blood loss was minimal, which contributed to a sudden large redistribution of her blood volume. The uterus was receiving about 20% of the cardiac output, which after delivery fell to 3%–5%. This resulted in a dilated cardiomyopathy, which resolved with aggressive chronotropic and inotropic support. This complication was always a theoretical risk, but this was the first time we actually observed its occurrence.

VII. Summary

Multifetal gestations are more common in the United States, with twins representing almost 3.5% of births occurring each year. Twins account for a disproportionate amount of morbidity and mortality in the population due to PTL and problems related to poor growth and placentation. HOM gestations will deliver prematurely, but management of these pregnancies must be focused on achieving the optimum gestation for elective birth.

Pharmacologic intervention in these pregnancies must be modified to account for the effects of the anatomy and physiology of the multifetal gestation. Larger doses of drugs are necessary to achieve the same effect as is achieved in a nonpregnant individual. This is true for tocolytic drugs ($MgSO_4$, terbutaline, nonsteroidal anti-inflammatory agents, or nifedipine [Procardia]), antibiotics, antiepileptics, antihypertensive drugs, etc. Assessment of the patient and proper treatment will minimize the complications that are inherent in these very special pregnancies.

VIII. References

1. Blickstein I, Kieth LG, eds. *Multiple Pregnancy—Epidemiology, Gestation, and Perinatal Outcome.* 2nd ed. London: Taylor and Francis, 2005.

2. Guttmacher AF. The incidence of multiple births in man and some of the other unipara. *Obstet Gynecol.* 1953;2:22–35.

3. National Vital Statistics Report. 2005.

4. Scholtz T, Bartholomaus S, Grimmer I, et al. Problems of multiple births after ARTT: medical, psychological, social and financial aspects. *Hum Reprod.* 1999;14:2932–2937.

5. Elliott JP, Radin TG. The effect of corticosteroid administration on uterine activity and preterm labor in high order multiple gestation. *Obstet Gynecol.* 1995; 85:250–254.

6. Christ K, Yarkoni A, Byrne T, et al. Rapidly resolving cardiomyopathy in a mother of sextuplets. *J Repro Med.* (Submitted May 2008).

7. Pritchard JA. Changes in the blood volume during pregnancy and delivery. *Anesthesiology*. 1965;26:393–399.

8. Veille JC, Morton MJ, Burry KJ. Maternal cardiovascular adaptations to twin pregnancy. *Am J Obstet Gynecol*. 1985;153:261–263.

9. Cunningham FG, Gant NF, Leveno KG, et al. editors. *Williams Obstetrics*. 22nd ed. New York,: McGraw-Hill, 2005.

10. Bleyl J. [Personal Communication]. Director, The Triplet Connection. Support group for multiple gestation families. (http://www.tripletconnection.org)

11. Spellacy WN, Handler A, Ferre CD. A case-controlled study of 1253 twin pregnancies from a 1982–1987 database. *Obstet Gynecol*. 1990;75:168–171.

12. Campbell DM. Maternal adaptation in twin pregnancy. *Semin Perinatol*. 1986; 10:14–18.

13. Coonrod DV, Hickok DE, Zhu K, et al. Risk factors for preeclampsia in twin pregnancies: a population-based cohort study. *Obstet Gynecol*. 1995;85:645–650.

14. Francois K, Sears C, Wilson R, et al. Maternal morbidity and obstetrical complications of quadruplet pregnancy: twelve year experience at a single institution (abstract). *Am J Obstet Gynecol*. 2001;184:S174.

15. Corrada F, Caputo F, Facciola G, et al. Gestational glucose intolerance in multiple pregnancy (abstract). *Diabetes Care*. 2003;26:1646.

16. Malone FD, Kaufman GE, Chelmow D, et al. Maternal morbidity associated with triplet pregnancy. *Am J Perinatol*. 1998;15:73–77.

17. Van Hoeven KH, Kitsis RN, Katz SD, et al. Peripartum versus idiopathic dilated cardiomyopathy in young women—a comparison of clinical pathologic, and prognostic features. *Int J Cardiol*. 1993;40:57–65.

18. Elliott, JP. Unpublished data of the author.

19. Malone FD, D'Alton MF. Multiple gestation. In Creasy RK, Resnik R, eds. *Maternal Fetal Medicine*. 5th ed. Philadelphia: Saunders, 2004;513–536.

20. Onyskowova Z, Dolezal A, Jedlicka V. The frequency and the character of malformations in the multiple birth. *Teratology*. 1971;4:496–501.

21. Garite TJ, Clark RH, Elliott JP, et al. Twins and triplets: the effect of plurality and growth on neonatal outcome compared with singleton infants. *Am J Obstet Gynecol*. 2004;191:700–707.

22. Elliott JP, Miller HS, Coleman S, et al. Indicated and non-indicated preterm delivery in twin gestations: impact on neonatal outcomes and cost. *J Perinatol*. 2005;25:4–7.

23. Bejar R, Vigliocci G, Gramajo H. Antenatal origin of neurologic damage in newborn infants: II. Multiple gestations. *Am J Obstet Gynecol*. 1990;162:1230–1236.

24. Monteagudo A, Timor-Tritsch IE, Sharma S. Early and simple determination of chorionic and amniotic type in multiple gestations in the first fourteen weeks by high frequency transvaginal ultrasonography. *Am J Obstet Gynecol*. 1994;170:824–829.

25. Cooperman AB, Benaceraf B. Early first-trimester ultrasound provides a window through which the chorionicity of twins can be diagnosed in an in vitro fertilization (IVF) population. *J Assist Reprod Genet*. 1995;12:693–697.

26. Finberg H. The "twin peak" sign: reliable evidence of dichorionic twinning. *J Ultrasound Med.* 1992;11:571–577.

27. Winn HN, Gabrietti S, Reece EA, et al. Ultrasonographic criteria for the prenatal diagnosis of placental chorionicity in twin gestations. *Am J Obstet Gynecol.* 1989;161:1540–1542.

28. Heyborne KD, Porreco RP, Garite TJ, et al. Improved perinatal survival of monoamniotic twins with intensive inpatient monitoring. *Am J Obstet Gynecol.* 2005;192:96–101.

29. Luke B, Eberlein T. *When You Are Expecting Twins, Triplets, or Quads.* New York: HarperCollins, 2004.

30. Elliott JP. Management of high-order multiple gestation. *Clin Perinatol.* 2005; 32:387–402.

31. Elliott JP, Urig MA, Clewell WH. Aggressive therapeutic amniocentesis for treatment of twin-twin transfusion syndrome. *Obstet Gynecol.* 1991;77:537–540.

32. Quintero RA, Dickinson JE, Morales WJ, et al. Stage-based treatment of twin-twin transfusion syndrome. *Am J Obstet Gynecol.* 2003;188:1333–1340.

33. Senat MV, Deprest J, Boulvain M, et al. Endoscopic laser surgery versus serial amnioreduction for severe twin-twin transfusion syndrome. *N Engl J Med.* 2004;351:136–144.

34. Grimes DA, Nanda K. Magnesium sulfate tocolysis time to quit. *Obstet Gynecol.* 2006;108:986–989.

35. Elliott JP, Lewis DF, Morrison JC, et al. In defense of magnesium sulfate. *Obstet Gynecol.* 2009; in press.

36. Elliott JP, Radin TG. Serum magnesium level during magnesium sulfate tocolysis in high order multiple gestations. *J Reprod Med.* 1995;40:450–452.

37. NIH Consensus Development Panel. Antenatal corticosteroids revisited: repeat courses. National Institutes of Health Consensus Development Conference Statement, August 17-18, 2000. *Obstet Gynecol.* 2001;98:144–150.

38. Yeast J, Halberstadt C, Meyer BS, et al. The risk of pulmonary edema and colloid osmotic pressure changes during magnesium sulfate infusion. *Am J Obstet Gynecol.* 1993;169:1566–1571.

QUESTIONS AND ANSWERS

1. Physiologic changes in multifetal gestations that affect pharmacology include which of the following?

   a. a significant increase in the intravascular blood volume, lowering the peak concentration of drugs

   b. alteration in clotting factors, which results in protection of the pregnant female against spontaneous clotting (deep venous thrombosis or pulmonary embolism)

   c. a significant increase in the glomerular filtration rate, which causes more rapid excretion of many drugs

   d. a and c

   e. a, b, and c

2. Each additional fetus that a woman is carrying will decrease the average gestational age at delivery by:

   a. 6 weeks

   b. 3.5 weeks

   c. 1 week and 1 day

   d. 31 hours

3. Important factors that contribute to the development of pulmonary edema in pregnancy include which of the following?

   a. multifetal gestation, fluid overload, anemia

   b. corticosteroids, cardiac disease, hypertension

   c. magnesium sulfate, chronic liver disease, infection

   d. all of the above

4. Which drugs cause an increase in contractions when given to patients with multifetal gestations?

   a. antibiotics

   b. narcotics

   c. corticosteroids

   d. antihypertensives

Answers:

1. d; 2. b; 3. a; 4. c

Gestational Hypertension, Preeclampsia, and Eclampsia

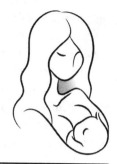

Julie Scott and Michael R. Foley

CHAPTER

11

LEARNING OBJECTIVES

1. Compare the definitions for gestational hypertension, preeclampsia, and eclampsia.

2. List three clinical scenarios classified as hypertensive emergencies.

3. Describe the typical screening tools used in the obstetrician's office for preeclampsia.

4. Summarize the basic management of preeclampsia in the antepartum and intrapartum periods.

I. Introduction

Pregnancy-related hypertension includes a spectrum of hypertensive disorders that contribute to both maternal and fetal morbidity and mortality. In the United States, 16% of pregnancy-related deaths are attributed to pregnancy-induced hypertension.[1] The National High Blood Pressure Education Program Working Group on High Blood Pressure in Pregnancy provides the accepted definitions for characterization of blood pressure in pregnancy. These categories include chronic hypertension, preeclampsia, chronic hypertension superimposed with preeclampsia, gestational hypertension, and transient hypertension.[2] Both chronic hypertension and chronic hypertension with superimposed preeclampsia are discussed in Chapter 22, Chronic Hypertension. All pregnancy-related hypertensive disorders discussed are defined by blood pressure elevations in systolic blood pressure ≥140 mmHg and/or diastolic blood pressure ≥90 mmHg measured in the sitting position at a minimum of 6 hours apart with Korotkoff phase I and V (disappearance) defining the blood pressure measurements.

The most frequent cause of hypertension in pregnancy is gestational hypertension affecting 6%–17% of nulliparous and 2%–4% of multiparous women.[3] Gestational hypertension is hypertension that occurs after 20 weeks' gestation in women known to be normotensive before pregnancy, without any other associated features, and resolves in the postpartum period. Mild gestational hypertension that develops late in the

177

pregnancy has similar outcomes as normotensive pregnancies except for a high rate of cesarean delivery that results from failed induction of labor. Gestational hypertension may be categorized as severe if there are sustained elevations in systolic blood pressure to at least 160 mmHg and/or diastolic blood pressure to at least 110 mmHg demonstrated on two separate occasions at least 6 hours apart. Progression to preeclampsia may occur in up to 50% of women who are diagnosed with gestational hypertension before 30 weeks' gestational age.[4] These pregnancies do have increased perinatal morbidities similar to severe preeclamptic pregnancies.[5]

Preeclampsia complicates between 2% and 8% of pregnancies.[6,7] Preeclampsia is hypertension with proteinuria of 300 mg or more in a 24-hour period that develops after 20 weeks gestational age in a previously normotensive woman. If a urine dipstick is used on a random sample, then a 1+ reading (at least 30 mg/dL) must be achieved on two separate occasions at least 6 hours apart. Urine dipstick evaluations are highly variable and have been shown to not correlate well with a 24-hour collection for protein and should not be used to diagnose severe proteinuria.[8] The gold standard for measurement of protein content in the urine is a 24-hour collection. Preeclampsia is severe if the hypertension present is ≥160 mmHg systolic or ≥110 mmHg diastolic or there are any associated symptoms or features consistent with organ involvement. These associated symptoms may be neurologic, including headache and visual disturbances, epigastric or right upper quadrant pain indicating impaired liver function (or changes noted by liver function tests), renal impairment demonstrated by oliguria of ≤500 cc/24 hours or severe proteinuria of ≥5 g/24 hours, respiratory complaints of shortness of breath from pulmonary edema detailing pulmonary involvement, hematologic involvement demonstrated by thrombocytopenia and/or hemolysis, and even placental involvement detailed by fetal growth restriction, oligohydramnios, abruption, or nonreassuring fetal status detailed by antenatal surveillance.

HELLP syndrome is considered a severe form of preeclampsia. The word HELLP is descriptive of the metabolic derangements: *h*emolysis, *e*levated *l*iver function tests, and *l*ow *p*latelets. The level of laboratory abnormalities to make the diagnosis of HELLP syndrome remains controversial. Based on expert opinion, hemolysis is evidenced by a declining hemoglobin and hematocrit level with evidence of microangiopathic anemia with a breakdown of cells on a peripheral smear. Elevated liver function tests are typically set at levels of transaminases >70 units/L and low platelets evidenced by thrombocytopenia of <100,000/mm³. Additionally, elevations of LDH and bilirubin with decreased haptoglobin levels further detail the potential end organ damage attributed to HELLP syndrome.

Eclampsia is considered one of the most severe manifestations of preeclampsia, and it is marked by seizures. This is a rare complication occurring in approximately 1% of preeclamptic pregnancies. These seizures can occur before pregnancy, during delivery, and also in the postpartum period. Most often, eclampsia occurs in the third trimester or within 48 hours of delivery. The majority of the cases reported occur in the third trimester of pregnancy. Perinatal morbidities are related to gestational age at delivery, abruption of the placenta yielding hypoxia, and placental insufficiencies thereby impacting growth. Intracranial hemorrhage, neurologic sequelae from recurrent seizure activity and edema, pulmonary complications such as pulmonary edema and aspiration pneumonia, cardiovascular injuries including ischemia, and acute hypertensive emergencies may result with the development of eclampsia, contributing to its significant impact on maternal mortality.

II. PATIENT CASE (PART 1)

Mrs. Upton is a 36-year-old African American gravida 1 para 0 at 36 5/7 weeks' gestation, based on her last menstrual period, who presents for routine prenatal care to her obstetrician's office. Her pregnancy has been complicated by gestational diabetes that has been well controlled with a diabetic diet. Her medical history is significant for an elevated body mass index of 29 kg/m³ and seasonal allergies. An appendectomy was performed at age 16. Her family history is significant for both diabetes and hypertension on both sides of her family, with her father suffering a heart attack at age 53. She is a nonsmoker, drank socially before pregnancy, and has never tried any illicit drugs. At today's office visit she complains of lower back pain, swelling, and a mild headache. She otherwise feels well and reports good fetal movement. On physical examination, the physician has noted a blood pressure of 142/88 and continued lower extremity edema with pitting edema to the knees (this has been persistent at the last three office visits). Notably, her patellar reflexes are brisk and she does not exhibit clonus. She also denies any tenderness to palpation of her abdomen and demonstrates fetal heart tones at 145 with palpable fetal movement. Her routine urinalysis is negative for evidence of infection and details an increased specific gravity, no glucose, and +2 protein.

III. Clinical Presentation

Hypertensive disorders may not necessarily be symptomatic unless they complicate or increase the severity of a preexisting condition. A great majority of women will present to their physician's office unaware of their blood pressure elevations and/or proteinuria. This is why there is such tremendous value in screening for its occurrence as a means to prevent further obstetric complications. Women who receive prenatal care will have regularly scheduled office visits temporally spaced throughout their pregnancy, with increased frequency beginning at 28 weeks with visits every 2 weeks. These visits will then be scheduled on a weekly basis from about 35 weeks on until delivery occurs. Included in every obstetric visit are blood pressure measurement, urinalysis, and a gross evaluation of the fetus for well-being. It is within the last third of pregnancy when the vast majority of gestational hypertension, preeclampsia, and eclampsia occur (concurrent with increased visits to the physician). Women exhibiting symptoms related to pregnancy-related hypertension by definition have severe disease and warrant further detailed evaluation. Physicians should always be cognizant of risk factors to offer earlier diagnosis and interventions to limit potential complications with ongoing disease (Table 1).

Table 1 Risk Factors for Developing Preeclampsia

Age
Nulliparity
Black race, especially Nigerian
Low socioeconomic status
Multiple gestation
Personal or family history of preeclampsia, HELLP syndrome, or eclampsia
Maternal chronic disease: chronic hypertension, diabetes, collagen vascular disease,
    metabolic syndrome
Antiphospholipid syndrome
Current gestational hypertension
Increased body mass index
Hypercoagulability (thrombophilias)
Renal disease
Hydatidiform mole

HELLP = hemolysis, elevated liver enzymes, and low platelets.

Acute presentations of hypertensive disease are typically urgent in nature, with severe elevations of blood pressure yielding clinically relevant disease manifestations. Hypertensive urgencies are severely elevated blood pressures *without* signs or symptoms of acute target organ damage, whereas hypertensive emergencies do have associated end organ damage of the central nervous system, the heart, or the kidneys (Table 2). Systemic vascular resistance related to humoral vasoconstrictors is thought to be the cause of hypertensive crises. Endothelial injury altering normal autoregulatory function of the vessel results in ischemic injury and further release of vasoactive substances. Thus continues a cascade of vasoconstriction.[9] Successful management and evaluation of the gravida with elevated pressures requires a targeted history and physical examination supported by appropriate laboratory studies. A necessary portion of the physical examination is an evaluation of the fetus for evidence of complications from hypertensive disease. This includes assessment of growth, amniotic fluid

Table 2 Hypertensive Emergencies

Hypertensive encephalopathy
Acute aortic dissection
Acute pulmonary edema with respiratory failure
Acute myocardial infarction/unstable angina
Eclampsia
Acute renal failure
Microangiopathic hemolytic anemia

Acute Management of Hypertensive Emergencies
Hydralazine: 5 mg IV bolus, then 10 mg every 20–30 min to a maximum dose of 30 mg
Labetalol: 10 mg IV test dose, then 20 mg given 10 min later, can be followed by 40 mg
    given 10 min later, followed by 80 mg 10 min thereafter for a total dose of 220 mg. Also
    can be used as a continuous infusion at 1–2 mg/min.
Nifedipine: 10 mg orally, can be repeated up to 30 mg total at 20-min intervals. Severe
    hypotension may result with concurrent use of magnesium sulfate.
Sodium nitroprusside: 0.25 µg/mg/min to 5 µg/mg/min titrated. Long-term administration
    may result in fetal cyanide poisoning.

volume, and specific antepartum testing for in utero well-being, such as the nonstress test or biophysical profile.

IV. Pathophysiology

The precise etiology of preeclampsia remains an extensive area of research and is most likely multifactorial. Accepted models for preeclampsia consistently detail abnormal placentation with failure to modify the uterine circulation with maternal immunomodulatory dysregulation as paramount to the disease process. This maladaptive process producing hypoxia and, ultimately, oxidative stress leads to the release of vasoactive mediators, pro- and antiangiogenic in nature.[10] Endothelial dysfunction ensues, with responses generated from the maternal immune system.[11] Data support that the clinical manifestations of preeclampsia are a late sign of the disease process that has been ongoing since placentation. Normal placentation requires the embryo to provide a differentiated trophoblast lineage capable of providing not only a means of low capacitance attachment to the uterus via the spiral arteries for trophic needs, but also a barrier to prevent release of trophoblastic materials into the maternal circulation, which could stimulate the maternal immune response.[12]

The pro- and antiangiogenic factors produced by the placenta that enter the maternal vascular system to exert their actions are among the exciting new molecules discovered to potentially play an important role in the clinically relevant features of preeclampsia. Soluble fms-like tyrosine kinase-1 (sFlt-1) is a placentally derived antagonist of vascular endothelial growth factor (VEGF). sFlt-1's actions are mediated through binding of VEGF receptor-1 and VEGF receptor-2. Its interaction with these receptors blocks the potent angiogenic and mitogenic properties of VEGF for endothelial cells. Similarly, sFlt-1 also inhibits placental growth factor (PlGF), which is a member of the VEGF family of growth factors chiefly produced by the placenta. Decreased circulating levels of VEGF and PlGF are contributory to the endothelial dysfunction seen in the clinically apparent features of preeclampsia. The vascular tone mediated by the endothelium is lost, which leads to hypertension (via the activities of angiotensin II), vascular permeability (of the glomerulus yielding proteinuria), and upregulation of coagulation factors results in coagulopathy.[10,13] Further, circulating factors induced by the relative hypoxic state and oxidative stress activate the placental renin-angiotensin system, which also damages the endothelium.

The maternal immune response may also contribute to the disease process. Cytokines such as tumor necrosis factor-α and interleukin-6 have been reported to be elevated in preeclamptic pregnancies. In vivo modeling has shown these inflammatory cytokines to cause increases in arterial pressure and to decrease renal plasma flow and glomerular filtration rate.[14,15] Maternal adaptations of the immune response are crucial not only in overall immune health, but also play a distinct role in responsiveness to disease states.[11]

V. Detection, Screening, and Diagnosis

Gestational hypertension and preeclampsia are hypertensive disorders of pregnancy that are routinely screened for as a regular part of prenatal care. Blood pressure monitoring and urine sampling occur at each office visit with an obstetric provider. Careful history and examination skills may provide clues as to changes in the overall health of the patient, who may not realize she has elevated pressures, including new onset head-aches and visual disturbances marked by diplopia and scotomata, nausea and vomiting with abdominal pain, swelling especially of the hands and face, and increased brisk responses of the reflexes. These symptoms are nonspecific, but present as a constella-tion of findings with elevated blood pressures and proteinuria, provide much concern for underlying pathology.

Presently, there are no acceptable screening tests that can accurately predict pre-eclampsia with enough sensitivity to make them widely accepted in clinical practice. Promising serum markers include sFlt-1, soluble endoglin (sEng), and PlGF, which have been shown to be altered in the sera of preeclamptic women.[16–18] Both sFlt-1 and sEng are antiangiogenic, whereas PlGF is a growth factor supporting vascular growth and remodeling. Various studies have investigated these markers with attempts to pro-vide cut-off levels predictive of disease, but reproducibility and prospective applicabil-ity remain difficult.

VI. Prevention

Strategies to prevent preeclampsia continue to be investigated in clinical trials. How-ever, because the exact etiopathogenesis of the disease is yet to be fully defined, a true cure or means of prevention has not been found. Disparate results of clinical trials exist because of wide variations in methodologies applied. As with most human research, larger multicenter prospective trials must be completed before therapies are instituted.

Calcium supplementation has been proposed as a dietary supplement that may play a role in vascular tone, based on earlier work linking hypocalciuria to preeclam-psia and its known involvement in calcium-dependent smooth muscle contraction. However, in a large multicenter trial involving healthy nulliparous women given 2 grams of elemental calcium versus placebo, there were no significant differences in the incidence and severity of preeclampsia. In women at high risk for preeclampsia there may be some benefit based on the data from recent trials. Further work needs to occur to validate these results.[3,19]

The benefit of low-dose aspirin is still under investigation. Aspirin inhibits throm-boxane synthesis, thereby affecting platelet aggregation. Platelet disturbances and endothelial dysfunction are key findings in preeclampsia. Several large studies failed to demonstrate efficacy in the reduction of incidence in preeclampsia or by improvement in perinatal outcomes. These studies included women deemed to be at high risk for the disease and still did not show any therapeutic response. These data are problem-atic in that the studies were underpowered and therefore potentially could not dem-onstrate significant benefits. Based on the available data, routine recommendation of low-dose aspirin for the prevention of preeclampsia should not be done until there are convincing data of its proven benefit.[3,19]

Other dietary factors, including the antioxidants vitamins C and E, zinc, and omega-3 fatty acids, have all been investigated in clinical trials with no proven benefit on perinatal outcomes. These agents also should not be routinely recommended for supplementation for the prevention of preeclampsia. Certain risk factors may be modifiable for the gravid patient including weight management with diet and exercise to limit comorbid medical diseases, such as obesity, diabetes, and hypertension.

VII. Treatment

A. Antepartum Management

Diagnosis typically occurs based on the suspicions of the practitioner. Elevated blood pressures and examination of the urine for protein ultimately provide the disease label. Currently, the only cure for preeclampsia is delivery. Yet this may be deleterious for a fetus who has not reached full maturation at a minimum of 37 weeks' gestation, thereby increasing the risks for neonatal morbidity and mortality secondary to prematurity. Depending on the severity of the disease and any other concomitant illnesses, a woman may be considered as a candidate for temporization of the pregnancy until either the disease state warrants delivery or an appropriate gestational age is reached. Typically, the blood pressures must be mild, the woman demonstrates no severe symptoms, and there is no evidence of fetal jeopardy in utero. Often, the gravid patient will be admitted to the hospital for a 24-hour observation period where serial blood pressures, baseline laboratory tests (complete blood count with platelets, creatinine, liver function studies, lactate dehydrogenase), and fetal surveillance can occur to make an appropriate decision for continuation of the pregnancy with either an outpatient status or inpatient monitoring.

Optimal management for gestational hypertension and preeclampsia in the antepartum setting is multimodal. Lifestyle choices are typically modified even though there is little supporting evidence of its efficacy in pregnancy. Women are routinely placed on modified bed rest and given instructions to reduce stress and eliminate strenuous exercise. Dietary adjustments are also offered for the woman with significant lower extremity edema by means of reduced sodium intake. Antepartum testing to monitor fetal status should be scheduled regularly. Most authorities agree that, at a minimum, weekly to two times a week antenatal surveillance is appropriate once there is a diagnosis. The nonstress test evaluates fetal heart rate patterns and biophysical profile testing, which is an ultrasound-based tool, evaluates fetal parameters, such as muscle tone, movement, and breathing, along with a calculation of the amniotic fluid volume to assess for the possibility of hypoxemia and acidemia in utero. The ultimate goal of antenatal testing is to prevent fetal death.[20] If any of these tests are abnormal, further testing and/or delivery may be necessary. Antenatal steroids (either betamethasone or dexamethasone) should be considered for those women with pregnancies between the gestational ages of 24 and 34 weeks who are at risk of premature delivery to promote fetal maturation.[21]

Pharmaceutical management of hypertension is critically important to prevent maternal sequelae for women with severe elevations of blood pressure. Most practitioners would agree to treatment of mean arterial pressures ≥125 mmHg with systolic blood pressure >155 mmHg and diastolic blood pressure ≥100 mmHg. Important to the management of these pressures is the continued desire to maintain uteroplacental blood flow for fetal well-being. The exact pressure level is variable from patient to patient where maximal benefit would be achieved, but typically blood pressures from the 130s to 150s/80s to 100s are tolerated well for both the mother and her baby. The ultimate goal for blood pressure management is to prevent acceleration of blood pressures to dangerous levels and to permit continuation of the pregnancy for fetal growth and development. For asymptomatic women with only mildly elevated blood pressure there appears to be no improvement in perinatal outcomes with pharmaceutical management and there may even be an increased risk of small for gestational age infants in women who receive treatment.[19,22]

Methyldopa is a first-line antihypertensive agent that has been extensively studied for efficacy and safety in pregnancy.[23] It is a centrally acting α_2-agonist acting through neurotransmitter pathways to decrease sympathetic outflow to the heart, kidneys, and peripheral vasculature. Initial starting doses are 250 mg BID with typical onset of action in 3–6 hours. Dosing parameters should be changed at 2-day intervals to a maximal dose of 1000 mg BID. Tolerance may occur after 2 months of therapy, requiring titration of the medicine. Typical side effects include somnolence, depression, orthostatic hypotension, and worsening of peripheral edema. This medication is considered safe for breastfeeding.

Nifedipine is another widely used medication in pregnancy, not only for hypertension but also for management of symptomatic preterm contractions. Available evidence has detailed that it is safe in pregnancy during any trimester. It is a calcium channel blocker that blocks calcium from entering the voltage-gated channels of vascular smooth muscle, thereby causing relaxation. Abrupt and severe maternal hypotension results from sublingual dosing of this medication and therefore should never be administered by this route. Flushing, headache, and peripheral edema (onset 2–3 weeks after administration) are among the common side effects. Typical dosing is 10–30 mg TID or via a sustained daily release formulation with maximal dosing between 120 and 180 mg daily. Tablets over capsule formulations may be better for the pregnant patient as they have been shown to cause fewer hypotensive episodes.[24] Care in prescribing this medication is important as it interacts with many others that are hepatically metabolized.

Labetalol has become increasingly the drug of choice for treatment of preeclampsia, especially its parenteral administration for severe preeclampsia. It is an α/β-blocker that provides a reliable reduction in blood pressure with fewer side effects than other antihypertensive agents. Fetal risks are also thought to be lower as fetal heart rate and uteroplacental blood flow demonstrate little change with its administration.[19] Dosing intervals are twice daily, with typical starting doses of 200–800 mg/d to a maximum daily dose of 2400 mg.

Hydralazine is a direct vasodilator of arterioles with a long history of safety and efficacy in pregnancy. Its parenteral administration for acute hypertension control is more common than chronic oral therapy. Typical dosing parameters require four times a day dosing, which can lead to compliance problems with this medication. Usual doses are 25–100 mg/d divided dosing. Maternal and neonatal lupuslike syndrome has occurred with this medication and is more common with larger doses or prolonged administration.

Both angiotensin-converting enzyme inhibitors and angiotensin-receptor blockers are to be avoided in pregnancy secondary to their fetotoxic effects. When used in the second and third trimesters, these classes of agents induce fetal and neonatal renal failure, probably related to fetal hypotension and decreased renal blood flow. Subsequent amniotic fluid abnormalities ensue, including oligohydramnios and anhydramnios, yielding other morbidities, including pulmonary hypoplasia and limb contractures. Fetal calvarial hypoplasia probably results from a combination of hypotension and deformation from lack of amniotic fluid.[25] Use of these agents poses calculated risks to the fetus and with other potential medication options available should not be used.

Diuretic therapy is also to be avoided as a treatment option for hypertension acutely compromising pregnancy. During the antenatal period, unless the patient is suffering from florid cardiac or respiratory failure, diuretics are essentially contraindicated in the treatment of preeclampsia. Acute diuresis will adversely affect the uterine blood flow, resulting in potentially dramatic reduction in placental perfusion. This can have a direct effect on the fetal physiologic status and further exacerbate compromised uteroplacental function.

B. Intrapartum and Postpartum Management

The one medication with a proven track record to prevent worsening of preeclampsia to eclampsia is magnesium sulfate ($MgSO_4$).[26] The exact mechanism of action is still unknown for the prevention of seizure activity, but is believed to be related to its ability to cause cerebral vascular dilation.[27] Typical management protocols include a 4- to 6-gram IV loading dose given over 20–30 minutes with a continuous IV infusion of 2 g/h. If an IV has not been established, then a total dose of 10 grams of a 50% $MgSO_4$ solution (divided to 5 g/buttock) can be administered IM. Care must be taken for patients with renal insufficiency as clearance is decreased, which could lead to toxicities, including respiratory depression and cardiac arrest. Toxicities require immediate management with advanced life support skills and the administration of calcium gluconate (10 mL of 10% solution) infused over 3 minutes to combat dangerous levels. Although delivery is the primary treatment of preeclampsia/eclampsia, this does not necessarily mean that one must deliver operatively. Clinical judgment and the usual obstetric indications for operative delivery will determine the route of delivery. Often, the vaginal route proves to be the safest for the mother without the additional surgical risks. $MgSO_4$ should be continued for at least 24 hours into the postpartum period. Postpartum eclampsia should also be treated with a 24-hour maintenance dose of $MgSO_4$, timed from the onset of the seizure activity.

The preeclamptic gravida who has been receiving the appropriate seizure prophylaxis with $MgSO_4$ may still progress to having convulsions. In addition to basic life support skills during the seizure episode, it is important to rebolus the $MgSO_4$ to a total of 6 grams from the continuous infusion level (ie, continuous infusion rate is 2 grams/h and the patient seizes, then bolus with 4 grams of $MgSO_4$ over 15 minutes). If the seizure activity is ongoing despite treatment, sodium amobarbital, phenytoin, and diazepam are alternative agents. This would be an extremely rare situation as most eclamptic seizures are self-limited, resolving typically within 5–10 minutes of onset.

VIII. PATIENT CASE [PART 2]

The decision is made to admit the patient to the hospital for further evaluation and bed rest with serial blood pressure measurements and continuous electronic fetal monitoring. Obstetric ultrasound is performed, revealing an appropriately grown fetus with adequate amniotic fluid in vertex presentation. A 24-hour urine is performed, detailing 412 mg/d protein, and laboratory studies as follows: hemoglobin/hematocrit 14 g/dL and 46%, respectively; platelets 158,000/mm³; creatinine 0.8 mg/dL; aspartate aminotransferase 28 IU/L; and alanine aminotransferase 32 IU/L. Fetal monitoring is reassuring and the maternal blood pressures range from the 130s to 150s/80s to 100s. The patient continues to complain of headache intermittently, but is reported with increased frequency compared to the day before.

Mrs. Upton is diagnosed with preeclampsia and concern for evolution to severe preeclampsia with continued reports of headache (considered a severe symptom). As she has achieved an acceptable gestational age when the neonatal morbidity is far less than the maternal morbidity associated with continuation of the pregnancy, her physician plans for delivery via an induction of labor. Intrapartum management includes seizure prophylaxis with MgSO$_4$ loaded at a 4-gram IV bolus with maintenance of 2 g/h and adequate pain management to decrease blood pressure elevations secondary to catecholamine release from pain. A female child is born weighing 3300 grams with Apgar scores of 8 and 9 at 1 minute and 5 minutes, respectively, and transitions well to newborn life. Mrs. Upton is stable after delivery with blood pressures remaining elevated in the 140s to 150s/90s, but no further symptoms. She is transitioned to postpartum care with continued maintenance of the MgSO$_4$ infusion for the next 24 hours for continued seizure prophylaxis. This medication is then discontinued on postpartum day 2 and she is feeling well and meeting all appropriate postpartum milestones.

IX. Summary

Pregnancy-related hypertensive disorders are commonly encountered in obstetric medicine. Recognition of problematic blood pressures and symptoms prompts the practitioner to evaluate for preeclampsia. Preeclampsia, unique to pregnancy, can only be treated by delivery. Temporization of pregnancy may be achievable in certain clinical situations even in specific patients with evidence of severe disease. Progression to eclampsia necessitates intervention to treat the seizure focus and plan for delivery to prevent further maternal and fetal morbidities and mortality. Early diagnosis and treatment of preeclampsia to maintain pregnancy will be one of the greatest achievements in obstetric medicine, with many working diligently toward this goal.

X. References

1. Chang J, Elam-Evans L, Berg CJ, et al. Pregnancy-related mortality surveillance— United States, 1991–1999. *MMWR Surveill Summ.* 2003;52:1–8.

2. U.S. Department of Health and Human Services. National High Blood Pressure Education Program. *The Seventh Report of the Joint National Committee on Prevention, Detection, Evaluation and Treatment of High Blood Pressure.* U.S. Department of Health and Human Services. National Institutes of Health. National Heart, Lung and Blood Institutes. NIH Publication Number 04-5230. 2004:48–53.

3. Sibai, BM. Diagnosis and management of gestational hypertension and preeclampsia. *Obstet Gynecol.* 2003;102:181–192.

4. Barton JR, O'Brien JM, Bergauer NK, et al. Mild gestational hypertension remote from term: progression and outcome. *Am J Obstet Gynecol.* 2001;184:979–983.

5. Buchbinder A, Sibai BM, Caritis S, et al. Adverse perinatal outcomes are significantly higher in severe gestational hypertension than in mild preeclampsia. *Am J Obstet Gynecol.*2002;186:66–71.

6. Saftlas AF, Olson DR, Franks AL, et al. Epidemiology of preeclampsia and eclampsia in the United States, 1979–1986. *Am J Obstet Gynecol.* 1990;163:460–465.

7. American College of Obstetricians and Gynecologists. Diagnosis and management of preeclampsia and eclampsia. *ACOG Practice Bulletin.* Number 33. January 2002. *Obstet Gynecol.* 2002;99:158–167.

8. Meyer NL, Mercer BM, Friedman SA, et al. Urinary dipstick protein: a poor predictor of absent or severe proteinuria. *Am J Obstet Gynecol.* 1994;170:137–141.

9. Varon J, Marik PE. The diagnosis and management of hypertensive crises. *Chest.* 2000;118:214–227.

10. Lam C, Lim K, Karumanchi SA. Circulating angiogenic factors in the pathogenesis and prediction of preeclampsia. *Hypertension.* 2005;46:1077–1085.

11. Visser N, van Rijn BB, Rijkers GT, et al. Inflammatory changes in preeclampsia: current understanding of the maternal innate and adaptive immune response. *Obstet Gynecol Survey.* 2007;62:191–200.

12. Huppertz B. Placental origins of preeclampsia challenging the current hypothesis. *Hypertension.* 2008;51:970–975.

13. Shah D. Preeclampsia: new insights. *Curr Opin Nephrol Hypertens.* 2007;16:213–220.

14. LaMarca BB, Bennett WA, Alexander BT, et al. Hypertension produced by reductions in uterine perfusion in the pregnant rat: role of tumor necrosis factor-α. *Hypertension.* 2005;46:1022–1025.

15. Gadonski G, LaMarca BB, Sullivan E, et al. Hypertension produced by reductions in uterine perfusion in the pregnant rat: role of IL 6. *Hypertension.* 2006;48:711–716.

16. Levine RJ, Maynard SE, Qian C, et al. Circulating angiogenic factors and the risk of preeclampsia. *N Engl J Med.* 2004;350:673–683.

17. Chaiworapongsa T, Romero R, Kim YM, et al. Plasma soluble vascular endothelial growth factor receptor-1 concentration is elevated prior to the clinical diagnosis of preeclampsia. *J Matern Fetal Neonatal Med.* 2005;17:3–18.

18. Hertig A, Berkane N, Lefevre G, et al. Maternal serum sFlt-1 concentration is an early and reliable predictive marker of preeclampsia. *Clin Chem.* 2004;50:1701–1703.

19. Frishman WH, Schlocker SJ, Awad K, et al. Pathophysiology and medical management of systemic hypertension in pregnancy. *Cardiol Rev* 2005;13:274–284.

20. American College of Obstetricians and Gynecologists. Antepartum fetal surveillance. *ACOG Practice Bulletin.* Number 9. October 1999.

21. American College of Obstetricians and Gynecologists. Antenatal corticosteroid therapy for fetal maturation. *ACOG Committee Opinion.* Number 273. May 2002. *Obstet Gynecol.* 2002;99:871–873.

22. Von Dadelszen P, Magee LA. Antihypertensive medications in management of gestational hypertension-preeclampsia. *Clin Obstet Gynecol.* 2005;48:441–459.

23. James PR, Nelson-Piercy C. Management of hypertension before, during and after pregnancy. *Heart.* 2004;90:1499–1504.

24. Montan S. Drugs used in hypertensive diseases in pregnancy. *Curr Opin Obstet Gynecol.* 2004;16:111–115.

25. Briggs GG, Freeman RK, Yaffe SJ. *Drugs in Pregnancy and Lactation: A Reference Guide to Fetal and Neonatal Risk.* 8th ed. Philadelphia: Lippincott Williams & Wilkins, 2008.

26. Magpie Trial Collaborative Group. Do women with preeclampsia, and their babies, benefit from magnesium sulfate? The Magpie Trial: a randomized placebo-controlled trial. *Lancet.* 2002;359:1877–1890.

27. Aagaard-Tillery KM, Belfort MA. Eclampsia: morbidity, mortality and management. *Clinical Obstet Gynecol.* 2005;48:12–23.

QUESTIONS AND ANSWERS

1. The most frequent cause of hypertension is:

   a. chronic hypertension

   b. preeclampsia

   c. gestational hypertension

   d. nephropathy

2. Preeclampsia is defined by:

   a. systolic blood pressure (BP) ≥140 or diastolic BP ≥90 mmHg measured at two different times at least 6 hours apart with proteinuria of 300 mg in a 24-hour collected sample.

   b. systolic BP ≥160 or diastolic BP ≥110 mmHg measured at two different times at least 6 hours apart with proteinuria of 5 grams in a 24-hour collected sample.

    c. systolic BP ≥130 or diastolic BP ≥80 mmHg measured at two different times at least 6 hours apart.

    d. systolic BP ≥140 or diastolic BP ≥90 mmHg measured at two different times at least 6 hours apart with lower extremity edema pitting +2.

    e. systolic BP ≥140 or diastolic BP ≥90 mmHg measured at two different times at least 6 hours apart with scotomata and right upper quadrant pain.

3. Definitive treatment of preeclampsia requires:

    a. strict control of blood pressure with magnesium sulfate

    b. delivery

    c. strict control of blood pressure with hydralazine

    d. delivery followed by curettage of the uterus for all placental tissue

4. The following two medications should be strictly avoided in pregnancy secondary to their fetotoxic effects:

    a. hydralazine and methyldopa

    b. lisinopril and losartan

    c. labetalol and metoprolol

    d. nifedipine and labetalol

Answers:

1. c; 2. a; 3. b; 4. b

Abruptio Placentae

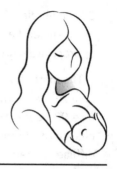

Tamerou Asrat

LEARNING OBJECTIVES

1. State the incidence and importance of abruptio placentae.

2. Describe the pathophysiology of abruptio placentae.

3. Summarize the diagnosis of abruptio placentae.

4. Outline the management of abruptio placentae.

I. Introduction

Abruption of the placenta refers to the premature separation of a normally implanted placenta before the delivery of the fetus.[1] Although there are no strict criteria for the diagnosis of placental abruption, the clinical findings of vaginal bleeding and pain arising from uterine contractions and, at times, fetal heart rate tracing abnormalities are the hallmarks of placental abruption. The vaginal bleeding seen in placental abruption results from the rupture of maternal vessels in the decidua basalis. This blood in turn causes a separation of the placenta from the uterus and, most commonly, escapes through the cervix. However, in about 20% of the cases when abruptio placentae is diagnosed, the blood does not escape through the cervix, giving rise to a "concealed" abruptio placentae.[2] The hematoma may be small and contained, leading to a partial abruption, or at times the dissection can lead to a complete separation of the placenta (total abruption), leading to fetal compromise and/or death.

II. PATIENT CASE [PART 1]

A 37-year-old gravida 5 para 4 African American patient presents to the labor and delivery unit at 29 weeks' gestation complaining of vaginal bleeding that began earlier that morning. She is in moderate distress, but reports normal fetal movements. The patient's pregnancy has been uncomplicated except for the finding of an unexplained elevation of the maternal serum alpha fetoprotein (MSAFP) at

3.96 multiple of the median at 17 weeks' gestation. The patient's four previous pregnancies have been uneventful, all ending in successful vaginal deliveries of appropriately grown newborns.

The maternal examination reveals her to be in moderate distress, with persistent complaints of lower abdominal pain. Her blood pressure is 151/92 mmHg, pulse rate 98 beats/min, and respiratory rate 18 breaths/min. There is no antecedent history of chronic hypertension. The abdominal examination is normal with mild diffuse tenderness. The fundal height is 28 centimeters, suggesting an appropriately grown fetus. A speculum examination shows a small amount of fresh blood in the posterior vaginal vault. There is no active bleeding emanating from the cervical os. There are no lesions or tears of the cervix or vaginal walls. The fetal heart rate tracing is reassuring with frequent accelerations, normal variability, and no decelerations. There are irregular uterine contractions that are perceived as painful by the patient.

An ultrasound evaluation is ordered to identify the cause of the patient's abdominal pain and vaginal bleeding. The placenta is not a previa and is implanted in the posterior fundal area. There are no retroplacental or subchorionic hematomas. A central cord insertion is documented. The fetus appears to be appropriately grown and the amniotic fluid volume is normal. The patient is left on continuous fetal monitoring and laboratory tests are ordered.

III. Differential Diagnosis

The patient case described above exemplifies a frequent presentation of pregnant women in the second and third trimesters. Once the initial evaluation confirms that bleeding did not emanate from the cervix or vaginal walls, the clinician must assume that the bleeding originated from above the cervix, somewhere inside the uterus. After establishing that both the mother and fetus are stable, an ultrasound examination is undertaken to rule out or rule in the diagnosis of placenta previa. When placenta previa has been conclusively ruled out, then one has to conclude that the bleeding originated from some degree of separation of the placenta from the wall of the uterus, or abruption placenta. Rarely, hemorrhage may result from a ruptured fetal vessel coursing across the internal os of the cervix. This is termed a *vasa previa*. Vaginal bleeding from a vasa previa usually occurs during labor following rupture of the membranes, and commonly results in fatal fetal exsanguination.[3] Patients with vaginal bleeding arising from a separation of the placenta need to be advised that there is a high risk for poor obstetric outcomes such as preterm births, premature rupturing of the membranes, and increased perinatal morbidity and mortality even if the bleeding resolves.[4]

IV. Incidence

Obstetric hemorrhage both antepartum and postpartum is a leading cause of maternal mortality and a major reason for admission of pregnant women to intensive care units.[5,6] Abruption of the placenta is the most common cause of antepartum bleeding, with a peak occurrence at 24–26 weeks' gestation. According to the U.S. birth certificate data of 2001, placental abruption occurs in about one in 185 deliveries.[7] However, histologic evidence of decidual hemorrhage, suggesting a diagnosis of abruptio placentae, has been noted in 2%–4% of term deliveries; hence, most cases are not associated with a clinical diagnosis of abruptio placentae.[8] Placental abruption severe enough to result in stillbirth occurs in about one in 1600 deliveries.[9]

V. Pathophysiology

The etiology of placental abruption is unknown. However, there are both acute and chronic pathologic processes that are associated with placental abruption. Although acute events, such as maternal trauma from a motor vehicle accident or a fall, may result in a clinically significant abruption of the placenta, it appears that the majority of cases of placental abruption result from a chronic vasculopathy at the placental–maternal interface.[10] This assertion is supported by clinical observations and histologic findings. For instance, several studies have demonstrated a higher occurrence of fetal growth restriction, hypertensive disorder, and preterm birth in pregnancies complicated by placental abruption.[11] Similarly, histologic examinations of the placenta in patients with abruption have revealed placental/decidual lesions including utero-placental arterial thrombosis, incomplete or failed transformations of utero-placental vessels, chronic inflammatory lesions, such as decidual necrosis, and chorionic plate neutrophil infiltration. These types of vascular lesions are also encountered at a higher frequency in pregnant patients with fetal growth restriction or hypertensive disorders.[12,13]

Thrombin appears to play a key role in the pathogenesis and clinical consequences of abruptio placentae.[14,15] When decidual hemorrhage occurs, tissue factor is released from the damaged decidual cells. The release of tissue factor engenders the formation of thrombin. Thrombin formation can also result from decidual hypoxia. Decidual hypoxia generates vascular endothelial growth factor, which can act directly on decidual endothelial cells to induce the expression of tissue factor, which, in turn, results in the generation of thrombin.[15] Thrombin has several actions; it is a potent direct uterotonic agent that leads to uterine contractions. It induces expressions of matrix metalloproteinases, upregulates genes involved in apoptosis, and induces expression of inflammatory cytokines, predominantly interleukin-8.[16] These actions lead to tissue necrosis and degradation of the extracellular matrix. A vicious cycle is created that results in further vascular disruption, rupturing of the membranes, and initiation of labor.[17]

Histologic evaluations of the placenta in patients with abruptio placentae have revealed typical lesions of decidual hemorrhage, inflammation and tissue hypoxia such as vascular thrombosis, abnormal spiral artery remodeling, villous hypovascularity, villous fibrosis, circulating nucleated red blood cells, and villous infarcts. Thus, it appears that both acute and chronic events are closely intertwined in the pathophysiology of placental abruption, and the consequences thereof, such as preterm births, premature rupture of membranes, and fetal growth restriction.[14–17]

VI. Clinical Manifestations

Placental abruption may be acute or chronic, concealed or clinically evident, and mild or severe. As detailed in the illustrative case, presentation of an acute clinical abruption typically presents with painful vaginal bleeding with uterine contractions and varying degree of abdominal pain. The uterus may be rigid and tender. Depending on the degree of the placental separation, fetal heart rate abnormalities may be seen. It is important to note that the amount of vaginal bleeding is not indicative of the degree of placental separation or the risk of fetal death.

Concealed hemorrhage, when all or most of the blood is trapped between the fetal membranes and decidua, rather than being expressed through the cervix and vagina, may be seen in as many as 20% of abruptions.[18] In such cases, the patient may present with only preterm uterine contractions. Thus, even in the presence of minimal vaginal bleeding or uterine contractions and abdominal pain, the clinician should look closely for placental abruption. Concealed hemorrhage carries with it much greater maternal and fetal hazards, not only because of the possibility of a consumptive coagulopathy, but also because the extent of the hemorrhage is not appreciated and the diagnosis is typically made late.

When the separation of the placenta involves >50% of the placental mass, the abruption is considered severe and is often accompanied by both maternal and fetal compromise.[11,18] In severe abruption, blood is exposed to large amounts of tissue factor over a short period of time, resulting in the massive expression of thrombin, which triggers the coagulation cascade. Systemic bleeding diathesis may result, leading to bleeding and hypovolemic shock. As this acute process unfolds, there is widespread intravascular fibrin deposition, tissue ischemic injury occurs, leading to disseminated intravascular coagulopathy (DIC). If prompt correction of the hypovolemia and tissue hypoxia does not occur, the patient begins to manifest failure or dysfunction of various organs such as the kidneys, liver, lungs, and central nervous system.

Placental abruption can also be a chronic process and a manifestation of ischemic placental disease.[12,13] Commonly, these women will present with chronic and intermittent bleeding. Patients with chronic abruption may also present with evidence of chronic uteroplacental insufficiency such as oligohydramnios, fetal growth restriction, and preterm premature rupture of membranes.

Bleeding with placental abruption is almost always maternal in origin. Rarely, fetal bleeding results from a tear or fracture of a fetal vessel within the placenta rather than from a separation of the placenta from the decidua. This type of feto-maternal hemorrhage is more common with traumatic abruption.[19]

VII. Diagnosis

The diagnosis of placental abruption is primarily clinical, but radiologic, laboratory, and postpartum histologic examination of the placenta can support the clinical diagnosis. The signs and symptoms of abruptio placentae can vary considerably. For example, external bleeding can be profuse, yet placental separation may not be so extensive that it compromises the status of the fetus. Conversely, there may be no external bleeding but the placenta may be completely separated with the fetus dead and the mother in extremis due to severe DIC. Bleeding and abdominal pain are the most frequent findings in patients who present with placental abruption. Many cases are misinterpreted as preterm labor.[18]

Ultrasound examination is an important adjunct to the clinical diagnosis of placental abruption. The principle use of an ultrasound evaluation in a patient who presents with vaginal bleeding and uterine contractions is to exclude a placenta previa. The sensitivity of ultrasound in confirming the clinical diagnosis of abruptio placentae ranges between 2% and 25%.[18,20,21] Overall, ultrasound has a low sensitivity for ruling in the diagnosis of abruptio placentae; however, the presence of sonographic features of abruption, such as retroplacental hematomas, has a very high positive predictive value.[20,21] Importantly, negative findings with ultrasound examinations do not exclude placental abruption. When present, the classic ultrasound description of a placental abruption is a retroplacental blood clot. Other findings include subchorionic collections of fluid, even remote from the attachment site of the placenta, a thickened placenta, and echogenic debris in the amniotic fluid. These ultrasound findings depend on the extent and severity of the hemorrhage, the chronicity of the bleeding, and whether this is a concealed hemorrhage.

There are no laboratory tests useful in making the diagnosis of abruptio placentae, but coagulopathy, particularly hypofibrinogenemia, supports a diagnosis of severe abruption. DIC occurs in 10%–20% of cases of severe abruption with death of the fetus.

It is noteworthy that in some patients, even before clinical or sonographic findings, there may be early markers of ischemic placental disease, including unexplained elevation in the MSAFP. Such patients have up to a 10-fold risk of subsequent abruption and should be followed closely.[22,23]

VIII. Risk Factors

The etiology of placental abruption is unknown, but there are several associated conditions. Risk factors can be categorized into those associated with acute etiology, medical or obstetric factors, sociodemographic, and behavioral.[24]

A. Acute Events

Acute events associated with placental abruption include blunt force trauma to the maternal abdomen or a rapid acceleration-deceleration situation such as a motor vehicle accident leading to a shearing of the placenta.[25,26] Rapid uterine decompression following the rupture of membranes in the setting of polyhydramnios or after delivery of a first twin can also result in placental abruption. Finally, at times when a placenta is implanted over a uterine septum or fibroid, a placental abruption can result from inadequate decidualization or torsion of the fibroid.[27]

B. Medical and Obstetric

The medical and obstetric risk factors include hypertensive disorders, premature rupture of membranes, chorioamnionitis, ischemic placental diseases either in the current or previous pregnancy including previous placental abruptions, fetal growth restriction, preeclampsia, and inherited thrombophilia. Of the above cited risk factors, hypertensive disorders complicating pregnancy, including chronic hypertension, preeclampsia, or gestational hypertension, have the strongest association with placenta abruption.[28-32] Hypertensive women have a fivefold increased risk of severe abruption compared with normotensive women. Antihypertensive therapy does not seem to reduce the risk of placental abruption among women with chronic hypertension.[32] Similarly, placental abruption occurs in 2%–5% of patients with preterm premature rupture of membranes. This increased risk of placenta abruption is enhanced further if the patient has oligohydramnios or evidence of an intrauterine infection associated with the rupture of membranes.[33]

Patients with a history of pregnancies complicated by ischemic placental diseases, such as preeclampsia, small for gestational age neonates, or abruptio placentae, are at an increased risk for having placental abruption in subsequent pregnancies. Furuhashi and colleagues analyzed subsequent pregnancy outcomes from 27 women who had a prior placental abruption. Of the six (22%) recurrences, four were at a gestational age of 1–3 weeks earlier than the first abruption.[34] Several other studies have shown that women with a history of placental abruption have a 5%–15% risk of recurrent abruption in a subsequent pregnancy, compared with a background incidence of 0.4%–1.3% in the general population. If the patient has had two consecutive episodes of placental abruption, her risk of a third episode of abruption increases to 25%.[35,36]

Over the past decade a number of inherited or acquired thrombophilic disorders have been described. These disorders have been associated with an increased incidence of venous thromboembolic complications during pregnancy. Similarly, the presence of thrombophilic mutations such as the factor V Leiden mutations and prothrombin gene mutations has been associated with an increased incidence of abruptio placentae, compared with normal controls. In addition, it appears the more mutations a pregnant patient has, the higher her risk of placental abruption.[37,38]

C. Sociodemographic

The incidence of placental abruption appears to increase with age. In addition, it appears that African American and white women have a higher incidence of abruptio placentae (1 in 200) than Asian (1 in 300) or Latin American (1 in 450) women.[39]

D. Behavioral

Maternal behavioral factors, particularly cocaine use and cigarette smoking, are associated with an increased risk of placental abruption. Ananth and colleagues found a twofold risk for abruption in smokers.[40,41] This was increased to five- to eightfold if smokers had chronic hypertension, severe preeclampsia, or both.[42] As many as 10% of women using cocaine in the third trimester will suffer placental abruption. The abruption may be caused by cocaine-induced acute vasoconstriction leading to vascular injury and disruption.[43]

IX. PATIENT CASE [PART 2]

During the next several hours of observation and fetal monitoring, the patient continues to have vaginal bleeding and her contractions became more painful and more regular. A pelvic examination is repeated and the patient is noted to be 2 centimeters dilated, approximately 50% effaced with a tense amniotic sac at the external os. Her hematocrit is 34%, and the platelet count is 245,000/μL. The serum fibrinogen is 420 mg/dL. The management questions that arise include the issue of tocolysis and administration of corticosteroids for fetal lung maturity. Should the patient be managed expectantly or aggressively with augmentation of labor?

X. Management and Outcome of Pregnancies Complicated by Placental Abruption

There are no outcome-based protocols to guide the management of patients with placental abruption. Thus, guidelines regarding management of placental abruption are based on published case series, anecdotal experience, and good clinical sense.

Maternal complications result from hypovolemia related to blood loss and the consequences of DIC. The fetal complications of placental abruption result from both acute and chronic hypoxemia and preterm birth. Placental abruption is the leading cause of stillbirths. The high mortality is due in part to the strong association between placental abruption and preterm delivery. However, even if the fetus is delivered at term, the perinatal mortality is 25-fold higher with placental abruption.[44] Moreover, in those infants who survived the placental abruption, the incidence of subsequent neurologic sequelae within the first years of life is markedly increased. Matsuda and coworkers followed 39 survivors delivered between 26 and 36 weeks, and reported a 20% incidence of cerebral palsy compared with 1% in gestational age–matched controls.[45]

A. Initial Management

Patients with suspected placental abruption should undergo a rapid initial evaluation to ascertain the stability of the mother. Subsequent management can be decided on a case-by-case basis based on the severity of the abruption, the gestational age, and the status of the mother and fetus. The steps of the acute management of patients with abruptio placentae include:

- institute continuous fetal monitoring
- establish at least one, preferably two, wide-bore intravenous lines
- closely monitor maternal hemodynamic status (pulse and blood pressure)
- closely monitor maternal urine output; it should be maintained at approximately 30 mL/h
- a complete blood count, blood type, and Rh, coagulation profile (PT, PTT, INR, serum fibrinogen, platelet count), and a complete metabolic panel (including serum calcium and glucose) are obtained.

Hypofibrinogenemia (<150 mg/dL) is the most sensitive indicator of coagulopathy related to abruption. A crude clotting test can be performed by placing 5 mL of the patient's blood in a nonheparinized tube for 10 minutes. Failure to clot within this time implies coagulopathy.

The issue of tocolysis in patients with placental abruption and in preterm labor is controversial. Expectant management and tocolysis to prolong the gestation may promote further separation of the placenta and seriously compromise or even kill the fetus unless delivery is performed immediately. On the other hand, delaying the delivery may prove beneficial when the fetus is immature. Towers and coworkers administered magnesium sulfate, terbutaline, or both to 95 of 131 women with placental abruption diagnosed before 36 weeks. There was no difference in the perinatal mortality rate in those given tocolysis versus the nontreated group.[46]

Combs and coworkers also provided data in support of tocolysis in a selected group of patients complicated by placental abruption.[47] If a short course of tocolytics is administered, it may be prudent to avoid β-sympathomimetics because of potentially adverse cardiovascular effects in bleeding patients.

B. Subsequent Management

Subsequent management of pregnancies complicated by abruption of the placenta depends on whether the fetus is alive or dead and maternal status. If the fetus is alive, then gestational age and fetal status determine the management scheme.

If the fetus is at least 34 weeks of gestation and abruption of the placenta is suspected, the fetus should be delivered expeditiously. Vaginal delivery is a reasonable option if the fetal heart rate tracing is reassuring. These patients may be contracting frequently, and often amniotomy and oxytocin infusion will result in a rapid delivery. Should there be a deterioration of either the maternal or fetal status, a prompt cesarean delivery should be done.

A cesarean delivery is indicated if the fetal heart tracing is nonreassuring or there is ongoing major blood loss or other serious maternal complication. Some experts recommend that operative intervention should not begin until the maternal coagulopathy is corrected, if waiting longer does not further compromise the fetal status. At cesarean delivery, one may encounter widespread extravasation of blood into the uterine musculature and underneath the uterine serosa. This is called a *Couvelaire uterus*, which was previously reported to be associated with an increased risk of uterine atony.

Postpartum, there is an increased risk of hemorrhage; therefore, uterotonic agents such as oxytocin (Pitocin), methylergonovine (Methergine) (in the absence of preeclampsia or hypertension), carboprost (Hemabate), and misoprostol (Cytotec) should be used after the delivery of the placenta (see also Chapter 17, Postpartum Obstetric Hemorrhage).

When the fetus is remote from term, delaying delivery is reasonable if fetal well-being tests are reassuring and there is no evidence of maternal coagulopathy, hypotension, or ongoing major blood loss. Glucocorticoids (eg, betamethasone) to promote fetal lung maturation should be administered, given the increased risk of preterm delivery. There are no guidelines as to how long the patient should be admitted. A reasonable approach is to monitor the patient in the hospital until the bleeding has subsided and the patient has normal hematologic parameters. Fetal assessment consisting of two times per week nonstress testing or biophysical profiles should be instituted. Serial sonographic assessments of the fetal weight to document normal interval growth should be done every 3 weeks. It is reasonable to consider delivering the patient by 37–38 weeks because of the increased risk of stillbirth.

When fetal demise has occurred, a vaginal delivery should be attempted unless the patient is unstable and rapid delivery is necessary. If a cesarean delivery is contemplated, the patient's coagulopathy should be corrected before or during the operative delivery.

XI. Summary

Placental abruption is a partial or complete premature separation of a normally implanted placenta. Chronic vascular changes appear to be the main pathophysiologic mechanism involved, although certain acute events can also lead to placental abruption.

There are various risk factors associated with an increased risk of placental abruption, but it appears that the strongest association is with maternal hypertensive disorders.

The diagnosis of abruption placenta is primarily clinical, with the classic symptoms and signs of vaginal bleeding, uterine contractions, abdominal-pelvic pain, and varying degrees of fetal heart tracing abnormalities.

Placental abruption is an obstetric emergency. All patients with suspected abruption of the placenta should undergo a rapid evaluation of the mother and fetus. The mother's hemodynamic status should be evaluated and immediate steps should be taken to correct hypovolemia and coagulopathy, if present, with aggressive fluid resuscitation and transfusion with red blood cells and blood by-products, such as platelets, fresh frozen plasma, and cryoprecipitate, as determined by the patient's coagulation profile. The fetal heart rate should be monitored continuously.

Once the mother has been stabilized, further management, expectant versus immediate delivery, cesarean section versus vaginal delivery, depends on the gestational age of the fetus, whether or not the fetus is alive, and the severity of the abruption.

Patients with abruptio placentae need to be informed that they are at an increased risk of recurrence of placental abruption in their subsequent pregnancies.

XII. References

1. Cunningham FG, Leveno KJ, Bloom SL, et al. Obstetrical hemorrhage. In *Williams Obstetrics*. 22nd ed. New York: McGraw-Hill, 2005:810.

2. Chang YL, Chang SD, Cheng PJ. Perinatal outcome in patients with placental abruption with and without antepartum hemorrhage. *Int J Gynecol Obstet*. 2001;75:193–194.

3. Fung TY, Lau TK. Poor perinatal outcome associated with vasa previa: is it preventable? A report of three cases and review of the literature. *Ultrasound Obstet Gynecol*. 1998;12:430–433.

4. Lipitz S, Admon D, Menczer J, et al. Midtrimester bleeding—variables which affect the outcome of pregnancy. *Gynecol Obstet Invest*. 1991;32:24–27.

5. Berg CJ, Chang J, Callaghan WM, et al. Pregnancy-related mortality in the United States, 1991–1997. *Obstet Gynecol*. 2003;101:289–296.

6. Gilbert TT, Smulian JC, Martin AA, et al. Obstetric admissions to the intensive care unit: outcomes and severity of illness. *Obstet Gynecol*. 2003;102:897–903.

7. Martin JA, Hamilton BE, Ventura SJ, et al. Births: final data for 2001. *National Statistics Reports*. Vol. 51, No. 2. Hyattsville, MD: National Center for Health Statistics, 2002.

8. Salafia CM, Lopez-Zeno JA, Sherer DM, et al. Histologic evidence of old intrauterine bleeding is more frequent in prematurity. *Am J Obstet Gynecol*. 1995; 173:1065–1070.

9. Pritchard JA, Cunningham FG, Prasad V, et al. On reducing the frequency of severe abruptio placentae. *Am J Obstet Gynecol*. 1991;165:1345–1351.

10. Ananth CV, Oyelesse Y, Prasad V, et al. Evidence of a placental abruption as a chronic process: associations with vaginal bleeding early in pregnancy and placental lesions. *Eur J Obstet Gynecol Reprod Biol*. 2006;128:15–21.

11. Ananth CV, Berkowitz GS, Savitz DA, et al. Placental abruption and adverse perinatal outcomes. *JAMA*. 1999;282:1646–1651.

12. Ananth CV, Peltier MR, Kinzler WL, et al. Chronic hypertension and risk of placental abruption: is the association modified by ischemic placental disease? *Am J Obstet Gynecol*. 2007;197:273.e1–7.

13. Ananth CV, Vintzileos AM. Maternal fetal conditions necessitating a medical intervention resulting in preterm birth. *Am J Obstet Gynecol*. 2006;195:1557–1563.

14. Mackenzie AP, Schatz F, Krikun G, et al. Mechanisms of abruption-induced premature rupture of the fetal membranes: thrombin enhanced decidual matrix metalloproteinase-3 (stromelysin-1) expression. *Am J Obstet Gynecol*. 2004;191:1996–2001.

15. Krikun G, Huang ST, Schatz F, et al. Thrombin activation of endometrial endothelial cells: a possible role in intrauterine growth restriction. *Thromb Haemost*. 2007;97:245–253.

16. Lockwood CJ, Toti P, Arcuri F, et al. Mechanisms of abruption-induced premature rupture of the fetal membranes: thrombin-enhanced interleukin-8 expression in term decidua. *Am J Pathol*. 2005;167:1443–1449.

17. Salafia CM, Minior VK, Pezzulio JC, et al. Intrauterine growth restriction in infants of less than thirty-two weeks' gestation: associated placental pathologic features. *Am J Obstet Gynecol*. 1995;173:1049–1057.

18. Oyelese Y, Ananth CV. Placental abruption. *Obstet Gynecol*. 2006;108:1005–1016.

19. Pearlman MD, Tintinalli JE, Lorenz RP. A prospective controlled study of outcome after trauma during pregnancy. *Am J Obstet Gynecol*. 1990;162:1502–1507.

20. Sholl JS. Abruptio placenta: clinical management in non acute cases. *Am J Obstet Gynecol*. 1987;156:40–51.

21. Glantz C, Purnell L. Clinical utility of sonography in the diagnosis and treatment of placental abruption. *J Ultrasound Med*. 2002;21:837–840.

22. Katz VL, Chescheir NC, Cefalo RC. Unexplained elevations of maternal serum alpha-fetoprotein. *Obstet Gynecol Surv*. 1990;45:719–726.

23. Tikkanen M, Hamalainen E, Nuutila M, et al. Elevated maternal second-trimester serum alpha-fetoprotein as a risk factor for placental abruption. *Prenat Diagn.* 2007;27:240–243.

24. Ananth CV, Getahun D, Peltier MR, et al. Placental abruption in term and preterm gestations: evidence for heterogeneity in clinical pathways. *Obstet Gynecol.* 2006;107:785–792.

25. Kettel LM, Branch DW, Scott JR. Occult placental abruption after maternal trauma. *Obstet Gynecol.* 1988;71:449–453.

26. Stafford PA, Biddinger PW, Zumwalt RE. Lethal intrauterine fetal trauma. *Am J Obstet Gynecol.* 1988;159:485–489.

27. Rice JP, Kay HH, Mahony BS. The clinical significance of uterine leiomyomas in pregnancy. *Am J Obstet Gynecol.* 1989;160:1212–1216.

28. Ananth CV, Savitz DA, Williams MA. Placental abruption and its associations with hypertension and prolonged rupture of membranes: a methodologic review and meta-analysis. *Obstet Gynecol.* 1996;88:309–318.

29. Ananth CV, Smulian JC, Demissie K, et al. Placental abruption among singleton and twin births in the United States: risk factor profiles. *Am J Epidemiol.* 2001; 153:771–778.

30. Kramer MS, Usher RH, Pollack R, et al. Etiologic determinants of abruptio placentae. *Obstet Gynecol.* 1997;89:221–226.

31. Williams MA, Mittendorf R, Monson RR. Chronic hypertension, cigarette smoking and abruptio placentae. *Epidemiology.* 1991;2:450–453.

32. Sibai BM, Mabie WC, Shamsa F, et al. A comparison of no medication versus methyldopa or labetalol in chronic hypertension during pregnancy. *Am J Obstet Gynecol.* 1990;162:960–966.

33. Major CA, de Veciana M, Lewis DF, et al. Preterm premature rupture of membranes and abruptio placentae: is there an association between these pregnancy complications? *Am J Obstet Gynecol.* 1995;172:672–676.

34. Furuhashi M, Kurauchi O, Suganuma N. Pregnancy following placental abruption. *Arch Gynecol Obstet.* 2002;267:11–13.

35. Toivonen S, Heinonen S, Anttila M, et al. Obstetric prognosis after placental abruption. *Fetal Diagn Ther.* 2004;19:336–341.

36. Tikkanen M, Nuutila M, Hiilesmaa V, et al. Prepregnancy risk factors for placental abruption. *Acta Obstet Gynecol Scand.* 2006;85:40–44.

37. Gherman RB, Goodwin TM. Obstetric implications of activated protein C resistance and factor V Leiden mutations. *Obstet Gynecol Surv.* 2000;55:117–122.

38. Kupferminc MJ, Eldor A, Steinman A, et al. Increased frequency of genetic thrombophilia in women with complications of pregnancy. *N Engl J Med.* 1999; 340:9–13.

39. Cunningham FG, Leveno KJ, Bloom SL, et al. Obstetrical hemorrhage. In *Williams Obstetrics.* 22nd ed. New York: McGraw-Hill, 2005:813.

40. Ananth CV, Savitz DA, Bowes WA Jr, et al. Influence of hypertensive disorders and cigarette smoking on placental abruption and uterine bleeding during pregnancy. *Br J Obstet Gynaecol*. 1997;104:572–578.

41. Misra DP, Ananth CV. Risk factor profiles of placental abruption in the first and second pregnancies: heterogeneous etiologies. *J Clin Epidemiol*. 1999;52:453–461.

42. Odendaal HJ, van Schie DL, de Jeu RM. Adverse effects of maternal cigarette smoking on preterm labor and abruptio placentae. *Int J Gynaecol Obstet*. 2001;74:287–288.

43. Addis A, Morretti ME, Ahmed Syed F, et al. Fetal effects of cocaine: an updated meta-analysis. *Reprod Toxicol*. 2001;15:341–369.

44. Ananth C, Wilcox AJ. Placental abruption and perinatal mortality in the United States. *Am J Epidemiol*. 2001;153:332–337.

45. Matsuda Y, Maeda T, Kouno S. Comparison of neonatal outcome including cerebral palsy between abruptio placentae and placenta previa. *Eur J Obstet Gynecol Reprod Biol*. 2003;106:125–129.

46. Towers CV, Pircon RA, Heppard M. Is tocolysis safe in the management of third trimester bleeding? *Am J Obstet Gynecol*. 1999;180:1572–1578.

47. Combs CA, Nyberg DA, Mack LA, et al. Expectant management after sonographic diagnosis of placental abruption. *Am J Perinatol*. 1992;9:170–174.

QUESTIONS AND ANSWERS

1. Abruptio placentae is a serious complication of pregnancy because:

   a. there is significant maternal and fetal mortality

   b. it increases the risk for a similar complication in a subsequent pregnancy

   c. it is related to significant neonatal morbidity

   d. all of the above

2. Most cases of abruptio placentae result from:

   a. motor vehicle accidents

   b. vascular abnormalities at placental–maternal interface

   c. fetal growth restriction

   d. unknown causes

3. The diagnosis of abruptio placentae is usually made by:

   a. clinical judgment

   b. postpartum examination of the placenta

   c. ultrasound

   d. laboratory tests

4. The management of abruptio placentae includes all of the following except:

   a. electrolytes and renal function tests

   b. coagulation tests

   c. monitoring of hemodynamic status of the mother

   d. monitoring of the fetus

Answers:

1. d; 2. b; 3. a; 4. a

Placenta Previa

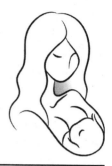

David Lagrew, Jr.

LEARNING OBJECTIVES

1. Describe the classifications of placenta previa and their potential clinical implications.

2. List the complications that occur in pregnancies complicated by placenta previa.

3. Outline the frequency of the risk factors for placenta previa and their changing nature.

4. Compare and contrast the various pharmacologic and other therapies required for management of placenta previa.

I. Introduction

Placenta previa is a complication in pregnancy that is defined as the placental tissue overlying the cervical os, which can lead to significant vaginal bleeding and morbidity. While definitions and incidences are variable, the impact on pregnancy is significant and can easily escalate to maternal and neonatal death in some cases. In a large respective review, the incidence of placenta previa was 2.8 per 1000 live births,[1] and others have found higher rates to 6.0 per 1000 deliveries.[2] This variation may be secondary to variable reporting or the variable definitions that accompany this diagnosis.[3] With the advent of modern obstetric ultrasound techniques, we have discovered the placenta seemingly migrates away from the internal cervical os with differential uterine stretching with advancing gestation. Comeau and coworkers noted that a placenta previa at 20 weeks had only a 2.3% chance of remaining at term, versus at 32 weeks, 23.9% of such placentas persisted to delivery.[4] Thus, the incidence of placenta previa is variable with gestational age.

Most authors believe the actual incidence is rising due to the increase in patients with risk factors, such as the rising number of cesareans, mature gravidas, and multiple gestations.[5] In 1985, Clark and coworkers described the correlation between prior cesarean section and placental abnormalities.[6] They found that, with four prior cesareans, 10% of women would have a placenta previa and two thirds of those would have placenta accreta (invasion of the uterine musculature) requiring hysterectomy.[6] These findings have been confirmed by other authors. In a recent study of more than 30,000 patients who had cesarean delivery without labor, the risk of placenta accreta ranged from 0.2% to 7.7% for women with zero to five cesareans. In the subgroup with placenta previa present, the risk of having accreta increased from 3% to 67%.[7] The combination of increased cesareans, coupled with increases in the traditional risk factors of advancing maternal age and multiple gestations, portends a continued rise in the risk of placenta previa complicating future pregnancies.[8] Such statistics are important because postpartum hemorrhage is one of the top five causes of maternal mortality in developed and developing countries, and placenta previa is one of the leading causes of serious hemorrhage.[9] Maternal morbidity is also markedly increased with requirement for cesarean hysterectomy,[10] blood transfusion, maternal shock, disseminated intravascular coagulation, acute renal failure, and other complications of massive hemorrhage (see Chapter 17, Postpartum Obstetric Hemorrhage). Rouse found transfusion was increased by the presence of placenta previa in primary cesareans fourfold and repeat cesareans 16-fold.[11] The children of these pregnancies are also at increased risk; Ananth and colleagues found that the neonatal mortality rate was 10.7 per 1000 with previa, compared with 2.5 per 1000 among other pregnancies without placenta previa.[1] Prematurity rates are also increased in mothers with placenta previa.[2] Both maternal and neonatal outcomes can be improved with early detection, careful planning, and prompt surgical and medical support.

II. PATIENT CASE [PART 1]

The patient is a 27-year-old married gravida 5 para 2 female with two prior cesarean sections with a known complete placenta previa by screening ultrasound at 20 weeks presents with painless vaginal bleeding and contractions at 28 weeks' gestation. During the antepartum period, the placenta is noted in the lower segment and extends from the posterior aspects to the anterior lower uterine segment. She is noted to have a blood clot of approximately 500 mL in the vagina, but minimal active bleeding from the cervix. Ultrasound confirms an anterior placenta previa, which is covering the internal os and extending past by 4 centimeters. Her admission hemoglobin is 9.0 and vital signs are stable, but with a pulse of 110 beats per minute.

III. Clinical Presentation

Placenta previa occurs in approximately 0.3%–0.6% of pregnancies.[1,2,6] The classic clinical presentation is bright red vaginal bleeding without any associated significant cramping or discomfort. The time of onset of bleeding is variable, but typically occurs in the later part of the second trimester and throughout the third trimester. The degree of bleeding can range from spotting to massive hemorrhage with large clots flowing from the vagina. The bleeding can be intermittent in nature or continuous. Vital signs of possible developing shock, such as a falling blood pressure and elevated pulse, should be checked. Most patients in developed countries will have the diagnosis made before clinical symptoms appear by the finding on prenatal ultrasound. However, placenta previa must be excluded in patients with little or no prenatal care who have not had an ultrasound after the first trimester and present with vaginal bleeding. Visualization of the placental location is typically easy from the abdominal approach but may require transvaginal visualization in marginal cases, since the latter can more easily delineate the internal cervical canal.

IV. Pathophysiology

Placenta previa is caused by the placenta embedding itself in the lower segment of the uterus. Implantation usually occurs in the wall of the uterus above the lower segment, but can occasionally make its way to the lower segment. Clinical risk factors include advanced maternal age, Asian race, increased parity, illicit drug use, history of spontaneous abortion, and prior cesarean deliveries.[12] These various clinical conditions have been associated, but the highest risk is prior uterine surgery in the lower segment, such as previous cesarean section with an increasing risk with multiple past surgeries.[13]

As discussed earlier, prior uterine surgery is a serious risk factor and multiple studies have confirmed this phenomenon.[6,14] The increase can be explained by the tendency of uterine scar tissue to be more adherent to invading chorionic tissue at embryonic implantation. Additionally, the less distensible previously scarred lower uterine segment is less likely to stretch with advancing gestation and prevents placental "migration" away from the internal cervical os.[4,15]

Bleeding can precede the onset of contractions as the placental attachment is disrupted as the lower uterine segment gradually thins with uterine growth. When this occurs, bleeding can occur at the implantation site, as the uteroplacental bed and intervillous space are disrupted. Once disruption occurs thrombin release from the bleeding sites promotes uterine contractions and a vicious cycle of bleeding–contractions–placental separation–bleeding can begin.

V. Detection, Screening, and Diagnosis

The classic clinic presentation of placenta previa is the onset of bright red painless bleeding in the second or third trimester, which may be light to heavy in amount. Typically heavy or life-threatening hemorrhage will not occur unless there has been cervical manipulation from intercourse, trauma, or examination. For this reason, while careful speculum examination can be safe, digital examination in light of known placenta previa should be avoided. The classic "double set-up examination" in which the patient is digitally examined in the operating room with the operating team standing by is rarely used since the advent of ultrasound in clinical practice. While the bleeding is usually as described, darker bleeding with clots can also be seen, and therefore the diagnosis must also be suspected in such presentations. The diagnosis is usually made in the asymptomatic patient during ultrasound performed for other purposes before the onset of vaginal bleeding.[16] Recording of the fetal heart rate can exclude fetal compromise from the effects of placental disruption and/or maternal hypotension with resultant diminished utero-placental perfusion.

Ultrasound is the most reliable diagnostic tool in the management of placenta previa. The placenta is usually easy to visualize abdominally and the placental location is a standard part of routine imaging. Placental location can be fairly reliably determined by the second trimester; however, because of differential growth of the uterus with more expansion of the lower uterine segment, the findings can change with advancing gestational age. Such changes commonly occur when the main body of the placenta is implanted away from the internal cervical os. In cases of central previa (placental implantation directly over the cervix) or where more than 2 centimeters of placenta covers the internal cervical os, this phenomenon is unlikely to occur.[15] Therefore, most recent management schemes are based on recommendations built around this distance when planning for route of delivery and possible complications.[17]

When the diagnosis cannot be clearly excluded on transabdominal ultrasound, proceeding to evaluation by transperineal or transvaginal ultrasound is indicated. Translabial/transperitoneal ultrasound can image the cervix and lower uterine segment and is considered a better predictor of placenta previa.[18] Even clearer images are obtained by transvaginal ultrasound, can very reliably identify placental location, and should be considered the best modality for assessing the placenta location in the lower uterus.[19] The high-frequency transvaginal probe allows for a more discrete view of the finer aspects of the endocervical canal and signal loss is minimal compared to other techniques. This becomes particularly helpful in later gestation when the fetal head and other structures obscure the posterior uterine wall and make visualization of a posterior placenta very difficult abdominally.

The descriptions used for placenta previa have had some variance since the addition of ultrasound diagnosis. Before ultrasound, the forms of previa were divided by the amount of placenta overlying the internal cervical os. These were made by palpation or direct visualization, often with a cervix open a few centimeters. In this setting, placenta previa was described as complete in those cases in which the placenta completely crossed the internal os, partial in cases in which the placenta partially crossed the internal os, and marginal where the placenta reached but did not cross the os. The differentiation with a closed internal cervical os between marginal and partial is less than a couple of millimeters, making differentiation very difficult. In addition, placentas close to the os but not over are described as low lying and despite not being over the os, are more prone to vaginal bleeding, particularly posterior implantations.

Newer classifications use the distance by ultrasound between the closest lower placental edge and the start of the endocervical canal (see Figure 1A–D). In these schemes, marginal placenta previa is described as those cases in which the distance is less than 2 centimeters.[20] Complete and central placenta previa should still be delineated, as these are less likely to "resolve" as gestation advances. Using this approach, the likelihood of long-term resolution of the previa is unlikely if the placenta overlays more than 2 centimeters.

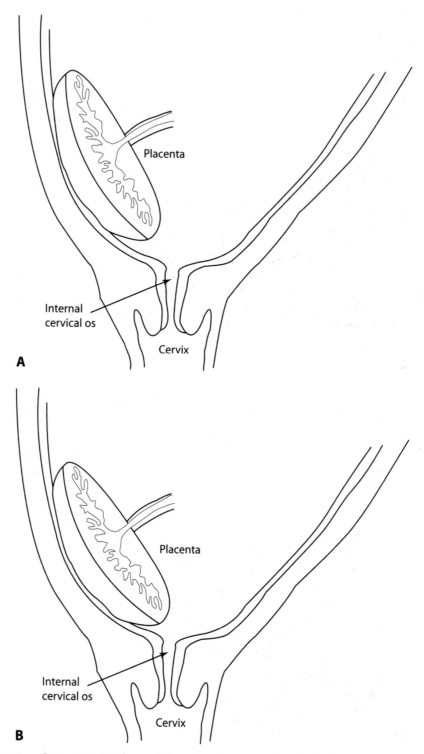

Figure 1. Classic Definitions of Placenta Previa. **A.** Normal Placental Location (>2 Centimeters Edge to Internal Os). **B.** Marginal Placenta Previa (<2 Centimeters Edge to Internal Os). (*continued*)

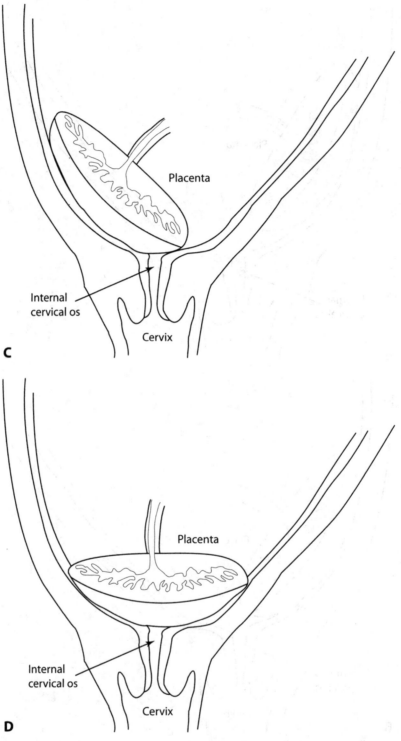

Figure 1. (Continued) **C.** Complete Placenta Previa. **D.** Central Placenta Previa.

Additional assessment is required in patients with low-lying placenta with anterior implantation and prior cesarean section to exclude possible placenta accreta. The old cesarean section scar sites should be examined with color Doppler flow patterns of lacunar flow, invasion into adjacent pelvic structures, and other signs to exclude placenta accreta (invasion of placenta into the myometrium) and percreta (full-thickness invasion).[21] When suspected, an MRI examination has been proposed by some authors to further investigate invasion of the myometrium.[22] Regardless, all techniques can fail to determine placenta accreta, and therefore special preparations are made for all prior uterine surgery cases that have the scar possibly overlaid with placenta.

Laboratory studies should be used to screen for the amount of hemorrhage and to rule out coagulation disorders. Measurement of hemoglobin/hematocrit values must be interpreted with the normal values of pregnancy being slightly less, with normal hemoglobin ranges (10.5–11.5 g/dL) and hematocrit levels (31%–33%) found in normal patients at term. Coagulation testing with the amount of fibrinogen, platelet count, INR/PT, and aPTT should be obtained where moderate to heavy bleeding is suspected. The normal nonpregnant values of these tests can be used for management, whereas other testing, such as D-dimer, is not helpful since values are elevated with normal pregnancy and is not an accurate determinant of fibrinolysis.[23] Routine type and cross to have adequate red blood cells, platelets, and fresh frozen plasma is indicated.

VI. Guidelines and/or Position Statements

The American College of Obstetrics and Gynecology has a bulletin for providers about maternal hemorrhage and uses the classic definition of excessive hemorrhage at delivery of 500 mL for vaginal deliveries and 1000 mL for cesarean deliveries.[24] The document reviews the contribution of placenta previa/accreta to hemorrhage risk, and reviews the current methods of management. It stresses the necessity of a multidisciplinary approach and stresses to clinicians the importance of early recognition and planning.

The bulletin also covers the proper management and planning for the Jehovah's Witness beliefs and reviews the necessity of careful discussion between patient and physician in making plans to achieve a successful outcome. It reviews the "approved" therapies and strategies that are acceptable to members of that religion. Special documentation and counseling are indicated in such patients since, despite modern measures, the mortality risk is increased significantly.[24]

VII. Prevention

Prevention of placenta previa is not clinically possible given the random chances of embryonic implantation. Reducing the chances for future pregnancy is possible by avoiding unnecessary uterine surgeries and supporting efforts to lower cesarean section rates. Avoidance of serious sequelae can occur if accurate and timely diagnosis is made, if logistical preparations for the timing, location, and support are made, and patients follow common sense precautions when the diagnosis of placenta previa is made to reduce the risk of serious sequelae.[24]

VIII. Treatment

The goals of treatment can be summarized into several stages. Patients significantly remote from term where neonatal outcome is poor should be stabilized with volume replacement, blood products if indicated, and then the pregnancy prolonged by tocolysis. Careful monitoring of the mother and fetus are indicated, along with medications to prepare the baby in case the maternal/fetal condition requires delivery. Once stable, medications and support to keep the uterus quiescent and replacement of maternal iron stores is indicated. For most clinicians, significant bleeding after 34 weeks indicates delivery and for asymptomatic patients, amniocentesis and planned cesarean section. After delivery, replacement of blood loss and prevention of further bleeding are indicated to prevent significant postpartum hemorrhage and possible hysterectomy.

Stabilization of the patient with acute heavy hemorrhage requires immediate isotonic crystalloid fluids given at rapid rates through a large bore IV. Use of other agents, such as Hespan, can be helpful to maintain maternal blood pressure. In the antepartum period, pressor agents, such as dobutamine, epinephrine, or dopamine, would be unlikely to be used since such significant hemorrhage would result in delivery. Blood replacement with packed red blood cells (PRBC) should be given for patients with active bleeding and hemoglobin/hematocrit levels less than 10 mg/dL or 30%. Most regimens include replacement of calcium after 6 units of PRBCs.[25] Survival statistics in combat trauma protocols have demonstrated that the concomitant use of fresh frozen plasma at a ratio of 1:1.5 PRBC/fresh frozen plasma improves survival and, given that most maternal hemorrhages simulate such hemorrhage patterns, should be followed.[26] If the patient has a coagulopathy, the replacement of choice is fresh frozen replacement since, compared to cryoprecipitate, it offers volume replacement. Coagulopathy treatment should be guided by laboratory values of INR, aPTT, and fibrinogen levels. Attempts to fully correct in the presence of active bleeding is indicated. Replacement of platelets is similarly dictated by laboratory values. Replacement for active bleeding or planned surgery is indicated when levels fall below 50,000 platelets/mm^3. In the 50,000–100,000 platelets/mm^3 range, replacement may be indicated, and values above 100,000 usually indicate expectant management. For further descriptions of the treatment of severe hemorrhage refer to Chapter 17, Postpartum Obstetric Hemorrhage.

As replacement and stabilization occur, tocolysis of magnesium sulfate should be started. Efficacy of magnesium sulfate therapy has been shown to be reasonably safe and helps prolong the pregnancy. Such therapy helps calm the uterus and break the cycle of contractions that are causing further bleeding. A 4- to 6-gram loading dose followed by an infusion rate of 2 g/h is standard therapy.[27] Flushing, nausea, and feeling of warmth is usually felt by most patients during bolus therapy, and diplopia, malaise, and weakness during prolonged infusion. The patient should be kept at 5–8 mg/dL, with infusion rates guided by serial magnesium levels. Careful monitoring of maternal urinary output, usually requiring monitoring by Foley catheter, is recommended. Because the major serious complication is pulmonary edema, careful clinical examination of maternal breath sounds, cardiac sounds for gallop, and pulse oximetry is indicated. In the acute setting, restricting oral intake is indicated in these patients as acute surgery is possible and the patient on intravenous magnesium is frequently nauseated.

Steroid administration with betamethasone (12 mg IM q24h times two doses) or dexamethasone (8 mg IV q8h times 3 doses) to promote lung maturation is indicated in pregnancies at 23–34 weeks.[28] Great controversy currently exists around the safety and efficacy of repeat doses and this practice is being studied in multiple clinical trials.[29]

The maternal and fetal condition should be carefully assessed, and careful monitoring for potential complications is indicated. Monitoring of the maternal vital signs, pulmonary status with pulse oximetry and breath sounds, and intake/urinary output will prevent the patient from suffering from significant hypotensive periods and/or pulmonary overload from excessive intravenous replacement. Fetal well-being is best assessed by continuous fetal heart rate monitoring and, if equivocal, assessment by ultrasound biophysical profile parameters. The latter surveillance consists of assessing the fetal movement, body tone, presence of breathing, and amniotic fluid volume. Aminiocentesis to determine fetal lung maturation can be undertaken if the fetus is at a gestational age at which lung maturity is possible and if delivery would be considered if mature.

IX. PATIENT CASE [PART 2]

The patient responds to conservative measures, the bleeding ceases, and by postadmission day 5 decisions regarding long-term planning, such as inpatient/ outpatient management, fetal surveillance, and medication therapy, are needed.

Once the acute episode of bleeding is stabilized, the patient must be watched closely for recurrent bleeding and contractions. Monitoring of the fetus can be changed to intermittent nonstress tests, usually performed daily to twice weekly, depending on maternal stability. Maintenance of uterine quiescence with oral terbutaline (2.5–5.0 mg q4–6h) or nifedipine (10–20 mg q4–6h) can be given. Monitoring of the maternal hemoglobin status and its recovery should be done, particularly if there is any residual bleeding or after significant replacement since hemodilution and hemoconcentration with fluid replacement can skew results. Chronic iron supplementation with equivalent of 60 mg elemental iron is recommended.

Patient education revolves around explaining the therapy and pathophysiology in understandable terms so she can participate in her own management and alert caregivers in a timely fashion. The patient should be instructed to carefully monitor herself for any signs of vaginal bleedings, excessive discharge, abdominal or back cramping, and signs of labor. In addition, fetal movement counting, to assess fetal well-being, should be carefully reviewed and the patient encouraged to perform this on a twice daily basis. Clear-cut instructions of the degree of ambulation, daily activities, weight lifting, traveling, and pelvic rest should be reviewed and understood by the patient. Discharge from the hospital, undelivered after acute bleeding, can be possible after the compliant patient demonstrates a protracted period of no further bleeding, understanding of instructions, and living a reasonably close distance from the hospital. Some studies have shown benefit to hospitalization and it may be appropriate in patients who do not fully meet these criteria.[30]

Patients who are discharged home should be followed with twice-weekly modified biophysical profiles consisting of nonstress testing and amniotic fluid assessments. In addition, given the increased incidence of fetal growth restriction, monthly ultrasound measurements of growth should be performed.[31] At 36–37 weeks, an amniocentesis for documenting maturity should be performed. This has been demonstrated to reduce the total blood loss, and allows for special preparations for inoperative complications with special equipment and blood product availability.[32]

Several medications and procedures for postpartum hemorrhage should be made available. Before surgery, placement of iliac occlusion balloons have been advocated, particularly in placenta previa/previous cesarean section patients.[33] Others have noted a high incidence of complications without significant documented benefits, so that the decision must be made based on institutional experience and availability.[34] Intraoperative aggressive treatment of uterine atony that is failing standard intravenous oxytocin infusion can usually be accomplished with IM carboprost (Hemabate) 250 µg or methylergonovine (Methergine) 0.2 mg. The latter should not be used in patients with prior or current history of hypertension. Repeated doses can be used, but problems with loose stools may occur with repeat prostaglandin F2α administration. Autologous blood collection autotransfusion during cesarean section has been used in obstetric cases, and filtration appears to safely return the patient blood cells while filtering out amniotic fluid and other contaminants.[35]

Frequently, the placental implantation site in the lower uterine segment will require special measures to combat the effect of lack of sufficient uterine musculature to contract the open blood vessels, or partial accreta effect. Packing of the uterus or inflation of a balloon catheter has been described.[36] Other surgical measures such as B-Lynch suturing or square suturing to keep the uterus contracted or reduce uterine blood flow with internal iliac ligation or O'Leary sidewall suturing can also be used.[37] These conservative measures usually work, but failure is possible, and the surgeon must be prepared to perform a hysterectomy if necessary; therefore, appropriate equipment and expertise should be readily available. It cannot be overstressed that patients with prior cesarean section or antepartum suspicion of placenta accreta may need many or all of these modalities and are always to be considered at risk for possible massive hemorrhage with complications similar to trauma patients.

It is critical that the patient with placenta previa have the risk of postpartum hemorrhage minimized by prophylactic measures immediately after delivery, and prompt intervention at the first signs of excessive bleeding. All postpartum patients should receive intravenous oxytocin at approximately 125 mL/h of 20 Units/L solutions after delivery of the placenta. In the postpartum period, the patient with uterine atony can be augmented with prostaglandins with the above medications as well as rectal miso-prostol (600–1000 µg), oral misoprostol (600 µg q6h), and oral methergine (0.2 mg q6h).[38] Oral misoprostol as an adjunct has been proposed by some authors, but there is less experience. Careful monitoring of the uterine tone and amount of bleeding is indicated for at least 24 hours in these patients.

Excessive bleeding should be suspected in all patients with heavy lochia, low blood pressure, or increased pulse. Massaging of the fundus and consideration of a bimanual exam to exclude retained blood clots and uterine atony should occur. If bleeding is confirmed, the prompt use of rectal misoprostol or intramuscular carbo-prost or methylergonovine as described for intrapartum bleeding cannot abate signifi-cant blood loss. Careful monitoring of hemoglobin measurement and coagulation studies should be performed and repeated as appropriate. Monitoring of the intake/output is important in preventing pulmonary overload, and watching for renal compli-cations of acute renal failure is indicated in these patients.

X. Summary

Patients with placenta previa comprise an important portion of pregnancies compli-cated by postpartum hemorrhage. They demand careful attention and expertise to prevent significant maternal and neonatal morbidity and mortality. Numerous studies have shown that risk factors of modern obstetric measures will lead to increasing num-bers of these patients and therefore all hospitals need to develop protocols for caring for such patients. Prenatal diagnosis and classification can be made in the majority of these patients. Well-planned antenatal management with prompt intervention can often prevent premature delivery and inherent risks. Intrapartum measures to mini-mize bleeding can reduce the need for transfusion and hysterectomy. Postpartum patients should be followed closely and managed aggressively to reduce blood loss from uterine atony and placental implantation site bleeding.

XI. References

1. Ananth CV, Smulian JC, Vintzileos AM. The effect of placenta previa on neona-tal mortality: a population-based study in the United States, 1989 through 1997. *Am J Obstet Gynecol.* 2003;188:1299–1304.

2. Zlatnik MG, Cheng YW, Norton ME, et al. Placenta previa and the risk of pre-term delivery. *J Matern Fetal Neonatal Med.* 2007;20:719–723.

3. Lu MC, Fridman M, Korst LM, et al. Variations in the incidence of postpartum hemorrhage across hospitals in California. *Matern Child Health J.* 2005;9:297–306.

4. Comeau J, Shaw L, Marcell CC, et al. Early placenta previa and delivery outcome. *Obstet Gynecol.* 1983;61:577–580.

5. Miller DA, Chollet JA, Goodwin TM. Clinical risk factors for placenta previa/placenta accreta. *Am J Obstet Gynecol.* 1997;177:210–214.

6. Clark SL, Koonings PP, Phelan JP. Placenta previa/accreta and prior cesarean sec-tion. *Obstet Gynecol.* 1985;66:89–92.

7. Silver RM, Landon MB, Rouse DJ, et al., and the National Institute of Child Health and Human Development Maternal-Fetal Medicine Units Network. Maternal morbidity associated with multiple repeat cesarean delivery. *Obstet Gynecol.* 2006;107:1226–1232.

8. Martin JA, Kung HC, Mathews TJ, et al. Annual summary of vital statistics: 2006. *Pediatrics.* 2008;121:788–801.

9. Jansen AJ, van Rhenen DJ, Steegers EA, et al. Postpartum hemorrhage and transfusion of blood and blood components. *Obstet Gynecol Surv.* 2005;60:663–671.

10. Castaneda S, Karrison T, Cibils LA. Peripartum hysterectomy. *J Perinat Med.* 2000;28:472–481.

11. Rouse DJ, MacPherson C, Landon M, et al., and the National Institute of Child Health and Human Development Maternal-Fetal Medicine Units Network. Blood transfusion and cesarean delivery. *Obstet Gynecol.* 2006;108:891–897.

12. Odibo AO, Cahill AG, Stamilio DM, et al. Predicting placental abruption and previa in women with a previous cesarean delivery. *Am J Perinatol.* 2007;24:299–305. Epub 2007 May 18.

13. Wu S, Kocherginsky M, Hibbard JU. Abnormal placentation: twenty-year analysis. *Am J Obstet Gynecol.* 2005;192:1458–1461.

14. Gilliam M, Rosenberg D, Davis F. The likelihood of placenta previa with greater number of cesarean deliveries and higher parity. *Obstet Gynecol.* 2002;99:976–980.

15. Predanic M, Perni SC, Baergen RN, et al. A sonographic assessment of different patterns of placenta previa "migration" in the third trimester of pregnancy. *J Ultrasound Med.* 2005;24:773–780.

16. Cunningham FG, MacDonald PC. Obstetrical hemorrhage. In Cunningham FG, Gilstrap LC, Gant NF, et al., eds. *Williams Obstetrics.* 20th ed. New York: McGraw-Hill, 1997:755–760.

17. Oppenheimer L, the Society of Obstetricians and Gynaecologists of Canada. Diagnosis and management of placenta previa. *J Obstet Gynaecol Can.* 2007;29:261–273.

18. Rani PR, Haritha PH, Gowri R. Comparative study of transperineal and transabdominal sonography in the diagnosis of placenta previa. *J Obstet Gynaecol Res.* 2007;33:134–137.

19. Mustafa SA, Brizot ML, Carvalho MH, et al. Transvaginal ultrasonography in predicting placenta previa at delivery: a longitudinal study. *Ultrasound Obstet Gynecol.* 2002;20:356–359.

20. Bhide A, Prefumo F, Moore J, et al. Placental edge to internal os distance in the late third trimester and mode of delivery in placenta praevia. *BJOG.* 2003;110:860–864.

21. Chou MM, Ho ES, Lee YH. Prenatal diagnosis of placenta previa accreta by transabdominal color Doppler ultrasound. *Ultrasound Obstet Gynecol.* 2000;15:28–35.

22. Warshak CR, Eskander R, Hull AD, et al. Accuracy of ultrasonography and magnetic resonance imaging in the diagnosis of placenta accreta. *Obstet Gynecol.* 2006;108(Pt 1):573–581.

23. Paniccia R, Prisco D, Bandinelli B, et al. Plasma and serum levels of D-dimer and their correlations with other hemostatic parameters in pregnancy. *Thromb Res.* 2002;105:257–262.

24. American College of Obstetricians and Gynecologists. Postpartum hemorrhage. *ACOG Practice Bulletin.* Number 76, October 2006. *Obstet Gynecol.* 2006;108:1039–1047.

25. Wilson RF, Binkley LE, Sabo FM Jr, et al. Electrolyte and acid-base changes with massive blood transfusions. *Am Surg.* 1992;58:535–544.

26. Burtelow M, Riley E, Druzin M, et al. How we treat: management of life-threatening primary postpartum hemorrhage with a standardized massive transfusion protocol. *Transfusion.* 2007;47:1564–1572.

27. Besinger RE, Moniak CW, Paskiewicz LS, et al. The effect of tocolytic use in the management of symptomatic placenta previa. *Am J Obstet Gynecol.* 1995;172:1770–1775.

28. National Institutes of Health Consensus Development Panel. Antenatal corticosteroids revisited: repeat courses—National Institutes of Health Consensus Development Conference Statement, August 17–18, 2000. *Obstet Gynecol.* 2001;98:144–150.

29. Wapner RJ, Sorokin Y, Mele L, et al., and the National Institute of Child Health and Human Development Maternal-Fetal Medicine Units Network. Long-term outcomes after repeat doses of antenatal corticosteroids. *N Engl J Med.* 2007;357:1190–1198.

30. Wing DA, Paul RH, Millar LK. Management of the symptomatic placenta previa: a randomized, controlled trial of inpatient versus outpatient expectant management. *Am J Obstet Gynecol.* 1996;175(Pt 1):806–811.

31. Ananth CV, Demissie K, Smulian JC, et al. Relationship among placenta previa, fetal growth restriction, and preterm delivery: a population-based study. *Obstet Gynecol.* 2001;98:299–306.

32. Cotton DB, Read JA, Paul RH, et al. The conservative aggressive management of placenta previa. *Am J Obstet Gynecol.* 1980;137:687–695.

33. Ornan D, White R, Pollak J, et al. Pelvic embolization for intractable postpartum hemorrhage: long-term follow-up and implications for fertility. *Obstet Gynecol.* 2003;102(Pt 1):904–910.

34. Shrivastava V, Nageotte M, Major C, et al. Case-control comparison of cesarean hysterectomy with and without prophylactic placement of intravascular balloon catheters for placenta accreta. *Am J Obstet Gynecol.* 2007;197:402.e1–5.

35. Rebarber A, Lonser R, Jackson S, et al. The safety of intraoperative autologous blood collection and autotransfusion during cesarean section. *Am J Obstet Gynecol.* 1998;179(Pt 1):715–720.

36. Bakri YN, Amri A, Abdul Jabbar F. Tamponade-balloon for obstetrical bleeding. *Int J Gynaecol Obstet.* 2001;74:139–142.

37. Allam MS, B-Lynch C. The B-Lynch and other uterine compression suture techniques. *Int J Gynaecol Obstet.* 2005;89:236–241.

38. Caliskan E, Dilbaz B, Meydanli MM, et al. Oral misoprostol for the third stage of labor: a randomized controlled trial. *Obstet Gynecol.* 2003;101(Pt 1):921–928.

QUESTIONS AND ANSWERS

1. Most authors consider a "complete" placenta previa to be best described as:

   a. the placental edge reaches the internal cervical os

   b. placental tissue covers the cervical os

   c. the placental edge comes within 2 centimeters of the internal cervical os

   d. placental tissue is noted on both the anterior and posterior wall

   e. none of the above

2. Which of the following clinical conditions has been associated with placenta previa?

   a. prior cesarean section

   b. increased maternal age

   c. vaginal bleeding

   d. multiple gestation

   e. all of the above

3. Which of the following would be the best way to clearly diagnose placenta previa?

   a. digital examination

   b. speculum exam with direct visualization

   c. transvaginal ultrasound

   d. transabdominal ultrasound

   e. none of the above

4. Which of the following describes significant vaginal bleeding associated with placenta previa?

   a. large vaginal clots with associated abdominal cramping

   b. dark red blood

   c. painless, bright red bleeding

   d. small amount of spotting with mucous discharge

   e. none of the above

5. Considering the use of intravenous magnesium sulfate in patients with placenta previa:

   a. it is strictly contraindicated since the tocolytic effect will increase hemorrhage

   b. can be carefully titrated with serum levels

   c. can be carefully titrated by monitoring with clinical signs of toxicity

   d. often causes respiratory depression

   e. rarely is associated with flushing and nausea with bolus dosing

Answers:

1. b; 2. e; 3. c; 4. c; 5. b

Fetal Arrhythmias

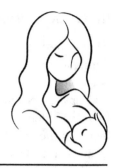

Anjan S. Batra and John-Charles Loo

LEARNING OBJECTIVES

1. List the types of common fetal arrhythmias.

2. Describe the treatment strategies for fetal arrhythmias.

3. Identify side effects of the medical therapies for fetal arrhythmias.

I. Introduction

The normal fetal heart rate ranges between 110 and 160 beats per minute. A fetal heart rate is considered abnormal if the heart rate is beyond the normal ranges or the rhythm is irregular. The rate, duration, and origin of the rhythm and degree of irregularity usually determine the potential for hemodynamic consequences. Most of the fetal rhythm disturbances are the result of premature atrial contractions (PACs) and are of little clinical significance. Other arrhythmias include tachyarrhythmias (heart rate >160 beats/min) such as supraventricular tachycardia (SVT), atrial flutter, and ventricular tachycardia, and bradyarrhythmias (heart rate <110 beats/min) such as sinus node dysfunction and complete heart block (CHB). Fetal arrhythmias can be detected in approximately 1% of all fetuses[1-4] and up to 49% of all referrals for fetal echocardiography.[5] In approximately 10% of pregnancies complicated by fetal arrhythmias, the arrhythmia may be life-threatening.[2]

II. PATIENT CASE (PART 1)

A 22-year-old gravida 2 para 1 with an intrauterine pregnancy at 32 weeks' gestation presented to her obstetrician for a routine visit. On presentation, she had no complaints. In clinic, fetal heart rate by Doppler was 240 beats per minute. Bedside ultrasound was then performed and tachycardia was confirmed. Questionable ascites were also noted. The patient's pregnancy until this point had been without complications. She had good prenatal care since the first trimester and denied contractions, vaginal bleeding, or loss of fluid.

III. Clinical Presentation

Fetal arrhythmias are usually detected during routine auscultation of the fetal heart or during an obstetric scan. The pregnancy is otherwise unremarkable. If the arrhythmia is sustained, there is a greater risk of fetal hemodynamic compromise leading to hydrops fetalis and fetal demise. Intermittent tachycardias can also be associated with hydrops.[6] Hence, patients with hydrops and a normal heart rate warrant repeat assessments of the fetal heart rate to detect intermittent arrhythmias. Earlier onset in gestation of a tachyarrhythmia and a higher ventricular rate[7] are other risk factors associated with a greater risk for development of hydrops fetalis.

In fetuses with bradycardia, a slow ventricular escape rate of less than 55 beats per minute appears to be a poor prognostic factor.[8] Fetuses of mothers suffering from a connective tissue disease (commonly Sjögren's syndrome or systemic lupus erythematosus) are at risk for developing isolated complete heart block. Both fetal brady- and tachyarrhythmias can be associated with structural heart disease and warrant a thorough echocardiogram and evaluation by a pediatric cardiologist. The combination of a sustained arrhythmia, structural heart disease, and hydrops fetalis is an ominous sign carrying a poor prognosis.

IV. Pathophysiology

A. Nonsustained Arrhythmias

PACs represent by far the single most common arrhythmia in fetuses referred for an arrhythmia. PACs are usually clinically insignificant, although approximately 1% of fetuses with PACs will have significant structural heart disease and 0.5% will develop supraventricular tachycardia.[9] Isolated premature ventricular contractions (PVCs) are far less common compared with PACs. The prevalence of fetal PACs to PVCs has been estimated at approximately 10:1.[2] PVCs may suggest a dilated or dysfunctional ventricle, intracardiac rhabdomyomas, or other anatomic abnormalities. However, in utero PVCs are difficult to distinguish from PACs. Premature atrial and ventricular contractions can be easily identified using Doppler or M-mode echocardiography.

B. Sustained Tachycardia

A pathologic tachycardia in the fetus is described as a sustained heart rate of more than 180 beats per minute. Sustained tachyarrhythmias are much more common than sustained bradyarrhythmias. Atrial tachyarrhythmias are much more common than ventricular tachyarrhythmias. The most common form of atrial tachyarrhythmias involves a reentry mechanism either within the atrium (atrial flutter) or between the atrium and the ventricle via an accessory pathway (supraventricular tachycardia).

C. Sustained Bradycardia

Fetal bradycardia that is nonsustained may be secondary to an exaggerated variability of the sinus rhythm. Sustained fetal bradycardia is most commonly secondary to congenital CHB. The incidence of CHB at birth has been reported to be approximately 1 in 20,000.[10] In patients presenting with fetal CHB, complex structural heart defects have been reported in up to 53% of the patients.[11] The combination of CHB and structural heart disease is usually an ominous sign with a high likelihood of hydrops leading to fetal or neonatal death. Isolated CHB in the absence of structural heart disease is usually well tolerated in utero and does not lead to hemodynamic consequences unless the heart rates are consistently less than 60 beats per minute. There is a high association of isolated CHB with maternal lupus, and all gravid mothers with fetal CHB should undergo testing for autoantibodies. The presence of maternal anti-SS-A/Ro or anti-SS-B/La antibodies has been associated with an increased risk for fetal CHB.[12] Autoantibody-associated CHB is not coincident with major structural abnormalities, is most often identified in the late second trimester, carries a higher mortality, and frequently requires a pacemaker in the neonatal period. The recurrence rate of CHB is at least two to three times higher than that of the first affected pregnancy, supporting the need for close echocardiographic monitoring in all subsequent pregnancies, with heightened surveillance between 18 and 24 weeks of gestation.

V. Diagnosis

The diagnosis of fetal arrhythmias remains challenging. Routine obstetric evaluation relies on auscultation and Doppler detection of pulsatile flow within the fetal heart. These techniques allow determination of the ventricular rate, but are incapable of evaluating the atrioventricular relationship or the origin of the rhythm. M-mode echocardiography with simultaneous recording of the atrial and ventricular contractions is the primary modality for determining the atrial and ventricular relationship and rates.

Atrial flutter usually has atrial rates between 300 and 500 beats per minute with variable conduction to the ventricle leading to ventricular rates between 200 and 250 beats per minute. In SVT, although the atrial rates are relatively slower, the 1:1 atrioventricular conduction leads to faster ventricular rates in the vicinity of 250–350 beats per minute. Episodes of abrupt onset and termination of tachycardia frequently help confirm the diagnosis of a reentry tachycardia. Sustained tachycardia can lead to hydrops. M-mode echocardiography can help in differentiating between atrial flutter (variable atrioventricular conduction), SVT (1:1 atrioventricular conduction) and ventricular tachycardia (complete atrioventricular dissociation). Fetal bradycardia can be determined by routine Doppler auscultation. The diagnosis of CHB can be made by fetal echocardiography.

Fetal magnetocardiography is the magnetic analog of fetal electrocardiogram (ECG), and currently is the most effective means of assessing fetal arrhythmias. It is done using external leads affixed to the maternal abdomen and detects magnetic fields caused by the external excitation of the fetal heart. These magnetic fields are plotted against time, resulting in information equivalent to the surface ECG. This technique has proved useful in the detection of fetal arrhythmias, particularly those not detectable by other diagnostic tools, such as in fetuses with long QT intervals.[13] However, fetal magnetocardiography is not routinely available for clinical use.

VI. Treatment

A precise assessment of the fetal arrhythmia is essential to administer the appropriate therapy. Prenatal therapy to treat the fetus can be administered through the maternal or direct fetal route. Initiation of antiarrhythmics should be done in an inpatient setting. The mother should be examined with a 12-lead ECG to exclude maternal diseases, such as Wolff-Parkinson-White syndrome, prolonged QT interval, or myocarditis, that may contraindicate certain antiarrhythmic therapies. Serial ECG monitoring for possible side effects to the mother is indicated. Serum drug concentrations may also be helpful. High concentrations may reflect potential for drug toxicity, and low levels may indicate sub-therapeutic treatment. An understanding of the half-life for each medication is essential, as it is important to allow for sufficient time for the drug to reach therapeutic levels before deciding to switch to or add another agent. Concentrations of the antiarrhythmic drugs measured in maternal blood may differ from that in the fetal blood. The transplacental transfer of each drug varies and is further influenced by fluid status of the fetus, gestational age, development of the villous placenta, and other physiologic changes.

A. Treatment of Premature Beats

In the setting of a structurally normal heart, both PACs and PVCs are benign, require no specific therapy, and usually resolve spontaneously before or shortly after birth. A complete fetal echocardiogram and Doppler assessment is indicated in these patients to rule out the associated risk of congenital heart disease, decrease in ventricular function, and other sustained arrhythmias. In rare cases, frequent PACs may lead to nonconducted beats and present as a bradycardic rhythm called *blocked atrial bigeminy*. These patients require close monitoring with weekly visits. The authors are unaware of isolated premature beats leading to hemodynamic compromise or hydrops and hence do not recommend any medical therapy or premature delivery for these patients.

B. Treatment of Tachyarrhythmias

Intermittent fetal tachycardias may require only close observation of the fetal heart rates during the remainder of the pregnancy. Sustained fetal tachycardias, however, usually require treatment (Figure 1 and Table 1).

1. Digoxin
Digoxin remains the initial drug treatment of choice for fetal tachycardia due to its safety profile and long track record. It acts by inhibiting the sodium-potassium ATPase and is classified as an inotrope rather than an antiarrhythmic drug. Simpson et al., in a review of 127 consecutive fetuses, showed that digoxin monotherapy converted most (62%) of the treated nonhydropic fetuses with atrial tachycardias, and 96% survived through the neonatal period.[14] However, the response rates to digoxin in the hydropic fetuses were only 20%, suggesting that it is a poor choice in this setting. Serum levels in the fetus range from 70%–100% of the maternal serum levels. The target maternal digoxin serum levels should be relatively high, between 2.0 and 2.5 ng/mL, mostly because of the higher glomerular filtration rate near term. The measurement of digoxin levels should be performed 6–8 hours after the last dose of digoxin. Digoxin therapy is usually initiated with a loading dose either intravenously (over 48–72

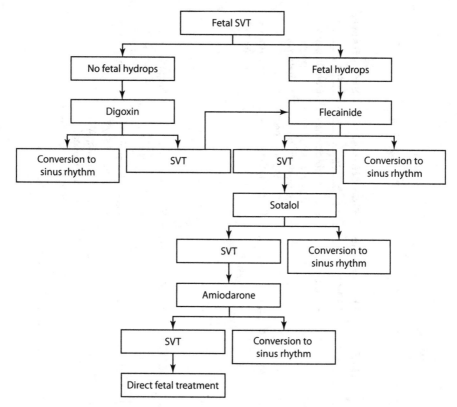

Figure 1. Protocol: Fetal Supraventricular Tachycardia (SVT).

hours) or orally (over 6–7 days). This is followed by maintenance dosing. Lower doses are indicated in the presence of maternal renal failure.

2. Flecainide

When digoxin fails to restore sinus rhythm or in a hydropic fetus with SVT, flecainide is a good next drug of choice. Flecainide can be used in conjunction with digoxin. It has been shown to successfully convert up to 92% of the nonhydropic[11] and 59% of the hydropic fetuses[15] to sinus rhythm. It is a class I C antiarrhythmic agent and acts by blocking the fast sodium channel and slowing conduction velocity in cardiac pathways. Its therapeutic range for serum drug levels lies between 200 ng/mL and 1000 ng/mL. Flecainide has an excellent bioavailablity, with 95% of the maternal plasma levels achieved in the nonhydropic fetus and 80% of the maternal plasma levels achieved in the hydropic fetus. Therapeutic serum levels are achieved after approximately 3 days. Hence, conversion into sinus rhythm can be expected 72 hours after initiation of therapy but may take up to 14 days.[16] Therapy should be continued beyond 72 hours, especially when an initial decrease of fetal heart rate is observed, which may represent an early therapeutic response. Paradoxic proarrhythmic effects can be seen with this drug. Initial studies reported proarrhythmic effects with this drug in adults with myocardial infarction[17] and in children with underlying congenital heart defects.[18] However, in the setting of an otherwise normal heart, this remains a good choice for fetal tachyarrhythmias.

Table 1. Drugs Used for Fetal Tachyarrhythmias

Drug	Class	Use	Dose	Metabolism	Half-life	Therapeutic range	Side effects, maternal	Side effects, fetal
Flecainide	1C	SVT, AF, VT	PO: 100–400 mg bid	Hepatic excretion 67%, renal excretion 33%	13–19 h	<1 µg/mL	Proarrhythmia, vertigo, nausea, headache, disturbed vision, paresthesia	Negative inotrope, proarrhythmia
Amiodarone	III	SVT, AF, VT	IV: 5 mg/kg over 20 min; 500–1000 mg over 24 h; PO: 1200–1600 mg/d for 7–14 d (loading), then 200–400 mg/d (maintenance)	Hepatic metabolism; renal excretion	25–110 d	1.0–2.5 µg/mL	Proarrhythmia risk	Proarrhythmia, hypothyroid
Sotalol	III	SVT, AF, VT	PO: 80–160 mg q12h; increase to 160 mg q8h	Renal excretion	15–17 h	1.5–2.5 µg/mL	Proarrhythmia risk	Negative inotrope, proarrhythmia
Adenosine	IV	SVT	IV: 100–200 µg/kg (into umbilical vein)	Throughout body	10–30 s	NA	Useful for acute termination of SVT	Proarrhythmia
Digoxin	Cardiac glycoside	SVT, AF	IV: 1 mg divided over 24 h; PO: 0.5–1.0 mg daily in 2 divided doses	Renal excretion	36 h	1–2 ng/mL	Proarrhythmia, AV block, nausea, anorexia, vomiting	

AF = atrial flutter, AV = atrioventricular, NA = not available, SVT = supraventricular tachycardia, VT = ventricular tachycardia.

3. Sotalol

Just as with flecainide, sotalol is a consideration for therapy when digoxin fails to restore sinus rhythm or in a hydropic fetus with SVT and can be used in conjunction with digoxin.[19] However, at least one study with sotalol reported good success rates in fetuses with atrial flutter but a relatively high mortality in the fetus with SVT.[20] These results may support initiating therapy with flecainide before sotalol. Sotalol is a class III antiarrhythmic drug with an additional β-adrenergic blocking effect. It acts on the potassium channels by prolonging the action potential. Its bioavailability and placental passage are excellent, with fetal serum levels approaching 70%–100% of maternal levels within 48–72 hours of initiation of therapy. It is exclusively excreted renally and adjustment of dosage is necessary in the presence of maternal renal failure. This drug is associated with a proarrhythmic risk. It prolongs the QT interval, which puts the mother at risk for life-threatening ventricular arrhythmias, such as torsades de pointes. Serial ECGs to monitor the QT intervals should be performed before and at regular intervals (daily until therapeutic levels are reached) after initiating therapy with sotalol.

4. Amiodarone

When therapy with digoxin, sotalol, or flecainide fails to restore sinus rhythm in hydropic fetuses with SVT, amiodarone therapy should be considered, as it allows a substantial number of these fetuses to be converted prenatally.[21] Amiodarone is a class III antiarrhythmic drug and acts on the potassium channels, resulting in prolongation of the action potential and repolarization. It has a very long half-life of 1–3 months and has an active hepatic metabolite, desethylamiodarone. Amiodarone has relatively low fetal bioavailability. It is administered as a loading dose of 1200 mg/d through the intravenous or oral route followed by a maintenance dose of 600–900 mg/d. The transplacental transfer is poor, with fetomaternal ratios for amiodarone between 10% and 40%, with even lower ratios in hydropic fetuses. Side effects of amiodarone therapy in the fetus that have been reported include hypothyroidism.[22,23] The hypothyroidism is usually transient and resolves after a few months of discontinuing therapy. Monitoring thyroid function of the mother and of the newborn is therefore necessary when administering amiodarone.

5. Adenosine

Adenosine is an endogenous purine nucleoside with a very short-lasting effect mediated by A1-purine receptors. Intravenous application of 100–200 µg/kg estimated fetal weight resulted in cardioversion within 15–30 seconds.[24] Adenosine acts by blocking conduction across the atrioventricular node and hence terminates SVTs that use the atrioventricular node, but fails to terminate atrial tachycardias, atrial flutter, and ventricular tachycardias. However, the failure to terminate these arrhythmias may aid in narrowing the differential diagnosis for the tachyarrhythmia. Direct fetal adenosine administration might be helpful in the treatment of fetal reentry tachycardias if the sinus rhythm achieved quickly can be preserved by long-acting antiarrhythmic drugs. Such a combined therapeutic approach might be especially advantageous in hydropic fetuses.

C. Treatment of Bradyarrhythmias

Fetal bradycardia rarely warrants intervention. Fetuses with heart rates above 60 beats per minute generally do well and do not require premature delivery or medical intervention in the neonatal period. On the other hand, sustained fetal heart rates of 55 beats per minute, in association with complex congenital heart disease or hydrops, may warrant early delivery and immediate intervention in the neonatal period. This intervention may be medical, using drugs that have a positive chronotropic effect, such as isoproterenol, or surgical with placement of a pacemaker.

Intervention with medications for treatment of fetal bradycardia is controversial. Isolated reports of therapy with corticosteroids for treatment of immune-mediated fetal CHB have been reported, but the evidence favoring this therapy is far from conclusive. Dexamethasone crosses the placenta well and has been associated with the resolution of fetal hydrops. Copel et al. evaluated the response of oral dexamethasone, 4 mg daily, administered to mothers.[25] They reported improvement from complete heart block to second-degree heart block or sinus rhythm in five cases, resolution of second-degree heart block in two patients, and no response in two patients. A subsequent larger series incorporating pregnancies reported to the National Lupus Registry failed to show any change in the degree of heart block among those fetuses exposed to steroids, but did show a tendency toward improvement in fetal hydrops.[26]

Maternal administration of sympathomimetic therapy with terbutaline, ritodrine, isoprenaline, or albuterol has also been advocated.[27,28] Although these drugs tend to increase the fetal heart rates, their effect on fetal mortality appears to be unchanged. Plasmapheresis has been postulated to decrease the transplacental delivery of maternal lupus antibodies, but its use is controversial as the efficacy is not proven, and it carries a significant risk to the mother.[29]

VII. PATIENT CASE [PART 2]

Plan of care was discussed with a pediatric cardiologist, and it was decided to proceed with attempted conversion of SVT using digoxin. Baseline ECG was performed and was within normal limits. The patient was then loaded with 0.5 mg IV digoxin and then started on oral digoxin, 0.25 mg three times a day, with a plan to check digoxin level in 24 hours. The plan was also made to do a fetal echocardiogram and complete fetal ultrasound the following morning. The patient remained on continuous monitoring, and fetal heart rates remained in the 240s.

The following morning a fetal echocardiogram revealed fetal hydrops with ascites and pleural effusion, moderate to severe tricuspid valve insufficiency, mild mitral insufficiency, and decreased cardiac function. After the echocardiogram was completed the pediatric cardiologist recommended adding flecainide, 100 mg twice a day. On the third day after starting flecainide, the fetal heart rates were in the 140s. The patient was maintained on digoxin and flecainide as an outpatient, and by the following week, the fetal echocardiogram returned to normal. At 40 weeks' gestation, a newborn was delivered by normal spontaneous vaginal delivery in no distress.

VIII. Summary

It is essential to have a thorough understanding of the mechanism of arrhythmia, treatment options, knowledge of drugs being used, and awareness of side effects from these drugs for mother and fetus. Paroxysmal tachycardias such as PACs and PVCs are common and do not warrant any therapy. Sustained SVT in the nonhydropic fetus can be treated initially with digoxin. In cases where digoxin fails to treat the tachycardia, flecainide and sotalol can be used, and if these drugs are not successful, amiodarone can be used. Digoxin is rarely successful in a hydropic fetus.

Fetuses with heart block generally carry a good prognosis, especially in the absence of structural heart disease or hydrops. Intervention is rarely indicated. Therapy with steroids, sympathomimetic agents, and plasmapheresis has been described in small case series of fetuses with heart block and hydrops, but verification with larger series of patients has not been done. The risks of premature delivery should be weighed with those of transplacental therapy when treating fetal arrhythmias.

IX. References

1. Ferrer PL. Fetal arrhythmias. In Deal B, Wolff GS, Gelband H, eds. *Current Concepts in Diagnosis and Treatment of Arrhythmias in Infants and Children.* Armonk, NY: Futura Publishing Company, Inc.; 1998:17.
2. Strasburger JF. Fetal arrhythmias. *Prog Pediatr Cardiol.* 2000;11:1–17.
3. Simpson LL. Fetal supraventricular tachycardias: diagnosis and management. *Semin Perinatol.* 2000;24:360–372.
4. Allan LD, Hornberger L, Sharland G. *Textbook of Fetal Cardiology.* London: Greenwich Medical Media; 2000:423–431.
5. Calvin SE, Gaziano EP, Bendel RP, et al. Evaluation of fetal cardiac arrhythmias. Ultrasound findings and neonatal outcome. *Minn Med.* 1992;75:29–31.
6. Simpson JM, Milburn A, Yates RW, et al. Outcome of intermittent tachyarrhythmias in the fetus. *Pediatr Cardiol.* 1997;18:78–82.
7. Van Engelen AD, Weijtens O, Brenner JI, et al. Management outcome and follow-up of fetal tachycardia. *J Am Coll Cardiol.* 1994;24:1371–1375.
8. Zhao H, Cuneo BF, Strasburger JF, et al. Electrophysiological characteristics of fetal atrioventricular block. *J Am Coll Cardiol.* 2008;51:77–84.
9. Rowland DG, Wheeler JJ. Congenital heart disease and arrhythmia in the fetuses. In Allen HD, Gutgesell HP, Clark EB, et al., eds. *Heart Disease in Infants, Children and Adolescents.* Philadelphia: Lippincott Williams & Wilkins; 2001:57.
10. Michaëlsson M, Engle MA. Congenital complete heart block: an international study of the natural history. *Cardiovasc Clin.* 1972;4:85–101.
11. Schmidt KG, Ulmer HE, Silverman NH, et al. Perinatal outcome of fetal complete atrioventricular block: a multicenter experience. *J Am Coll Cardiol.* 1991;17:1360–1366.
12. Buyon JP, Hiebert R, Copel J, et al. Autoimmune-associated congenital heart block: demographics, mortality, morbidity and recurrence rates obtained from a national neonatal lupus registry. *J Am Coll Cardiol.* 1998;31:1658–1666.

13. Schmitz L, Burghoff M. Images in cardiovascular medicine. Magnetocardiography in a fetus with long-QT syndrome. *Circulation.* 2005;112:e68–69.

14. Simpson JM, Sharland GK. Fetal tachycardias: management and outcome of 127 consecutive cases. *Heart.* 1998;79:576–581.

15. Ebenroth ES, Cordes TM, Darragh RK. Second-line treatment of fetal supraventricular tachycardia using flecainide acetate. *Pediatr Cardiol.* 2001;22:483–487.

16. Krapp M, Baschat AA, Gembruch U, et al. Flecainide in the intrauterine treatment of fetal supraventricular tachycardia. *Ultrasound Obstet Gynecol.* 2002;19:158–164.

17. Echt DS, Liebson PR, Mitchell LB, et al. Mortality and morbidity in patients receiving encainide, flecainide, or placebo. The Cardiac Arrhythmia Suppression Trial. *N Engl J Med.* 1991;324:781–788.

18. Fish FA, Gillette PC, Benson DW Jr. Proarrhythmia, cardiac arrest and death in young patients receiving encainide and flecainide. The Pediatric Electrophysiology Group. *J Am Coll Cardiol.* 1991;18:356–365.

19. Sonesson SE, Fouron JC, Wesslen-Eriksson E, et al. Foetal supraventricular tachycardia treated with sotalol. *Acta Paediatr.* 1998;87:584–587.

20. Oudijk MA, Michon MM, Kleinman CS, et al. Sotalol in the treatment of fetal dysrhythmias. *Circulation.* 2000;101:2721–2726.

21. Jouannic JM, Delahaye S, Fermont L, et al. Fetal supraventricular tachycardia: a role for amiodarone as second-line therapy? *Prenat Diagn.* 2003;23:152–156.

22. Laurent M, Betremieux P, Biron Y, et al. Neonatal hypothyroidism after treatment by amiodarone during pregnancy. *Am J Cardiol.* 1987;60:942.

23. Matsumura LK, Born D, Kunii IS, et al. Outcome of thyroid function in newborns from mothers treated with amiodarone. *Thyroid.* 1992;2:279–281.

24. Kohl T, Tercanli S, Kececioglu D, et al. Direct fetal administration of adenosine for the termination of incessant supraventricular tachycardia. *Obstet Gynecol.* 1995;85:873–874.

25. Copel JA, Buyon JP, Kleinman CS. Successful in utero therapy of fetal heart block. *Am J Obstet Gynecol.* 1995;173:1384.

26. Saleeb S, Copel J, Friedman D, et al. Comparison of treatment with fluorinated glucocorticoids to the natural history of autoantibody associated complete heart block: retrospective review of the Research Registry for Neonatal Lupus. *Arthritis Rheum.* 1999;42:2335.

27. Groves AM, Allan LD, Rosenthal E. Therapeutic trial of sympathomimetics in three cases of complete heart block in the fetus. *Circulation.* 1995;92:3394–3396.

28. Schmidt KG, Ulmer HE, Silverman NH, et al. Perinatal outcome of fetal complete atrioventricular block: a multicenter experience. *J Am Coll Cardiol.* 1991;17:1360–1366.

29. Aslan E, Tarim E, Kilicdag E, et al. Sjögren's syndrome diagnosed in pregnancy: a case report. *J Reprod Med.* 2005;50:67–70.

QUESTIONS AND ANSWERS

1. The normal fetal heart rate ranges between:

   a. 110 and 160 beats per minute

   b. 80 and 150 beats per minute

   c. 150 and 250 beats per minute

   d. 120 and 200 beats per minute

2. The most common arrhythmia in fetuses that leads to a referral for an arrhythmia is:

   a. premature atrial contractions

   b. premature ventricular contractions

   c. supraventricular tachycardia

   d. atrial flutter

3. The drug of first choice for treatment of nonhydropic fetal supraventricular tachycardia is:

   a. sotalol

   b. amiodarone

   c. flecainide

   d. digoxin

4. The presence of maternal anti-SS-A/Ro or anti-SS-B/La antibodies has been associated with an increased risk in the fetus for

   a. supraventricular tachycardia

   b. complete heart block

   c. ventricular tachycardia

   d. premature atrial contractions

5. The level of drug in the fetus is influenced by all of the following except:

   a. transplacental transfer

   b. dosage of drug

   c. maternal serum levels

   d. type of arrhythmia

Answers:

1. a; 2. a; 3. d; 4. b; 5. d

Induction of Labor

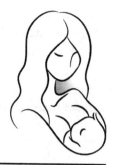

Anna M. Galyean

CHAPTER
15

LEARNING OBJECTIVES

1. List common indications for induction of labor.

2. Describe the difference between cervical ripening and labor induction.

3. Describe a "favorable" cervix.

4. Identify the most common ways to induce labor.

I. Introduction

Induction of labor is the purposeful stimulation of uterine contractions for the goal of delivery. Labor induction is one of the most commonly practiced procedures in obstetrics, occurring in more than 20% of pregnancies, and the incidence has been climbing steadily over the past 20 years. Specifically, the rate of induction has more than doubled from 1990 (9.5%) to 2005 (22.3%). These numbers vary greatly among geographic regions, institutions, and patient populations.[1] The potential explanations for this trend include physician/patient convenience, improved induction agents, and increased medical indications in high risk populations.

Just as the rate of induction varies among populations so does the reason for induction. Labor induction may be indicated or elective. The rate of indicated inductions has risen more slowly than that of overall inductions, demonstrating that elective inductions (with possibly marginal indications) are becoming more frequent. Elective inductions currently account for at least half of all inductions.[2]

II. PATIENT CASE (PART 1)

Mrs. T.S. is a 38-year-old gravida 1 para 0 with an intrauterine pregnancy at 40 weeks who presented to her doctor's office for a routine prenatal care visit. The patient had felt good fetal movement over the past week and had no uterine contractions or vaginal bleeding. The patient had noted significantly increased swelling in her hands, feet, and face. She had been experiencing a headache for 2 days that was not relieved with acetaminophen. Her physical examination revealed the following: blood pressure 172/100 mmHg and 174/102 mmHg when repeated, urine dip test 3(+) protein, pedal edema 3(+), and fundal height 40 centimeters. A sterile vaginal examination revealed the cervix to be 1 centimeter dilated, 50% effaced, and 0 station/soft/anterior. Fetal heart tones were 125 beats per minute. She was promptly sent to labor and delivery for induction of labor for preeclampsia.

III. Indications for Induction

Labor induction is indicated when the maternal or fetal benefits from delivery outweigh the risks of prolonging the pregnancy. Indications for induction vary in acuity and may be for elective or medical reasons. The indication for delivery includes, but is not limited to, those described in the American College of Obstetricians and Gynecologists (ACOG) Technical Bulletin number 10 (Table 1).[3] The indication and plan for delivery should be clearly outlined with the patient and documented in the medical record. Induction of labor has its own inherent risks, and these should be discussed with the patient before initiation of the induction.

IV. Risks of Induction

The risks of induction include chorioamnionitis (infection involving the placenta and amniotic fluid), cesarean delivery, iatrogenic prematurity, and respiratory morbidities

Table 1. Patient Selection for Induction of Labor

Indications
  Preeclampsia, eclampsia
  Gestational hypertension
  Chorioamnionitis
  Suspected fetal jeopardy, evident by biochemical or biophysical indications (eg, fetal growth restriction, isoimmunization)
  Maternal medical problems (eg, diabetes mellitus, renal disease, chronic hypertension, chronic obstructive pulmonary disease)
  Fetal demise
  Logistic factors (eg, risk of rapid labor, distance from hospital)
  Postterm gestation
Contraindications
  Placenta or vasa previa
  Abnormal fetal lie
  Funic presentation/cord prolapse
  Prior classical uterine incision
  Active genital herpes infection
  Pelvic structural deformities
  Invasive cervical carcinoma

Adapted from American College of Obstetricians and Gynecologists. Induction of labor. ACOG Practice Bulletin, Number 10, November 1999. Reaffirmed in 2006.

in the newborn. The risk of chorioamnionitis is directly related to the length of labor. This effect has been demonstrated in both nulliparous and multiparous women.[4]

Elective inductions are associated with a twofold increase in cesarean delivery. This is seen more dramatically in the nulliparous patient with an unfavorable cervix.[5]

To reduce the risk of iatrogenic prematurity (delivery of a premature infant by health care member), the pregnancy must be at least 39 weeks by strict dating criteria. These criteria include[6]:

1. Fetal heart tones have been documented for 20 weeks by nonelectronic fetoscope or for 30 weeks by Doppler.

2. It has been 36 weeks since a positive serum or urine human chorionic gonadotropin pregnancy test was performed by a reliable laboratory.

3. An ultrasound measurement of the crown–rump length, obtained at 6–12 weeks, supports a gestational age of at least 39 weeks.

4. An ultrasound obtained at 13–20 weeks confirms the gestational age of at least 39 weeks determined by clinical history (last menstrual period) and physical exam.

The largest neonatal risk after elective induction at term is related to retained lung fluid. The spontaneous onset of labor seems to be important in preparing the lungs for extrauterine respiration.[7] Risk can range from minor, resolving without intervention shortly after birth, to severe, requiring respiratory assistance.

V. Patient Selection

As can be seen from the potential risks associated with labor induction, patient selection is an important aspect of successful inductions. Appropriate patient selection can assist in lowering the likelihood of the aforementioned risks. The mode of induction may be selected by assessing the patient's cervical status. Cervical readiness for labor is determined by using the Bishop score (Table 2). The Bishop score, first described in 1964 in multiparous women, is a methodical and efficient way to document cervical status. This score can facilitate choosing an induction agent (see section VII. Labor Inducing Agents, below) and predicting induction success.[8] A Bishop score of <6 indicates an unfavorable cervix that may require a prelabor induction agent to "ripen" the cervix. This is in contrast with a Bishop score >6, which indicates the cervix is more likely ready for labor and an agent that induces contractions should be used. A bishop

Table 2. Bishop Score

	0	1–2	3–4	5–6
Dilation (cm)	0	1–2	3–4	5–6
Effacement (%)	0–30	40–50	60–70	80
Station	–3	–2	–1 to 0	+1 to +2
Consistency	Firm	Medium	Soft	—
Position	Posterior	Mid	Anterior	—

Adapted from Bishop EH. Pelvic scoring for elective induction. *Obstet Gynecol.* 1964;24:266–268.

score of 9 suggests a high likelihood of success and a score of <4 has a high probability of induction failure. In the latter case, a cervical ripening agent (described in section VI. Cervical Ripening Agents, below) may increase the "favorability" of the cervix and thus increase the likelihood of induction success.

There are a variety of induction agents to choose from, some mechanical and others pharmacologic. Patient selection, indication for induction, and the Bishop score are the primary components of induction success. Tables 1 and 2 can be used to determine appropriate management algorithms for your patients.

VI. Cervical Ripening Agents

A. Mechanical

1. Membrane Stripping
Induction of labor by "stripping" the amniotic membranes is a common practice. The majority of studies have found membrane stripping to be safe and result in fewer postdate inductions being required. This entails an examiner's finger being placed in the cervix and then revolving the finger around the cervix between the interior of the cervix (internal os) and the fetal membranes. More specifically, the "stripping" of membranes refers to separating the membranes from the lower uterine segment that results in an increase in phospholipase A_2 and prostaglandin $F_{2\alpha}$ which releases prostaglandins known to be important for the onset of labor.[9,10] In patients undergoing labor induction, the use of membrane stripping is associated with a decreased need for oxytocin and an increased vaginal delivery rate.[11] A randomized controlled trial of postterm pregnancies demonstrated that a statistically significant number of patients went into spontaneous labor within 72 hours after membrane stripping compared with those who did not have membrane stripping.[12] To reduce the risk of iatrogenic prematurity, membrane stripping is not recommended before 39 weeks. The only down side of this form of cervical ripening is temporary mild patient discomfort.

2. Transcervical Catheter (Foley Balloon)
Mechanical dilation of the cervix with a balloon catheter was first described in 1863. Since then there have been variations; however, the basic concept remains the same. The Foley balloon catheter is the most commonly used instrument in this class. The Foley bulb is used as a mechanical method of cervical ripening. This is achieved by placing the balloon into the endocervix and then filling the balloon with saline. This causes an increase in local pressure inside the cervical canal. This pressure facilitates cervical ripening by stimulating the release of local prostaglandins and triggering the Ferguson reflex. The Ferguson reflex refers to the phenomenon of the body releasing oxytocin to stimulate uterine contractions when pressure is applied inside the cervix or as the cervix starts to open. A recent randomized controlled trial found the intracervical Foley catheter to be comparable to misoprostol for preinduction cervical ripening.[13] Placement of the catheter requires some skill, but generally can be placed without difficulty (Table 3).

B. Pharmacologic

Prostaglandins are hormonelike, fat soluble, regulatory molecules that are derived from fatty acids and have abundant physiologic actions. They are important in inflam-

Table 3. Technique for Intracervical Balloon Catheter Placement

Instruments
  Sterile speculum and gloves
  26 French (or 30 mL balloon catheter)
  Ring forceps (2)
  Sterile scissors
  50 mL saline
Procedure
  A 26 French catheter is placed into the endocervical canal using a sterile speculum and
    direct visualization or manual palpation
  The tip of the catheter may be shortened using sterile scissors to facilitate placement (cut
    distal to the balloon)
  Test inflating balloon before placement
  Tip of catheter may be placed in endocervix
  Insufflate balloon with 30–50 mL saline
  Withdraw balloon slightly until it rests in the canal at the internal os
  Tape catheter to leg with traction
  Remove if membranes rupture or after 12 hours

mation, contraction of smooth muscle, and maintenance of body temperature. They have also been used extensively for reproductive reasons, namely cervical ripening and labor induction. Numerous randomized controlled trials have demonstrated prostaglandins (PGE_1 and PGE_2) to be effective in both preparing the cervix for induction and induction of labor.[14,15]

1. Prostaglandin E$_1$

Misoprostol (Cytotec) is a synthetic form of PGE_1 that is labeled for use by the U.S. Food and Drug Administration (FDA) for prevention of peptic ulcer disease. However, in obstetrics, misoprostol has been used (off label) as an effective and inexpensive cervical ripening agent. Misoprostol is available in tablet form and can be administered intravaginally or by mouth. Misoprostol is dispensed in 100 μg tablets that can be cut in quarters for convenient use. The optimal dose for a term pregnancy is 25 μg every 3–6 hours placed in the posterior vaginal fornix. Administration or repeat dosing is not recommended if there are ≥3 contractions in 10 minutes. Many clinical trials have documented the safety of using misoprostol for cervical ripening and labor induction. Studies evaluating misoprostol uniformly demonstrated a decreased cesarean section rate and higher incidence of vaginal delivery within 24 hours of initiation and a decreased need for oxytocin.[15] When used in higher doses (≥50 μg), misoprostol has been correlated with a higher rate of tachysystolic uterine contractions (6 or more contractions in 10 minutes in two consecutive 10 minute periods) than placebo or PGE_2.[3]

An alternative route is oral administration. This course of therapy is typically 50 μg orally every 4 hours. The oral route of delivery is not the preferred regimen, as it has been shown to be less successful in cervical preparation or induction than the vaginal route.[16]

The most significant risk from using misoprostol is the increased occurrence of uterine hyperstimulation and the potential for disruption of the uterine scar in patients with a previous cesarean delivery.[3] Induction of labor in patients with a prior cesarean delivery is not discussed as it is beyond the scope of the focus of this chapter.

2. Prostaglandin E₂

Dinoprostone, the naturally occurring form of PGE$_2$, is a low-dose cervical preparation that is approved for cervical ripening and induction of labor. Ideally, PGE$_2$ alters the cervical collagen fibers, which results in separation of the closely knit collagen bundles and an increase in the intervening ground substance by increasing the submucosal water content.

The FDA has approved two low-dose preparations of dinoprostone: Prepidil, 0.5 mg gel, placed intracervical, and Cervidil, 10 mg vaginal insert, placed transversely in the posterior fornix of the vagina. The vaginal insert releases dinoprostone at approximately 0.3 mg/h for 12 hours and the attached retrieval system allows rapid removal if uterine hyperstimulation occurs. Alternatively, a 1- to 3-mg gel can be made from 20-mg suppositories (Prostin E2) and placed in the posterior vaginal fornix. With any of the products, PGE$_2$ enhances cervical ripening, increasing the likelihood of successful initial induction, decreases the incidence of prolonged labor, increases uterine contractions, and lowers oxytocin requirements.[17] In the nulliparous patient, who usually has an unfavorable cervix, the enhancement of contractility mimics spontaneous labor more closely than oxytocin or amniotomy.[18] PGE$_2$ is recommended for use in the patient with a low Bishop score (≤6).

After placement of PGE$_2$, the patient should remain recumbent for 30–60 minutes followed by observation for 1–2 hours. If uterine activity does not change, the patient can be transferred to an antepartum floor or possibly discharged. If there is an increase in uterine activity, the fetal heart rate and contraction pattern should be continuously monitored for 4–6 hours. A second dose of gel can be placed 6 hours after the initial dose, if necessary.

Prostaglandins are rarely used in the setting of frequent fetal heart rate decelerations because of an inability to quickly terminate the possible long-acting effects on uterine contractility. If uterine hyperstimulation occurs, the administration of subcutaneous or intravenous terbutaline (0.25 mg) will often result in quiescence of uterine activity. When used appropriately, the incidence of uterine hypertonicity with prostaglandin use is low, and maternal side effects are essentially negligible.

VII. Labor-Inducing Agents

A. Amniotomy

Amniotomy can safely and effectively induce or augment labor. The mechanism of action of amniotomy stems from the release of prostaglandins, which stimulate uterine contractions. Endogenous oxytocin production does not seem to be involved in this beneficial effect.

In the patient with a Bishop score >8, artificial rupture of membranes induces labor successfully, with only an occasional need for oxytocin augmentation.[8] Amniotomy also produces beneficial effects for the augmentation of labor. Proponents of the active management of labor protocol hold amniotomy as a key component for induction success. Studies have shown there is a significant shortening of labor when amniotomy is performed in the setting of cervical dilation of 3 centimeters or more.[19]

Before performing amniotomy, care should be taken to ensure the fetal head is well applied to the cervix and the Group B *Streptococcus* status has been confirmed. The fetal heart rate should be recorded immediately after amniotomy. If labor does not follow, oxytocin augmentation may be added to the treatment algorithm to assist in initiating uterine contractions. This regimen has been shown to be more effective than amniotomy alone.[20]

B. Oxytocin

Oxytocin, an octapeptide, can be used for augmentation (as mentioned above) or for induction of labor. Oxytocin is one of the most studied and used methods of labor induction. Theobald first described the continuous infusion of oxytocin in 1948.[21] More than a half-century of use has confirmed its safety, but the precise dosing protocol and interval is debatable. This ambiguity stems from the fact that oxytocin has different responses in several subpopulations of patients (ie, nulliparous vs multiparous; elective induction vs augmentation). The 1999 ACOG Technical Bulletin (reaffirmed in 2006) lists two intervals for the administration of oxytocin.[3] One is considered to be low dose (physiologic) with longer dosing intervals and the other, high dose (pharmacologic), with intervals that are closer. In 1984, Seitchik et al. published research that demonstrated the pharmacokinetics of oxytocin.[22] They showed that a 40-minute period is needed to reach steady-state concentrations, but uterine response occurs rapidly, within 3–5 minutes.

Recommendations for selection of a particular regimen (high dose vs low dose) vary. Multiple studies have found both protocols effective in establishing adequate labor patterns, but when focusing on outcomes, the high-dose protocol has consistently demonstrated a faster induction time and fewer failed inductions. Lopez-Zeno et al. found, in a select patient population (nulliparous), that high-dose oxytocin, in the setting of an active management protocol, decreased cesarean section rate, time in labor, and maternal infectious morbidity.[23]

For a brief summary of the various protocols for oxytocin delivery, refer to Table 4.

Table 4. Use of Oxytocin

Indications
  For the induction or augmentation of labor
Contraindications
  Those patients in whom a vaginal delivery is contraindicated
Administration
  15 Units of oxytocin in 250 mL IV fluid = 60 mU/mL (rate of 1 mL/h = 1 mU/min)
    Induction
      Start at a rate of 1 mU/min and increase by 1–2 mU/min q40–60min to a maximum of 20–30 mU/min
    Augmentation
      Multiparae (low dose)
        Start at a rate of 1 mU/min and increase by 1–2 mU/min q40–60min to a maximum of 20–30 mU/min
      Nulliparae (low versus high dose)
        Can use low-dose protocol (above)
        High-dose protocol: Start at 6 mU/min and increase by 6-mU increments q15min to a maximum of 36 mU/min until adequate labor reached (defined as 7 uterine contractions in 15 min)

Adapted from Lopez-Zeno JA, Peaceman AM, Adashek JA, et al. A controlled trial of a program for the active management of labor. *N Engl J Med.* 1992;326:450–454.

VIII. PATIENT CASE [PART 2]

After admission to labor and delivery, the patient's cervical examination was confirmed and her Bishop score assessed (Bishop score 8). Given that her cervix was slightly dilated, the decision was made to place a mechanical dilator (Foley bulb). Due to her preeclampsia, IV magnesium sulfate was started for seizure prophylaxis.

Eight hours following placement, the Foley bulb dislodged. The patient was reexamined and noted to be 3 centimeters/80%/0 station/soft/anterior. She was having uterine contractions every 8–10 minutes. The decision was made to continue the induction with oxytocin. Oxytocin was started at 6 mU/min and increased by 6 mU every 15–20 minutes. The patient was reexamined in 2 hours and amniotomy was performed. Oxytocin was continued at 20 mU/min when a regular contraction pattern of 2 minutes was achieved.

The patient proceeded to progress through labor normally and subsequently delivered a viable male infant with Apgar scores of 8 and 9 at 1 and 5 minutes, respectively.

IX. Summary

One out of five pregnancies undergoes induction of labor. There are numerous indications and management options for labor induction. Cervical status, patient selection, and management algorithm are imperative in success of induction. Before labor induction, the pregnancy must be well dated, have an indication for induction, and be a candidate for vaginal delivery. Understanding the various modalities for induction and being able to appropriately assign them clinically will aid in patient satisfaction and induction success.

X. References

1. Martin JA, Hamilton BE, Sutton PD. National Vital Statistics Reports. 2005;56:6.

2. Moore LE, Rayburn WF. Elective induction of labor. *Clinic Obstet Gynecol.* 2006; 49:698–704.

3. American College of Obstetricians and Gynecologists. Induction of labor. *ACOG Practice Bulletin.* Number 10. Washington, DC: ACOG. November 1999.

4. Cheng YW, Hopkins LM, Laros RK Jr, et al. Duration of the second stage of labor in multiparous women: maternal and neonatal outcomes. *Am J Obstet Gynecol.* 2007;196:585.e1–6.

5. Cheng YW, Hopkins LM, Caughey AB. How long is too long: does a prolonged second stage of labor in nulliparous women affect maternal and neonatal outcomes? *Am J Obstet Gynecol.* 2004;191:933–938.

6. Maslow AS, Sweeny AL. Elective induction of labor as a risk factor for cesarean delivery among low-risk women at term. *Obstet Gynecol.* 2000;95(Part 1):917–922.

7. McCray PB Jr, Bettencourt JD. Prostaglandins stimulate fluid secretion in human lung fluid. *J Devel Physiol.* 1993;19:29.

8. Bishop EH. Pelvic scoring for elective induction. *Obstet Gynecol.* 1964;24:266–268.

9. Adair CD. Nonpharmacologic approaches to cervical priming and labor induction. *Clin Obstet Gynecol.* 2000;43:447–454.

10. Hadi H. Cervical ripening and labor induction: clinical guidelines. *Clin Obstet Gynecol.* 2000;43:524–536.

11. Foong LC, Vanaja K, Tan G, et al. Membrane sweeping in conjunction with labor induction. *Obstet Gynecol.* 2000;96:539–542.

12. Allot HA, Palmer CR. Sweeping of membranes: a valid procedure in stimulating the onset of labour? *Br J Obstet Gynaecol.* 1993;100:898–903.

13. Chung JA, Huang WH, Rumney PJ, et al. A prospective randomized controlled trial that compared misoprostol, Foley catheter, and combination misoprostol-Foley catheter for labor induction. *Am J Obstet Gynecol.* 2003;189:1031–1035.

14. Alfirevic Z, Weeks A. Oral misoprostol for induction of labor. *Cochrane Database Syst Rev.* 2006;CD001338.

15. Hofmeyr GJ, Gulmezoglu, AM. Vaginal misoprostal for cervical ripening and induction of labour. *Cochrane Database Syst Rev.* 2003;(1):CD000941.

16. Alfirevic Z, Weeks A. Oral misoprostol for induction of labor. *Cochrane Database Syst Rev.* 2006;CD001338.

17. Rayburn WF. Prostaglandin E2 gel for cervical ripening and induction of labor: a critical analysis. *Am J Obstet Gynecol.* 1989;160:529–534.

18. Lamont RF, Neave S, Baker AC, et al. Intrauterine pressures in labours induced by amniotomy and oxytocin or vaginal prostaglandin gel compared with spontaneous labor. *Br J Obstet Gynaecol.* 1991;98:441–447.

19. Fraser WD, Marcoux S, Moutquin JM, et al. Effect of early amniotomy on the risk of dystocia in nulliparous women. *N Engl J Med.* 1993;324:1145–1149.

20. Howarth GR, Botha DJ. Amniotomy plus intravenous oxytocin for induction of labor. *Cochrane Database Syst Rev.* 2001;CD003250.

21. Theobald GW, Graham A, Campbell J, et al. The use of post-pituitary extract in physiological amounts in obstetrics. *BMJ.* 1948;2:123–127.

22. Seitchik J, Amico J, Robinson AG, et al. Oxytocin augmentation of dysfunctional labor. *Am J Obstet Gynecol.* 1984;150:225–228.

23. Lopez-Zeno JA, Peaceman AM, Adashek JA, et al. A controlled trial of a program for the active management of labor. *N Engl J Med.* 1992;326:450–454.

QUESTIONS AND ANSWERS

1. Which of the following is an indication for labor induction?

    a. gestational hypertension

    b. chorioamnionitis

    c. insulin-dependent diabetes

    d. all of the above

2. What can be done to the cervix to increase the success of labor induction?

    a. membrane stripping

    b. intravaginal misoprostol

    c. oxytocin infusion

    d. all of the above

3. The name of the scoring system used to assess and describe the status of the cervix is _____ .

4. A common intravenous agent used for labor induction is _____ .

Answers:

1. d; 2. b; c. Bishop score; d. oxytocin

Pain Control in Labor

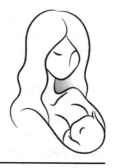

Michael Haydon

LEARNING OBJECTIVES

1. Describe etiologies of pain in labor.

2. Compare methods of analgesia available to women in labor.

3. Evaluate the effects of labor analgesia on the fetus.

4. Identify the possible maternal complications of labor analgesia.

I. Introduction

Dr. James Simpson, a Scottish obstetrician, used ether to treat labor pain as early as 1847.[1] Today there are numerous modalities used to minimize or alleviate pain associated with labor contractions. Nonpharmacologic means include hypnotherapy, massage, acupuncture, and breathing techniques performed with the help of a labor coach. Systemic pharmacologic treatments include oral, intravenous, or intramuscular narcotics or sedatives. More recently, nerve blocking approaches have been adopted including a neuraxial epidural block and regional pudendal block.

II. CASE HISTORY [PART 1]

A 32-year-old gravida 1 para 0 presents to the labor and delivery suite in early labor. Her cervix is noted to be 3 centimeters dilated, and she is having regular uterine contractions. Her chief complaint is labor pain. She notes that the fetus is actively moving and she has not had any vaginal bleeding. She denies fever, chills, nausea, or vomiting. She has a history of asthma, which is controlled with albuterol as needed. The only other medications she is taking are prenatal vitamins, iron sulfate, and folic acid. She denies the use of alcohol and tobacco. She has no surgical history and her family history is noncontributory. The vital signs on presentation are temperature 36.7°C (98°F), heart rate 110 beats/min, blood pressure systolic 130 mmHg/diastolic 84 mmHg. The relevant admission laboratory results are hemoglobin 10.2, hematocrit 31.4, and platelets 168,000.

III. Pathways of Labor Pain

Labor pain is primarily the result of uterine contractions. Uterine contractions cause uterine muscle ischemia, which in turn mediates the release of bradykinin, serotonin, and histamine. Additionally, cervical dilatation causes stretching of the lower uterine segment, which refers noxious pain stimuli through mechanoreceptors. Pain in the first stage of labor is mediated through sympathetic nerves, specifically thoracic and lumbar spinal nerves (T10 through T12 and L1). During the pushing phase of labor (stage 2), the fetal head stretches the vagina and perineum. Pain due to this distention of the pelvic floor is mediated through sacral spinal nerves S2-S4, also referred to as the *pudendal nerve* (Figure 1).

IV. Systemic Analgesia

A. Intravenous Narcotics

IV opium derivatives (narcotics) for pain control during labor have been used for decades.[2] Morphine, a natural derivative of opium initially used for this purpose, has fallen out of favor due to its side effect profile, including respiratory depression. Meperidine (Demerol) also is less commonly used due to its delayed metabolism and extended half-life in newborns. Synthetic compounds such as fentanyl and butorphanol are more commonly used today. Butorphanol (Stadol) is a mixed agonist/antagonist and has the advantage of a ceiling effect on respiratory depression. The most common side effect of all systemic narcotics is nausea, and, therefore, the concomitant use of antiemetics is recommended.

All systemic opioids are known to cross the placenta and exert physiologic effects on the fetus. Specifically, opioids have been shown to decrease the changes in the fetal heart rate that are critical to evaluating fetal well-being during labor. A recent randomized controlled trial compared the effects of IV meperidine versus epidural analgesia on the fetal heart rate. Meperidine was associated with statistically significant heart rate changes compared to epidural administration of narcotics.[3] An additional concern of systemic opioids is their association with neonatal respiratory depression. In this case, the use of naloxone to reverse the opioid may be necessary to resuscitate the newborn. A recent prospective study reviewing neonatal resuscitation guidelines found that proper resuscitation techniques can dramatically reduce or eliminate the need for naloxone (Narcan) use in this regard.[4] Moreover, there do not appear to be any long-term neurobehavioral effects of opioids on the newborn. However, to minimize fetal effects and immediate neonatal effects, current recommendations are to use synthetic opioids, such as fentanyl (Sublimaze), which are short acting and have no active metabolite.

B. Patient-Controlled Intravenous Analgesia

Similar to their use in nonobstetric populations, opioids for patient-controlled IV analgesia, commonly called *PCA*, have been used for pain relief in labor. This technique uses a standard infusion pump that allows the laboring patient to administer IV

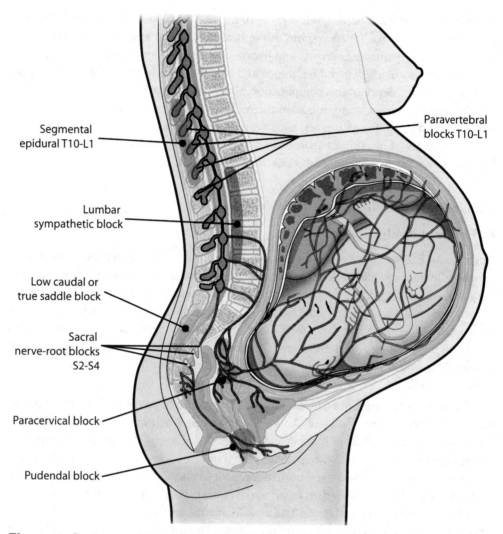

Segmental epidural T10-L1

Paravertebral blocks T10-L1

Lumbar sympathetic block

Low caudal or true saddle block

Sacral nerve-root blocks S2-S4

Paracervical block

Pudendal block

Figure 1. Pathways of Labor Pain. From Eltzschig HK, Lieberman ES, Camann WR. Regional anesthesia and analgesia for labor and delivery. N Engl J Med 2003;348: 319–322. Copyright © 2003 Massachusetts Medical Society. All rights reserved, with permission.

boluses of narcotic at preset dosages and time intervals. Initial aims were to provide patient autonomy and avoid prolonged waiting times for nursing administration of pain relief during labor. Most studies have shown that this approach provides equivalent pain control to narcotics administered by a nurse or anesthesiologist. Additional benefits to this approach are the efficiency it provides in a busy labor and delivery ward, as well as a reduction in total narcotic used by the patient. However, its use is diminishing, as maternal nausea and neonatal respiratory depression are still concerns.

V. Regional Anesthesia: Pudendal Block

A pudendal block can be administered to provide safe and effective pain relief for a vaginal delivery. The block should also provide sufficient pain control to repair an episiotomy or routine vaginal lacerations. Lidocaine, 5–10 mL of 1% solution, is injected below and posterior to the ischial (sciatic) spine through a transvaginal approach. As with spinal anesthesia, toxicity including seizure and hypotension can be encountered if the injection is placed intravascularly. Careful technique and detailed knowledge of the vascular anatomy make the incidence of this complication extremely rare. It is also important to quantify the amount of local anesthetic administered. It is recommended not to exceed a total dose of lidocaine of 4 mg/kg when used without epinephrine, and 7 mg/kg when used with epinephrine. This form of analgesia may also provide pain control for a vacuum- or forceps-assisted delivery if epidural is not used during labor.

VI. Neuraxial Analgesia

A. Epidural Analgesia

Approximately 60% of pregnant women, or 2.4 million, in the United States each year choose epidural analgesia for labor.[4] Epidural analgesia works by blocking labor pain arising from the lower thoracic, lumbar, and sacral nerve roots. Epidural analgesia was traditionally given as an intermittent bolus by a nurse midwife or anesthesiologist. A continuous epidural infusion by a mechanical pump is now more commonly used. This advancement has improved sterility and decreased toxicity associated with large single boluses. It is widely accepted as the most effective form of analgesia for labor pain with minimal side effects.

The procedure is performed by placing the patient upright on the bed or table and having her lean forward from the waist. An aseptic technique is performed and 1% lidocaine is first used for local anesthetic of the skin and interspinous ligament. A large-bore needle (16–18 gauge) is then directed into the epidural space (Figure 2). Once the proper needle placement is confirmed with a small test dose of local anesthetic, a catheter is threaded into the epidural space. The catheter is then taped to the patient's back to prevent it from being dislodged during labor. The catheter is traditionally placed into the lower lumbar spine (L2-L4) to predominantly exert its effects on the sympathetic nerves associated with early labor pain. Low-dose local anesthetic (0.125% bupivacaine or 0.2% ropivacaine) is commonly used; however, many practitioners also include a small amount of fentanyl (2 µg/mL). The addition of a small amount of fentanyl allows for a lower concentration of maintenance local anesthetic. The lower concentration of local anesthetic decreases the amount of motor block encountered and allows for more effective pushing during the second stage of labor.

B. Combined Spinal Epidural Analgesia

A common form of epidural analgesia is referred to as a *combined spinal epidural*. This allows for rapid onset of a spinal block (placed in the intrathecal space) followed by an epidural that can be titrated for long-term labor pain. The technique uses a needle through needle approach. A 16- to 18-gauge needle is first advanced into the epidural space. A 25-gauge spinal needle is then advanced through the large-bore needle farther into the intrathecal space. Placement is confirmed once spinal fluid is identified. A small amount of local anesthetic plus narcotic (0.125% bupivacaine plus 2 µg fentanyl) is placed into this intrathecal space for a fast and predictable sympathetic block. The fine spinal needle is then removed and the epidural catheter is guided into the epidural space for continuous epidural infusion.

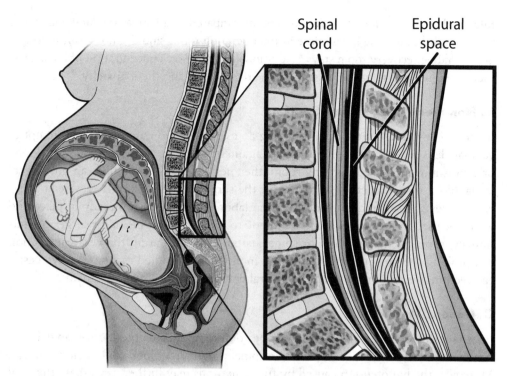

Figure 2. Location of Epidural Analgesia. From Sharma SK, Leveno KJ. Regional analgesia and progress of labor. Clin Obstet Gynecol 2003;46:633, with permission.

C. Patient-Controlled Epidural Analgesia

A significant advance in labor pain relief is the patient-controlled epidural analgesia. This provides the most effective form of labor analgesia combined with patient autonomy. The most common approach is to initially place a combined spinal epidural for immediate pain relief. Once the patient is comfortable, the epidural catheter is activated and administered as needed by the patient. The most common protocol is to have a continuous epidural infusion for maintenance. In addition to this continuous infusion, the patient has the ability to provide additional epidural boluses every 10 to 30 minutes as needed. Patients are able to personally provide pain relief during the active phase of labor. They may then reduce these boluses when directed to push, to allow for more explosive expulsion efforts in the second stage of labor. A recent meta-analysis including 640 patients compared patient-controlled epidural anesthesia to traditional continuous epidural infusion. Investigators found those patients receiving patient-controlled epidural analgesia required less intervention from anesthesia personnel, had less motor block, and used less total anesthetic in labor.[5]

VII. Anesthesia for Cesarean Section

A. Scheduled Cesarean Section

If a patient has a scheduled cesarean section, the use of a regional anesthesia is preferred. The most commonly used regional method in this case is a short-acting spinal block.

Riley and colleagues found this approach, as compared to a lumbar epidural, was easier to accomplish, resulting in less time in the operating room, and did not result in longer postoperative recovery room stays.[6] Additionally, the lower concentration of local anesthetic required in a spinal block reduces the risk of local anesthetic toxicity.

B. Non-Elective Cesarean Section

In the event that a patient is undergoing a cesarean section after a failed attempt at vaginal delivery, a spinal block would again be the preferred method. Once the patient is moved to the operating room, the anesthesiologist will place an intrathecal spinal block that will act long enough for the surgeons to perform the cesarean delivery. However, if an epidural is used during labor, this catheter is already in place and would be used for a bolus of local anesthetic to create a dense block for surgery. Additionally, supplemental epidural or spinal narcotics given during the cesarean section can prolong the postoperative analgesia. In either a scheduled or non-elective cesarean section, the patient will need IV or oral narcotics for postoperative pain.

C. General Anesthesia

In certain situations, the fetal status may be compromised and urgent cesarean delivery may be necessary. In this case, placing a spinal or epidural block could delay delivery. Moreover, the hypotension caused by these methods may further exacerbate the fetal stress. Each of the inhaled and IV medications used in general anesthesia is considered safe for the fetus. Initially, a short-acting IV barbiturate is used to put the patient to sleep. After the endotracheal tube is noted to be properly placed, a mixture of oxygen and nitrous oxide are provided for analgesia. The addition of a halogenated agent, such as isoflurane, can provide additional analgesia. Benefits to this approach are complete analgesia and amnesia. One of the most concerning complications of general anesthesia is aspiration. Several factors associated with pregnancy place the patient at risk for aspiration of gastric contents. The lower esophageal sphincter is relaxed, gastric emptying is delayed, and the pregnant uterus increases intra-abdominal pressure. Therefore, in all cases of cesarean section, an antacid is provided before surgery to decrease to the risk of complications if aspiration occurs.

VIII. Concerns about Epidural Analgesia

A. Effect of Epidural on Progression of Labor

Early observational studies indicated that the use of an epidural was associated with an increase in the cesarean section rate. The difficulties in analyzing these data are the various patient populations and physician practice styles that can affect the rate of cesarean section.[7,8] A meta-analysis comprised of 37,000 patients from a variety of practice settings did not find an increased cesarean section rate with use of epidural.[9] Some practitioners were also concerned about the placement of an epidural before a certain point in labor had been achieved—engagement of the fetal head or a certain cervical dilation. However, two randomized controlled trials did not show an increase in cesarean section when epidural was administered early in labor.[10,11] Moreover, a large randomized controlled trial was performed studying 750 women having their first child to evaluate the effects of early epidural use on the cesarean section rate. All of the women were dilated less than 4 centimeters. One arm of the study (early epidural group) was provided a combined spinal epidural at first request for pain. The second arm received IV hydromorphone. The IV hydromorphone group was later provided an epidural after reaching 4 centimeters cervical dilation. The authors concluded that the cesarean section rate was similar between the groups (17.8% early epidural vs 20.7% early IV hydromorphone [Dilaudid]).[12] They also found that the epidural provided better analgesia and a more rapid progression of labor. These findings further support a joint statement by the American College of Obstetricians and Gynecologists and the American Society of Anesthesiologists in 2002 stating that a woman's request for pain relief is sufficient medical indication for its use.[13]

B. Hypotension

Decrease in blood pressure is common after the placement of an epidural or spinal anesthesia. The sympathetic nervous system is important for maintaining vascular tone. The effects of local anesthetics in the intrathecal or epidural space will decrease vascular tone and possibly result in decreased maternal cardiac output. Uterine blood flow may be compromised with resultant effects on the fetus. This possibility can be diminished with the use of intravenous volume expansion with crystalloids before neuraxial anesthesia. If encountered, first-line treatment of anesthesia-related hypotension is a vasoconstrictive agent. IV ephedrine in 5- to 10-mg increments is effective in increasing blood pressure in most cases. Rarely, with severe hypotension and delay in resuscitative measures, a profound fetal bradycardia may be encountered, necessitating an emergent cesarean section for nonreassuring fetal status.

C. Spinal Headache

Women receiving an epidural catheter must be counseled regarding the possibility of an epidural needle accidentally entering the intrathecal space, causing leakage of a small amount of cerebral spinal fluid. Often, this will result in a severe headache that is worse when sitting up and markedly improved when lying down. It is estimated to occur in up to 3% of procedures.[14] This is much less likely to occur with a combined spinal epidural, as the needle used to perforate the dura for intrathecal administration is extremely small and atraumatic. Pain is thought to result from loss of cerebral spinal fluid and stretching of the meninges. Mild symptoms can be treated with intravenous caffeine or narcotics. For severe cases, approximately 20–30 cc of the patient's blood can be placed into the epidural space. This treatment, a "blood patch," is the gold standard for treatment of a severe spinal headache.

D. High Spinal Block

Rarely, neuraxial anesthesia will cause a spinal block that is too high in the spinal cord. This may block the cervical spine nerves, including C3-C5, which innervate the diaphragm. Patients may complain of difficulty breathing or tingling in the hands and fingers. Severe hypotension and cardiovascular collapse have been reported. The complication results from miscalculated spinal doses, inadvertent intrathecal placement of epidural dose of a local anesthetic, or improper positioning of patients with hyperbaric local anesthetic solutions. If symptoms persist, intubation to protect the airway may be necessary.

E. Anesthetic Toxicity

During placement of an epidural or spinal block, the anesthesiologist uses a small test dose to be sure the medication is not being injected directly into a blood vessel. If accidentally administered into the vasculature, the patient may experience nervous system findings (ringing in ears, agitation, seizure) followed by cardiovascular symptoms (hypertension and tachycardia). Treatment includes antiepileptics or benzodiazepines for convulsions and supportive measures, including oxygen and vasopressors.

F. Contraindications to Epidural Anesthesia

Absolute contraindications to epidural anesthesia include coagulopathy, infection at injection site, raised intracranial pressure, and hypovolemia. Coagulopathy (clotting abnormalities) may lead to the development of a large hematoma due to needle placement causing spinal cord compression. Infection at the insertion site could result in meningitis or epidural abscess. Placing an epidural with increased intracranial pressure could result in brain herniation. The sympathetic blockade produced by epidurals, in combination with uncorrected hypovolemia, may cause profound circulatory collapse. Relative contraindications include fixed cardiac output states (ie, aortic stenosis) and vertebral anatomic abnormalities. Patients with fixed cardiac output are unable to increase their cardiac output in response to the peripheral vasodilatation caused by epidural blockade, and may develop profound circulatory collapse. Anatomic abnormalities may preclude the placement of an epidural.

IX. CASE HISTORY [PART 2]

Assessment

Considering that the patient is in early labor with her first pregnancy, some form of long-acting pain relief is preferred. Although previously thought to delay labor if given early, neuraxial analgesia should be offered in this case. The patient's vital signs are stable. However, her increased pulse rate is consistent with worsening labor pain. The platelet count is normal and, therefore, there is no risk of epidural hematoma that can be caused by thrombocytopenia.

Plan

To provide immediate pain relief, a combined spinal epidural should be placed. Once the patient is comfortable due to the spinal anesthetic, a patient-controlled epidural can be activated for pain relief throughout labor. In order to decrease the risk of hypotension, the patient should be prehydrated with crystalloid. Hypotension should be aggressively treated with an IV pressor agent, such as ephedrine. Continuous fetal monitoring should be performed during and after the regional anesthesia is placed to evaluate fetal well-being.

X. Summary

Pain control during labor must be individualized for each patient. Pain thresholds, cultural differences, and personal expectations all make each patient's assessment of pain in labor unique. Nonpharmacologic methods assist patients in minimizing and coping with the pain of labor. Systemic pharmacologic approaches can lessen pain through the sedative and analgesic effects of intravenous narcotics. Epidural analgesia is the most common form of analgesia for labor pain and patient-controlled options improve satisfaction through increased autonomy. As pain is the fifth vital sign, effective and immediate pain relief should be offered at the patient's first request at any point in labor.

XI. References

1. Simpson W. *The Works of Sir J.Y. Simpson*. Edinburgh, Scotland: Adam and Charles Black, 1871.

2. Hill JB, Alexander JM, Sharma SK, et al. A comparison of the effects of epidural and meperidine analgesia during labor on fetal heart rate. *Obstet Gynecol*. 2003; 102:333–337.

3. Box D, Cochrane D. Safe reduction in administration of naloxone to newborn infants: an observational study. *Acta Paediatr*. 2006;95:1083–1086.

4. Hawkins JL, Beaty BR, Gibbs CP. Update on U.S. OB practice. *Anesthesiology*. 1999;91:436–441.

5. Van der Wyer M, Halpern S, Joseph G. Patient-controlled epidural analgesia versus continuous infusion for labour analgesia: a meta-analysis. *Br J Anaesthesia*. 2002;89:459–465.

6. Riley E, Cohen S, Macario A, et al. Spinal versus epidural anesthesia for cesarean section: a comparison of time efficiency, costs, charges, and complications. *Anesth Analg*. 1995;80:709–712.

7. Rogers R, Gilson G, Kammerer-Doak D. Epidural analgesia and active management of labor: effects on length of labor and mode of delivery. *Obstet Gynecol*. 1999;93:995–998.

8. Lieberman E, Lang JM, Cohen A, et al. Association of epidural analgesia with cesarean delivery in nulliparas. *Obstet Gynecol*.1996;88:993–1000.

9. Segal S, Su M, Gilbert P. The effect of a rapid change in availability of epidural analgesia on the cesarean section rate: a meta-analysis. *Am J Obstet Gynecol*. 2000;183:974–978.

10. Chestnut DH, McGrath JM, Vincent RD Jr, et al. Does early administration of epidural analgesia affect obstetric outcome in nulliparous women who are in spontaneous labor? *Anesthesiology*. 1994;80:1201–1208.

11. Luxman D, Wohlman I, Groutz A, et al. The effect of early epidural block administration on the progression and outcome of labor. *Int J Obstet Anesth*. 1998;7:161–164.

12. Wong CA, Scavone B, Peaceman A, et al. The risk of cesarean delivery with neuraxial analgesia given early versus late in labor. *N Engl J Med*. 2005;352:655–665.

13. American College of Obstetricians and Gynecologists. Analgesia and cesarean delivery rates. *ACOG Committee Opinion.* Number 269. February 2002. *Obstet Gynecol.* 2002;99:369–370.

14. Turnbull DK, Shepherd DB. Post-dural puncture headache: pathogenesis, prevention, and treatment. *Br J Anaesth.* 2003;91:718–729.

QUESTIONS AND ANSWERS

1. In the event a severe spinal headache is diagnosed, what is the gold standard treatment?

   a. acetaminophen

   b. IV meperidine

   c. "blood patch"

   d. IM morphine

2. What is the most common side effect of IV narcotics in labor?

   a. fever

   b. bleeding

   c. nausea

   d. shortness of breath

3. What is a major maternal complication of general anesthesia in pregnancy?

   a. weakness

   b. aspiration of gastric contents

   c. nerve injury

   d. hypotension

4. Which type of labor analgesia is the most effective for immediate relief and long-term labor pain?

   a. IV narcotics

   b. pudendal block

   c. patient-controlled intravenous analgesia

   d. combined spinal epidural block

Answers:

1. c; 2. c; 3. b; 4. d

Postpartum Obstetric Hemorrhage

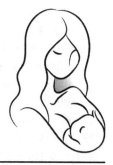

Jennifer McNulty

LEARNING OBJECTIVES

1. List the causes of postpartum hemorrhage.

2. Summarize the maternal physiologic changes that are important in preparation for blood loss at childbirth.

3. Describe the pharmacologic treatment of postpartum hemorrhage due to uterine atony.

4. Summarize the use of recombinant factor VIIa in postpartum hemorrhage.

5. List the treatment options available for postpartum anemia.

I. Introduction

Obstetric hemorrhage remains one of the top three causes of maternal mortality in the United States, and it is estimated that mortality due to hemorrhage is a largely preventable event. According to data from the U.S. Centers for Disease Control and Prevention (CDC), obstetric hemorrhage was the cause of 17% of maternal deaths in the United States between 1991 and 1999, second only to thromboembolism. When stillbirth was the outcome of the pregnancy, hemorrhage was the leading cause of maternal death, in 21% of cases. In contrast, when the outcome was a liveborn infant, hemorrhage was the cause of 2.7% of maternal deaths.[1] Case fatality rates for women who experience obstetric hemorrhage differ significantly among white and African American women, with overall mortality three-fold higher among African Americans.[2] Among white women in the United States older than 40 years of age, hemorrhage was the number one cause of mortality, followed by pulmonary embolism. Among African American women older than 40 years of age, hemorrhage was the second leading cause of death, following mortality due to preeclampsia and eclampsia. Worldwide, it is estimated that approximately 14 million cases of postpartum hemorrhage occur annually, with a case fatality rate of 1%. Thus, 140,000 women die annually of postpartum hemorrhage, resulting in a death every 4 minutes. Obstetric hemorrhage is responsible overall for 13% of maternal deaths in developed countries, compared to 20% of deaths in Latin American countries and 30%–34% of deaths in Asia and Africa.[3]

The definition of postpartum hemorrhage varies, but has traditionally been defined as blood loss at the time of a vaginal delivery of greater than 500 mL. The *International Statistical Classification of Diseases and Related Health Problems*, Tenth Revision (ICD-10) describes postpartum hemorrhage as blood loss greater than 500 mL for vaginal delivery and 750 mL for cesarean delivery. It has been demonstrated, however, that 500 mL is the average blood loss after vaginal delivery. Furthermore, the loss of this amount of blood does not result in significant morbidity for most women. In 1996, the World Health Organization suggested that in a healthy population, blood loss up to 1000 mL could be considered physiologic. They suggested that blood loss estimated at greater than 500 mL be considered an "alert line," with an "action line" reached when the vital signs of the woman become affected, usually at 1000 mL.

Data from a large population-based Dutch study of almost 3500 vaginally delivered women demonstrated that 4.2% experienced severe blood loss of more than 1000 mL. Furthermore, of the 2.7% of women who were given a red cell transfusion, 84% were in this group.[4] Estimation of blood loss by clinical providers is notoriously imprecise, and tends toward underestimation when larger amounts are lost. In an evaluation of 228 vaginally delivered women, for example, 3.5% of women lost more than 1000 mL by direct measurement, yet only 0.44% were reported to have lost this much by visual estimation of the clinician.[5] Similarly, a study of more than 4500 women vaginally delivered found that 5.2% had blood loss of greater than 1000 mL when measured directly.[6] Although the threshold for transfusion may also be variable across patient populations, the incidence of transfusion with childbirth may provide some practical information. Reported rates of transfusion in obstetric populations in the United States range from 0.13% to 3.2%.[7,8]

Postpartum hemorrhage occurs within the first 24 hours in more than 95% of cases and is termed *primary* or *early hemorrhage*. The remaining hemorrhage cases are defined as *secondary* or *late*, and occur after 24 hours but within 6 weeks of delivery.[9] The peak time of onset of secondary hemorrhage is about 2 weeks postpartum.

Risk factors for postpartum hemorrhage are multiple and can be divided into historical, antepartum, intrapartum, and postpartum risks (Table 1). Prolonged labor is associated with an increased risk of hemorrhage, including the second stage of labor exceeding 3 hours (time from complete cervix dilatation to infant delivery) or the third stage of labor longer than 30 minutes (time for placental delivery). It is impor-

Table 1. Risk Factors for Postpartum Hemorrhage

Historical	Antepartum	Intrapartum	Postpartum
Prior postpartum hemorrhage	Placenta previa	Induction of labor	Infant birth weight >4000 grams
Obesity	Antepartum bleeding	Chorioamnionitis	Genital tract trauma
Increasing maternal age	Multifetal pregnancy	Prolonged second stage of labor	Prolonged third stage of labor
	Twin to twin transfusion syndrome	Rapid labor	
	Intrauterine fetal death	Cesarean section	
	Preeclampsia	Instrumental vaginal delivery	
		Episiotomy	

tant, however, for clinicians and health care facilities to always be prepared to rapidly and efficiently deal with unexpected catastrophic bleeding, as up to one-third of patients will have no identified risks.[6,10]

A multipronged approach is required to prevent postpartum hemorrhage and reduce related maternal morbidity and mortality. Given that at least one third of women who experience hemorrhage have no risk factors, all clinicians and hospitals that provide medical care to pregnant women must be well versed in the prompt evaluation and stabilization of this obstetric emergency. This requires a multidisciplinary approach involving at a minimum staff from obstetrics, anesthesia, labor and delivery, surgical services, pharmacy, the laboratory, and the blood bank. Strategies at the hospital level may include training staff to recognize hemorrhage risk factors and to actively manage the third stage of labor, creation of a massive transfusion protocol in conjunction with blood bank staff, and creation of an obstetric hemorrhage tool kit that includes relevant equipment, such as appropriate vaginal retractors and suture materials, uterine packing balloons and gauze, and large bore intravenous start kits and fluid pressure bags.[11,12] Identification of antepartum risk factors in advance is crucial, particularly if abnormal placentation is identified, to ensure that delivery occurs at a tertiary hospital where the most skilled individuals can be prepared for complications.

II. PATIENT CASE [PART 1]

D.L. is a 39-year-old gravida 4 para 3 woman who presents to labor and delivery at 40 weeks' gestational age with regular painful contractions and cervix dilation of 6 centimeters. She is obese, with a body mass index of 32. The birth weights of her three other children were 3800–4400 grams. She has no medical problems except for mild anemia (hematocrit of 30%) identified at the time of her negative diabetic screen at 27 weeks' gestational age. Two hours after arrival, she vaginally delivers a healthy 4252-gram infant. Thirty-five minutes later, the placenta is still retained within the uterus and is manually extracted by her physician. Heavy vaginal bleeding is subsequently noted.

III. Clinical Presentation

Most patients with postpartum hemorrhage have obvious heavy vaginal bleeding that is apparent within minutes to hours after delivery. Patients who first develop abnormal bleeding hours after delivery may have already lost a significant amount of their blood volume before recognition of a problem, because of the collection of large clots within the uterus and distensible upper vagina. Some patients have recurrent episodic bleeding, both immediately postpartum and over the next several hours. Although each episode may resolve with treatment, the cumulative blood loss may also be unappreciated and substantial, particularly if different clinicians are involved in the care of the patient over time.

IV. Pathophysiology

There are a number of maternal adaptations that occur in preparation for physiologic blood loss during childbirth. Maternal hypervolemia develops, with a 45% increase in plasma volume by 30–32 weeks. The increase is greater for multifetal pregnancies. The primary mechanism for this is renal sodium and water retention, which results from increased mineralocorticoid activity in pregnancy. Overall, intravascular volume expands by 1–2 liters and extravascular volume increases by 4–7 liters. Maternal blood volume is approximately 4.5–5.5 liters. Importantly, women with preeclampsia have significantly less intravascular volume and are much less able to tolerate blood loss at delivery. They may have deceptively high hemoglobin values, however, due to lack of the normal increase in plasma volume.

Maternal red blood cell volume increases by approximately 25% due to increased erythropoiesis. This increases maternal iron requirements by 500 mg, in addition to 300 mg needed for transfer to the fetus, and 200 mg needed for maternal maintenance during the course of the pregnancy. There is an obligatory transfer of iron from the mother to her fetus, even if iron deficiency is present. Without supplemental iron during pregnancy, maternal iron stores typically become exhausted by the early third trimester.

Other important maternal cardiovascular changes include a decrease in systemic vascular resistance, which peaks at about 24 weeks, and an increase in cardiac output due to increasing stroke volume and heart rate. By term, the increased cardiac output is due primarily to the increase in heart rate. However, during labor, stroke volume increases, further raising cardiac output, which peaks just after delivery.

The uterus significantly increases in size from a nonpregnant weight of 40–70 grams and volume capacity of 10 mL, to 1200 grams with a volume capacity averaging 5000 mL. Uterine blood flow increases from 2% of total cardiac output before pregnancy to 17% in a term pregnancy. Typical blood flow through the uterus at term is 600–800 mL/min.[13] The potential, therefore, to rapidly lose a substantial and catastrophic portion of the total maternal blood volume through the pregnant uterus is remarkable.[14]

After the infant is delivered, the uterus continues to contract and the placenta cleaves along the decidua basalis as the surface area of the underlying uterine attachment site decreases. Thickening and shortening of myometrial fibers surrounding the exposed bleeding vessels limits blood loss. Coagulation and thrombus formation at the placental attachment site are of only secondary importance in this process.[15] This explains why women with inherited and acquired clotting deficits or thrombocytopenia commonly do not experience postpartum hemorrhage in the absence of significant birth canal lacerations or cesarean delivery.

Significant increases in clotting factors including VII, VIII, IX, X, and XII and fibrinogen develop early in pregnancy. In addition, there is a decrease in overall fibrinolytic activity. These result in improved clotting during pregnancy, which is thought to minimize blood loss at delivery, although there are also associated risks of thromboembolism during pregnancy and the puerperium.

V. Etiology of Postpartum Hemorrhage

A commonly used pneumonic to classify the causes of primary postpartum hemorrhage is "the four Ts," which includes tone, tissue, trauma, and thrombin (Table 2). *Tone* refers to the ability of the uterus to contract, and *tissue* refers to retained placental material, including abnormalities of placentation, such as placenta accreta. *Trauma* includes lacerations of any portion of the birth canal, including uterine rupture, and *thrombin* refers to disorders of coagulation, either congenital, such as von Willebrand's disease, or acquired, such as disseminated intravascular coagulopathy (DIC). Many patients will develop a combination of these factors. For example, retained placenta will lead to uterine atony by preventing adequate contraction of the uterus, and inadequate replacement of clotting factors with plasma transfusion during subsequent red cell transfusion will lead to so-called wash-out coagulopathy. A patient with a prolonged second stage delivering a macrosomic infant may experience both uterine atony and vaginal laceration, especially if instrumental delivery is performed.

By far the most common cause of primary postpartum hemorrhage is uterine atony, occurring in 75% of cases.[9] Retained placental material is reported as the principle cause in approximately 15% of cases, and coagulation defects reported in 0.5%–1% of cases. Additionally, genital tract trauma is found in up to 20% of women experiencing postpartum hemorrhage, as either a primary or contributing cause.[6] An invasive placental attachment due to a defect in the decidua basalis is called a *placenta accreta* and is usually associated with a placenta previa covering the cervix. This entity is discussed in greater detail in Chapter 13, Placenta Previa. Placental abruption occurs when the placenta prematurely separates from the decidua basalis before delivery of the fetus. Resulting hemorrhage into the decidua basalis can be extensive, but may not manifest as visible vaginal bleeding. If separation of the placenta from the uterus is sufficient to kill the fetus, then up to 50% of maternal blood volume can be lost, resulting in hypovolemic shock and the release of thromboplastin, triggering DIC. This entity as a cause of obstetric hemorrhage is discussed in detail in Chapter 12, Abruptio Placentae.

Table 2. Causes of Postpartum Hemorrhage

Tone	Primary uterine atony
Tissue	Retained placenta
	Abnormal placentation (placenta accreta, placenta previa)
Trauma	Lacerations of perineum, vagina, cervix
	Hematomas of vulva, vagina, broad ligament
	Uterine rupture
	Uterine inversion
Thrombin (coagulopathy)	Dilutional coagulopathy (after intravenous fluid and red cell transfusion)
	Disseminated intravascular coagulopathy (anaphylactoid syndrome of pregnancy, placental abruption, sepsis)
	Obstetric thrombocytopenia (HELLP syndrome)
	Obstetric coagulopathy – liver failure (acute fatty liver of pregnancy)
	Inherited (von Willebrand's disease, hemophilia)
	Anticoagulant therapy (mechanical valve replacement)

HELLP = hemolysis, elevated liver enzymes, and low platelets.

VI. Prevention

A. Antepartum Anemia

Women who enter the process of childbirth already significantly anemic are at greater risk for morbidity and the need for transfusion should postpartum hemorrhage occur. Attention should therefore be given in the antepartum period to prevention, identification, and treatment of iron deficiency anemia in all women. Iron deficiency has been strictly defined as a serum ferritin level <12 ng/dL; however, levels <30 ng/dL indicate low iron reserves that are too small to cover the combined fetal and maternal iron requirements in pregnancy. There is a broad overlap in measured hemoglobin between women with and without iron deficiency. Furthermore, a decrease in the mean corpuscular volume of red cells is a relatively late finding in iron deficiency anemia. Studies of large numbers of reproductive age women have demonstrated that, at most, 15%–20% have ferritin levels consistent with adequate iron reserves sufficient for a pregnancy. While only 2%–4% had overt iron deficiency anemia, 10% had evidence of complete iron depletion (ferritin <15 ng/dL) and 42% had very small iron reserves (ferritin <30 ng/dL).[16] The incidence of iron deficiency anemia is greater among women of lower socioeconomic status, and U.S. studies demonstrate that more than one third are anemic by the third trimester of pregnancy.[17]

Supplementation with elemental iron is recommended for all pregnant women, at a dose of 30 mg/d, by both the American College of Obstetrics and Gynecology (ACOG) and the CDC, and dietary iron intake and absorption is inadequate to meet this need. This recommendation recognizes that, although a woman may enter pregnancy with normal hemoglobin levels, inadequate total body iron reserves sufficient to cover the total pregnancy needs are common. The recommendation of 30 mg of iron daily is not sufficient, however, in women with iron deficiency anemia, and the CDC recommends 60–120 mg elemental iron daily for these women during pregnancy.

Iron absorption is affected by many variables and is best with an empty stomach. In particular, iron absorption is inhibited by antacids, polyphenols found in coffee and especially tea, phytate found in breads and cereals, oxalic acid in spinach and rice, and calcium found in milk, cheese, and vitamin supplements. Improved absorption with an empty stomach is most notable in women who have had gastric bypass surgery, and up to half of whom are iron deficient outside of pregnancy. Concomitant vitamin C ingestion improves iron absorption. Women taking levothyroxine for hypothyroidism should be told to take the iron separately, as it will decrease the absorption of their thyroid hormone. Iron may decrease the absorption of methyldopa, often used in pregnancy to treat mild chronic hypertension. Although much has been reported about gastrointestinal symptoms with oral iron therapy, high-quality trials involving more than 500 women found no difference in gastrointestinal side effects between placebo and iron-treated patients (21% vs 28%). A more recent study of 427 women found no dose-related correlation to gastrointestinal side effects among pregnant women taking 20, 40, 60, or 80 mg doses of elemental iron daily.[18]

It is important to note that although higher maternal hemoglobin levels in the third trimester are reported in association with low infant birth weights, this appears to be due to the association of preeclampsia with low birth weight and inappropriate maternal hemodilution. Meta-analysis of placebo-controlled trials in healthy pregnant women does not show a decrease in infant birth weight in women taking iron supplementation. Furthermore, the incidence of iron deficiency at term decreased from 55% to 31% and the incidence of actual iron deficiency anemia decreased from 15% to 5% at term in women taking supplementation.[19] One randomized controlled trial of 30 mg daily elemental iron supplementation from weeks 12 through 29 in 429 women with normal iron stores (ferritin >40 ng/dL) and hemoglobin >11 g/dL, found fewer preterm births and associated higher birth weights in those who received iron compared to placebo.[20]

The iron found in oral supplements comes in multiple forms and each contains a different percentage of elemental iron (Table 3). It is important for clinicians to be aware of the potential risk for lethal iron overdose in a young child who consumes as few as 6–8 high-dose iron supplements intended for an adult. Patient education is important, as young children are commonly in the households of pregnant women. Iron supplements should be packaged in childproof containers or individual blister packs and in all cases kept from children. Occasionally, due to lack of compliance with oral iron therapy or need for a more rapid correction of anemia, consideration should be given to parenteral treatment of iron deficiency anemia, and is discussed later in this chapter (see Table 3). Recombinant human erythropoietin has also been evaluated in very small studies for the treatment of antepartum iron deficiency anemia, in combination with parenteral iron. This expensive agent, however, has recently been associated with an increased risk of thromboembolism in treated subjects who had cancer, were undergoing spinal surgery, or were undergoing coronary bypass.[21] Erythropoietin has also been evaluated for management of postpartum anemia and is discussed later in this chapter.

Table 3. Iron Preparations

Oral	Contents	Product Examples
Ferrous sulfate	20% elemental iron	Ferrous sulfate 325 mg = 65 mg elemental iron
Dried ferrous sulfate	33% elemental iron	SlowFe (dried ferrous sulfate 160 mg) = 50 mg elemental iron Feosol tablets (dried ferrous sulfate 200 mg) = 65 mg elemental iron
Ferrous fumarate	33% elemental iron	Ferrous fumarate 324 mg = 106 mg elemental iron Maternal prenatal vitamin (ferrous fumarate 84 mg) = 27 mg elemental iron
Ferrous gluconate	12% elemental iron	Fergon (ferrous gluconate 240 mg) = 28 mg elemental iron
Carbonyl iron	100% elemental iron	Feosol caplets (carbonyl iron 45 mg) = 45 mg elemental iron
Parenteral		**Comments**
Iron dextran (Infed®)	1 mL = 50 mg elemental iron	1%–2% incidence of anaphylaxis
Iron sucrose (Venofer®)	1 mL = 20 mg elemental iron	No need for test dose

B. Management of the Third Stage of Labor

Active management of the third stage of labor has clearly and consistently been demonstrated to decrease the risk of postpartum hemorrhage in large randomized controlled trials. Active management generally includes early clamping and cutting of the umbilical cord, maternal administration of a prophylactic uterotonic agent after delivery of the infant, and facilitation of placental delivery by controlled cord traction. Expectant management, conversely, relies on spontaneous delivery of the placenta, and no uterotonic agents are given unless abnormal bleeding develops. The most recent Cochrane review of randomized controlled trials of management of the third stage of labor included more than 6000 women. It found that active management reduced the proportion of women experiencing blood loss of more than 500 or 1000 mL, the numbers of women with postpartum hemoglobin levels lower than 9 g/dL, the need for transfusion, and the need for therapeutic oxytocics to treat abnormal bleeding. These findings were consistent across all individual trials included in the larger analysis, and were both statistically and clinically significant. Oxytocin is as effective as ergometrine for prophylaxis, but without the side effects of nausea, emesis, headaches, or elevated blood pressure. One randomized trial of 600 women that specifically excluded those with hypertension or preeclampsia found a nearly 18% incidence of elevated blood pressure after treatment with ergometrine, compared to none in the group given oxytocin for third stage of labor prophylaxis.[22] Misoprostol given orally or rectally has also been studied for prophylaxis in the third stage of labor. Overall, studies suggest that oxytocin is more effective in decreasing the risk of hemorrhage of more than 1000 mL and the need for additional therapeutic uterotonic agents, compared to misoprostol. In addition, common side effects of misoprostol include shivering, nausea, diarrhea, and pyrexia.[23]

VII. Treatment

A. Initial Resuscitation and Evaluation

Management of the patient experiencing postpartum hemorrhage requires prompt attention to resuscitation of the patient, simultaneously with efforts to treat the cause of bleeding. Additional personnel must be immediately recruited to assist the bedside clinician. These patients typically will require placement of additional IV lines, delivery of blood samples to the laboratory, transport of blood products from the blood bank, administration of uterotonic agents, which must be retrieved from a refrigerated unit, placement of warming blankets, and mobilization of adequate lighting and instruments for vaginal exploration and repair of lacerations. In addition, these patients will often need to be transported to another location, such as the operating room, radiology embolization suite, or intensive care unit. It is in this potentially chaotic setting that advance training of staff and physicians via education and drills can be helpful in improving patient outcome.

Establishing adequate IV access early with large bore peripheral IVs is critical. If the patient becomes hypovolemic, placement of such IVs will become difficult or impossible due to constriction of the peripheral veins, which occurs as the body attempts to preserve volume in the central circulation. The importance of IV cannula size cannot be overstated. Flow of crystalloid by gravity through a 20- or 18-gauge cannula, both typical for a labor and delivery unit, is only approximately 65 or 140 mL/min, respectively.[24] Gravity flow through a 16- or 14-gauge cannula, in contrast, is approximately 190 or 300 mL/min, respectively, and can be further increased to 350 or 500 mL/min using a rapid infuser system.[25]

Establishing bladder drainage is important, to monitor urine output as well as to allow for better visual and manual examination of the adjacent uterus, cervix, and vagina. A full bladder may also contribute to uterine atony and preclude adequate uterine massage. A urinary catheter with an attached urometer is preferred to allow accurate measurement of milliliters of urine produced over short time intervals.

Avoidance of patient hypothermia is important to preserve platelet function and avoid pathologic microvascular bleeding. The interaction of von Willebrand's factor with platelet glycoprotein Ib/IX is important for platelet adhesion and activation, and is steadily diminished with decreasing body temperatures.[26] In addition, administering cold blood at more than 100 mL/min can induce cardiac arrhythmias and arrest.[27] Maintaining a euthermic environment can be accomplished in part by using warming devices for blood and crystalloid products, and by using warming blankets or other specially designed devices about the patient's head, trunk, and extremities.

Additionally, acidosis resulting from profound hypotension and poor tissue perfusion leads to coagulopathy by marked reduction in the activity of clotting factor VIIa, complexes of VIIa with tissue factor, and complexes of Xa with Va.[26] Once begun, this type of coagulopathy is very difficult to reverse. Therefore, early recognition of abnormal bleeding, anticipation of volume replacement needs, appropriate resuscitation, and, ideally, avoidance of hypotension are important in improving patient outcomes. Because of the importance of hypothermia and acidosis in coagulopathy, it has been suggested that patient temperature and pH are parameters that should be tracked as part of quality improvement programs for management of obstetric hemorrhage within hospital systems.[28]

B. Pharmacologic Therapy for Uterine Atony

In the meantime, a simultaneous search must be made for uterine atony, by far the most common cause of postpartum hemorrhage. Uterine atony is diagnosed by bimanual evaluation of the uterine tone, by compressing the uterus between the clinician's hand on the mother's abdomen and the other hand within the upper vagina. Often, the upper uterus will be well contracted, but the lower uterus will be soft and yielding and filled with blood clots. Thus, evaluation of uterine tone in a patient with abnormal bleeding by only an abdomen examination is insufficient. Exclusion of retained placenta and membranes can be made by complete evaluation of the placenta after delivery, which should be routine, and by manual exploration of the internal uterine cavity by the vaginal hand of the clinician. Bimanual massage of the uterus between the abdomen and vaginal hands of the clinician can increase uterine tone and improve atony. If available, bedside ultrasound can assist in the evaluation by excluding grossly obvious placenta cotyledons. If uterine massage is not immediately successful in resolving the atony and there are no retained fragments of placenta, therapeutic uterotonic medication is initiated. Available agents are outlined in Table 4,

Table 4. Uterotonic Drugs for Postpartum Hemorrhage

Drug	Brand Name	Dispensed	Dose	Route	Frequency of Dose	Absolute Contraindications	Relative Contraindications	Comments
Oxytocin	Pitocin®	10 IU in 1 mL vial	20–40 IU in 1 liter crystalloid at 250 mL/min	IV as dilute solution, or 10 IU given IM	Continuous IV infusion or single IM injection	None	None	Should not be given as undiluted IV bolus due to hypotension
Methylergonovine maleate (same as methylergometrine)	Methergine®	0.2 mg in 1 mL ampul, stored at 36°F–46°F, protect from light	0.2 mg	IM; onset 2–5 min	Every 2–4 h, clinical action sustained for 3 h or more	Hypertension, Raynaud's phenomenon, coronary artery disease, peripheral vascular disease, arteriovascular shunts	IV administration (slowly over 60 s) has greater risk of sudden hypertension and stroke and is generally avoided	Can be given as 0.2 mg oral tablet (onset 5–10 min) every 6–8 h postpartum; outside of United States parent compound is available ergonovine/ergometrine maleate
Carboprost tromethamine (same as 15-methyl $PGF_{2\alpha}$)	Hemabate®	0.25 mg in 1 mL ampul, stored at 36°F–46°F	0.25 mg	IM, onset	Every 15–90 min, no more than 8 doses total	Intravascular injection	Asthma, cardiac disease	Can also be given as 0.25 mg directly intramyometrial (during cesarean or transabdominal into the uterus after vaginal delivery)

| Misoprostol prostaglandin E$_1$ analog | Cytotec® | 200 µg tablets, long shelf life | 600 µg orally or sublingually, also reported as 600, 800, or 1000 µg rectally | Oral, sublingual, rectal, onset 4–11 min | Usually given once, could repeat 2 h later if no fever | None except known allergy | — | Studies in progress to determine best route and dose, suggested as a second-line agent until more data available |
| Dinoprostone prostaglandin E$_2$ | Prostin® | 20 mg frozen vaginal suppository | 20 mg after defrosting | Intrauterine, vaginal, rectal | Every 2 h | Hypotension | Asthma | — |

and include oxytocin, methylergonovine (Methergine), and prostaglandin agents such as carboprost (Hemabate) and prostaglandin E$_1$ (misoprostol [Cytotec]). Prostaglandin E$_2$ (dinoprostone [Prostin E2]) also has been used, although with limited available information.

Oxytocin (Pitocin) is a hypothalamic polypeptide hormone released by the posterior pituitary. It was discovered in 1909 and later synthesized in 1954. The drug induces rhythmic uterine contractions and, because of its half-life of just 3 minutes, must be given by continuous IV infusion. Its onset of action when given this way is immediate. The drug is supplied in 1 mL vials containing 10 international units (IU). It is usually administered as 20–40 IU mixed in 1 liter of crystalloid, at a rate of 250 mL/min. It may also be given as a 10-IU IM injection, with a time of onset of 3–8 minutes. Rapid IV bolus of the undiluted drug can result in hypotension due to vasodilatation.

Methylergonovine maleate, also known as methylergometrine (Methergine), is from a class of compounds known as ergot alkaloids. They were identified as a product of the fungus *Claviceps purpurea*, which grows on rye. This fungus has been long been recognized for its uterotonic properties. The parent compound of methylergometrine is ergometrine, which was first isolated in 1935, and is available in countries outside of the United States. Although first used in the 19th century to stimulate labor, recognition of associated uterine hyperstimulation and intrauterine fetal deaths led to the use of these compounds instead for postpartum hemorrhage. These drugs are sensitive to both heat and light. The parenteral preparation (1 mL ampul containing 0.2 mg) must be refrigerated and the oral preparation (0.2-mg tablets) should be stored at less than 77°F. Because of their α-adrenergic actions, they cause vasoconstriction of vascular smooth muscle, which can in turn elevate both systemic blood pressure and central venous pressure. The most common side effect is hypertension, and these drugs should not be given to those who already have hypertension, either preexisting or pregnancy-related, or those with vascular disease. More severe side effects have been reported rarely, including hypertension associated with seizures, encephalopathy, stroke, myocardial infarction, and pulmonary edema. Nausea, vomiting, and headaches occur commonly. The clinical onset of action is within 2–5 minutes if given intramuscularly and within 5–10 minutes if given orally. The drug can be given intravenously with immediate onset of action. However, this should generally be avoided due to more severe side effects, especially of significant hypertension.

Carboprost, also known as 15-methyl PGF$_{2\alpha}$ (Hemabate), is a member of the family of prostaglandins that were discovered in 1935. They were originally believed, incorrectly, to occur only in tissues of the prostate gland, hence their name. Carboprost is a potent smooth muscle stimulant that has a longer duration of action, because of the methyl group, compared with the parent compound PGF$_{2\alpha}$. It is supplied in a 1-mL ampul containing 0.25 mg and is given as a deep IM injection. It has also been given as an intramyometrial injection, either at the time of cesarean section, or directly through the abdomen wall into the uterus after vaginal delivery. The intramyometrial route may result in quicker absorption and onset of action in a patient with hypotension and poor peripheral circulation. The drug should not be given IV. The dose can be repeated every 15–90 minutes up to 8 total doses; however, in clinical trials, the vast majority of patients responded after just a single dose. Carboprost causes bronchoconstriction and vasoconstriction, and there are reported cases of intrapulmonary shunting with clinically significant arterial oxygen desaturation occurring within 5–10 minutes of administration.[29] Bronchospasm has occurred in patients with and without asthma and has been life-threatening on occasion.[30] Diarrhea is common, as are nausea and pyrexia. It is the most expensive of the uterotonic agents available in the United States.

Misoprostol (Cytotec) is a synthetic analog of prostaglandin E_1. The drug is available as 100- or 200-µg tablets intended for oral use, and is currently approved by the U.S. Food and Drug Administration (FDA) for the treatment of gastric ulcers. It is rapidly metabolized to misoprostol acid. It has potent uterotonic and cervix softening effects and has been widely adopted for use in reproductive medicine for prevention and treatment of postpartum hemorrhage, labor induction, medical treatment of early pregnancy failure, and pretreatment before intrauterine gynecologic procedures. Unlike methylergonovine and carboprost, the drug is heat and temperature stable with no special storage precautions needed. It is an inexpensive, safe, and well-tolerated drug, without clinically significant cardiovascular or respiratory complications, and can be administered to patients in whom methylergonovine or carboprost are relatively or absolutely contraindicated. The only known contraindication to use is a history of allergy to misoprostol. Pyrexia occurred in approximately 4% of nearly 400 women receiving treatment with misoprostol for postpartum hemorrhage prophylaxis, and diarrhea occurred in approximately 3%.[31] Shivering and chills occur more commonly, in up to 30%–50% of patients.[32] There is growing literature supporting its use for treatment of postpartum hemorrhage; however, the optimal dose and route of delivery remain unclear. Furthermore, misoprostol has not yet been directly compared to other uterotonic agents for treatment of uterine atony in published trials with significant numbers of patients. Absorption of the medication occurs across all mucosal surfaces and the tablets have been administered by the sublingual, buccal, vaginal, and rectal route, in addition to orally. Vaginal administration is generally not chosen for treatment of postpartum hemorrhage due to concerns about the tablet washing out with ongoing bleeding.

Pharmacokinetic and pharmacotherapeutic data for misoprostol in stage three of labor are limited. One small study of postpartum women given 400 µg of misoprostol by various routes determined both serum levels of misoprostol and the amount of uterine activity by intrauterine pressure catheters for 2 hours after administration of the drug. Onset of action was fastest when the drug was given orally dissolved in water (4 minutes), followed by oral tablets (6 minutes), and then by rectal administration (11 minutes). Mean uterine activity was highest in the first 15 minutes after the oral solution was given, with declines thereafter, but highest in the second 15-minute time period for oral tablet and rectal routes. Mean cumulative uterine activity was greatest in the oral solution group, as were the side effects of pyrexia and maximum temperature. Mean cumulative uterine activity and side effects were lowest in the rectal group.[33] It is unknown how this information directly translates to clinical efficacy in the treatment of postpartum hemorrhage due to uterine atony.

ACOG, in their most recent Practice Bulletin on the management of postpartum hemorrhage, suggests using misoprostol 800–1000 µg given per rectum.[34] Recently, an international group of physicians convened by the World Health Organization presented a consensus guideline for the use of misoprostol in a variety of reproductive settings. Based on the current available and limited data, they suggested reserving misoprostol for use as an adjunct after other uterotonic agents had already been used, and in a dose of 600 µg given orally or sublingually. A repeat dose is not recommended unless at least 2 hours have passed from the first dose, or 6 hours if the patient had side effects of pyrexia or shivering.[32] Large studies are needed to better address the role, route, and dose of misoprostol in the management of postpartum hemorrhage due to atony.

Fortunately, pharmacologic therapy of uterine atony is quickly successful in the vast majority of cases, either using a single agent, or with more than one drug in combination. Often success becomes apparent, even as preparations are being made for more aggressive patient resuscitation. Patients with a less than satisfactory immediate response, or in whom atony recurs soon after the initial therapy, will require more aggressive treatment. It is critical at this juncture to again be certain that there are no other contributing factors that should be addressed and were not appreciated at the initial patient evaluation or have newly developed. Moving the patient to an operating room setting should be strongly considered at this point. Bimanual examination should continue to be used to confirm that atony is still present. Reevaluation of the birth canal with adequate assistance, lighting, and retraction to exclude any undetected lacerations of the cervix or uterus is important. Genital tract injury should be especially suspected in all cases of instrumental vaginal delivery (with forceps or vacuum extraction) and in women who have undergone vaginal birth after cesarean section. If there is evidence of retained placental material by ultrasound or manual evaluation that was previously missed, careful uterine curettage with a large blunt Sims curette (sometimes called a banjo curette) can be undertaken. Ideally, this is performed with bedside ultrasound visualization and downward traction on the cervix with a ring forceps to lessen the significant risk of perforation of the soft postpartum uterus.

Definitive treatment for persistent uterine atony is ultimately a hysterectomy. There are several conservative options that can be considered before performing a hysterectomy for uterine atony, however. These include intrauterine tamponade, either with gauze packing or inflatable balloon devices, suturing techniques performed during laparotomy, which are intended to either mechanically compress the uterus or decrease its blood flow, and pelvic vessel embolization performed by an interventional radiologist. Ultimately, performance of a hysterectomy can be life saving, however, and although conservative methods are attractive, the available data on their role remain limited to case reports and collected case series. Randomized controlled trials of these various options will be difficult if not impossible to perform, however, and with increasing experience, conservative techniques will likely play an increasingly important role in the management of postpartum hemorrhage.[35]

C. Uterine Tamponade for Uterine Atony

Uterine tamponade can be accomplished in two ways; by tightly packing a gauze roll into the cavity or by inserting and inflating a balloon device within the cavity. Either is intended to provide direct pressure against bleeding vessels of the uterine lining. Uterine packing with gauze fell out of favor in the 1950s in part because of concern about concealed hemorrhage above the packing that could be detected only after blood soaks through yards of gauze. However, there has been new interest in this technique, beginning in the 1970s and 1980s. Generally, a long gauze roll is used and typically 5 or more yards are required. If needed, two rolls can be knotted together end to end to provide enough length. Some have reported using povidone iodine–soaked gauze to decrease infection, and others, including ACOG in the 2006 Practice Bulletin, have suggested soaking the gauze in a solution of 5000 units of thrombin in 5 mL of sterile saline to improve local hemostasis.[34] Regardless, tight packing with a back and forth layering of the uterus from the fundus to the cervix is stressed, and some have suggested packing of the entire vagina as well to facilitate retention of the packing material within the uterus. Consideration of prophylactic antibiotics while the packing is in place (generally no more than 24 hours) has also been suggested.[13,36]

Because of concern about concealed hemorrhage and because it has been reported to be difficult to achieve sufficiently tight intrauterine packing with gauze, recent attention has been turned to inflatable balloons as a way to quickly and easily tamponade the uterus. Reported devices have included a Rüsch bladder balloon (which holds more than 500 mL), a Sengstaken-Blakemore tube which has two linked balloons originally designed to tamponade gastroesophageal varices, and multiple Foley balloons inflated simultaneously into the uterine cavity (each filled with 60 mL). In 2002, the FDA granted clearance of the SOS Bakri Tamponade Balloon Catheter® specifically for use in postpartum hemorrhage. It consists of a silicone rubber balloon device, packaged with a syringe for inflation with up to 500 mL, and can be used in patients with latex allergies. The device has an open inner lumen, which was designed to allow intrauterine blood to escape while the balloon is within the uterus. It is simple to place either transvaginal, or at the time of cesarean section through the uterine incision before closure. A vaginal gauze pack soaked in povidone iodine can be simultaneously packed in the vagina to assist in maintaining the balloon within the uterus. After a vaginal delivery and initial pharmacologic treatment for atony, the balloon can be quickly placed while preparing the patient for laparotomy and definitive hysterectomy. If the balloon appears to be working during that time, then hysterectomy might be avoided. As with intrauterine gauze packing, prophylactic antibiotics should also be considered while an intrauterine balloon is in place, although there are no data on which to base firm recommendations in this regard. Generally, the balloon is removed within 24 hours, after gradual deflation. The success rates of an intrauterine balloon as a single measure for treatment of postpartum hemorrhage pharmacologic therapy was reported to be 84% in a recent compilation of 164 published cases.[35]

The usual next step for treatment of uterine atony is laparotomy. Continued attention to mobilization of adequate personnel, acquisition of blood products if not already started, patient warming, and all the other components of resuscitation are critical at this junction. Immediate operative intervention is also indicated for patients with suspected or diagnosed uterine rupture or abnormal placentation such as placenta accreta, increta, or percreta. Patients with uterine rupture will require surgical repair and in a minority of cases, hysterectomy, and those with an abnormally adherent placenta (either the entire placenta or focal areas) will require hysterectomy except in rare cases. Massive transfusion needs should be anticipated, including replacement of clotting factors. In addition, intraoperative blood salvage can be considered in patients undergoing laparotomy for postpartum hemorrhage, as well as at the time of initial cesarean section if hemorrhage is encountered.

D. Intraoperative Blood Salvage

Intraoperative blood salvage, also known as cell salvage, was first reported with an automated device in 1968 and multiple improvements in the technology have been made since then. Current devices use a suction catheter treated with heparin to aspirate blood from the surgical field and collect it within a centrifuge bowl. As the bowl fills, red cells are spun out to the periphery and the lighter free hemoglobin, plasma, and platelets are discarded through a center exit. When the bowl is filled with red cells, they are automatically washed with saline to remove the heparin and concentrated. The resulting product typically has a hematocrit of 60% and is devoid of coagulation factors and platelets. The process is efficient, yielding a volume of about 50% of what is aspirated. Contraindications to the use of salvaged blood have included cases in which the aspirated blood is expected to contain malignant cells or be heavily contaminated with bowel bacteria or amniotic fluid. In obstetrics, cell saver technology therefore has been used infrequently due to concern about the potential risks of anaphylactoid syndrome of pregnancy (ASP). This commonly lethal condition was originally believed to be due simply to entry of amniotic fluid containing fetal skin cells, fetal hair, and other particulate matter into the maternal circulation. However, the exact nature of ASP (previously known as amniotic fluid embolism) is unknown, and it is now understood that some quantity of amniotic fluid probably normally enters the maternal circulation during or after every delivery, almost always without harm.[37] In extremely rare cases, a maternal anaphylactoid reaction will occur after exposure to an unknown component of amniotic fluid. This anaphylactoid response results in transient catastrophic pulmonary vasoconstriction, right heart failure, profound hypoxia, and cardiovascular collapse. These individuals typically develop DIC, of which the etiology also remains uncertain.

Current autotransfusion devices combined with leukodepletion filters appear to efficiently clear measurable elements of amniotic fluid from salvaged blood.[38] There are currently approximately 400 reported cases of blood salvage with autotransfusion in obstetrics.[39] There has been just a single case of cell salvage in obstetrics in which maternal death occurred and was attributed by the author to ASP.[40] The patient, who refused blood products due to her Jehovah's Witness beliefs, had preeclampsia complicated by HELLP (hemolysis, elevated liver enzymes, and low platelets) syndrome, coagulopathy, and anemia, and others have argued that ASP was not likely the cause of her death.[39] Currently, ACOG suggests that women at known risk for massive obstetric hemorrhage due to suspected placenta accreta should be candidates for cell saver technology where available.[41] It is an attractive option for many patients who experience hemorrhage but will not accept autologous blood products due to religious beliefs. One study found that 55% of pregnant women who were Jehovah's Witnesses would accept cell saver technology in the event of operative hemorrhage.[42]

E. Surgical Treatment of Uterine Atony

Hysterectomy is usually considered the definitive treatment for persistent postpartum hemorrhage and can indeed be life saving. Often, a subtotal hysterectomy is performed, leaving all or some of the cervix because this is usually a simpler procedure. The junction between the cervix and vagina can be difficult to identify after labor and delivery have occurred, and removing the cervix completely may require greater mobilization of the bladder, which can further complicate the surgery. If the hysterectomy is being performed because of a placenta previa with associated placenta accreta or increta, then complete hysterectomy including the cervix will likely be needed to completely control the bleeding. There are, however, three additional surgical techniques that can be used in the hope of avoiding hysterectomy, particularly in cases of uterine atony.

The first consists of uterine sutures designed to compress the uterus top to bottom in an accordion style, and, when placed, have the appearance of vertical suspenders or braces running from the "waist" of the uterus at the cervix/uterine corpus junction, over the "shoulders" of the top of the uterus. This technique was first described by a British obstetrician and is called the B-Lynch compression suture.[43] The uterus must be open (via a cesarean incision) to place the B-Lynch suture. A modification was later described that would allow vertical compression stitches to be placed without having an open uterine incision.[44]

The second technique consists of suturing the uterus front to back in several locations from top to bottom, thereby directly juxtaposing and compressing the anterior wall against the posterior wall.[45] In both cases, absorbable sutures are used to minimize the risk of subsequent complications such as erosion of suture material into the cavity, collections of pus within the cavity, or intrauterine scarring. Either uterine suture compression technique may be considered if bimanual compression of the uterus during surgery results in near cessation of bleeding while evaluating both the abdomen and vagina. There is, however, greater published experience with uterine brace sutures.

A third suture technique is designed to reduce overall blood flow to the uterus by sequentially ligating the uterine arteries adjacent to the lower uterine segment, followed by ovarian vessel ligation near the uterine cornua and medial to the ovary. The technique is reported to be successful after just bilateral uterine artery ligation in about three fourths of cases because the uterus receives 90% of its blood supply via these vessels.[46] Suture ligation of the uterine vessels was described by O'Leary and O'Leary in 1974, and the technique is often referred to as placement of "O'Leary stitches."[47]

F. Recombinant Activated Factor VIIa

The newest pharmacologic agent available for off-label management of massive hemorrhage is recombinant activated factor VII (rFVIIa). Factor VII is a vitamin K–dependent coagulation protein produced by the liver, and it initiates hemostasis by combining with tissue factor present at the site of blood vessel damage. This stimulates the generation of thrombin, which results in formation of a stable fibrin clot. RFVIIa (NovoSeven®) is also able to bind directly to the surface of locally activated platelets, further enhancing coagulation at the site of local vascular injury. The drug, created by DNA technology, is not derived from blood and is therefore acceptable to Jehovah's Witness patients who refuse blood products. Because it is produced using bovine albumin in the cell culture medium, it cannot be used for patients with hypersensitivity to bovine proteins. The FDA approved rFVIIa in March 1999 for the treatment of acute bleeding episodes in patients with hemophilia A or B with antibody inhibitors to factor VIII or IX. The recommended dose for treatment of bleeding episodes in those with hemophilia is 90 µg/kg. The drug is supplied as a powder, packaged in a vial with a 3-year expiration time, which must be refrigerated until reconstituted with sterile water. The reconstituted product is then given as an IV bolus over 2–5 minutes. In addition, in 2008, a room temperature stable formulation of the drug that requires no refrigeration received FDA approval (NovoSeven RT®).

The medical literature has reported increased off-label use of rFVIIa in nonhemophilic patients with massive bleeding. Most have been surgical patients undergoing cardiothoracic, liver transplant, and trauma procedures, but has also been tried in cases of postpartum hemorrhage. Most of the obstetric patients were undergoing emergent peripartum hysterectomy; however, some were treated with rFVIIa after vaginal delivery and before operative intervention.

The largest case series reported to date comes from the Northern European Registry, which reported on 108 women treated with rFVIIa between 2000 and 2004. Of those cases, 92 (the "treatment" group) were given the drug after all standard therapies had failed with a median blood loss of 5.8 liters when administered. Those women had a median of 13 units of transfused packed cells, and coagulopathy was reported in 70%. An additional 16 women were given the drug as an adjunct to standard therapy, which was judged to be working at the time rFVIIa was given, with a median blood loss at the time of 2.5 liters (the "prophylactic" group). The most common etiology of hemorrhage was atony, followed by birth canal injuries, retained placenta, and placenta previa. Most women (91%) were given a dose ≤90 µg/kg, and this is consistent with previously reported cases in which doses have typically been between 60 and 100 µg/kg. In the "treatment" group, 14 women (15%) received a second dose and just 3 women were given three or more doses. Overall, of 108 women given rFVIIa, 76% had a response noted with observed reduction in bleeding after a single dose. The drug was believed to have failed in 15 cases (13.8%).[48]

Studies have suggested that the efficacy of rFVIIa is diminished when used in the setting of acidemia and correction of the pH to greater than or equal to 7.2 with sodium bicarbonate has been recommended.[49,50] Hypothermia does not appear to affect the function of rFVIIa. It also appears that adequately correcting coagulopathy with appropriate transfusions of fresh frozen plasma (FFP), cryoprecipitate, and platelets is important in the patient response to rFVIIa. Achieving fibrinogen levels of at least 50 mg/dL, preferably greater than 100 mg/dL and platelet levels of at least 50,000/µL and preferably greater than 100,000/µL has been suggested.[49,51] There are currently no laboratory assays available to monitor rFVIIa therapy. Because the drug has a half-life of 2.3 hours, in a small number of cases the dose was repeated empirically in those judged to be at high risk of ongoing bleeding. RFVIIa is relatively expensive, and the current cost for a typical 90-µg/kg dose given to a 70-kilogram pregnant woman would be approximately $9000. It has been suggested that rFVIIa should be reserved for cases in which all else has failed due to uncertainty about efficacy, dosing, and safety. However, it is also possible that waiting for severe derangement of the coagulation system before giving the drug may compromise its efficacy. There is a randomized clinical trial currently in progress in Europe to determine if there is a role for rFVIIa in the early treatment of postpartum hemorrhage before proceeding with uterine artery embolization, laparotomy, or hysterectomy.

The greatest safety concern regarding rFVIIa is the potential risk of more widespread coagulation beyond the site of vessel injury. Between 1996 and 2003, more than 700,000 doses of rFVIIa had been given in patients with hemophilia, and a total of 16 thromboembolic events, including myocardial infarction, stroke, and deep venous thrombosis, were reported. Of those cases, the majority had known risks for thromboembolism, such as obesity, coronary artery disease, and previous myocardial infarction.[52] Review of 5 years of data from the FDA's adverse event reporting system after initial licensure of rFVIIa indicates that the majority of the 185 reported thromboembolic events were seen in patients without hemophilia who were treated off-label for bleeding.[53] Approximately half of these thromboembolic events occurred within 24 hours of the administration of the drug, and 16% occurred within 2 hours. However, this report is unable to provide any information about actual rates of thromboembolism because the total number of treated patients was unknown. In addition, patients treated for massive bleeding likely have inherently high background risks for thromboembolism due to other factors, such as pregnancy or trauma, making assessment of drug safety in such patients difficult. One review of pooled data from reported single cases, case series, and clinical trials of patients without hemophilia who were treated with rFVIIa noted an incidence of thromboembolism of approximately 1.4%.[54] In the Northern European Registry, of 108 treated women there were four thromboembolic events and one myocardial infarction (in a woman who had a cardiac arrest before administration of rFVIIa). Randomized clinical trials will be needed to determine the safety and efficacy of rFVIIa for postpartum hemorrhage but may be difficult to accomplish.

G. Uterine Artery Embolization

One additional method of management of postpartum obstetric hemorrhage is angiographic uterine artery embolization (UAE), performed by an interventional radiologist. First reported in 1979, this technique has seen increasing experience. UAE can be considered in primary postpartum hemorrhage before resorting to laparotomy, in the treatment of delayed or secondary postpartum hemorrhage, and has also been used specifically to treat expanding genital tract hematomas of the upper vagina above the levator ani muscle, which would otherwise require laparotomy. It is probably best suited to a patient who is hemodynamically stable. UAE typically involves rapid transport of a bleeding patient to the interventional radiology suite and immediate involvement of radiologic staff in an emergent setting. Because postpartum hemorrhage is typically not anticipated, occurring at any time of the day or night, use of this technique requires the advance development of a protocol and close coordination between obstetric and radiologic personnel. These logistical issues have likely limited more widespread use of this technique. Obvious advantages include the avoidance of surgery and the associated complications, particularly in a patient who may have developed coagulopathy, as well as the ability to preserve the uterus if future fertility is desired.

UAE involves accessing the femoral artery by a Seldinger technique and injecting contrast material first into the aorta and then selectively into the internal iliac arteries. This arteriogram may allow identification of a specific location of bleeding. However, particularly in the case of uterine atony, and overall in approximately 50% of cases, a specific bleeding vessel will not be visualized and therefore embolization of the uterine artery or the anterior branch of the internal iliac artery is performed.[55] Embolization can be repeated on the opposite site if needed. The choice of material for embolization is commonly cut particles of gelatin sponge. Gelatin sponge has the advantage of being a temporary agent and recanalization of the occluded vessel occurs within 1–3 weeks. Other permanent materials have also been used, including micro coils and polyvinyl alcohol, which scleroses the vessel. High success rates have been reported among case series in the literature, most in excess of 90%.

A recent report of 36 cases of UAE for postpartum hemorrhage, 28 who had uterine atony, demonstrated success in all. One case was complicated by a femoral vein thrombus and one case by inadvertent creation of a local false aneurysm.[56] Another series of 49 patients, 24 of whom had uterine atony, achieved success in all with UAE. In this center, 69% of the cases were successfully treated within 60 minutes and the remaining cases with one exception were completed within 90 minutes.[55] They experienced one complication of a vessel dissection. A third series of 29 patients reported success in 26 (90%). Of the patients treated, 62% had uterine atony, and in 90% of cases the patient was stable at the time of the procedure. Median estimated blood loss at the time embolization was started in these patients was 3500 mL. One third of the patients were treated within 30 minutes and the other two thirds were treated within 60 minutes of starting the procedure. One patient experienced transient unilateral leg claudication, and six experienced transient pyrexia afterward. Of the patients with postpartum hemorrhage in the treating hospitals during the time of this report, only a very small proportion, 0.4%, actually underwent UAE.[57]

Reported complications after UAE to treat postpartum hemorrhage have included local vessel thrombosis or trauma such as dissection, perforation, or creation of a false aneurysm. Postembolic ischemia appears to be very uncommon, probably due to the large collateral blood flow in the pelvis during pregnancy; however, it could result from overflow of embolization material into vessels not intended for occlusion. In addition, infarction and necrosis of the uterus requiring later hysterectomy, the cervix, upper vagina, and bladder have been reported. Postprocedure infection as well as pyrexia and pain have been reportedly managed with anti-inflammatory medications and antibiotics.

Fertility and childbearing after UAE for postpartum hemorrhage have been reported in small numbers. In one series of 37 women treated with UAE who had not had a hysterectomy, 36 resumed regular menstrual cycles and 9 became pregnant again. Of these women, six had uncomplicated deliveries and three had early miscarriage.[55] Review of multiple other cases of pregnancy after UAE suggests that fertility is probably not adversely affected after UAE specifically for postpartum hemorrhage.[58]

H. Transfusion

Clinicians caring for pregnant women need to be very familiar with the appropriate use of blood products in the resuscitation and ongoing management of those experiencing hemorrhage. This knowledge should include the available products and the usual time frame they can be made available from the blood bank in their particular hospital (Table 5). Transfusion with packed red blood cells will likely be needed in those with tachycardia and hypotension, which suggests that 40% of blood volume has been lost. It takes approximately 45 minutes to cross match the first unit of blood requested. Therefore, in a patient experiencing catastrophic hemorrhage, the clinician should be prepared to request type-specific blood if the blood bank already has a record of the patient's blood type, or O negative blood if this information is not documented at the blood bank. While it is common practice to forego a routine type and screen for a low-risk woman presenting in labor, it should be obtained in a high-risk woman because the time for delivery of blood will be reduced to 15–20 minutes. Deciding when to transfuse packed red blood cells (PRBCs) can be a difficult task and in the setting of an acute massive blood loss must be based in part on knowledge of the patient's initial hemoglobin and hematocrit, assessment of the patient's current hemodynamic status, in particular evaluation for hypotension and tachycardia, and judgment as to the likely time frame when bleeding will be halted. It has been increasingly recognized that when profound blood loss occurs and massive transfusion is anticipated, generally defined as replacement of one blood volume within 24 hours or need for 8–10 units of blood, that dilutional coagulopathy should also be anticipated and avoided if possible. In the massively bleeding patient there appears to be a role for formulaic transfusion of FFP along with PRBCs until the situation is more stable or lab-

Table 5. Blood Transfusion Products

Product	Volume (mL)	Expected Result	Storage, Approximate Preparation Time	Comments
Packed red blood cells	250–400	Increases hemoglobin 1–1.5 g/dL	Refrigerated; cross match takes 45 min, only 15–30 min preparation if type and screen already in blood bank	Can be leukocyte reduced to minimize number of white cells, decreases risk of cytomegalovirus infection and immune-mediated side effects of transfusions such as febrile nonhemolytic reactions
Fresh frozen plasma	250	Increases fibrinogen 10 mg/dL/unit	Frozen; 30 min thaw plus 15 min prep time	Contains all clotting factors in addition to fibrinogen
Cryoprecipitate	40	Increases fibrinogen 10 mg/dL/unit	Frozen; 15–20 min thaw plus 15 min prep time	Contains fibrinogen and factor VIII, not commonly used in obstetrics except for isolated fibrinogen depletion
Single donor platelet apheresis unit (equivalent of 6 single donor units)	300	Increases platelets 30,000–50,000/apheresis unit	Room temperature; 10 min prep time	Can be leukocyte reduced

oratory data return to better guide the use of individual blood components. Suggested guidelines in this specific setting have included ratios from 1:1 to 2:3 units of FFP to PRBCs.[12,59] Guidelines for transfusion based on available laboratory data have varied; however, administration of 4 units of FFP for an international normalized ratio of >1.5 and one platelet apheresis unit for a platelets count of <25,000–50,000 in an actively bleeding patient have been suggested.[12,60]

Ongoing care and monitoring of the patient with postpartum hemorrhage includes close vital sign monitoring, including urinary output on an hourly basis, monitoring of laboratory parameters particularly hemoglobin, prothrombin (PT), partial thromboplastin time (PTT), fibrinogen, and platelets. Monitoring of ionized calcium is also important in the patient undergoing transfusion. This is because the anticoagulant preservative citrate phosphate dextrose used for PRBCs can bind plasma calcium, and in massive transfusions this can lead to hypocalcemia with associated hypotension, tetany, and cardiac arrhythmias. Hypocalcemia should be treated with parenteral calcium chloride. Hyperkalemia can also occur because potassium diffuses out of PRBCs during storage. Although potassium is usually excreted by the kidneys or reabsorbed intracellularly, patients who have undergone massive transfusion should have their potassium levels evaluated. Patients with uterine atony that has resolved with initial pharmacologic therapy need to have the uterine tone monitored frequently. Prophylactic antibiotics may be needed in those with intrauterine packing or an intrauterine balloon as noted previously. Patients with limited mobility or obesity, those who are older, and those who have had a laparotomy should have deep venous thrombus prophylaxis. In the patient with postpartum hemorrhage, especially if there has been coagulopathy or recent cesarean section or laparotomy, use of an intermittent pneumatic compression device is an attractive option in lieu of prophylactic anticoagulation.

VIII. Therapy of Postpartum Anemia

The mainstay of therapy for the postpartum woman with anemia is oral iron, similar to the pregnant woman with anemia. Women with anemia often have headaches, tiredness, dizziness, and a reduction in exercise tolerance. Only approximately 25% of women are able to meet their body's maintenance needs for iron through diet alone, and diet alone is insufficient to make up actual iron deficits in the setting of postpartum anemia. Compliance with oral iron therapy is a frequent problem.[21] One study of oral iron therapy to treat postpartum anemia in which compliance was stressed and pill counts were performed found that approximately 15% of patients self-discontinued or took less than two thirds of the prescribed iron tablets.[61] Compliance in actual practice is likely substantially lower. Therapeutic effect with oral iron therapy is slow, and in a study group with high compliance and a dose of 200 mg ferrous sulfate twice daily, the median observed increase in hemoglobin was only 1.5 g/dL by 2 weeks. By 6 weeks, the hemoglobin had increased by 4 g/dL.[62] Of note however, there was almost no increase in serum ferritin by this time, indicating minimal effect on total iron body stores. In contrast, patients in that study who received parenteral iron sucrose in two doses of 200 mg had an increase in hemoglobin by 2 g/dL at 5 days, and 4 g/dL at 2 weeks. In addition, although at 6 weeks the increase in hemoglobin was the same as in the oral iron therapy group, serum ferritin levels were normalized for the parenteral iron group.

Parenteral iron sucrose has an excellent safety record in obstetrics, both antepartum and postpartum. One report of experience with more than 2500 ampoules administered in pregnancy observed no side effects, no anaphylaxis symptoms, and no cases in which discontinuation was required.[63] In contrast, parenteral iron dextran, which has a very high molecular mass of more than 100,000 Daltons, has been associated with a significant risk of anaphylaxis of 0.6%–2.3%, caused by antibodies to dextran. Iron sucrose can cause minor anaphylactoid-type reactions due to histamine release, but these are without significant consequence and a test dose is not indicated.[64] Iron sucrose is removed from the plasma within 24 hours after administration, incorporated into the bone marrow, and used for erythropoiesis. The dose of iron needed for a given patient can be calculated by the following formula where "deposit iron" is 500 mg in patients with a weight of more than 35 kilogram, and the "hemoglobin deficit" is the difference between the actual and target hemoglobin in g/L: iron deficit (mg) = 0.24 × body weight (kilogram) × "hemoglobin deficit" (g/L) + "deposit iron" (mg).

Recombinant erythropoietin (rEPO) has also been studied for the treatment of severe postpartum anemia combined with iron sucrose compared to iron sucrose alone. A small study of rEPO 300 U/kg daily for 4 days demonstrated statistically significant improvement in hemoglobin levels at day 7, but not at day 14, compared with patients who received only iron sucrose.[65] A recent study found no difference in hemoglobin levels at day 7 or day 14 in patients receiving iron sucrose alone or combined with two doses of either 10,000 U or 20,000 U rEPO.[66] Given the expense, the role of rEPO in the treatment of postpartum anemia remains to be determined.[67]

IX. PATIENT CASE [PART 2]

When D.L.'s physician and nurse observe her brisk bleeding after delivery of the placenta, they immediately call for assistance from other personnel on the labor and delivery unit. She has multiple risk factors for both uterine atony as well as genital tract laceration. Her nurse adds an additional 20 IU of oxytocin to the liter of lactated Ringer's, which already contained 20 IU of oxytocin, and checks to be sure that the IV line is running wide open. While her nurse places a second antecubital IV line using a 16-gauge catheter, her physician massages her uterus between two hands and reports that she indeed has atony. Additional uterotonic agents are requested. A second nurse arrives in the room with a vial of methylergonovine from the unit refrigerator and 0.20 mg is given IM after confirming with the team already present in the room that she does not have a history of hypertension. Pressure sleeves are placed on her two bags of IV fluids to increase flow. Five minutes later, the physician notes continued atony, although slightly improved, and the patient is given one dose of carboprost IM. Manual exploration of the poorly contracted uterine cavity confirms that no retained placental tissue is present.

A phone call is made to the hospital blood bank and 4 units of packed red blood cells are requested for cross match. Uterine massage continues. The physician also notes a vaginal side wall laceration that is bleeding and needs repair, but because of continued uterine bleeding, visualization is poor and the decision is made to move the patient to the operating room on the unit. Before moving the patient, an intrauterine balloon (SOS Bakri Intrauterine Balloon®) is manually inserted by the physician and filled with 400 mL of sterile saline by the nurse. The upper vagina is quickly packed with an iodine-soaked vaginal pack. A second dose of IM carboprost is given 15 minutes after the first and the patient is transported.

In the operating room, the patient is again placed in the lithotomy position and a bladder catheter with attached urometer is inserted. Operating room personnel prepare for laparotomy and a second physician arrives. Meanwhile, the patient's nurse notifies the team that elapsed time since delivery of the placenta and the beginning of the hemorrhage has been 50 minutes. Estimated blood loss by the team is approximately 2000 mL at this point, and because her starting hematocrit was known to be only 30% and laparotomy may be needed, uncrossmatched type-specific blood is requested for immediate release from the hospital blood bank while waiting for the previously requested cross matched units. Four units of FFP are also ordered because they will take 45 minutes to defrost, and laboratory studies (complete blood count with platelet count, fibrinogen, and PT/PTT) are drawn and sent. The patient's pulse is 120 beats per minute, her blood pressure is 110/62 mmHg, and she had 400 mL of urine output from her catheter. At this time, with the intrauterine balloon in place, bleeding seems to have diminished some and only a mild to moderate amount of blood is returning from the side channel of the uterine balloon catheter. With good lighting, use of the retractors available in the operating room and assistance of the second physician, the patient's deep vaginal laceration is sutured closed. The first unit of type-specific uncross matched blood is started using a rapid infuser with a warming unit and a heated air blanket is placed on the patient's chest and arms. Bedside ultrasound demonstrates no evidence of blood collecting within the uterus and blood flow from the side channel of the intrauterine balloon catheter has begun to decrease.

Results of the initial blood work include a hemoglobin of 7.8, hematocrit of 23%, fibrinogen of 175, and platelets of 110,000. At this time, cross matched blood arrives in the operating room and a second unit of blood is started, anticipating that those laboratory values are not yet reflective of her actual blood loss. Continued observation of the patient while in the operating room suggests that the atony has resolved, and the patient is moved 30 minutes later back to labor and delivery for the next 12 hours for close monitoring. Because of her urinary catheter and vaginal and uterine packing, mobility will be limited for some period of time and so sequential pneumatic compression devices are placed on her legs. Blood work is repeated 4 hours after the first set was drawn, and close monitoring of her uterine tone by palpation of her abdomen and vaginal bleeding by inspection of the perineum and blood flow from the uterine catheter continues.

Her next hematocrit, after the 2 units of packed cells, is 26% and remains stable thereafter. Her fibrinogen and platelet counts remain normal. Her vital signs are monitored, including hourly assessment of urine output. Prophylactic antibiotics are started because of the indwelling intrauterine balloon. Eight hours later, with resolution of her tachycardia and no evidence of further significant vaginal bleeding, 100 mL are removed from the uterine balloon, and by 18 hours after placement, the balloon has been deflated completely and is removed. She is able to be discharged home 3 days after her delivery. Before discharge, D.L. is counseled regarding the two-fold increased risk of recurrent postpartum hemorrhage in future pregnancies. In addition, she is informed of the importance of iron therapy for resolving her postpartum anemia and replacing her total body iron stores. She is started on oral ferrous sulfate, 325 mg, daily with an empty stomach and will see her obstetrician for follow-up in 4 weeks.

X. Summary

Postpartum obstetric hemorrhage remains a significant cause of both maternal mortality and morbidity. Significant blood loss is usually defined as greater than 1000 mL, and approximately 4%–5% of women will experience this during childbirth. Risk factors should be identified in all patients if present; however, a significant number of women who experience obstetric hemorrhage will have no such risk factors. Therefore, all clinicians and hospitals that care for obstetric patients must be prepared to deal with this complication of pregnancy in a timely and efficient manner. Screening for and treatment of iron deficiency anemia during pregnancy, and active management of the third stage of labor are strategies designed to limit anemia and blood loss. Uterine atony is by far the most common cause of postpartum hemorrhage. Uterine massage and pharmacologic uterotonic agents are the most important therapies and are usually effective. Adjunctive measures that can be employed include internal uterine tamponade, compression suture techniques during laparotomy, uterine artery embolization, and hysterectomy. Additional therapies that may be helpful include intraoperative cell salvage and, in selected cases, recombinant factor VIIa. Clinicians must also be able to direct transfusion therapy in the acute massive hemorrhage situation as well as based on laboratory values in the more stable patient. In the stable patient who has significant postpartum anemia, therapy should be directed toward correcting anemia as well as replenishing body iron stores.

XI. References

1. Chang J, Elam-Evans LD, Berg CJ, et al. Pregnancy-related mortality surveillance—United States, 1991–1999. *MMWR Morb Mortal Wkly Rep*. 2003;52:1–8.

2. Tucker MJ, Berg CJ, Callaghan WM, et al. The Black-White disparity in pregnancy-related mortality from 5 conditions: differences in prevalence and case-fatality rates. *Am J Public Health*. 2007;97:247–251.

3. Kahn KS, Wojdyla D, Say L, et al. WHO analysis of causes of maternal death: a systematic review. *Lancet*. 2006;367:1066–1074.

4. Bais JMJ, Eskes M, Pel M, et al. Postpartum haemorrhage in nulliparous women: incidence and risk factors in low and high risk women. A Dutch population-based cohort study on standard ($\geq$500 ml) and severe ($\geq$1000 ml) postpartum haemorrhage. *Eur J Obstet Gynecol Reprod Biol*. 2004;115:166–172.

5. Prasertcharoensuk W, Swadpanich U, Lumbiganon P. Accuracy of the blood loss estimation in the third stage of labor. *Int J Gynaecol Obstet*. 2000;71:69–70.

6. Magann EF, Evans S, Hutchinson M, et al. Postpartum hemorrhage after vaginal birth: an analysis of risk factors. *South Med J*. 2005;98:419–422.

7. Rouse DJ, MacPherson C, Landon M, et al. Blood transfusion and cesarean delivery. *Obstet Gynecol*. 2006;108:891–897.

8. Lu MC, Fridman M, Korst LM, et al. Variations in the incidence of postpartum hemorrhage across hospitals in California. *Matern Child Health J*. 2005;9:297–306.

9. Joseph KS, Rouleau J, Kramer MS, et al. Investigation of an increase in postpartum haemorrhage in Canada. *BJOG*. 2007;114:751–759.

10. Reyal F, Sibony O, Oury J, et al. Criteria for transfusion in severe postpartum hemorrhage: analysis of practice and risk factors. *Eur J Obstet Gynecol Reprod Biol*. 2004;112:61–64.

11. Baskett TF. Surgical management of severe obstetric hemorrhage: experience with an obstetric hemorrhage equipment tray. *J Obstet Gynaecol Can*. 2004;26:805–808.

12. Burtelow M, Riley E, Druzin M, et al. How we treat: management of life-threatening primary postpartum hemorrhage with a standardized massive transfusion protocol. *Transfusion*. 2007;47:1564–1572.

13. Burton R, Belfort MA. Etiology and management of hemorrhage. In Dildy GA, Belfort MA, Saade GR, et al, eds. *Critical Care Obstetrics*. Malden, MA: Blackwell Science, 2004:298–311.

14. Monga M. Maternal cardiovascular and renal adaptation to pregnancy. In Creasy RK, Resnik R, Iams JD, eds. *Maternal-Fetal Medicine: Principles and Practice*. Philadelphia: Saunders, 2004;111–120.

15. Bowes WA, Thorp JM. Clinical aspects of normal and abnormal labor. In Creasy RK, Resnik R, Iams JD, eds. *Maternal-Fetal Medicine: Principles and Practice*. Philadelphia: Saunders, 2004:671–705.

16. Milman N. Iron and pregnancy—a delicate balance. *Ann Hematol*. 2006;85:559–565.

17. Centers for Disease Control and Prevention. Recommendations to prevent and control iron deficiency in the United States. Available at http://www.cdc.gov/mmwr/preview/mmwrhtml/00051880.htm. Accessed June 2, 2008.

18. Milman N, Bergholt T, Eriksen L, et al. Iron prophylaxis during pregnancy—how much iron is needed? A randomized dose-response study of 20–80 mg ferrous iron daily in pregnant women. *Acta Obstet Gynecol Scand*. 2005;84:238–247.

19. Pena-Rosas JP, Viteri FE. Effects of routine oral iron supplementation with or without folic acid for women during pregnancy. *Cochrane Database Syst Rev*. 2006, Issue 3. Art. No:CD004736.

20. Siega-Riz AM, Hartzema AG, Turnbull C, et al. The effects of prophylactic iron given in prenatal supplements on iron status and birth outcomes: a randomized controlled trial. *Am J Obstet Gynecol.* 2006;194:512–519.

21. United States Food and Drug Administration. Information on erythropoiesis stimulating agents. Available at http://www.fda.gov/cder/drug/infopage/RHE/default.htm. Accessed June 1, 2008.

22. Orji E, Agwu F, Loto O, et al. A randomized comparative study of prophylactic oxytocin versus ergometrine in the third stage of labor. *Int J Gynecol Obstet.* 2008;101:129–132.

23. Villar J, Gülmezoglu AM, Hofmeyr GJ, et al. Systematic review of randomized controlled trials of misoprostol to prevent postpartum hemorrhage. *Obstet Gynecol.* 2002;100:1301–1312.

24. Cowen MJ. Resuscitation. In B-Lynch C, Keith LG, Lalonde A, et al, eds. *A Textbook of Postpartum Hemorrhage.* Duncow, UK: Sapiens Publishing, 2006:170–178.

25. Barcelona SL, Vilich F, Coté CJ. A comparison of flow rates and warming capabilities of the Level 1 and Rapid Infusion System with various-size intravenous catheters. *Anesth Analg.* 2003;97:358–363.

26. Hess JR, Lawson JH. The coagulopathy of trauma versus disseminated intravascular coagulation. *J Trauma.* 2006;60:S12–S19.

27. Sacks DA. Blood component replacement therapy. In Dildy GA, Gelfort MA, Saade GR, et al, eds. *Critical Care Obstetrics.* Malden, MA: Blackwell Science, 2004:162–183.

28. Skupski DW, Eglinton S, Lowenwirt IP, et al. Building hospital systems for managing major obstetric hemorrhage. In B-Lynch C, Keith LG, Lalonde A, et al, eds. *A Textbook of Postpartum Hemorrhage.* Duncow, UK: Sapiens Publishing, 2006:183–191.

29. Hankins GD, Berryman GK, Scott RT, et al. Maternal arterial desaturation with 15-methyl prostaglandin F2 alpha for uterine atony. *Obstet Gynecol.* 1988;72:367–370.

30. Harber CR, Levy DM, Chidambaram S, et al. Life-threatening bronchospasm after intramuscular carboprost for postpartum haemorrhage. *BJOG.* 2007;114:366–368.

31. Çalikan E, Meydanli MM, Dilbaz B, et al. Is rectal misoprostol really effective in the treatment of third stage of labor? A randomized controlled trial. *Am J Obstet Gynecol.* 2002;187:1038–1045.

32. Blum J, Alfirevic Z, Walraven G, et al. Treatment of postpartum hemorrhage with misoprostol. *Int J Gynaecol Obstet.* 2007;99:S202–S205.

33. Chong Y, Chua S, Shen L, et al. Does the route of administration of misoprostol make a difference? The uterotonic effect and side effects of misoprostol given by different routes after vaginal delivery. *Eur J Obstet Gynecol Reprod Biol.* 2004;113:191–198.

34. American College of Obstetricians and Gynecologists. Postpartum hemorrhage. ACOG Practice Bulletin Number 76, October 2006. *Obstet Gynecol.* 2006;108:1039–1047.

35. Doumouchtsis SK, Papageorghiou AT, Arulkumaran S. Systematic review of conservative management of postpartum hemorrhage: what to do when medical treatment fails. *Obstet Gynecol Surv.* 2007;62:540–547.

36. Shevell T, Malone F. Management of obstetric hemorrhage. *Semin Perinatol.* 2003; 27:86–104.

37. Waters JH, Biscotti C, Potter PS, et al. Amniotic fluid removal during cell salvage in the cesarean section patient. *Anesthesiology.* 2000;92:1519–1522.

38. Catling S, Thomas D. Intraoperative autologous blood transfusion. In B-Lynch C, Keith LG, Lalonde AB, et al, eds. *A Textbook of Postpartum Hemorrhage.* Duncow, UK: Sapiens Publishing, 2006:421–426.

39. Allam J, Cox M, Yentis SM. Cell salvage in obstetrics. *Int J Obstet Anesth.* 2008; 17:37–45.

40. Oei SG, Wingen CB, Kerkamp HE. Cell salvage: how safe in obstetrics? (letter) *Int J Obstet Anesth.* 2000;19:143.

41. Anonymous. Placenta accreta. ACOG Committee Opinion No. 266. *Obstet Gynecol.* 2002;99:169–170.

42. Gyamfi C, Berkowitz RL. Responses by pregnant Jehovah's Witnesses on health care proxies. *Obstet Gynecol.* 2004;104:541–544.

43. B-Lynch C, Coker A, Lawal AH, et al. The B-Lynch surgical technique for the control of massive postpartum haemorrhage: an alternative to hysterectomy? Five cases reported. *Br J Obstet Gynaecol.* 1997;104:372–375.

44. Hayman RG, Arulkumaran S, Steer PJ. Uterine compression sutures: surgical management of postpartum hemorrhage. *Obstet Gynecol.* 2002;99:502–506.

45. Cho JH, Jun HS, Lee CN. Hemostatic suturing technique for uterine bleeding during cesarean delivery. *Obstet Gynecol.* 2000;96:129–131.

46. AbdRabbo SA. Stepwise uterine devascularization: a novel technique for management of uncontrollable postpartum hemorrhage with preservation of the uterus. *Am J Obstet Gynecol.* 1994;171:694–700.

47. O'Leary JL, O'Leary JA. Uterine artery ligation for control of postcesarean section hemorrhage. *Obstet Gynecol.* 1974;43:849–853.

48. Alfirevic Z, Elbourne D, Pavord S, et al. Use of recombinant activated factor VII in primary postpartum hemorrhage. The Northern European Registry 2000–2004. *Obstet Gynecol.* 2007;110:1270–1278.

49. Martinowitz U, Michaelson M. Guidelines for the use of recombinant activated factor VII (rFVIIa) in uncontrolled bleeding: a report by the Israeli Multidisciplinary rFVIIa Task Force. *J Thromb Haemost.* 2006;3:640–648.

50. Sobieszczyk S, Breborowicz GH. The use of recombinant factor VIIa. In B-Lynch C, Keith LG, Lalonde A, et al, eds. *A Textbook of Postpartum Hemorrhage.* Duncow, UK: Sapiens Publishing, 2006:170–178.

51. Lam MS, Sims-McCallum RP. Recombinant factor VIIa in the treatment of non-hemophiliac bleeding. *Ann Pharmacother.* 2005;39:885–891.

52. Abshire T, Kenet G. Recombinant factor VIIa: review of efficacy, dosing regimens and safety in patients with congenital and acquired factor VIII or IX inhibitors. *J Thromb Haemost.* 2004;2:899–909.

53. O'Connell KA, Wood JJ, Wise RP, et al. Thromboembolic adverse events after use of recombinant human coagulation factor VIIa. *JAMA*. 2006;295:293–298.

54. Levi M, Peters M, Büller HR. Efficacy and safety of recombinant factor VIIa for treatment of severe bleeding: a systematic review. *Crit Care Med*. 2005;33:883–890.

55. Shim J, Yoon H, Won H, et al. Angiographic embolization for obstetrical hemorrhage: effectiveness and follow-up outcome of fertility. *Acta Obstet Gynecol*. 2006;85:815–820.

56. Boulleret C, Chahid T, Gallot D, et al. Hypogastric arterial selective and superselective embolization for severe postpartum hemorrhage: a retrospective review of 36 cases. *Cardiovasc Intervent Radiol*. 2004;27:344–348.

57. Yong SB, Cheung KB. Management of primary postpartum haemorrhage with arterial embolization in Hong Kong public hospitals. *Hong Kong Med J*. 2006;12:437–441.

58. Kachura JR. The role of interventional radiology in obstetrics. *Fetal Matern Med Rev*. 2004;15:145–180.

59. Gonzalez EA, Moore FA, Holcomb JB, et al. Fresh frozen plasma should be given earlier to patients requiring massive transfusion. *J Trauma*. 2007;62:112–119.

60. Sacks DA. Blood component replacement therapy. In Dildy GA, Belfort MA, Saade GR, et al, eds. *Critical Care Obstetrics*. Malden, MA: Blackwell Science, 2004:162–183.

61. Van Wyck DB, Martens MG, Seid MH, et al. Intravenous ferric carboxymaltose compared with oral iron in the treatment of postpartum anemia. A randomized controlled trial. *Obstet Gynecol*. 2007;110:267–278.

62. Bhandal N, Russell R. Intravenous versus oral iron therapy for postpartum anaemia. *BJOG*. 2006;113:1248–1252.

63. Perewusnyk G, Huch R, Huch A, et al. Parenteral iron therapy in obstetrics: 8 years experience with iron-sucrose complex. *Br J Nutr*. 2002;88:2–10.

64. Bashiri A, Burstein E, Sheiner E, et al. Anemia during pregnancy and treatment with intravenous iron: review of the literature. *Eur J Obstet Gynecol Reprod Biol*. 2003;110:2–7.

65. Breymann C, Richter C, Hüttner C, et al. Effectiveness of recombinant erythropoietin and iron sucrose vs. iron therapy only, in patients with postpartum anaemia and blunted erythropoiesis. *Eur J Clinic Investig*. 2000;30:154–161.

66. Wågström E, Åkesson A, Van Rooijen M, et al. Erythropoietin and intravenous iron therapy in postpartum anaemia. *Acta Obstet Gynecol*. 2007;86:957–962.

67. Dodd J, Dare MR, Middleton P. Treatment for women with postpartum iron deficiency anaemia. *Cochrane Database Syst Rev*. 2004, Issue 4 Art. No:CD004222.

QUESTIONS AND ANSWERS

1. The most common cause of postpartum hemorrhage is:

   a. vaginal lacerations

   b. uterine atony

    c. disseminated coagulopathy

    d. uterine rupture

2. All of the following are physiologic adaptations in pregnancy except:

    a. increased systemic vascular resistance

    b. increased blood volume

    c. increased clotting factors

    d. increased heart rate

3. The pharmacologic treatment of postpartum uterine atony in a patient with asthma can include all of the following except:

    a. methylergonovine

    b. oxytocin

    c. misoprostol

    d. carboprost

4. Treatment with recombinant factor VIIa

    a. is an option if a patient is a Jehovah's Witness

    b. likely requires correction of acidosis for optimal benefit

    c. may increase risks of thromboembolism

    d. all of the above

5. Disadvantages of iron sucrose for treatment of postpartum anemia include:

    a. risk of anaphylaxis of about 1%

    b. higher serum ferritin 6 weeks after treatment compared to oral iron therapy

    c. greater cost than oral iron therapy

    d. persistent gastrointestinal side effects

Answers:

1. b; 2. a; 3. d; 4. d; 5. c

SECTION 3
Treatment of Chronic Diseases in Pregnancy

Ambulatory Management of Asthma during Pregnancy

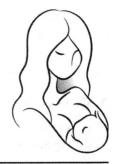

Leslie Hendeles and Michael Schatz

LEARNING OBJECTIVES

1. Describe maternal and fetal risks of poorly controlled asthma during pregnancy.

2. Analyze signs and symptoms of asthma and differences in clinical presentations.

3. Identify the National Asthma Education and Prevention Program's (NAEPP) preferred pharmacologic agents for treating exacerbations and for long-term control of persistent asthma, and their risks during pregnancy.

4. Outline how to assess and monitor asthma control.

5. Summarize what education and self-management skills need to be provided to patients.

PULMONARY ABBREVIATIONS

FEF_{25-75} Forced expiratory flow between 25% and 75% of vital capacity as measured by spirometry

FEV_1 Forced expiratory volume in the first second of exhalation measured by spirometry

FVC Forced vital capacity measured by spirometry

PEF Peak expiratory flow measured by peak flow meter

I. Introduction

Asthma is a chronic inflammatory disease of the airways that affects more than 20 million people in the United States. Symptoms vary in frequency and severity between patients, as well as within the same patient. Poorly controlled asthma is characterized by frequent symptoms; nighttime awakenings from cough, wheeze, and/or dyspnea; interference with normal activity (eg, missing work or school); overuse of short-acting β_2-selective agonists (SABA) to relieve symptoms, frequent use of short courses of oral corticosteroids, and reduced lung function.[1] It is likely to increase resource use, such

285

as unscheduled physician visits, emergency department (ED) visits, and hospitalizations for asthma,[2] all of which increase the economic burden of this disease. Inadequately treated asthma or poor adherence can result in death in approximately 5000 patients each year in the United States.[2]

A. Relevance to Pregnancy

There are very important additional risks for poorly controlled asthma during pregnancy. Asthma may worsen during pregnancy, resulting in increased ED visits, hospitalizations, and need for oral corticosteroids.[3] Also, poorly controlled asthma may be associated with increased preeclampsia, prematurity, need for cesarean delivery, low birth weight term deliveries,[4–8] and congenital malformations.[9] In contrast, mild or well-controlled more severe asthma has been associated with excellent maternal and perinatal outcomes.[10–12]

B. Epidemiology and Incidence in Pregnancy

Asthma may complicate 4%–8% of pregnancies.[13,14] In approximately 30% of pregnant patients with asthma, symptoms may become worse, whereas they may improve in 23% of women and remain unchanged in the remainder.[3] The frequency of exacerbations and hospitalizations increases with asthma severity during pregnancy. One large prospective study found that pregnant patients with mild asthma had exacerbation rates of approximately 12.6% and hospitalization rates of 2.3%, whereas patients with severe asthma had exacerbation rates of 52% and hospitalization rates of 27%.[3]

II. PATIENT CASE (PART I)

Kathy is a 28-year-old prima gravida in her first trimester. As a child, she had moderate persistent asthma, but by age 12 her disease became mild and intermittent. Subsequently, she had mild exacerbations a few times a year associated with viral respiratory tract infections. Most of these episodes were well controlled with as needed (PRN) use of albuterol metered-dose inhaler (MDI), and she rarely required a short course of oral corticosteroids. However, about 1 month after becoming pregnant, she began wheezing with vigorous exercise. This progressed to symptoms without exercise three times a week, along with waking up in the middle of the night from cough and wheeze once a week. She is now using albuterol about three times a week but gets complete relief after two puffs. At her prenatal visit today, spirometry revealed a FVC of 102% predicted and an FEV_1 of 81% that increased to 98% after two puffs of albuterol MDI. Pulse oximetry revealed an oxygen saturation of 97%. A radioallergosorbent test (RAST) indicated that she is not sensitive to dust mites or other indoor allergens and that her total immunoglobulin E (IgE) was 60 IU. Her chest was clear to auscultation. A chest x-ray was negative.

III. Clinical Presentation

Symptoms of asthma include wheeze, cough, chest tightness, and/or dyspnea. There are three distinct patterns of presentation:

A. Intermittent Asthma

Patients with intermittent asthma have extended periods (weeks or months) during which they are symptom-free.[1] However, when they are exposed to a trigger, such as a viral respiratory tract infection, exposure from an allergen, vigorous exercise, or a chemical irritant, such as cigarette smoke, they will begin to have symptoms that vary in severity and duration.

B. Persistent Asthma

Patients with persistent asthma do not have extended symptom-free periods and experience symptoms more than 2 days a week; they may wake up from asthma symptoms at night more than two times a month, and need an SABA to relieve symptoms more than twice a week.[1] In patients who are not taking a controller (preventer) medication the frequency of these symptoms and impairment in lung function determine whether they are classified as mild, moderate, or severe persistent asthma (Figure 1).

Components of Severity		Classification of Asthma Severity ≥12 years of age			
				Persistent	
		Intermittent	Mild	Moderate	Severe
Impairment Normal FEV₁/FVC: 8–19 yr 85% 20–39 yr 80% 40–59 yr 75% 60–80 yr 70%	Symptoms	≤2 days/week	>2 days/week but not daily	Daily	Throughout the day
	Nighttime awakenings	≤2x/month	3–4x/month	>1x/week but not nightly	Often 7x/week
	Short-acting β₂-agonist use for symptom control (not prevention of EIB)	≤2 days/week	>2 days/week but not daily, and not more than 1x on any day	Daily	Several times per day
	Interference with normal activity	None	Minor limitation	Some limitation	Extremely limited
	Lung function	• Normal FEV₁ between exacerbations • FEV₁ >80% predicted • FEV₁/FVC normal	• FEV₁ >80% predicted • FEV₁/FVC normal	• FEV₁ >60% but <80% predicted • FEV₁/FVC reduced 5%	• FEV₁ <60% predicted • FEV₁/FVC reduced >5%
Risk	Exacerbations requiring oral systemic corticosteroids	0–1/year (see note)	≥2/year (see note) ⟶		
		Consider severity and interval since last exacerbation. Frequency and severity may fluctuate over time for patients in any severity category. Relative annual risk of exacerbations may be related to FEV₁.			
Recommended Step for Initiating Treatment (See Figure 3 for treatment steps.)		Step 1	Step 2	Step 3	Step 4 or 5 and consider short course of oral systemic corticosteroids
		In 2–6 weeks, evaluate level of asthma control that is achieved and adjust therapy accordingly.			

Figure 1. Classifying Asthma Severity and Initiating Treatment in Youths ≥12 Years of Age and Adults. EIB = exercise-induced bronchospasm, FEV₁ = forced expiratory volume in the first second, FVC = forced vital capacity, ICU = intensive care unit. Adapted from EPR-3.[1]

C. Seasonal Allergic Asthma

The third clinical presentation is patients with seasonal allergic asthma. Their pattern of presentation is characterized by persistent asthma during a particular season when allergens to which they are sensitive are in the air (eg, the fall ragweed season) and intermittent symptoms during the rest of the year.

IV. Definition and Pathophysiology

Asthma symptoms are a result of airway obstruction caused by inflammation and airway hyperresponsiveness. The NAEPP's working definition of asthma is as follows:

"Asthma is a chronic inflammatory disorder of the airways in which many cells and cellular elements play a role: in particular, mast cells, eosinophils, neutrophils (especially in sudden onset, fatal exacerbations, occupational asthma, and patients who smoke), T lymphocytes, macrophages, and epithelial cells. In susceptible individuals, this inflammation causes recurrent episodes of coughing (particularly at night or early in the morning), wheezing, breathlessness, and chest tightness. These episodes are usually associated with widespread but variable airflow obstruction that is often reversible either spontaneously or with treatment."[1]

Airflow obstruction is a result of bronchial smooth muscle contraction (bronchoconstriction) and airway edema, which includes swelling of the airway walls, mucous hypersecretion and, during acute exacerbations, formation of inspissated mucous plugs. Airway hyperresponsiveness, an exaggerated response to a variety of stimuli (eg, cigarette smoke), is a major cause of bronchoconstriction in the patient with asthma.

In some patients with asthma, airway obstruction is not completely reversible after inhaled bronchodilators and systemic corticosteroids. This is a result of permanent structural changes in the airways and is referred to as *airway remodeling*.[1] There is no information on how pregnancy affects this process.

In patients with an allergic component to their asthma, IgE plays an important role in the pathogenesis of airway inflammation.[1] In the genetically predisposed patient, IgE production is increased and circulating IgE attaches to high affinity receptors on mast cells. Subsequent exposure to allergen results in activation of mast cells with the release of proinflammatory cytokines and mediators (eg, leukotrienes) that produce bronchospasm. The cytokines, such as interleukins, cause inflammatory cells, such as eosinophils, to migrate to the airways and become activated, releasing mediators of inflammation and causing increased airway responsiveness.

V. Diagnosis

The diagnosis of asthma in a pregnant patient is the same as for a nonpregnant adult. It is based on medical history, physical examination, spirometry, and exclusion of alternative diagnoses (eg, dyspnea of pregnancy).[15] A history of recurrent cough or wheeze, especially if worse at night, recurrent chest tightness, or difficulty breathing raises the possibility of asthma. Also, a history of symptoms that occur or worsen with exercise, viral infection, exposure to animals (eg, cats), irritants, and/or with strong emotional reactions increases the probability of asthma. The physical examination may reveal findings such as wheezing that support the diagnosis, but absence of these findings between episodes does not rule out asthma.

Spirometry is an essential objective measure to establish the diagnosis of asthma.[1,15,16] Even when a patient is symptom-free, spirometry may reveal an abnormal aspect, such as FEV_1 <80% predicted, FEV_1/FVC ratio <0.8, and/or a scooped flow-volume curve. Patients are given a bronchodilator and spirometry is repeated. Ideally, the FEV_1, if initially <80%, should increase by ≥12% to confirm the diagnosis, but inflammation may reduce bronchodilator responsiveness and it may only increase after institution of a short course of systemic corticosteroids and/or inhaled corticosteroids (ICS). If corticosteroids, especially when given systemically, do not improve spirometry and the patient has been adherent, the diagnosis should be reevaluated.

In patients with a history of symptoms consistent with persistent asthma and completely normal spirometry, a therapeutic trial with ICS is still warranted. If the patient does not become relatively symptom-free after 3 or more weeks of treatment with an ICS, referral to an asthma specialist to re-evaluate the diagnosis is indicated. In nonpregnant patients, a methacholine challenge is often used to confirm a diagnosis of asthma when pulmonary function testing and clinical responsiveness are not definitive.[17] However, methacholine challenges are contraindicated during pregnancy.

VI. National Guidelines

In 2005, NAEPP published an update on its 1993 recommendations for managing asthma during pregnancy. This document provides evidenced-based recommendations for the pharmacologic management of asthma during pregnancy and evaluation of the safety of asthma medications on pregnancy outcomes.[16]

In August 2007, NAEPP released its 487-page Expert Panel Report 3 (EPR-3), which provides newer guidelines on classifying asthma severity, a more extensive stepwise approach to pharmacologic therapy, and criteria for assessing asthma control and adjusting therapy.[1] Last, the American College of Obstetrics and Gynecology (ACOG) published clinical management guidelines that included features of the two NAEPP Guidelines.[15] This chapter relies heavily on these three national guidelines.

VII. Prevention

There is currently no known way of preventing the development of asthma. However, it is possible to prevent symptomatic episodes by avoiding or reducing exposure to triggers, such as tobacco smoke (see the section F. Nonpharmacologic Treatment, below).

VIII. Treatment

A. Goals and Overall Strategies

The ultimate goal of asthma therapy during pregnancy is to maintain adequate oxygenation of the fetus by preventing hypoxic episodes in the mother.[15] Thus, it is particularly important for asthma to be well controlled in the mother. The NAEPP Working Group has emphasized that *"it is safer for pregnant women with asthma to be treated with asthma medications than it is for them to have asthma symptoms and exacerbations."*[16]

Asthma is well controlled when patients have minimal or no chronic symptoms, infrequent use of SABAs, maintenance of normal or near normal lung function, no limitation of activities, and not more than one exacerbation requiring systemic corticosteroids in a year (Figure 2).

In a patient who previously has not been taking long-term control medication, asthma severity is classified and therapy initiated at one of six levels according to severity (Figure 1). In contrast, in a patient who is already taking a long-term control medication, asthma control is assessed (Figure 2). If the patient is not well controlled,

Components of Control		Classification of Asthma Control (≥12 years of age)		
		Well Controlled	Not Well Controlled	Very Poorly Controlled
Impairment	Symptoms	≤2 days/week	>2 days/week	Throughout the day
	Nighttime awakenings	≤2x/month	1–3x/week	≥4x/week
	Interference with normal activity	None	Some limitation	Extremely limited
	Short-acting β_2-agonist use for symptom control (not prevention of EIB)	≤2 days/week	>2 days/week	Several times per day
	FEV_1 or peak flow	>80% predicted/ personal best	60–80% predicted/ personal best	<60% predicted/ personal best

	Validated questionnaires
	
	    ATAQ
	    ACQ
	    ACT
		
		0
		≤0.75*
		≥20
			
			1–2
			≥1.5
			16–19
				
				3–4
				N/A
				≤15

Risk	Exacerbations requiring oral systemic corticosteroids	0–1/year	≥2/year (see note)	
		Consider severity and interval since last exacerbation		
	Progressive loss of lung function	Evaluation requires long-term follow-up care		
	Treatment-related adverse effects	Medication side effects can vary in intensity from none to very troublesome and worrisome. The level of intensity does not correlate to specific levels of control but should be considered in the overall assessment of risk.		
Recommended Action for Treatment (see Figure 3 for treatment steps)		• Maintain current step. • Regular follow-ups every 1–6 months to maintain control. • Consider step down if well controlled for at least 3 months.	• Step up 1 step and • Reevaluate in 2–6 weeks. • For side effects, consider alternative treatment options.	• Consider short course of oral systemic corticosteroids. • Step up 1–2 steps, and • Reevaluate in 2 weeks. • For side effects, consider alternative treatment options.

*ACQ values of 0.76–1.4 are indeterminate regarding well-controlled asthma.

Figure 2. Assessing Asthma Control and Adjusting Therapy in Youths ≥12 Years of Age and Adults. ACQ = Asthma Control Questionnaire©, ACT = Asthma Control Test™, ATAQ = Asthma Therapy Assessment Questionnaire©, EIB = exercise-induced bronchospasm, ICU = intensive care unit, N/A = not available. Minimal Important Difference: 1.0 for the ATAQ; 0.5 for the ACQ; not determined for the ACT. Adapted from EPR-3.[1]

therapy is increased to the next higher step (Figure 3). If the patient has been well controlled for ≥3 months, consideration is given to decrease therapy to the next lower step (Figure 3).

B. Quick-Relief Medications

Providing patients with a written asthma action plan and teaching them to use quick-relief medications early prevents exacerbations from becoming more severe and prevents or reduces the need for ED treatment or hospitalizations.[18] An inhaled SABA is the mainstay of self-management, and the initial response to this quick-relief medication indicates whether a short course of oral corticosteroids is required or whether the patient should seek ED treatment (Figure 4). Depending on the practice setting and experience with a particular patient, many clinicians will provide their patients with a supply of oral corticosteroids to keep on hand at home with the instruction to call them before taking it. Others may instruct their patients to take the first dose of oral corticosteroid based on symptoms and/or a decrease in PEF and then contact them.

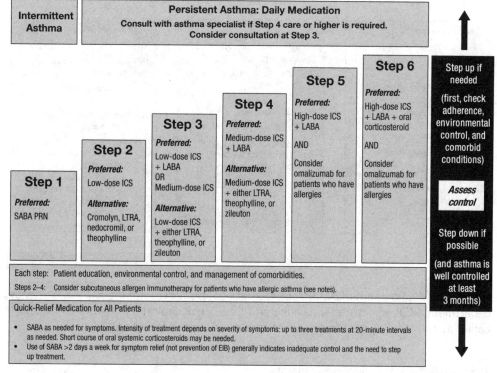

Figure 3. Stepwise Approach for Managing Asthma in Youths ≥12 Years of Age and Adults. *Alphabetical order is used when more than one treatment option is listed within either preferred or alternative therapy.* EIB = exercise-induced bronchospasm, ICS = inhaled corticosteroid, LABA = long-acting β₂-selective agonist, LTRA = leukotriene receptor antagonist, PRN = as needed, SABA = short-acting β₂-selective agonist. Adapted from EPR-3.[1]

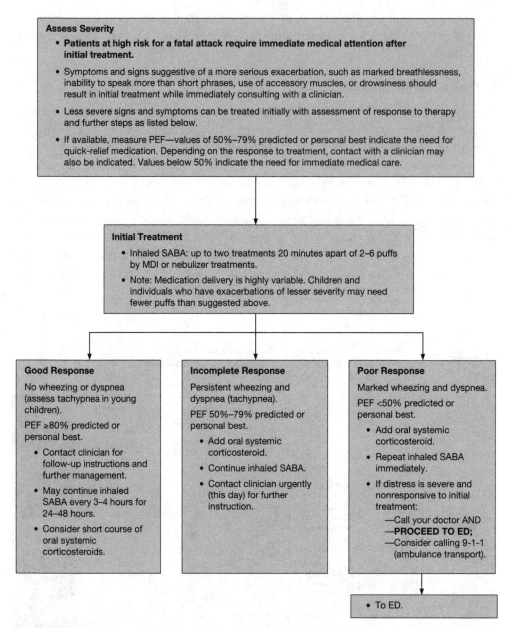

Assess Severity

- **Patients at high risk for a fatal attack require immediate medical attention after initial treatment.**

- Symptoms and signs suggestive of a more serious exacerbation, such as marked breathlessness, inability to speak more than short phrases, use of accessory muscles, or drowsiness should result in initial treatment while immediately consulting with a clinician.

- Less severe signs and symptoms can be treated initially with assessment of response to therapy and further steps as listed below.

- If available, measure PEF—values of 50%–79% predicted or personal best indicate the need for quick-relief medication. Depending on the response to treatment, contact with a clinician may also be indicated. Values below 50% indicate the need for immediate medical care.

Initial Treatment

- Inhaled SABA: up to two treatments 20 minutes apart of 2–6 puffs by MDI or nebulizer treatments.

- Note: Medication delivery is highly variable. Children and individuals who have exacerbations of lesser severity may need fewer puffs than suggested above.

Good Response

No wheezing or dyspnea (assess tachypnea in young children).

PEF ≥80% predicted or personal best.

- Contact clinician for follow-up instructions and further management.

- May continue inhaled SABA every 3–4 hours for 24–48 hours.

- Consider short course of oral systemic corticosteroids.

Incomplete Response

Persistent wheezing and dyspnea (tachypnea).

PEF 50%–79% predicted or personal best.

- Add oral systemic corticosteroid.

- Continue inhaled SABA.

- Contact clinician urgently (this day) for further instruction.

Poor Response

Marked wheezing and dyspnea.

PEF <50% predicted or personal best.

- Add oral systemic corticosteroid.

- Repeat inhaled SABA immediately.

- If distress is severe and nonresponsive to initial treatment:

  —Call your doctor AND

  —**PROCEED TO ED;**

  —Consider calling 9-1-1 (ambulance transport).

- To ED.

Figure 4. Management of Asthma Exacerbations: Home Treatment. ED = emergency department, MDI = metered-dose inhaler, PEF = peak expiratory flow, SABA = short-acting β_2-selective agonist (quick-relief inhaler). Adapted from EPR-3.[1]

1. Short-Acting β_2-Selective Agonists

This category includes albuterol and levalbuterol, available in hydrofluoroalkane (HFA) MDIs and nebulizer solutions, and pirbuterol, available in a breath-actuated chlorofluorocarbon (CFC) MDI. All patients with asthma, whether intermittent or persistent, should have an inhaled SABA to use PRN to provide quick relief of asthma symptoms. Albuterol is the preferred SABA during pregnancy because it has a good safety profile and there is more gestational safety data for this agent than for other

SABAs.[16] It provides symptom relief by stimulating β_2-adrenergic receptors, which, in turn, cause relaxation of airway smooth muscles. Also, pretreatment with a SABA before vigorous exercise prevents exercise-induced bronchospasm (EIB). Side effects are transient and dose dependent; they include tremors, headache, and, at higher doses, tachycardia and hypokalemia. There is no role for oral albuterol in the treatment of asthma as this mode of delivery is less effective and causes more systemic side effects than the inhaled route.[19]

Delivery of albuterol by MDI is the most convenient method, but patients must be taught the appropriate technique. The NAEPP's recommended dose for home management of exacerbations is 2–6 puffs every 20 minutes, until symptoms are relieved, for up to two doses. If symptoms do not resolve and PEF does not return to >80% of personal best, contacting the physician, going to the ED, or initiation of a short course of oral corticosteroids should be considered, depending on the severity of the exacerbation and the patient's individual written asthma action plan. Chronically, the frequency of use of a SABA is one clinical indicator of asthma control. Use of a SABA more often than twice a week should prompt reevaluation of therapy and consideration should be given to institute an increase in maintenance therapy (Figure 3).

In the ED, treatment of asthma via four puffs of albuterol MDI delivered by a valved holding chamber (VHC) is as effective and as safe as delivery of 2.5 mg by nebulization.[20] Thus, nebulizer delivery of albuterol offers no advantage in most circumstances. Because all of the beneficial and systemic effects of albuterol are related to the R-isomer, and the S-isomer is not deleterious in humans, there is no advantage in either efficacy or adverse effects to the single isomer product, levalbuterol.[21,22]

HFA MDIs and CFC MDIs are equivalent in efficacy and safety.[23] However, the orifice of the actuator is more likely to clog with the HFA formulation; patients should be taught to rinse the actuator once a week in warm water and allow it to air dry, to prevent clogging. Rinsing in this manner may unclog the actuator when the spray volume decreases.

2. Anticholinergics

Inhaled ipratropium bromide is available as a nebulizer solution and HFA MDI alone and a CFC MDI in combination with albuterol. It reduces vagal tone of the airways by competitively inhibiting muscarinic cholinergic receptors. The drug is approved by the U.S. Food and Drug Administration (FDA) only for reversing cholinergically medicated bronchospasm in chronic obstructive pulmonary disease (COPD) and not for asthma. However, there are data indicating that multiple doses of ipratropium provide added benefit to albuterol in the treatment of severe exacerbations in the ED.[24] There are no data on its use in the home management of exacerbations of asthma, and NAEPP does not recommend it in this situation. It may be an alternative for patients who do not tolerate a SABA, but the onset of action is much slower and the peak bronchodilator effect is less than albuterol MDI.[25] The most common side effects are drying of the mouth and respiratory secretions.

3. Oral Corticosteroids

Methylprednisolone, prednisone, or prednisolone are indicated for exacerbations of asthma that are not bronchodilator responsive. They prevent the progression of an exacerbation, reverse inflammation, speed recovery, and reduce the frequency of relapses.[26] Early intervention is likely to prevent ED visits and hospitalizations for asthma. Corticosteroids inhibit migration and activation of eosinophils and lymphocytes and thereby inhibit cytokine production. Also, within a few hours of administration, they increase the number of β_2-receptors and thereby increase response to subsequent doses of a SABA. The NAEPP's recommended dose for treating an exacerbation is 40–80 mg/d in single or 2 divided doses for 5–10 days, or less if the patient is symptom-free for 24 hours. Because the effects of a dose may dissipate within 12 hours,[27] 2 divided doses, approximately 12 hours apart, theoretically may provide greater benefit than taking the total daily dose only once a day.

Tapering the dose over several days provides no benefit.[28,29] Common adverse effects of a short course of oral corticosteroids include increased appetite, fluid retention, weight gain, and, less often, mood alteration. Less common adverse effects are decreased glucose metabolism or increased blood pressure in patients with latent or coexisting diabetes or hypertension.

4. Inhaled Corticosteroids

For the most part, the literature indicates that inhaled corticosteroids are much less effective than the oral route for the treatment of acute exacerbations.[30] Doubling the ICS dose in patients already taking maintenance therapy has not been effective in decreasing the severity of an exacerbation or preventing the progression.[31] However, one study suggested that increasing the maintenance dose four-fold for 7 days, starting at the first appearance of worsening symptoms, may decrease the need for systemic corticosteroids.[32] Therefore, for patients who have a history of substantial adverse effects (eg, mood changes), diabetes, or those who strongly object to taking a short course of oral corticosteroids, high-dose ICS (eg, 1600 μg/d of budesonide) may offer an alternative if the exacerbation is not severe.

It is noteworthy that ICSs with **negligible** oral bioavailability from the swallowed portion (eg, budesonide, ciclesonide, fluticasone, and mometasone) are absorbed from the lungs and high inhaled doses also may have systemic adverse effects,[33] although they will be less than with oral corticosteroids.

C. Long-Term Control Medications

In patients with intermittent asthma, long-term controller medications are not indicated. These patients are treated with SABA PRN and short courses of oral corticosteroids when indicated (see section B. Quick-Relief Medications, above). In contrast, in patients with persistent asthma, long-term control medications are used daily, even when the patient is symptom-free, to prevent and control symptoms, improve quality of life, reduce the frequency and severity of asthma exacerbations, and reverse airflow obstruction.[1] ICSs are the most effective control medications as they attenuate airway inflammation to the greatest extent.[34] Low-dose ICSs are preferred to other alternatives for mild persistent asthma, such as leukotriene receptor antagonists (LTRAs), cromolyn, or theophylline, as they are more effective.[1,35,36] If low or medium doses of ICSs are not sufficient to control asthma, the preferred medication to add is a long-acting β-agonist (LABA).[1,15,16]

1. Inhaled Corticosteroids

Several ICSs are available in the United States in different devices and strengths (Table 1). Based on the available evidence, NAEPP has concluded that ICSs are the most potent and consistently effective long-term control medication for asthma. They reduce the severity of symptoms, improve asthma control and quality of life, improve pulmonary function, decrease airway responsiveness, prevent exacerbations, and reduce the need for short courses of systemic corticosteroids, ED care, hospitalizations, and deaths due to asthma.[1,37] As a consequence, ICSs are recommended for all severity classifications of persistent asthma (Figure 3).

The anti-inflammatory effects of ICS are mediated through glucocorticoid receptors that modulate inflammatory gene expression. They suppress the generation of cytokines, recruitment of inflammatory cells into the airways, and release of inflammatory mediators. Several studies indicate that they improve asthma control more effectively than LTRAs or any other single long-term control medication. There is some variation in response. For example, ICSs are less effective in patients who smoke.[38] Also, some data suggest that there is variation in the sensitivity to ICS (ie, steroid resistance),[39,40] but the most common cause of treatment failure is poor adherence.[41] Budesonide is the preferred ICS during pregnancy because more data are available on its safety in pregnant women than are available for other ICSs.[16] However, there are no data indicating that other ICSs are unsafe during pregnancy. They are available as HFA MDIs, dry powder inhalers (DPIs; Table 1), and budesonide is available also as a

Table 1. Estimated Comparative Daily Dosages for Most Commonly Prescribed[a] Inhaled Corticosteroids for Youths ≥12 Years of Age and Adults

Drug	Low Daily Dose (μg)	Medium Daily Dose (μg)	High Daily Dose (μg)
Beclomethasone HFA, 40 or 80 μg/puff	80–240	>240–480	>480
Budesonide DPI, 90 or 180 μg/inhalation	180–600	>600–1200	>1200–1600
Ciclesonide HFA/MDI, 80 or 160 μg/puff	160	>160–640	>640
Fluticasone			
HFA/MDI, 44, 110, or 220 μg/puff	88–264	>264–440	>440
DPI, 50 μg/inhalation	100–300	>300–500	>500
Mometasone DPI,[b] 220 μg/inhalation	220	>220–440	>440

DPI = dry powder inhaler, HFA = hydrofluoroalkane, MDI = metered-dose inhaler.
[a]Flunisolide and triamcinolone are not included in this table since they are rarely prescribed. Both are available as a chlorofluorocarbon MDI, which will be withdrawn from the market in the near future. An HFA MDI of flunisolide is approved by the U.S. Food and Drug Administration (FDA) but not yet available.
[b]The only inhaled corticosteroid FDA-approved for once daily dosing at the lowest dose. Divide medium and high doses into 2 doses/d.
Adapted from EPR-3.[1]

nebulizer suspension. The DPI is more convenient and has fewer topical side effects, but the MDI is an acceptable alternative. There is no role for the nebulizer suspension in treating pregnant women because it is inconvenient, time consuming, and more costly than using a DPI or MDI alone or with a VHC.

The daily dose differs among ICSs and devices. On the basis of limited data, NAEPP has classified the dose into low, medium, and high daily doses (Table 1). It is noteworthy that mometasone DPI is the only ICS approved by the FDA for once-daily dosing. This is on the basis of pivotal studies demonstrating that dividing the dose twice daily was no more effective than once daily, but the patients in those studies had relatively mild asthma. In patients with more severe disease, mometasone may be required twice daily to achieve control.

Local side effects of ICS include thrush and dysphonia. Thrush may be prevented by mouth rinsing and spitting or use of a VHC, particularly with medium and high doses delivered by MDI. A VHC decreases dysphonia as well as local side effects, which are less common with DPIs than MDIs without VHC.[42]

The systemic effects of ICS relate to the dose, method of delivery, and affinity for the glucocorticoid receptor. As doses are increased, there is an increase in systemic effect. Those agents with higher receptor affinity, such as fluticasone and mometasone, have a steeper dose response curve for systemic effects than agents with lower affinity, such as budesonide.[33] These effects include decreases in bone mineral density and increased risk of osteoporosis, dermal thinning, and increased skin bruising, increased intraocular pressure, and altered glucose metabolism in susceptible individuals.[43] ICSs may also decrease hypothalamic-pituitary-adrenal (HPA) axis function, the most sensitive biomarker of systemic absorption,[44] but reports of Cushingoid symptoms are extremely rare with ICSs. One circumstance in which the risk of systemic adverse effects may be increased is in patients who require another medication that inhibits cytochrome P-450 3A4, the pathway through which ICSs are metabolized (eg, ritonavir, azole antifungal agents, and macrolide antibiotics, other than azithromycin).[45]

2. Long-Acting β-Agonists

Formoterol and salmeterol are the two LABAs available in the United States as a single DPI or in combination with an inhaled corticosteroid as a DPI or HFA MDI. The weight of evidence indicates that in a patient with asthma that is not well controlled on low-dose ICS alone, adding a LABA leads to greater improvement in lung function and decrease in exacerbations and SABA use than does increasing the dose of ICS[46,47] or adding a leukotriene receptor antagonist.[48] However, NAEPP still recommends increasing the dose of ICS as an equally acceptable option because of rare, serious safety concerns with LABAs and (during pregnancy) the paucity of gestational safety data available for LABA. In contrast, addition of a LABA to medium- or high-dose ICS is the preferred treatment for Steps 4–6 (Figure 3) in both pregnant and nonpregnant patients.

LABAs stimulate β$_2$-receptors, which increase cyclic adenosine monophosphate through a second messenger, adenylate cyclase, and thereby relax airway smooth muscle. Because of high lipophilicity that prolongs retention in the airways, both formoterol and salmeterol have a duration of 12 hours. In addition, formoterol has an onset of action as rapid as albuterol, whereas the onset of salmeterol is 15–30 minutes.[49]

LABAs should never be used alone for persistent asthma as they lack anti-inflammatory activity and may mask worsening asthma.[50] The maximum recommended daily dose of formoterol is 24 µg/d when delivered by DPI and 18 µg/d when delivered in combination with budesonide in an HFA MDI. The maximum recommended daily dose of salmeterol is 100 µg when delivered by DPI or in combination with fluticasone in either a DPI or an HFA MDI.

The most common adverse effects of LABAs are skeletal muscle tremor, headache, and tachycardia.[51] At high doses, they can cause hypokalemia and prolonged QT_c interval. All products containing a LABA have a boxed warning that severe, life-threatening, or fatal exacerbations may sometimes occur. This was largely the result of a single large study in which subjects were not carefully monitored and may not have been taking an inhaled corticosteroid.[52] Subsequent systematic reviews,[53] case control studies,[54] large year-long clinical trials,[46,47] and a large postmarketing study[55] failed to detect an increased risk of asthma exacerbations with LABAs in combination with ICS. Moreover, the death rate from asthma in the United States has actually decreased since the marketing of the combination of fluticasone and salmeterol.[2]

3. Leukotriene Modifiers
a. Leukotriene Receptor Antagonists

The two LTRAs available in the United States as oral tablets are montelukast and zafirlukast. NAEPP recommends them as alternative, but not preferred, therapy for mild persistent asthma and as nonpreferred adjunctive therapy in combination with an ICS. In addition to lower efficacy, nonpreferred status during pregnancy is based on there being only a small amount of available published gestational safety data.[56]

Cysteinyl leukotrienes are released from mast cells and eosinophils. They contract airway smooth muscle, increase mucous secretions, and attract and activate inflammatory cells in the airways of asthma patients. LTRAs are competitive inhibitors of leukotriene D_4 at the Cys LT_1 receptor. Because they inhibit only a single mediator involved in the pathogenesis of asthma, they have only modest efficacy. Several randomized controlled trials demonstrated that ICSs are more effective than LTRAs for most end points.[35,36] In fact, patients in pivotal trials of LTRAs, on average, would not have met criteria for well-controlled asthma. However, their mechanism of action makes LTRAs an attractive adjunctive therapy in a patient not well controlled by ICS alone when aspirin-, NSAID-, or exercise-induced bronchospasm is part of the clinical picture. Aspirin-induced bronchospasm involves increased conversion of arachidonic acid to cysteinyl leukotrienes,[57] and EIB is mediated, in part by cysteinyl leukotrienes released from mast cells.[58] Moreover, in EIB, the duration of protection with LABAs decreases with regular use, whereas tachyphylaxis does not occur with montelukast.[59]

The dose is 10 mg at bedtime for montelukast and 20 mg BID for zafirlukast taken fasting. Montelukast has several advantages over zafirlukast. It is effective with once-daily administration, has no clinically relevant food or drug interactions, and does not cause any specific adverse effects. In contrast, zafirlukast requires twice-daily administration, has decreased bioavailability when taken with food, inhibits the metabolism of warfarin and other drugs, can cause elevation of liver enzymes, and, on rare occasion, has been implicated in irreversible hepatic failure requiring a liver transplant or has resulted in death.[60]

b. 5-Lipoxygenase Inhibitors

Zileuton, a 5-lipoxygenase inhibitor, is available as a slow-release oral tablet and recommended by NAEPP as a "not preferred" alternative to be added to low-dose ICS in moderate persistent asthma for nonpregnant patients (Figure 3, Step 3). However, because animal data submitted to the FDA are not reassuring and there are no published human gestational data, NAEPP recommends avoiding zileuton during pregnancy.[16]

4. Anti-Immunoglobulin E

Omalizumab is a monoclonal anti-IgE antibody available as a subcutaneous injection. It is FDA-approved for patients with moderate or severe allergic asthma who are not well controlled with an ICS. However, NAEPP only recommends it for severe asthma that is not well controlled on the combination of ICS plus LABA (Figure 3, Steps 4 and 5). It decreases exacerbations and ED visits,[61] but only modestly improves lung function and allows a median ICS dose reduction of 25% over that of placebo.[62] Omalizumab binds circulating IgE and prevents attachment of IgE to its high affinity receptor on mast cells and basophils, and decreases the number of these receptors on basophils and submucosal cells. As a consequence, it decreases the release of mediators upon exposure to allergens.

The subcutaneous dose of omalizumab is based on total IgE and body weight; 0.016 mg/kg/IgE unit/month up to a maximum of 750 mg. When the monthly dose exceeds 375 mg, the total dose is divided into equal parts and administered at 2-week intervals. The maximum dose for each injection should not exceed 150 mg. Thus, 1–3 injections may be required at each visit. Because of a small risk of anaphylaxis, omalizumab should always be administered under direct medical supervision in a clinic or office.

Pain or bruising at the injection site was reported in 5%–20% of patients during pivotal trials, but in our experience it is less common when a skillful nurse administers the injections. Anaphylaxis has been reported in 0.2% of patients, most often within 2 hours of administration at the first three visits. Also, malignant neoplasms were reported during pivotal trials slightly more frequently than with placebo. This may be a chance finding and not caused by the drug, but surveillance for such an increased risk is ongoing.

Finally, in addition to being an inconvenient therapy, omalizumab is very expensive, costing $10,000–$30,000 per year for the drug plus the cost of office visits for each dose.[63]

5. Oral Systemic Corticosteroids

Long-term maintenance therapy with oral corticosteroids is only indicated for the most severe asthma that is not well controlled on high-dose ICS plus LABA (Figure 3, Step 5). Oral corticosteroids suppress, control, and reverse airway inflammation, but can cause severe adverse effects. It is only a rare patient who requires this extreme measure. Poor adherence to ICS plus LABA as a cause of difficult-to-control asthma should be excluded before initiating this intervention.

The dose of methylprednisolone, prednisolone, or prednisone is 7.5–60 mg daily or every other morning. Alternate morning therapy reduces the risks of some systemic adverse effects. There are some data indicating that if daily therapy is required, administration of the dose at 3 pm is associated with less HPA axis suppression,[64] but it is difficult for many patients to take medication consistently at this time of day.

The magnitude of adverse effects is related to dose, frequency of administration, and duration of therapy. They include HPA axis suppression, dermal thinning, osteoporosis, hypertension, Cushing's syndrome, glaucoma, cataracts, and muscle weakness. Also, there is an increased risk of suppression of the immune system, reactivation of latent tuberculosis, and possibly infection, especially disseminated varicella.[65] They have additional risks during pregnancy (see section D. Safety of Asthma Medications during Pregnancy, below).

6. Other "Not Preferred" Alternatives

Cromolyn, nedocromil, and theophylline are listed by the NAEPP as "not preferred" alternatives to low-dose ICS in mild persistent asthma (Figure 3, Step 2). Also, theophylline is listed as alternative adjunctive therapy to ICS for moderate persistent asthma (Figure 3, Step 3). Cromolyn is available as an MDI and nebulizer solution, while nedocromil is no longer manufactured. Theophylline is available as slow-release tablets and capsules.

a. Cromolyn

Cromolyn decreases symptoms and attenuates EIB and both the early and late responses to allergens. However, low doses of ICS are much more effective for maintenance therapy,[66] and albuterol is more effective at blocking EIB.[67] Cromolyn decreases mast cell release of mediators and eosinophil recruitment, probably by blocking chloride channels. The nebulizer solution delivers more drug to the airways than MDI and more effectively blocks EIB.[68] Both are inconvenient, requiring administration four times a day. Cromolyn has no adverse effects, with the exception of an occasional patient who coughs after taking an MDI dose.

b. Theophylline

Monotherapy with theophylline is less effective than low-dose ICSs in mild asthma,[69] and addition of theophylline to ICS is less effective than addition of a LABA in controlling symptoms.[70] It has both modest bronchodilator and anti-inflammatory actions, probably as a result of nonselective phosphodiesterase inhibition. Therapeutic serum concentrations attenuate EIB[71] and responses to allergen challenge as well as cromolyn MDI does.[72]

Because of a large interpatient variation in metabolism, theophylline serum concentrations must be measured to adjust dosage so that maximum potential benefit is obtained with minimal risk of adverse effects.[73] When serum concentrations exceed 20 µg/mL, the risks of acute theophylline toxicity include nausea, vomiting, headache, and, at high concentrations, cardiac arrhythmias, seizures, and death. Also, one slow-release formulation currently available in the United States, Theo-24, dose dumps when taken with food and, on average, releases the entire 24-hour dose within 4 hours.[74]

7. Anticholinergics

Ipratropium and tiotropium are not indicated for long-term asthma control. Ipratropium does not improve asthma control when added to ICSs[75] and does not attenuate airway responsiveness to exercise or allergens. There are no published studies on tiotropium in patients with asthma.

D. Safety of Asthma Medications during Pregnancy

An NAEPP Working Group conducted a systematic review of the evidence of the safety of asthma medications during pregnancy.[16] They concluded that the data were reassuring regarding the safety of SABAs, ICSs, cromolyn, and theophylline. More data were available for albuterol than other SABAs and for budesonide than other ICSs, but there is no evidence that other members of these pharmacologic groups pose additional risks. In fact, a 2008 large population-based cohort study of 4561 pregnancies from women with asthma concluded that use of medium-dose ICS during the first trimester was associated with a reduced risk of congenital malformations.[76] The risk was not significantly reduced in the low-dose cohort, whereas there was a trend toward increased risk in the cohort taking high-dose ICS (>1000 µg/d CFC beclomethasone equivalent).

In contrast, data on the safety of oral corticosteroids during pregnancy are conflicting. Their use, especially during the first trimester, was associated with an estimated excess risk of 0.2%–0.3% for isolated cleft lip with or without cleft palate, which is several times higher than the baseline risk.[16] However, few pregnant women with oral corticosteroid–dependent asthma were included in these studies, and extent of exposure was not described well. Long-term use during pregnancy was associated with an increased incidence of preeclampsia and the delivery of both preterm and low-birth-weight infants. However, it is difficult to separate the effects of corticosteroids on these outcomes from the effects of severe or uncontrolled asthma.

From the available data, it is not clear that an occasional short course of oral corticosteroids to treat exacerbations poses the above-mentioned risks, and the benefit to both mother and fetus outweighs the risks. Use of ICSs clearly reduces exacerbations and the need for short courses of oral corticosteroids, which will reduce the risk of adverse outcomes.

There are limited data on the safety of LABAs.[16] However, their pharmacologic and toxicologic profiles are similar to SABAs, so they should not be withheld, when indicated, for moderate and severe persistent asthma. Similarly, minimal human data are available for LTRAs, but reassuring animal studies have been submitted to the FDA for LTRAs.[16] Data from animal studies submitted to the FDA for zileuton are not reassuring and thus, this drug should be avoided during pregnancy.[16]

There are few or no human data on the safety of anticholinergics, ciclesonide, pirbuterol, or omalizumab during pregnancy. The manufacturer of omalizumab has established a registry to obtain data on pregnancy outcomes in women exposed to this drug.[77]

Ipratropium is a quaternary ammonium compound with poor membrane penetrability and very low systemic bioavailability. Thus, the short-term use of this drug in the treatment of acute exacerbations in the ED poses a low risk.

E. Monitoring and Assessing Asthma Control

ACOG recommends monthly evaluation of asthma control, including assessment of symptoms, spirometry, and fetal well-being[15] (Figure 2). This will provide an opportunity to step down therapy, if possible, or to increase it, if indicated (Figure 3). Before increasing therapy in a patient not well controlled on appropriate maintenance therapy, inhalation technique and adherence should be assessed. The latter can be obtained by calling the patient's pharmacy to obtain a prescription refill history.[78]

Although the guidelines indicate that measurement of PEF may be sufficient, spirometry provides more valuable information on small airway obstruction. It is not uncommon for a patient with moderate or severe asthma to have a peak flow >80% of personal best, while FEV_1 may be reduced. Also, FEV_1 may be >80%, while FEF_{25-75} and/or scooping of the flow-volume loop indicates continued obstruction. Impairment in FEV_1 or these other indices may be a harbinger of an exacerbation in the near future.[79]

Some clinicians ask patients to monitor PEF at home, but many patients are poorly adherent, and the available scientific evidence indicates that PEF monitoring generally does not add benefit to self-monitoring of symptoms and following a written asthma action plan.[1]

Ultrasound examinations and antenatal fetal testing should be considered for women who have poorly controlled asthma, for those with moderate-to-severe asthma, and for women recovering from a severe exacerbation.[15] Pregnant patients with moderate or severe asthma also should be under the care of an asthma specialist.[16]

F. Nonpharmacologic Treatment

Identifying and controlling or avoiding factors that contribute to asthma severity may reduce exacerbations or allow a lower step of pharmacologic therapy.[1] These include tobacco smoke, allergens, and exposure to indoor pollutants and irritants such as formaldehyde, volatile organic compounds, fumes from wood-burning appliances and fireplaces, sprays, and strong odors such as perfume and colognes. If the patient has not been previously tested, allergen testing (usually RAST) should be performed for indoor allergens such as dust mites, cockroaches, animals, if present, and molds. If positive, specific measures to reduce exposure should be instituted. These include dust mite–proof encasings of mattress and pillows and pest control for cockroaches. Animals to which a patient is sensitive should be removed from the home or at least kept out of the patient's bedroom.

Allergen immunotherapy ("allergy shots") should not be started during pregnancy because of the risk of anaphylaxis.[15] However, they can be continued in a patient who is receiving maintenance doses, not experiencing adverse reactions, and apparently deriving benefit.

Acupuncture is not recommended for the treatment of asthma.[1] There is insufficient evidence to recommend chiropractic therapy, homeopathy, herbal medicine, breathing techniques, or yoga.[1] Herbal remedies are not standardized and may contain harmful ingredients or ingredients that interact with medications.[1] In contrast, there are data from small studies indicating that relaxation techniques, such as biofeedback and hypnotherapy, may have some benefits,[80] but data from randomized controlled studies are required before these nonpharmacologic treatments can be recommended.

G. Patient Education

Education, including self-management skills, is an important component of asthma management that can improve patient outcomes.[1] Patients need to be informed about the basic facts of asthma, as well as how pregnancy can affect asthma control and how poor asthma control can affect pregnant women and fetuses.[15] Patients should be informed about their current level of control and what constitutes well-controlled asthma.

It is important to teach patients how to optimally use inhalers, VHCs, and peak flow meters. Since technique may decline with time, especially when using an MDI without an assist device, asking the patient to demonstrate her technique periodically will reinforce good technique or identify the need for repeat instruction. If an insufficient amount of drug reaches the airways, response to therapy may be inadequate.

Patients should be provided with a written asthma action plan that specifies the need to take control medications, such as ICS, daily, even when asymptomatic, how to recognize signs and symptoms of worsening asthma and decreased fetal activity, when and how to treat increasing symptoms, and when to seek medical advice.[15] Patients should also be given advice on how to reduce exposure to environmental triggers and what practical control measures are available.

For additional information on methods of providing asthma education and forms that can be used, refer to Section 3 of EPR-3.[1]

IX. PATIENT CASE (PART 2)

Kathy is started on budesonide DPI 180 µg/actuation, one actuation BID. She was instructed on how to use the device and her prescription for albuterol HFA MDI was renewed.

At her next visit, she reported no longer waking up with asthma and having transient daytime symptoms about once every 2 weeks. Also, she has not used albuterol in several weeks and is able to exercise without symptoms. She demonstrated good inhaler technique. Repeat spirometry indicated a FVC of 98% predicted and a FEV_1 of 90% predicted. Bronchodilator response was not measured. On the basis of these findings, her clinician assessed that her asthma was well controlled.

A. Case Discussion

This case demonstrates how pregnancy can change the clinical pattern of asthma, the characteristics of poor control, and how regular use of an ICS can result in well-controlled asthma. The increase in FEV_1 from 81% to 98% predicted (a 21% increase) and her response to budesonide confirms the diagnosis of asthma and rules out the diagnosis of dyspnea of pregnancy. Based on the NAEPP Guidelines, Kathy's asthma would be classified as mild persistent on her first visit since she was not previously taking control medication (Figure 1). She had symptoms more than two times a week, but less than daily, used albuterol more than twice a week, but less than daily, and had an FEV_1 of 81% predicted with an FEV_1/FVC ratio <85%. The recommended therapy for this classification is low-dose ICS daily as a control medication. Budesonide was chosen because there are more data on the safety of this medication during pregnancy than for other ICSs.[16]

As a result of low-dose budesonide, her symptoms markedly decreased and her prebronchodilator FEV_1 increased to 90% predicted. On the basis of the NAEPP Guideline, her asthma was assessed as well controlled (Figure 2). Thus, as a result of low-dose budesonide, she is less likely to have an exacerbation that would require a short course of oral corticosteroids. Given her lung function and asthma control, it is unlikely that oxygenation of her fetus will be compromised. However, maintenance therapy with an inhaled corticosteroid is unlikely to prevent a viral-induced exacerbation[81] and she may still require a short course of oral corticosteroids if this occurs.

X. Summary

Asthma, an inflammatory disease of the airways, complicates 4%–8% of pregnancies in the United States. In one third of women with asthma, the disease worsens during pregnancy. Poorly controlled maternal asthma increases the risks of perinatal morbidity and mortality as a result of poor oxygenation of the fetus. In addition, poorly controlled asthma creates serious risks for the mother. **Therefore, it is safer for pregnant women who have asthma to be treated with asthma medication than to have asthma symptoms and exacerbations.**

The NAEPP Guidelines recommend inhaled albuterol as the preferred SABA for quick relief. More data in pregnancy are available for this agent than others in this class, and the data are reassuring regarding its safety during pregnancy.

For patients with persistent asthma, budesonide is the preferred ICS. ICSs improve lung function, decrease symptoms, and decrease exacerbations. Budesonide is the only member of this class of drugs with substantial safety data during pregnancy. However, no data suggest that other inhaled corticosteroids are unsafe during pregnancy. A LABA should be added when medium-dose ICSs do not control symptoms.

A short course of oral corticosteroids is required for moderate-to-severe exacerbations of asthma that are unresponsive to bronchodilators. However, data on safety of oral corticosteroids are conflicting, and such therapy may increase the risk of preeclampsia, prematurity, or increased risk of cleft lip with or without cleft palate when used during the first trimester. Nevertheless, when clinically indicated, the benefit outweighs the risk.

Patients must be provided with a written asthma action plan outlining when and how to use medications, and their inhaler technique should be assessed periodically. Symptoms and spirometry should be assessed monthly and treatment increased if necessary or stepped down, if possible.

XI. References

1. National Asthma Education and Prevention Program. Expert Panel Report 3: Guidelines for the Diagnosis and Management of Asthma. NIH Publication # 08-4051, August 2007. Available at http://www.nhlbi.nih.gov/guidelines/asthma/asthgdln.htm. Accessed August 5, 2008.

2. Moorman JE, Rudd RA, Johnson CA, et al. National surveillance for asthma—United States, 1980–2004. *MMWR Surveill Summ*. 2007;56:1–54.

3. Schatz M, Dombrowski MP, Wise R, et al. Asthma morbidity during pregnancy can be predicted by severity classification. *J Allergy Clin Immunol*. 2003;112:283–288.

4. Demissie K, Breckenridge MS, Rhoads GG. Infant and maternal outcomes in the pregnancies of asthmatic women. *Am J Respir Crit Care Med*. 1988;158:1091–1095.

5. Perlow JH, Montgomery D, Morgan MA, et al. Severity of asthma and perinatal outcome. *Am J Obstet Gynecol*. 1992;167:963–967.

6. Kallen B, Rydhstroem H, Aberg A. Asthma during pregnancy—a population based study. *Eur J Epidemiol*. 2000;16:167–171.

7. Greenberger PA, Patterson R. The outcome of pregnancy complicated by severe asthma. *Allergy Proc*. 1988;9:539–543.

8. Bakhireva LN, Scharz M, Chambers CD. Effect of maternal asthma and gestational asthma therapy on fetal growth. *J Asthma*. 2007;44:71–76.

9. Blais L, Forget A. Asthma exacerbations during the first trimester of pregnancy and the risk of congenital malformations among asthmatic women. *J Allergy Clin Immunol*. 2008;121:1379–1384.

10. Schatz M, Zeiger RS, Hoffman CP, et al. Perinatal outcomes in the pregnancies of asthmatic women: a prospective controlled analysis. *Am J Respir Crit Care Med*. 1995;151:1170–1174.

11. Bracken MB, Triche EW, Belanger K, et al. Asthma symptoms, severity, and drug therapy: a prospective study of effects on 2205 pregnancies. *Obstet Gynecol*. 2003;102:739–752.

12. Dombrowski MP, Schatz M, Wise R, et al. Asthma during pregnancy. National Institute of Child Health and Human Development Maternal-Fetal Medicine

Units Network and the National Heart, Lung, and Blood Institute. *Obstet Gynecol.* 2004;103:5–12.

13. Alexander S, Dodds L, Armson BA. Perinatal outcomes in women with asthma during pregnancy. *Obstet Gynecol.* 1998;92:435–440.

14. Kwon HL, Belanger K, Bracken MB. Asthma prevalence among pregnant and childbearing-aged women in the United States: estimates from national health surveys. *Ann Epidemiol.* 2003;13:317–324.

15. American College of Obstetricians and Gynecologists. Asthma in pregnancy. *Obstet Gynecol.* 2008;111:457–464.

16. National Asthma Education and Prevention Program. Working Group Report on Managing Asthma During Pregnancy: Recommendations for Pharmacologic Treatment. NIH Publication # 05-5236, March 2005. Available at http://www.nhlbi.nih.gov/health/prof/lung/asthma/astpreg.htm. Accessed July 16, 2008.

17. American Thoracic Society. Guidelines for methacholine and exercise challenge testing—1999. *Am J Respir Crit Care Med.* 2000;161:309–329.

18. Gibson PG, Powell H, Coughlan J, et al. Self-management education and regular practitioner review for adults with asthma. *Cochrane Database Syst Rev.* 2003;(1): CD001117.

19. Larsson S, Svedmyr N. Bronchodilating effect and side effects of beta$_2$-adrenoceptor stimulants by different modes of administration (tablets, metered aerosol, and combinations thereof). *Am Rev Resp Dis.* 1977;116:861–869.

20. Hendeles L, Hatton RC, Coons TJ, et al. Automatic replacement of albuterol nebulizer therapy by metered-dose inhaler and valved holding chamber. *Am J Health-Syst Pharm.* 2005;62:1053–1061.

21. Asmus MJ, Hendeles L, Weinberger M, et al. Levalbuterol has not been established to have therapeutic advantage over racemic albuterol (letter). *J Allergy Clin Immunol.* 2002;110:325.

22. Barnes PJ. Treatment with (R)-albuterol has no advantage over racemic albuterol (editorial). *Am J Resp Crit Care Med.* 2006;174:969–972.

23. Hendeles L, Colice GL, Meyer RJ. Withdrawal of albuterol inhalers containing chlorofluorocarbon propellants. *N Engl J Med.* 2007;356:1344–1351.

24. Rodrigo GJ, Rodrigo C. The role of anticholinergics in acute asthma treatment—an evidence-based evaluation. *Chest.* 2002;121:1977–1987.

25. Easton PA, Jadue C, Dhingra S, et al. A comparison of the bronchodilating effects of a beta-2 adrenergic agent (albuterol) and an anticholinergic agent (ipratropium bromide), given by aerosol alone or in sequence. *N Engl J Med.* 1986;315:735–739.

26. Rowe BH, Spooner CH, Ducharme FM, et al. Corticosteroids for preventing relapse following acute exacerbations of asthma. *Cochrane Database of Systematic Reviews* 2007, Issue 3, Art. No.: CD000195. DOI: 10.1002/14651858.CD000195.pub2.

27. Ellul-Micallef R. Pharmacokinetics and pharmacodynamics of glucocorticosteroids. In Jenne JW, Murphy S, eds. *Drug therapy for asthma: research and clinical practice.* Vol 31. New York: Marcel Dekker Inc., 1987:492.

28. O'Driscoll BR, Kaira S, Wilson M, et al. Double-blind trial of steroid tapering in acute asthma. *Lancet.* 1993;341:324–327.

29. Hatton MQF, Vathenen AS, Allen MJ, et al. A comparison of 'abruptly stopping' with 'tailing off' oral corticosteroids in acute asthma. *Respir Med.* 1995;89:101–104.

30. Schuh S, Reisman J, Alshehri M, et al. A comparison of inhaled fluticasone and oral prednisone for children with severe acute asthma. *N Engl J Med.* 2000;343:689–694.

31. Harrison TW, Oborne J, Newton S, et al. Doubling the dose of inhaled corticosteroid to prevent asthma exacerbations: randomised controlled trial. *Lancet.* 2004;363:271–275.

32. Foresi A, Morelli MC, Catena E. Low-dose budesonide with the addition of an increased dose during exacerbations is effective in long-term asthma control. On behalf of the Italian Study Group. *Chest.* 2000;117:440–446.

33. Lipworth BJ. Systemic adverse effects of inhaled corticosteroid therapy: a systematic review and meta-analysis. *Arch Intern Med.* 1999;159:941–955.

34. Barnes PJ, Pedersen S. Efficacy and safety of inhaled corticosteroids in asthma. Report of a workshop held in Eze, France, October 1992. *Am Rev Respir Dis.* 1993;148:S1–S26.

35. Zeiger RS, Szefler SJ, Phillips BR, et al. Childhood Asthma Research and Education Network of the National Heart, Lung, and Blood Institute. Response profiles to fluticasone and montelukast in mild-to-moderate persistent childhood asthma. *J Allergy Clin Immunol.* 2006;117:45–52.

36. Sorkness CA, Lemanske RF, Mauger DT, et al for the Childhood Asthma Research and Education Network of the National Heart, Lung, and Blood Institute. Long-term comparison of 3 controller regimens for mild-moderate persistent childhood asthma: The Pediatric Asthma Controller Trial. *J Allergy Clin Immunol.* 2007;119:64–72.

37. Suissa S, Ernst P, Benayoun S, et al. Low-dose inhaled corticosteroids and the prevention of death from asthma. *N Engl J Med.* 2000;343:332–336.

38. Lazarus SC, Chinchilli VM, Rollings NJ, et al. Smoking affects response to inhaled corticosteroids or leukotriene receptor antagonists in asthma. *Am J Respir Crit Care Med.* 2007;175:783–790.

39. Leung DY, Bloom JW. Update on glucocorticoid action and resistance. *J Allergy Clin Immunol.* 2003;111:3–22.

40. Szefler SJ, Martin RJ, King TS, et al. Asthma Clinical Research Network of the National Heart, Lung, and Blood Institute. Significant variability in response to inhaled corticosteroids for persistent asthma. *J Allergy Clin Immunol.* 2002;109:410–418.

41. Milgrom H, Bender B, Acherson L, et al. Noncompliance and treatment failure in children with asthma. *J Allergy Clin Immunol.* 1996;98:1051–1057.

42. Dubus JC, Marguet C, Deschildre A, et al. Local side-effects of inhaled corticosteroids in asthmatic children: influence of drug, dose, age, and device. *Allergy.* 2001;56:944–948.

43. Allen DB, Bielory L, Derendorf H, et al. Inhaled corticosteroids: past lessons and future issues. *J Allergy Clin Immunol.* 2003;112(suppl):S1–S40.

44. Martin RJ, Szefler SJ, Chinchilli VM, et al. Systemic effect comparisons of six inhaled corticosteroid preparations. *Am J Respir Crit Care Med.* 2002;165:1377–1383.

45. Johnson SR, Marion AA, Vrchoticky T, et al. Cushing syndrome with secondary adrenal insufficiency from concomitant therapy with ritonavir and fluticasone. *J Pediatr.* 2006;148:386–388.

46. O'Byrne PM, Barnes PJ, Rodriquez-Roisin R, et al. Low dose inhaled budesonide and formoterol in mild persistent asthma—the OPTIMA randomized trial. *Am J Respir Crit Care Med.* 2001;164:1392–1397.

47. Bateman ED, Boushey HA, Bousquet J, et al; GOAL Investigators Group. Can guideline-defined asthma control be achieved? The Gaining Optimal Asthma Control Study. *Am J Respir Crit Care Med.* 2004;170:836–844.

48. Ram FS, Cates CJ, Ducharme FM. Long-acting beta$_2$-agonists versus anti-leukotrienes as add-on therapy to inhaled corticosteroids for chronic asthma. *Cochrane Database Syst Rev.* 2005;(1):CD003137.

49. Becker AB, Simons FER, McMillan JL, et al. Formoterol, a new long-acting selective beta$_2$-adrenergic receptor agonist: double-blind comparison with salbutamol and placebo in children with asthma. *J Allergy Clin Immunol.* 1989;84:891–895.

50. Lazarus SC, Boushey HA, Fahy JV, et al. Long-acting β-agonist monotherapy vs continued therapy with inhaled corticosteroids in patients with persistent asthma. *JAMA.* 2001;285:2583–2593.

51. Burgess C, Ayson M, Rajasingham S, et al. The extrapulmonary effects of increasing doses of formoterol in patients with asthma. *Eur J Clin Pharmacol.* 1998;54:141–147.

52. Nelson HS, Weiss ST, Bleecker ER, et al. The salmeterol multicenter asthma research trial. A comparison of usual pharmacotherapy for asthma or usual pharmacotherapy plus salmeterol. *Chest.* 2006;129:15–26.

53. Walters EH, Walters JA, Gibson MD. Inhaled long acting beta agonists for stable chronic asthma. *Cochrane Database Syst Rev.* 2003;(4):CD001385.

54. Anderson HR, Ayres JG, Sturdy PM, et al. Bronchodilator treatment and deaths from asthma: case-control study. *BMJ.* 2005;330:117.

55. Wolfe J, LaForce C, Friedman B, et al. Formoterol, 24 microg bid, and serious asthma exacerbations: similar rates compared with formoterol, 12 microg bid, with and without extra doses taken on demand, and placebo. *Chest.* 2006;129:27–38.

56. Bakhireva LN, Jones KL, Schatz M, et al; Organization of Teratology Information Specialists Collaborative Research Group. Safety of leukotriene receptor antagonists in pregnancy. *J Allergy Clin Immunol.* 2007;119:618–625.

57. Szczeklik A, Stevenson DD. Aspirin-induced asthma: advances in pathogenesis, diagnosis, and management. *J Allergy Clin Immunol.* 2003;111:913–921.

58. Reiss TF, Hill JB, Harman E, et al. Increased urinary excretion of LTE$_4$ after exercise and attenuation of exercise-induced bronchospasm by montelukast, a cysteinyl leukotriene receptor antagonist. *Thorax.* 1997;52:1030–1035.

59. Edelman JM, Turpin JA, Bronsky EA, et al. Oral montelukast compared with inhaled salmeterol to prevent exercise-induced bronchoconstriction. *Ann Intern Med.* 2000;132:97–104.

60. Reinus JF, Persky S, Burkiewicz JS, et al. Severe liver injury after treatment with the leukotriene receptor antagonist zafirlukast. *Ann Intern Med.* 2000;133:964–968.

61. Holgate ST, Chuchalin AG, Hebert J, et al; Omalizumab 011 International Study Group. Efficacy and safety of a recombinant anti-immunoglobulin E antibody (omalizumab) in severe allergic asthma. *Clin Exp Allergy.* 2004;34:632–638.

62. Busse W, Corren J, Lanier BQ, et al. Omalizumab, anti-IgE recombinant humanized monoclonal antibody, for the treatment of severe allergic asthma. *J Allergy Clin Immunol.* 2001;108:184–190.

63. Hendeles L, Sorkness CA. Anti-immunoglobulin E therapy with omalizumab for asthma. *Ann Pharmacother.* 2007;41:1397–1410.

64. Beam WR, Weiner DE, Martin RJ. Timing of prednisone and alterations of airways inflammation in nocturnal asthma. *Am Rev Respir Dis.* 1992;146:1524–1530.

65. Spahn JD, Covar R, Szefler SJ. Glucocorticoids: B. Clinical science. In Adkinson NJ, Bochner BS, Busse WW, Holgate ST, Simons FER, Yunginger JW, eds. *Middleton's Allergy Principles and Practice.* 6th ed. Philadelphia: Mosby, 2004:887–913.

66. Svendsen UG, Frolund L, Madsen F, et al. A comparison of the effects of sodium cromoglycate and beclomethasone dipropionate on pulmonary function and bronchial hyperreactivity in subjects with asthma. *J Allergy Clin Immunol.* 1987;80:68–74.

67. Rohr AS, Siegel SC, Katz RM, et al. A comparison of inhaled albuterol and cromolyn in the prophylaxis of exercise-induced bronchospasm. *Ann Allergy.* 1987;59:107–109.

68. Patel KR, Wall RT. Dose-duration effect of sodium cromoglycate aerosol in exercise-induced asthma. *Eur J Respir Dis.* 1986;69:256–260.

69. Reed CE, Offord KP, Nelson HS, et al. Aerosol beclomethasone dipropionate spray compared with theophylline as primary treatment for chronic mild-to-moderate asthma. The American Academy of Allergy, Asthma and Immunology Beclomethasone Dipropionate-Theophylline Study Group. *J Allergy Clin Immunol.* 1998;101:14–23.

70. Wiegand L, Mende CN, Zaidel G, et al. Salmeterol vs theophylline: sleep and efficacy outcomes in patients with nocturnal asthma. *Chest.* 1999;115:1525–1532.

71. Pollock J, Kiechel F, Cooper D, et al. Relationship of serum theophylline concentration to inhibition of exercise-induced bronchospasm and comparison with cromolyn. *Pediatrics.* 1977;60:840–844.

72. Hendeles L, Harman E, Huang D, et al. Theophylline attenuation of airway responses to allergen: comparison with cromolyn metered-dose inhaler. *J Allergy Clin Immunol.* 1995;95:505–514.

73. Hendeles L, Weinberger M. Theophylline Use in Asthma (CD Rom). Rose, BD (Ed). *UpToDate*, Waltham, MA. 2007.

74. Hendeles L, Weinberger M, Milavetz G, et al. Food-induced dumping from a "once-a-day" theophylline product as a cause of theophylline toxicity. *Chest*. 1985;87:758–765.

75. Kerstjens HA, Brand PL, Hughes MD, et al. A comparison of bronchodilator therapy with or without inhaled corticosteroid therapy for obstructive airways disease. *N Engl J Med*. 1992;327:1413–1419.

76. Blais L, Beauchesne M-F, Rey E, et al. Use of inhaled corticosteroids during the first trimester of pregnancy and the risk of congenital malformations among women with asthma. *Thorax*. 2007;62:320–328.

77. The Xolair Pregnancy Registry: An Observational Study of the Use and Safety of Xolair (omalizumab) During Pregnancy (EXPECT). Identifier NCT00373061. http://www.clinicaltrials.gov/ct/show/NCT00373061?order=1. Accessed March 26, 2007.

78. Sherman J, Hutson A, Baumstein S, et al. Telephoning the patient's pharmacy to assess adherence with asthma medications by measuring refill rate for prescriptions. *J Pediatr*. 2000;136:532–536.

79. Fuhlbrigge AL, Kitch BT, Paltiel AD, et al. FEV_1 is associated with risk of asthma attacks in a pediatric population. *J Allergy Clin Immunol*. 2001;107:61–67.

80. Loew TH, Tritt K, Siegfried W, et al. Efficacy of "functional relaxation" in comparison to terbutaline and a "placebo relaxation" method in patients with acute asthma. A randomized, prospective, placebo-controlled, crossover experimental investigation. *Psychother Psychosom*. 2001;70:151–157.

81. Doull IJM, Lampe FC, Smith S, et al. Effect of inhaled corticosteroids on episodes of wheezing associated with viral infection in school age children: randomised double blind placebo controlled trial. *BMJ*. 1997;315:858–862.

QUESTIONS AND ANSWERS

1. Which of the following is the most serious risk from poorly controlled asthma during pregnancy?

   a. It increases the risk of the mother developing long-term irreversible airway obstruction (eg, COPD).

   b. It causes gastroesophageal reflux, which may complicate the pregnancy.

   c. It increases the risk of isolated cleft lip with or without cleft palate.

   d. It decreases oxygen supply to the fetus, which increases the risk of perinatal mortality, preeclampsia, preterm birth, and low-birth-weight infants.

   e. It increases the risk of the baby developing asthma during infancy.

2. Which of the following is the most effective long-term controller medication for all levels of severity of persistent asthma during pregnancy?

   a. budesonide

   b. montelukast

   c. theophylline

   d. albuterol

   e. cromolyn

3. Which of the following has the highest risk of causing preeclampsia and delivery of both preterm and low-birth-weight infants?

   a. medium-dose inhaled corticosteroids

   b. a short course of oral corticosteroids (eg, 5 days)

   c. long-term use of oral corticosteroids

   d. theophylline

   e. long-acting β_2-selective agonists

4. In the case example of Kathy, which of the following would be the best choice if she caught a cold and began to wheeze and cough, waking several times during the night, obtained no relief from albuterol MDI, and had a peak flow of 60% of her personal best?

   a. Change the budesonide to a combination product containing both budesonide and formoterol (Symbicort) for 5 days.

   b. Add a short course of prednisone for 5 days.

   c. Double the dose of budesonide for 5 days.

   d. Switch the albuterol MDI to a nebulizer solution four times a day until symptom-free.

   e. Add montelukast for 5 days.

5. Assume that Kathy in the case example did not improve after several weeks of treatment with budesonide. You check her inhaler technique and it is excellent. Which of the following would be the most likely cause of this treatment failure?

   a. Poor adherence.

   b. The 180-μg dose was too low.

   c. Although budesonide is the safest ICS during pregnancy, it has low affinity for the glucocorticoid receptor (ie, lower potency than fluticasone or mometasone).

   d. Metabolism of budesonide is increased during pregnancy and the frequency of administration BID is insufficient.

   e. Steroid resistance due to polymorphism of the gene that expresses the glucocorticoid receptor.

Answers:

1. d; 2. a; 3. c; 4. b; 5. a

Depression in Pregnancy

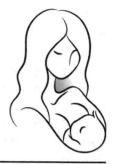

Lisa O'Brien and Gideon Koren

CHAPTER

19

LEARNING OBJECTIVES

1. Compare the symptoms of depression with the normal symptoms of pregnancy.

2. Identify predictors of depression in pregnancy.

3. Describe validated tools available to screen for depression in pregnancy.

4. Outline pharmacologic treatments available for depression and the teratogenic risk associated with their use in pregnancy.

5. Discuss the risks and benefits associated with antidepressant use in pregnancy.

I. Introduction

Major depressive disorder (MDD), commonly referred to as *depression*, is a chronic and recurrent mental illness. It is estimated that more than 100 million people worldwide are currently suffering from depression; it is predicted that by 2012, depression will be the leading cause of disease in the world.[1]

Depression affects both men and women; women, however, are disproportionately affected by this disorder. The lifetime occurrence of major depression is approximately 2–3 times higher in women than in men, regardless of ethnicity.[2] Annually, between 7% and 13% of women worldwide experience MDD.[3] Furthermore, depression is the leading cause of disease for women between 15 and 44 years of age, which approximates a woman's childbearing years.[4] Therefore, it is not surprising that depression is one of the most common conditions to complicate pregnancy. For many complex reasons, pregnancy represents a time in which women are more vulnerable to the onset of depression or its return.[5]

It has been estimated that as many as 30% of women suffer from some degree of depression during pregnancy. Some studies report the prevalence of depression in pregnancy to be between 25% and 35%, with approximately 10% of women meeting criteria for MDD.[6] A recent meta-analysis estimated the disease burden of depression in pregnancy by trimester. It was found that rates in the first, second, and third trimesters were 7.4%, 12.8%, and 12.0%, respectively.[7]

It is imperative that depression during pregnancy be recognized and managed in obstetric populations, as untreated depression is a significant risk factor for unfavorable pregnancy outcomes, such as prematurity, low birth weight, and increased admissions to neonatal care units.[8] Moreover, the consequences of untreated depression do not end with delivery—delays in the cognitive and emotional development of babies born to and cared for by depressed women have been demonstrated. Infants born to these mothers may be passive, withdrawn, and have dysregulated attention and arousal patterns; evidence of lower cognitive performance has also been reported in these babies.[9] This is due to the fact that depressed mothers are more likely to be disengaged and unresponsive to their newborn infants, unable to support the infants' activity or provide them with stimulation. If depression remains untreated and continues into toddlerhood, these children often display less creative play, continued lower cognitive performance, passive noncompliance, and lower interaction.[9] It is, therefore, very important that depression be recognized and treated at all stages of pregnancy and into the postpartum period.

It has been reported that pregnant women with depression are more likely to use alcohol or illicit drugs, which poses further risks to the developing fetus.[10] However, the unborn fetus is not the only one put at risk. There are risks to the mother that are associated with not treating depression in pregnancy, which include impaired self-care, failure to follow prenatal guidelines, suicidal ideations, self-injurious behaviors, and lower than expected weight gain. In addition, it has been shown that women who are depressed during pregnancy are at a greater risk for postpartum depression.[3]

Postpartum depression is a serious condition and occurs in up to 13% of women after delivery.[11] Symptoms usually appear after birth and should not be confused with the weeping, sadness, and irritability of the postpartum blues that appear during the first postpartum week and resolve within a few hours to days; no negative sequelae are associated with postpartum blues. Postpartum depression, however, lasts longer than the baby blues and its symptoms are more intense and mirror closely the signs and symptoms of major depression discussed below. This condition interferes with a mother's daily ability to adequately care for herself and her newborn infant.[12] Consequently, the overall objective of treating depression in pregnancy and the postpartum period is to maximize maternal health while minimizing the risk to the developing infant.

II. PATIENT CASE [PART 1]

A 30-year-old woman presents with symptoms of fatigue, nausea, and recent weight gain (6.8 kilograms over 2 months). She also discloses that for the past 5 weeks she has become uninterested in her daily activities and has had difficulty concentrating at work and at home. She attributes much of her mood and persistent somatic complaints to the fact that she is currently 9 weeks pregnant. She states that she is married; however, this pregnancy was unplanned. Obstetric history reveals this is her first pregnancy with no previous terminations or spontaneous abortions. Physical examination reveals she is healthy, and laboratory tests show normal thyroid function. The patient has a history of unipolar depression (ie, depression without manic episodes) with no other psychiatric comorbidities. Two years ago she had a major depressive episode and was treated with venlafaxine, 150 mg/d, which relieved her symptoms and returned her to normal functioning. She stopped taking the medication 1 year ago and has not experienced a relapse, so she is not currently taking any medication. A family history of depression also exists; her maternal grandmother and aunt were diagnosed with clinical depression many years ago. The patient has no known allergies to medication.

III. Clinical Presentation

Depression is a complex and heterogeneous disorder. Depressive symptoms often present with varying degrees of intensity and duration. Consequently, MDD can be classified as mild, moderate, or severe depending on the degree to which these symptoms impair an individual's daily functioning in social and/or occupational settings.[13]

Clinical depression is characterized by isolated or repeated major depressive episode(s) (MDE). An MDE is defined as a 2-week period or longer in which there is depression and/or a loss of interest or pleasure in usual activities.[14] In addition to prolonged depressed mood or loss of interest, the patient may also present with various clinical signs and symptoms of depression, which include, but are not limited to, anhedonia (inability to experience pleasure from normally pleasurable activities), significant fluctuations in weight, changes in appetite, insomnia or hypersomnia almost daily, fatigue, excessive or inappropriate feelings of worthlessness or guilt, diminished libido, observed psychomotor agitation/retardation, difficulty concentrating, and recurrent suicidal ideations. It is helpful to remember these clinical symptoms using the acronym SIGECAPS (sleep, interest, guilt, energy, concentration, appetite, psychomotor, suicide). An important caveat is that none of the above-mentioned symptoms can be due to direct physiologic effects of a substance or medical condition, be accounted for by bereavement, or meet the criteria for other psychiatric conditions (Table 1).[13]

Table 1. Symptoms of Major Depressive Disorder

Physical Symptoms	Psychological Symptoms
Appetite (increase or decrease)	Depressed mood
Sleep disturbances (insomnia or hypersomnia)	Loss of interest and/or pleasure in daily activities
Weight fluctuations	
Fatigue/decreased energy	Suicidal ideation (recurrent)
Psychomotor disturbances (agitation/retardation)	Guilt/worthlessness
Diminished concentration	Hopelessness
	Diminished libido

Depression often goes unrecognized in the obstetric population for a variety of reasons, including the overlap of the somatic symptoms of depression with those of pregnancy.[15] For instance, sleep and appetite disturbance, diminished libido, and low energy are symptoms of both conditions; this duplication of symptoms further impedes the accurate diagnosis of depression in pregnancy. Therefore, it is important to be aware of some of the distinguishing features of depression. The cognitive and affective aspects of depression, such as anhedonia, excessive or inappropriate feelings of guilt and hopelessness, and persistent thoughts of suicide or self-harm, allow symptoms of pregnancy to be discerned from those of depression. The symptoms of depression and pregnancy are most similar in the first and third trimesters of pregnancy.[16]

IV. Pathophysiology

The exact etiology of depression is unknown, but there is strong evidence of a genetic predisposition for depression. Epidemiologic studies have shown that approximately 40%–50% of the risk for depression is genetic.[17,18] The relative risk for the disorder is 1.5–3 times greater when a first-degree biological relative is diagnosed with depression than when not.[13] Biological, psychological, and sociocultural factors have also been implicated in shaping this disorder; stress (acute and chronic) may also play an important role in the development of MDD.[19]

Various theories exist that try to elucidate the biological origins of depression. The monoamine hypothesis of depression has been the leading theory for many years. It postulates that depression is caused by a deficiency in the biogenic monoamines, serotonin, norepinephrine, and/or dopamine, in synaptic clefts that results in interference to brain circuits involved in their signaling pathways.[20] The serotoninergic system is involved in modulating mood, appetite, and sleep, whereas norepinephrine plays a variety of roles, including regulating emotions, such as anxiety, aggression, and pleasure, and it is involved in the regulation of appetite, weight, sex drive, cognition, and attention.[21]

It is unlikely, however, that depression results solely from a depletion of monoamine transmitters. Stress and hormones that modulate the body's response to stress also appear to be involved in the pathophysiology of MDD. The hypothalamic-pituitary-adrenal (HPA) axis becomes activated during periods of acute and chronic stress. Current evidence suggests that increased levels of the glucocorticoid cortisol and corticotrophin-releasing factor (CRF) are linked to depression. It is proposed that the dysregulation of the HPA and hippocampus contributes to depression via hypercortisolism and enhanced hypothalamic CRF transmission.[22,23] Clinically, decreased activity of the HPA, including a reduction in CRF, has been found in patients who recovered from depression.[24] Other hypotheses exist that propose different etiologies of depression; these, however, are beyond the scope of this chapter; references for these can be found in the Suggested Readings section.

It was once assumed that pregnancy was a time of emotional well-being for women; however, it is now known that pregnancy may act as a trigger for the return of depressive symptoms in women who are susceptible to the disorder. Many hormonal changes are associated with pregnancy, including gradually increasing levels of estradiol, progesterone, CRF, corticotrophin, and cortisol. Because CRF and estrogen are principal regulators of the HPA, their increased levels result in the increased secretion of cortisol, which as discussed above, is associated with vulnerability to depression.[25]

It should be kept in mind that depression is often comorbid with other psychiatric illnesses and can also occur in the context of other medical conditions, such as diabetes, stroke, cancer and endocrine disturbances (ie, hypothyroidism).

V. Screening and Diagnosis

No reliable or practical biological marker currently exists that can predict those at risk for depressive disorders. At present, the diagnosis of depression is based on a core set of clinical signs and symptoms exhibited by the patient. The *Diagnostic and Statistical Manual of Mental Disorders*, fourth version (DSM-IV) has put forth the following criteria for the diagnosis of depression: a person must have an MDE **and** display five or more of the symptoms described by SIGECAPS.[14] This is the most widely accepted and used criteria for the diagnosis of depression; this descriptive approach facilitates a reproducible diagnosis regardless of the clinical or cultural setting. The diagnosis, therefore, relies on both patient self-report regarding the duration and severity of symptoms and the clinician's observations of behavioral and functional impairment. The DSM-IV does not have explicit criteria for the diagnosis of antenatal depression, nor does it address the confounding effect of pregnancy symptoms on those used to determine depression.

The diagnosis of depression by clinicians is costly and time-consuming, thus lay-administered screening tools and patient self-report questionnaires have been developed to aid in the identification of depressive symptoms. It is important to note that screening instruments and self-report questionnaires cannot diagnose depression; they can, however, provide an indication of the severity of depressive symptoms. Patients scoring above the cut-off value of any particular scale are more likely to be diagnosed with MDD, as higher scores are regularly associated with more severe symptoms.[26] Screening tools provide a simple mechanism to help increase the awareness of health care providers and aid in the early detection and diagnosis of depression.

Several factors need to be taken into consideration when deciding on an appropriate instrument for screening: the characteristics of the population to be screened, the psychometric properties of the tool, how straightforward it is to use, time required to administer and score the questionnaire, and the actual cost of obtaining the measure.

The Edinburgh Post Natal Depression Scale (EPDS), the Center for Epidemiologic Studies Depression Scale (CES-D), and the Beck Depression Inventory (BDI) are screening instruments that have been commonly used to screen for depression in obstetric populations.

The EPDS was originally designed to detect postnatal depression; the scale has since been validated for use in obstetric populations. The EPDS focuses on the cognitive and affective aspects of depression rather than the somatic symptoms due to the overlap of physiologic symptoms of depression and those of a typical pregnancy. The EPDS is a self-report scale that examines a person's mood in the last week; the scale has been found to have a sensitivity of 86% and a specificity of 78%.[27] The EPDS consists of 10 questions that are each assigned a score from 0–3; the maximum possible score is 30. A score above 12 is accepted to indicate probable depressive disorder.[28] The EPDS is currently available in 23 languages.

The CES-D has not been validated for use in pregnancy; however, it has been extensively used for research on depression in pregnancy.[29] It is a 20-item measure that examines mood in the past week. The total possible score is 60, with scores greater than or equal to 16 corresponding to depressive symptomology in the general population.

The BDI is a self-report questionnaire that has been validated for use in an obstetric population; however, it was initially designed to evaluate the intensity of depression in a psychiatric population.[30] The scale examines a person's mood for the present day and consists of 21 items that include questions regarding the somatic symptoms of depression. The maximum possible score that can be obtained with this measure is 63; scores greater than or equal to 16 are indicative of depression.

Not surprisingly, it has been found that when the BDI and the CES-D have been used on symptomatic pregnant women they generate higher scores and have a larger proportion of false positives, as the assessment by these scales relies in part on the somatic symptoms of depression.[31–33] This has not been found when using the EPDS in a similar population. This illustrates that there are certain inherent limitations present with the use of any screening tool. Depression screening instruments are limited in that they are not able to address the degree of impairment caused by the condition, nor are they able to ascertain the duration of symptoms or if a comorbid condition(s) exists. Therefore, if a positive result is produced by a screening measure, a clinical diagnosis should be made using DSM-IV criteria. Furthermore, depression may manifest itself differently depending on a person's age, gender, or cultural background[26]; hence, the value of sound clinical judgment should not be forgotten.

It may not be feasible to screen all obstetric patients for depression, but the literature suggests that certain women may be at higher risk for prenatal depression than others. This includes women with a history of depression, younger age, limited social support, living alone, a greater number of children, and comorbid illness. Depression has also been shown to be negatively correlated with socioeconomic status.[6,34] These women may benefit most from being screened for depression during the perinatal period (Table 2).

Table 2. Risk Factors for Depression in Pregnancy

Biological	Psychosocial
Prior history of depression or mood disorders	Unplanned pregnancy
Prior history of postpartum depression	Younger age
Prior history of premenstrual dysphoric disorder	Single motherhood
Family history of psychiatric illness	Limited social support
	History of child abuse
	Low level of education
	Unemployment
	Substance abuse and smoking

VI. Prevention

For women predisposed to MDD, there is no sure way to prevent the onset of depressive symptoms. However, if symptoms are normally minor, there are prevention strategies that can be employed to prevent the exacerbation of these symptoms. These strategies include an alcohol-, nicotine-, and caffeine-free diet and lifestyle. Regardless of depression status, the use of these substances should be limited in pregnancy. Nevertheless, it must be acknowledged that some women may have alcohol or nicotine dependencies, which are often found in women with depression, and, therefore, these women should be advised that a reduction in the intake of these substances is still helpful for their health and that of their developing child, even if they cannot quit completely.

It is also important to emphasize that lifestyle changes such as establishing consistent sleep-wake routines, finding ways to cope with stress (eg, yoga, enhancing time management skills), and incorporating regular and appropriate physical activities into their everyday schedules can provide relief from mild depression. Assisting women with recognizing and accessing support systems may also be a valuable prevention strategy for women who find themselves socially isolated.[35]

VII. Guidelines and/or Position Statements

There is a dearth of guidelines or consensus statements specifically pertaining to the treatment and management of depression in pregnancy. A small section is devoted to this topic in the Practice Guidelines of the American Psychiatric Association (APA). These guidelines briefly touch on three main treatment options for depression in pregnancy: psychotherapy, antidepressant medication, and electroconvulsive therapy (ECT). The guidelines suggest that, whenever possible, a pregnancy be planned in consultation with a psychiatrist (or health care provider); this may not always be feasible as up to 50% of pregnancies are unplanned. In regard to treatment, the guidelines advise that pregnancy, lactation, or the desire to become pregnant may be an indication for psychotherapy as an initial treatment. However, it cautions that there may be the risk for delayed effectiveness and onset of symptom alleviation; thus, these issues should be considered when choosing this as a treatment modality. Antidepressant treatment in pregnancy is recommended for women who have or are in remission from MDD, or for women who are on maintenance therapy and are deemed at high risk for reoccurrence of depression if pharmacotherapy is discontinued. In addition, if antidepressants are used during gestation, it is suggested that maternal weight gain be carefully monitored and that a gradual tapering off of medication be considered 10–14 days before the expected (or planned) date of delivery to circumvent any potential neonatal withdrawal symptoms. Antidepressant therapy may be resumed at the prepregnancy dose after delivery if the woman is deemed to be at risk from her MDD. The APA recommends ECT for patients who are unsuitable for or unresponsive to medication, who have MDD with psychotic features, or who have an individual preference for this treatment modality after being informed about its risks and benefits in pregnancy.[36]

Establishing the safety of medications is often difficult, as women of childbearing age are frequently excluded from participation in clinical trials due to concerns regarding potential teratogenicity, other adverse pregnancy outcomes, and ensuing liability and litigation issues. As such, agencies such as the U.S. Food and Drug Administration warn against the use of all psychotropic drugs in pregnancy, since limited data are available from randomized controlled trials.[37] This, however, creates further barriers to treatment for women who become pregnant and require treatment for their depressive disorder.

In 2001, the Canadian Psychiatric Association, in collaboration with the Canadian Network for Mood and Anxiety Treatments, developed recommendations for the treatment of depression in pregnancy.[38] They suggested that fluoxetine be the first-line treatment, while citalopram, fluvoxamine, paroxetine, and sertraline are second-line treatments. Finally, they recommended that tricyclic antidepressants (TCAs), ECT, and interpersonal therapy be used as third-line treatments for depression in pregnancy. However, it should be kept in mind that not all antidepressants are equally effective for everyone; there is variability in an individual's response to different medications. Therefore, if a patient has had success on a prior medication, it is best to try to restart her on that medication instead of trying a first-line treatment that may not work for her.

The American College of Obstetricians and Gynecologists recommend that the use of selective serotonin reuptake inhibitors (SSRIs) to manage depression in pregnancy should be individualized based on the specific risks and benefits to the patient. It also cautions against the use of Paxil® in pregnancy, when possible, due to reports of potential increased risk for fetal cardiac defects, persistent pulmonary hypertension of the newborn (PPHN), and other negative effects.[39]

VIII. Treatment

A. Nonpharmacologic Options

Depression is associated with significant morbidity and an increased risk of mortality if left untreated.[19] Approximately 15% of patients with a mood disorder commit suicide,[13] moreover, at least 66% of all suicides are preceded by depression.[40] Early identification and proper treatment significantly decrease the negative impact of depression in most patients. In obstetrics, there are two patients that must be taken into account when choosing treatment options—the mother and her developing fetus. Treatment should ultimately resolve the mother's condition without causing harm to the fetus.

Interventions that can be used to manage depression can take various forms, such as light therapy, ECT, psychotherapy, or pharmacotherapy. Psychotherapy, pharmacotherapy, and ECT have been shown to be the three most effective treatments for depression; these treatment modalities can be used alone or in combination with each other.[41] Alternative treatments, such as acupuncture, herbal remedies, and guided imagery, do exist; however, there is little to no scientific evidence that has established their efficacy and/or effectiveness. For example, St. John's wort (*Hypericum perforatum*) has been touted as a "natural" way to treat depression, and, because it is perceived as a nonpharmacologic agent, many pregnant women may feel it is a safer alternative to use in pregnancy than prescription medications. However, there is a paucity of scientific data regarding the safety and efficacy of St. John's wort in pregnancy. One case report describing the safety of its use in pregnancy found it to have minimal risk when used in pregnancy, as a normal health baby was born following gestational exposure. In terms of efficacy, studies in nonpregnant populations demonstrated that St. John's wort was no more effective than placebo in treating severe depression, while showing potential benefit in milder cases of depression. St. John's wort has also been shown to have many drug interactions that decrease the systemic exposure of many conventional drugs that may be concomitantly administered, thereby decreasing their effectiveness.[42] Due to the lack of safety and efficacy data, the use of St. John's wort cannot be recommended in pregnancy.

Factors that need to be taken into consideration when choosing a treatment option include patient preference, compliance, and treatment and resource availability. ECT in pregnancy is considered to be relatively safe; it has been used to treat severe, resistant depression in pregnant women for more than 50 years.[43] This treatment has been reported to be highly efficacious and low risk during all three trimesters of pregnancy and into the postpartum period. As with any treatment, there are potential risks associated with ECT during pregnancy; these include gastric reflux, aortocaval compression, spontaneous abortion, preterm labor, and placental abruption.[44] ECT is not a first-line treatment for depression in pregnancy due to the effectiveness and noninvasiveness of other methods.

Psychotherapy can take various forms, including the two most commonly used: interpersonal psychotherapy (IPT) and cognitive-behavioral therapy (CBT). IPT is a structured therapy that seeks to improve an individual's social interactions and coping skills for life transitions and conflict, whereas CBT aims to modify negative cognitive processes. One study found IPT to be effective at significantly improving mood in depressed pregnant women after 16 weeks of therapy.[45] There is a lack of data on the effectiveness of CBT during pregnancy, although it has been shown to be useful for postpartum depression.[46] It should be kept in mind that the usefulness of psychotherapy can be limited by its high resource consumption and costs as well as the availability of skilled therapists to provide the service.

B. Pharmacologic Treatment

Treatment with antidepressants is the most common form of therapy for depression regardless of pregnancy status; SSRIs and serotonin-norepinephrine reuptake inhibitors (SNRIs) are among the most widely used antidepressants, as they have a better side-effect profile than the older generation TCAs and monoamine oxidase inhibitors. It has been demonstrated that many medications, including antidepressants and their metabolites, cross the placenta, resulting in fetal exposure. The question then arises: Does fetal exposure equate to fetal harm? In the general population, the baseline risk for having a baby with a major malformation is 1%–3%; this occurs purely by chance and is not the result of exposure to teratogenic agents. There is a growing body of clinical evidence regarding the relative safety of antidepressants in all stages of pregnancy. No association has been found between TCAs and major fetal malformations.[47] A recent meta-analysis by Einarson et al. summarizes many of the studies undertaken to determine the safety of the newer antidepressants, including SSRIs and SNRIs, in pregnancy; these medications were not found to be associated with increased teratogenic risk.[48] It is also reassuring to note that in utero exposure to TCAs and fluoxetine have not been shown to effect the global IQ, language, temperament, or behavioral development of children followed up to 4 years of age.[49-51]

Concern still exists, however, regarding the use of antidepressants during pregnancy as data have been published suggesting an increased incidence of PPHN in infants whose mothers used SSRIs during late pregnancy (after 20 weeks)[52] and an increased risk for cardiac malformations in infants exposed to paroxetine (Paxil) during gestation.[53] Further research needs to be conducted to establish a causal relationship between SSRI medications and these negative outcomes.

Women who choose to continue using antidepressants during pregnancy should be cautioned that their infants may be at risk for poor neonatal adaptation syndrome (PNA), a condition that results from the use of antidepressants (SSRIs) in late pregnancy. It is characterized by self-limiting symptoms such as jitteriness, irritability, hypoglycemia, and respiratory distress; these symptoms typically appear within the first 48 hours after birth and resolve within 2–4 weeks after birth. The absolute risk for PNA ranges up to 30%.[54] It is important to note that no neonatal deaths have been reported in association with third trimester exposure to antidepressants.

Due to the complex and sometimes conflicting nature of the information available, many women who take antidepressants before conception are advised or choose to discontinue therapy upon confirmation of pregnancy due to perceptions of teratogenic risk.[55] Discontinuation of antidepressant medication during pregnancy has been associated with adverse maternal consequences. In a preliminary study, it was demonstrated that depressed women who abruptly discontinued their medication upon confirmation of pregnancy experienced both physical and psychological effects, including suicidal ideation.[55] Cohen et al. have shown that women who discontinued antidepressant medications before conception or during early pregnancy had an increased risk for depressive relapse during pregnancy compared with women who maintained therapy throughout pregnancy.[56] It has been shown that providing women with evidence-based counseling regarding the safety of medications in pregnancy is an effective means by which to lower fear of teratogenic risk and increase the likelihood of women maintaining needed pharmacotherapy during gestation.[55,57] It is important that depressed women who are planning to become or are pregnant receive evidence-based information that will equip them to make a decision, along with their health care provider, regarding their treatment options during this time. Women have terminated otherwise wanted pregnancies due to fear and misinformation.

Once the diagnosis of depression is made, the pivotal question then becomes how to go about choosing a treatment regimen for depression in pregnancy. Non-pharmacologic treatment is recommended for pregnant and depressed women with mild mood impairment who are able to function reasonably well in their day-to-day life, who do not experience sleep or appetite disturbances, and who are free from suicidal ideations. The decision surrounding commencing or continuing antidepressant treatment during pregnancy remains a common obstetric challenge. Pharmacologic treatment is appropriate for depressed and pregnant women who are unable to care for themselves in terms of their health and nutritional status and who have substantial anxiety, sleep disturbances, and thoughts of self-harm. Women who have experienced severe episodes of depression and who relapsed upon withdrawal of antidepressants are also good candidates for pharmacotherapy during gestation.

If antidepressant therapy is the chosen treatment modality, the question of exactly which medication to use then arises. This decision is guided by an individual's prior response or her family history of response (if applicable) to a specific therapeutic agent and her ability to tolerate its side effects. It is also a matter of clinician and patient preference. In trying to determine the correct dosage of medication to prescribe, it is suggested that the minimally effective dose be used; however, it should also be kept in mind that while minimizing fetal risk is paramount, there may be increased risks inherent in exposing the fetus simultaneously to subtherapeutic levels of medication and depression throughout pregnancy.[13] There have also been reports of the need for an increase in the daily dosage of certain SSRIs during pregnancy to keep depressive symptoms under control.[58] Regardless of dose, careful monitoring of women using antidepressants during pregnancy is essential; if adequate remission of symptoms is not being achieved, then the treatment plan must be revisited and adjusted accordingly. Since the onset of symptom relief is not immediate no matter which treatment modality is chosen, a brief follow-up with the patient every few weeks once treatment has commenced may be prudent, until her symptoms abate.

In identifying and subsequently discussing and choosing treatment options for women with depression in pregnancy, it is important to reassure them that they are not alone and that this is a common condition that many women experience. It should be emphasized that treatment for this condition, whatever form it may take, is imperative during this time as it benefits both her and her baby. Women with moderate-to-severe depression who are unsure or hesitant to commence pharmacotherapy should be reminded that often the risk of antidepressant medications in pregnancy is outweighed by the substantial morbidity associated with untreated or subtherapeutically treated depression. Although it does not change a woman's risk of having a baby with a major birth defect, women who are tentative about starting antidepressants during pregnancy can be advised to begin antidepressant therapy after the first trimester, as all the baby's major organs are already formed by this time. They should be reminded, however, that the brain is continually developing throughout pregnancy and, therefore, neurologic complications cannot be completely ruled out. These women, however, should receive some form of therapy during the first trimester if they refuse to use medication during that time period. Women with inadvertent exposure to antidepressants during pregnancy should be reassured that confirmation of pregnancy should not be a reason to terminate an otherwise wanted pregnancy, nor should they discontinue their medication abruptly; if they wish to discontinue, they should discuss it with their health care provider and taper off the medication gradually.

Figures 1 and 2 may be a useful guide when thinking about how to decide on a treatment option; these figures are not intended to be a comprehensive depiction of available treatment options as they only include the three most commonly used interventions for depression in pregnancy, nor are they intended to replace clinical judgment or patient preference.

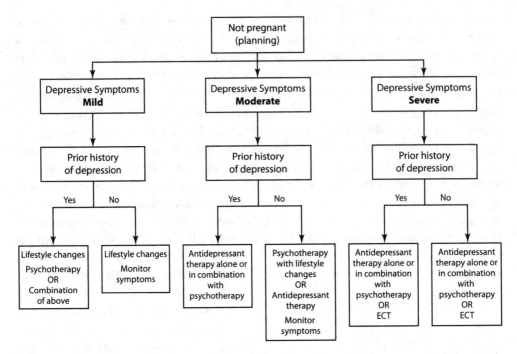

Figure 1. Determining Treatment Options for Depression in Nonpregnant (Planning) Women. ECT = electroconvulsive therapy.

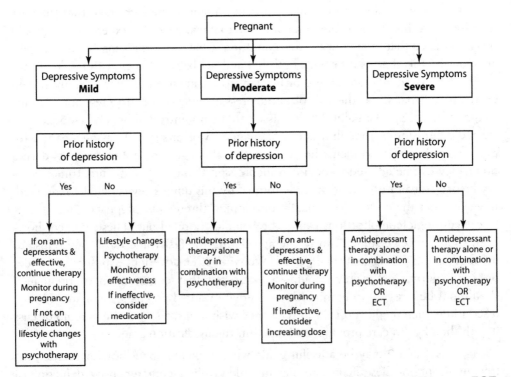

Figure 2. Determining Treatment Options for Depression in Pregnant Women. ECT = electroconvulsive therapy.

IX. PATIENT CASE [PART 2]

The patient complained of many of the somatic symptoms associated with pregnancy: fatigue, nausea and weight gain. However, when this is coupled with her loss of interest in her daily activities, inability to focus, and history of depression, it is a good indicator of antenatal depression. Normal thyroid function rules out that form of endocrine dysfunction.

Discuss with the patient her mood in the recent past, determine when she began having the symptoms she described, inquire about her past experience with depression, if she has recently experienced a large change or loss in her life, and how she is feeling about her current pregnancy. Smoking and alcohol status along with recreational drug use should be asked about. It would then be beneficial to screen the patient using the EPDS so that the severity of her symptoms could be determined. Depending on the severity of her symptoms and the information just obtained from her, a discussion regarding appropriate treatment options should occur. If her symptoms warrant starting medication, venlafaxine would be an appropriate option since she had a positive response to it previously; she could be restarted on her previous dosage (gradually dosed up). She would then be monitored to determine if the dose is still effective for her or if a dose adjustment is required; the EPDS could be used to check for depressive symptoms as pregnancy progresses. Safety considerations should be reviewed with the patient, including the risks of SNRIs in pregnancy. The patient should be advised that if at any time during her pregnancy she wishes to discontinue her medication, she should not stop taking it abruptly. She should contact her health care provider to design a tapering-off regimen.

X. Summary

Major depression is characterized by a 2-week period or longer during which an individual experiences depression and/or a loss of interest or pleasure in her usual activities; in addition, she must also exhibit several symptoms, such as fatigue, significant weight fluctuations, psychomotor retardation, sleep disturbances, or suicidal ideation. It is a complex and variable disorder, the management of which can be further complicated by pregnancy. At least 10% of women will experience MDD during gestation. It is important that depression during pregnancy be properly recognized, diagnosed, and treated to avoid negative maternal and fetal outcomes. The EPDS is a rapid and reliable screening tool that can easily be used in the obstetric setting. The treatment options most commonly used during pregnancy include psychotherapy and antidepressant medications; these may be used alone or in combination with each other. SSRIs are the most commonly prescribed antidepressants and have been shown to cross the placenta. The relative safety of these medications in pregnancy has been demonstrated; infants exposed to these medications in late pregnancy should be closely observed after birth for poor neonatal adaptability, which is a transient and self-limiting condition. A woman's depressive history, severity of symptoms, availability of resources, and personal preference must be taken into consideration when trying to decide on a treatment regimen. An individualized risk–benefit assessment should be conducted for each patient to determine the course of action that is most suitable for her and that will ensure effective treatment.

XI. References

1. World Health Organization. Mental health: depression. Available at http://www.who.int/mental_health/management/depression/definition/en/. Accessed April 20, 2008.

2. Macqueen G, Chokka P. Special issues in the management of depression in women. *Can J Psychiatry*. 2004;49:27S–40S.

3. Bennett HA, Einarson A, Taddio A, et al. Depression during pregnancy: overview of clinical factors. *Clin Drug Invest*. 2004;24:157–179.

4. Weissman MM, Olfson M. Depression in women: implications for health care research. *Science*. 1995;269:799–801.

5. Wisner KL, Gelenberg AJ, Leonard H, et al. Pharmacologic treatment of depression during pregnancy. *JAMA*.1999;282:1264–1269.

6. Noble RE. Depression in women. *Metabolism*. 2005;54(suppl 1):49–52.

7. Bennett HA, Einarson A, Taddio A, et al. Prevalence of depression during pregnancy: systematic review. *Obstet Gynecol*. 2004;103:698–709.

8. Bonari L, Pinto N, Ahn E, et al. Perinatal risks of untreated depression during pregnancy. *Can J Psychiatry*. 2004;49:726–735.

9. Psychosocial Paediatrics Committee, Canadian Paediatric Society. Maternal depression and child development. *Paediatrics and Child Health*. 2004;9:575–583.

10. Zuckerman B, Amaro H, Bauchner H, et al. Depressive symptoms during pregnancy: relationship to poor health behaviors. *Am J Obstet Gynecol*. 1989;160(Pt 1):1107–1111.

11. O'Hara MW, Swain AM. Rates and risk of postpartum depression: a meta analysis. *Int Rev Psychiatry*. 1996;8:37–54.

12. Wisner KL, Parry BL, Piontek CM. Postpartum depression. *N Engl J Med*. 2002;347:194–199.

13. Remick RA. Diagnosis and management of depression in primary care: a clinical update and review. *CMAJ*. 2002;167:1253–1260.

14. American Psychiatric Association. *Diagnostic and Statistical Manual of Mental Disorders*. 4th ed. Washington, DC: American Psychiatric Association, 1994.

15. Chokka P. Postpartum depression: part 1. *Can J CME*. 2002;14:37–48.

16. Nonacs R, Cohen LS. Assessment and treatment of depression during pregnancy: an update. *Psychiatr Clin North Am*. 2003;26:547–562.

17. Fava M, Kendler KS. Major depressive disorder. *Neuron*. 2000;28:335–341.

18. Sanders AR, Detera-Wadleigh SD, Gershon ES. Molecular genetics of mood disorders. In Charney DS, Nestler EJ, Bunney BS, eds. *Neurobiology of Mental Illness.* New York: Oxford. 1999:299–316.

19. Kalia M. Neurological basis of depression: an update. *Metabolism.* 2005;54(suppl 1):24–27.

20. Stahl S. Basic psychopharmacology of antidepressants, part 1: antidepressants have seven distinct mechanisms of action. *J Clin Psychiatry.* 1998;59(suppl 4):5–14.

21. Shelton R. The dual-action hypothesis: does pharmacology matter? *J Clin Psychiatry.* 2004;65(suppl 17):5–10.

22. Nestler EJ, Barrot M, DiLeone RJ, et al. Neurobiology of depression. *Neuron.* 2002;34:13–25.

23. Farvolden P, Kennedy SH, Lam RW. Recent developments in the psychobiology and pharmacology of depression: optimizing existing treatments and novel approaches for the future. *Expert Opin Investig Drugs.* 2003;12:65–86.

24. Holsboer F. Stress, hypercortisolism and corticosteroid receptors in depression: implications for therapy. *J Affect Disord.* 2001;62:77–91.

25. Chrousos GP, Torpy DJ, Gold PW. Interactions between the hypothalamic-pituitary-adrenal axis and the female reproductive system: clinical implications. *Ann Intern Med.* 1998;129:229–240.

26. Sharp LK, Lipsky MS. Screening for depression across the lifespan: a review of measures for use in primary care settings. *Am Fam Physician.* 2002;66:1001–1008.

27. Cox JL, Holden JM, Sagovsky R. Detection of postnatal depression: development of the Edinburgh Postnatal Depression Scale. *Br J Psychiatry.* 1987;150:782–786.

28. Evans J, Heron J, Francomb H, et al. Cohort study of depressed mood during pregnancy and after childbirth. *BMJ.* 2001;323:257–260.

29. Radloff LS. The CES-D scale: a self-report depression scale for research in the general population. *Appl Psychol Measure.* 1977;1:385–401.

30. Beck AT. An inventory for measuring depression. *Arch Gen Psychiatry.* 1961;4:53–61.

31. Myers JK, Weissman MM. Use of a self-report symptom scale to detect depression in a community sample. *Am J Psychiatry.* 1980;137:1081–1084.

32. Holcomb WL Jr, Stone LS, Lustman PJ, et al. Screening for depression in pregnancy: characteristics of the Beck Depression Inventory. *Obstet Gynecol.* 1996;88:1021–1025.

33. Salamero M, Marcos J, Gutierrez F, et al. Factorial study of the BDI in pregnant women. *Psychol Med.* 1994;24:1031–1035.

34. Boyd RC, Pearson JL, Blehar MC. Prevention and treatment of depression in pregnancy and the postpartum period—summary of a maternal depression roundtable: a U.S. perspective. *Arch Women Ment Health.* 2002;4:79–82.

35. Marcus SM, Barry KL, Flynn HA, et al. Treatment guidelines for depression in pregnancy. *Int J Gynaecol Obstet.* 2001;72:61–70.

36. American Psychiatric Association. *Practice Guidelines: Treatment of Patients with Major Depressive Disorder*, 2nd ed. April 2000. Available at http://www.psychiatryonline.com/pracGuide/loadGuidelinePdf.aspx?file=MDD2e_05-15-06. Accessed April 20, 2008.

37. Weissman MM, Olfson M. Depression in women: implications for health care research. *Science*. 1995;269:799–806.

38. Thorpe L, Whitney DK, Kutcher SP, et al. Clinical guidelines for the treatment of depressive disorders: VI. Special populations. *Can J Psychiatry*. 2001;46:647–768.

39. American College of Obstetricians and Gynecologists. The challenges of diagnosing and treating maternal depression: women's health experts weigh in. Available at http://www.acog.org/from_home/publications/press_releases/nr05-07-07-2.cfm. Accessed April 20, 2008.

40. Bostwick JM, Pankratz VS. Affective disorders and suicide risk: a re-examination. *Am J Psychiatry*. 2000;157:1925–1932.

41. Nemeroff CB. Recent advances in the neurobiology of depression. *Psychopharmacol Bull*. 2002;36:6–23.

42. Dugoua JJ, Mills E, Perri D, et al. Safety and efficacy of St. John's wort (*Hypericum*) during pregnancy and lactation. *Can J Clin Pharmacol*. 2006;13:e268–e276.

43. Miller LJ. Use of electroconvulsive therapy during pregnancy. *Hosp Community Psychiatry*. 1994;45:444–450.

44. Rabheru K. The use of electroconvulsive therapy in special patient populations. *Can J Psychiatry*. 2001;46:710–719.

45. Spinelli MG, Endicott J. Controlled clinical trial of interpersonal psychotherapy versus parenting education program for depressed pregnant women. *Am J Psychiatry*. 2003;160:555–562.

46. Zlotnick C, Johnson SL, Miller IW, et al. Postpartum depression in women receiving public assistance: pilot study of an interpersonal-therapy-oriented group intervention. *Am J Psychiatry*. 2001;158:638–640.

47. McEllhaton PR, Garbis HM, Elefant M, et al. The outcome of pregnancy in 689 women exposed to therapeutic doses of antidepressants. A collaborative study of the European Network of Teratology Information Services (ENTIS). *Reprod Toxicol*. 1996;10:285–294.

48. Einarson TR, Einarson A. Newer antidepressants in pregnancy and rates of major malformations: a meta-analysis of prospective comparative studies. *Pharmacoepidemiol Drug Saf*. 2005;14:823–827.

49. Casper RC, Fleisher BE, Lee-Ancajas JC, et al. Follow-up of children of depressed mothers exposed or not exposed to antidepressant drugs during pregnancy. *J Pediatr*. 2003;142:402–408.

50. Nulman I, Rovet J. Stewart D, et al. Neurodevelopment of children exposed in utero to antidepressant drugs. *N Engl J Med*. 1997;336:258–262.

51. Nulman I, Rovet J, Stewart D, et al. Child development following exposure to tricyclic antidepressants or fluoxetine throughout fetal life: a prospective controlled study. *Am J Psychiatry*. 2002;159:1889–1895.

52. Chambers CD, Hernandez-Diaz S, Van Marter LJ, et al. Selective serotonin-reuptake inhibitors and risk of persistent pulmonary hypertension of the newborn. *N Engl J Med.* 2006;354:579–587.

53. Bar-Oz B, Einarson T, Einarson A, et al. Paroxetine and congenital malformations; meta-analysis and consideration of potential confounding factors. *Clin Ther.* 2007;29:918–926.

54. Moses-Kolko EL, Bogen D, Perel J, et al. Neonatal signs after late in utero exposure to serotonin reuptake inhibitors: literature review and implications for clinical applications. *JAMA.* 2005;293:2372–2383.

55. Einarson A, Selby P, Koren G. Abrupt discontinuation of psychotropic drugs during pregnancy: fear of teratogenic risk and impact of counseling. *J Psychiatry Neurosci.* 2001;26:44–48.

56. Cohen LS, Altshuler LL, Harlow BL, et al. Relapse of major depression during pregnancy in women who maintain or discontinue antidepressant treatment. *JAMA.* 2006;295:499–507.

57. Bonari L, Koren G, Einarson TR, et al. Use of antidepressants by pregnant women: evaluation of perception of risk, efficacy of evidence based counseling and determinants of decision making. *Arch Women Ment Health.* 2005;8:214–220.

58. Hostetter A, Stowe ZN, Strader JR, et al. Dose of selective serotonin uptake inhibitors across pregnancy: clinical implications. *Depress Anxiety.* 2000;11:51–57.

XII. Suggested Readings

Altar CA. Neurotrophins and depression. *Trends Pharmacol Sci.* 1999;20:59–61.

Duman RS, Heninger GR, Nestler EJ. A molecular and cellular hypothesis of depression. *Arch Gen Psychiatry.* 1997;54:597–606.

Orr ST, Miller CA. Maternal depressive symptoms and the risk of poor pregnancy outcome: review of the literature and preliminary findings. *Epidemiol Rev.* 1995;17:165–171.

QUESTIONS AND ANSWERS

1. List four symptoms of pregnancy that can be confused with those of depression.

2. Discuss factors that should be included in a risk-benefit assessment for women interested in using antidepressants during pregnancy.

3. What are some of the predictors of depression in pregnancy?

4. Describe common treatment modalities for depression in pregnancy.

Answers:

1. Symptoms of pregnancy that can be confused with depression include fatigue, appetite disturbances, sleep disturbances, such as insomnia or hypersomnia, and diminished libido.

2. Factors that should be included in a risk-benefit assessment for women interested in using antidepressants in pregnancy include history of depression, including postpartum depression, the severity of depressive symptoms and resulting functional impairment, and previous response to antidepressant therapy.

3. Predictors of depression in pregnancy include history of depression, unplanned pregnancy, family history of psychiatric illness, limited social support, and single motherhood.

4. The most common treatment modalities for depression in pregnancy are psychotherapy and antidepressant therapy; ECT is used more rarely in pregnancy.

Management of Gestational Diabetes

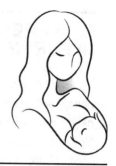

Kathleen M. Berkowitz

LEARNING OBJECTIVES

1. Describe the protocols for screening and diagnosis of gestational diabetes.

2. Formulate a plan for patient education concerning goals of therapy.

3. Evaluate the rationale for using oral agents or insulin during pregnancy.

I. Introduction

Diabetes is fast emerging as a health concern for people residing in developing countries and in the developing world. Increasing rates of obesity are linked to rising rates of insulin resistance, impaired glucose tolerance, and development of type 2 diabetes in many populations. As these conditions begin to afflict a younger cohort of people, the reproductive health issues associated with the diagnosis of diabetes become more important to address in a systematic manner. It is now estimated that 30% of the population in the "border regions" between California and Mexico have either impaired glucose tolerance or diabetes, and that 1 in 3 people in this region is obese.[1] Among women of reproductive age in the United States, approximately 4%–5% have either impaired glucose tolerance or diabetes.[2] The hormonal milieu of pregnancy potentiates this underlying insulin resistance. The hidden, chronic beta cell defect is revealed as the pregnancy progresses—usually, in the third trimester as insulin resistance peaks. Most patients revert to a state of normal glucose tolerance after delivery, but remain at risk to develop type 2 diabetes as they age or become more obese. Since today's pregnant population is, on average, older and heavier than that of just a decade ago, the development of gestational diabetes is occurring more frequently and at earlier gestational ages. Clinicians caring for pregnant women must be familiar with the diagnosis and management of this condition in pregnancy to prevent maternal and fetal morbidity. This chapter highlights the screening protocols for gestational diabetes and the needs assessment for patients diagnosed in early pregnancy and reviews the expanded range of therapeutic options available for treating gestational diabetes.

II. PATIENT CASE [PART 1]: CLINICAL INFORMATION

Y.L. is a 28-year-old patient, gravida 2 para 1-0-0-1, who presents at 14 weeks' pregnancy for her first visit. She received care with you 4 years ago during her last pregnancy, which was complicated by Class A1 diabetes, successfully controlled by diet. She had a vaginal delivery at term of a 9 pound, 2 ounce (approximately 4.143 kilograms) baby. Your notes reflect a mild shoulder dystocia, but the baby had no deficits at discharge. She has no other medical problems, with the exception of morbid obesity. Her only surgical procedure was a cholecystectomy, which was uncomplicated. She has a strong family history of diabetes, with three first-degree relatives already known to have diabetes. She has no allergies and is taking no medications. She does not smoke or drink and denies any drug use. She does not recall any recent exposure to any unusual substances or illnesses. The pregnancy, while unplanned, is desired.

She is 5'2" tall and weighs 208 pounds. Blood pressure is 120/78. Pulse is 82 and regular. Urine shows trace glucose, trace proteinuria, and moderate ketonuria. There is no thyromegaly noted and there are no clinically significant cardiovascular or pulmonary findings. The fundal height is consistent with her reported menstrual dates.

III. Screening Strategies

There are several screening strategies in use for the diagnosis of gestational diabetes. The American Diabetes Association and the American College of Obstetrics and Gynecology have published criteria for risk assessment and screening (Table 1). At the first visit, a risk assessment should be performed and the patient placed in a risk group.[3] Patients who fulfill all the criteria for inclusion in the low-risk group do not require screening. Patients who have any criteria that place them in the high-risk group should be screened at first visit. If that screening is normal, it should be repeated for high-risk patients in the third trimester. All other patients fall into a category of average risk and should be screened in the early third trimester. Screening can be performed using either the two-step or one-step method. In the one-step method, a fasting glucose level is obtained before administering 75 grams of oral glucose solution. One and two hours after ingestion, plasma glucose levels are obtained. In the two-step method, an oral solution of 50 grams glucose is given and plasma glucose is obtained 1 hour after ingestion. If the screening threshold of 140 mg/dL is exceeded,[4] the patient proceeds to a 3-hour test with administration of 100 grams glucose solution. The "cut-off" values for screening and diagnostic tests are listed in Table 2. Table 3 lists the characteristics used to classify gestational diabetic patients as well as pregestational diabetic patients. A retrospective review failed to identify any diagnostic advantage in choosing the one-step or the two-step method.[5] Physicians in the United States tend to favor the two-step model, while physicians in Europe favor the one-step model. Patients who have had gastric bypass should not be given osmotically active solutions of glucose, as this may induce severe gastrointestinal distress. A

Table 1. Screening for Gestational Diabetes. Assessment of Need for and Timing of Screening for Gestational Diabetes Based on Presence of Risk Factors

Risk Group	Patient Characteristics	Screening Recommendations
Low risk: Fulfills all listed criteria	Member of ethnic group with low prevalence of GDM, age <25 y, normal weight before pregnancy, normal weight at birth, no personal history of poor obstetric history or prior abnormal glucose metabolism, no first-degree relatives with diabetes	Blood glucose screening not routinely required
Average risk	Does not meet criteria for low or high risk	Screen at 24–28 wks' gestation using one-step or two-step method
High risk: At least one criteria is present	Severe obesity, strong family history of type 2 diabetes, history of GDM, glucosuria, or impaired glucose tolerance	Screen at first visit; repeat at 24–28 wk if initial screening is normal

GDM = gestational diabetes mellitus.
From Metzger BE, et al.[3]

Table 2. Recommended Criteria for Diagnosis of Gestational Diabetes by One-Step and Two-Step Methods

Test	Fasting	1 Hour	2 Hour	3 Hour	Comment
50-gram screening test	—	<140 mg/dL	—	—	A positive screen requires 100-gram, 3-h diagnostic testing
100-gram diagnostic test	<95 mg/dL	<180 mg/dL	<155 mg/dL	<140 mg/dL	Requires a 3-d unrestricted carbohydrate diet before performing test; any two abnormal values confirm diagnosis of GDM
75-gram diagnostic test	<95 mg/dL	<180 mg/dL	<155 mg/dL	—	Any two abnormal values confirm diagnosis of GDM

GDM = gestational diabetes mellitus.
Abnormal values = those exceeding the normal values above.
From Carpenter MW, Coustan DR.[4]

Table 3. Classification of Gestational Diabetes and Pregestational Diabetes

Class of Diabetes	Age at Onset	Duration of Disease	Presence of Vascular Complications
Class A1	First recognized during pregnancy	First recognized during pregnancy	None; fasting sugars <105 mg/dL
Class A2	First recognized during pregnancy	First recognized during pregnancy	None; at least one fasting sugar >105 mg/dL
Class B	>20 y	<10 y	None
Class C	10–19 y	10–19 y	None
Class D	<10 y	>20 y	Microalbuminuria or background retinopathy
Class F	Any age onset	Any duration	Nephropathy
Class R	Any age onset	Any duration	Retinopathy
Class H	Any age onset	Any duration	History of myocardial infarct

mixed-meal preparation or fasting glucose levels should be used for diagnosis of gestational diabetes in this population.

IV. PATIENT CASE [PART 2]: DIAGNOSIS AND INITIATION OF THERAPY

A. Diagnosis

Y.L. fulfills criteria for inclusion in a high-risk group and undergoes screening by the two-step method. Her 1-hour, 50-gram screen result is 182 mg/dL. Her 3-hour diagnostic test results are 108 mg/dL fasting, 212 mg/dL 1 hour, 185 mg/dL 2 hour, and 166 mg/dL 3 hour.

B. Initiation of Therapy

Before initiating therapy, it is important to review what normal glucose levels are in the pregnant population. These normal values serve as a reference point for the patient to understand her condition. Compliance with a difficult therapeutic regimen can be expected only when she understands the definition of "normal" glucose tolerance during pregnancy and the consequences to herself and her fetus if that baseline is significantly exceeded in a prolonged manner. Normal fasting glucose values during pregnancy are generally in the 60–90 mg/dL range; normal 1-hour postmeal glucose values should be below 120 mg/dL.[6,7] A discussion of glycemic targets and the rationale for choosing those targets should occur within a week of diagnosing gestational diabetes. The initial plan of management requires teaching the patient about diet therapy, exercise recommendations, and home glucose monitoring. Most general obstetricians find it time-consuming and difficult to provide these services in their offices, and thus use a team of professionals to assist in patient education and surveillance. Ideally, the team should consist of a physician with experience dealing with diabetes during pregnancy, a diabetic nurse educator, a specially trained nutritionist, and pharmacist clinical specialists.

Nutritional interventions are the primary focus for initial therapy. Emphasis must be placed on portion control, keeping diet logs, and maintaining a schedule of frequent meals and snacks. Carbohydrates should form about 35% of the caloric intake daily. The new regimen is most likely to be accepted and maintained if the patient finds it to be minimally disruptive. Thus, nutritional information must be tailored to a patient's cultural dietary preferences and flexible enough to help her make healthy choices when dining out in fast food establishments. The patient must also be made to feel that her team wishes to hear about the challenges she faces in initiating therapy. If she does not feel "safe" in reporting poor control, she is likely to adjust her glucose log to please her health care team. Findings and recommendations from the diabetes treatment team should be communicated promptly and in an ongoing manner to the obstetrician caring for the patient. Patients with pregestational diabetes usually require the same multidisciplinary approach. These patients pose additional challenges, as many have entrenched habits providing them with fair-to-poor glycemic control. It is an excellent time to highlight the life-long benefits of good glycemic control as the relatively long gestational period allows for reestablishing new mechanisms of coping with disease. Pregestational diabetes may also be complicated by vascular damage to major organs. Existence of comorbidities, such as hypertension, thyroid disease, or nephropathy, must be determined early in pregnancy, as the risk of maternal and fetal morbidity increases markedly in the presence of these conditions (see Table 3).

V. PATIENT CASE [PART 3]: ASSESSMENT OF COMPLIANCE

Y.L. has a 1-hour counseling session to discuss diet, exercise, and home glucose monitoring. She is asked to maintain a 2000-calorie diet divided into three meals and three snacks. She is asked to keep a diet log and begin home glucose monitoring. She is instructed to check fasting and 1-hour postmeal glucose values and record those values in her diet log. She is asked to begin a program of exercise, consisting of walking either 20–30 minutes a day or at least 10 minutes after each meal. She returns in 1 week with a diet and exercise log that is inadequately maintained. A review of the home blood glucose meter's memory feature reveals she is checking glucose levels at most twice a day and that the glucose values recorded in her log are 10%–30% lower than those stored in the meter's memory. Upon checking a random blood sugar in your office, the value is found to be 196 mg/dL. There has been a 3-pound weight gain in 1 week's time. A urine sample is obtained and reveals both ketonuria and glucosuria.

The initiation of therapy is an emotionally traumatic time. For some, it is the first time that their obesity and eating habits have been linked to the occurrence of an actual medical complication. Faced with a choice of complying with a difficult change in diet or being labeled as noncompliant, many patients will embellish on their ability to make these changes. Thus, the first return visit should occur within 1 week of initiation of therapy. Objective data, such as patient weight and urine sample, serve as independent markers for compliance and control. At this time, it is appropriate to have a more detailed discussion of the pregnancy risks and desired benefits of therapy. For the patient diagnosed in the third trimester, complications include macrosomia, preeclampsia, increased risk for stillbirth, and the occurrence of neonatal metabolic disturbances. The link between the effect of glycemic control and reduction in these risks must be clear to the patient. An evidence-based approach yields some basic tenets to adhere to. Therapy should be initiated before 30 weeks' gestation to minimize disruptions in fetal growth patterns and neonatal metabolic parameters. Patients should be performing home blood glucose monitoring and should be testing fasting and postprandial glucose levels.[8] There is no consensus concerning the use of 1-hour versus 2-hour postprandial monitoring, although physiologically the 1-hour values more closely reflect peak postprandial values. The optimal target values for glycemic control are a subject of much debate. Most treatment trials have proceeded by setting somewhat arbitrary target levels and then evaluating maternal and fetal complications rates based on compliance with those targets. Thus, there are nearly as many recommendations in the literature as there are publications. Indeed, the U.S. Preventative Health Services Task Force was unable to find consistent evidence that treating mild degrees of glucose intolerance improved the incidence of several short-term maternal and fetal health outcomes.[9] A practical way to evaluate a patient's response to therapy is to categorize her efforts at one of three levels: as achieving a level of glycemic control, which the majority of providers accept as being associated with decreased complication rates, achieving an inadequate level of glycemic control clearly associated with higher complication rates, or achieving a middle ground in which the evidence for benefit is mixed. A patient who has achieved fasting glucose levels in the 95–105 mg/dL range and postmeal glucose values in the 130–150 mg/dL range exemplifies this dilemma, as there is as much evidence to support intensifying therapy as there are data to support continuation of diet and exercise alone.[9]

The diabetes care team must work with the patient's primary care providers to maintain consistent advice to the patient concerning the desired frequency of home glucose monitoring, exercise recommendations, and whether she should test at 1 or 2 hours after meals. The team should also agree on parameters for success in glycemic control, as patients in the "middle ground" become confused and frustrated if they believe their caregivers cannot even agree on an optimal level of glycemic control to strive for. The Fifth International Congress on Gestational Diabetes Mellitus has proposed that fasting blood sugar levels be maintained between 90 and 99 mg/dL, that 1-hour postprandial targets be set at <140 mg/dL and that 2-hour postprandial values should not exceed 120–127 mg/dL.[3] Maintaining these levels will minimize the occurrence of macrosomia and neonatal metabolic complications.[10] However, these improvements are also associated with an increased risk for undergoing induction of labor and delivering by cesarean section.[11]

VI. Early Pregnancy Concerns about Diabetes

The case of Y.L. highlights additional concerns when gestational diabetes is diagnosed early in pregnancy. For those diagnosed very early in pregnancy, it is likely that poor glycemic control was present at the time of conception. Fasting sugars in excess of 120 mg/dL, or HbA1c values greater than 7.5%, have been associated with increased risks for miscarriage and major congenital malformations.[12] Patients with preexisting diabetes may also have end organ damage or be on medications that further exacerbate the risks for pregnancy complications. Women with preexisting hypertension or renal disease are at particularly high risk and should be evaluated for the severity of their comorbidities early. Preconception recognition of diabetes and attaining good glycemic control before conception significantly decreases the risk for these complications.[13] Medications such as angiotensin converting enzyme (ACE) inhibitors and angiotensin receptor blockers (ARBs) increase the incidence of fetopathy and fetal nephrotoxicity.[14] They can cause significant fetal and neonatal toxicity when used in the last half of pregnancy, but any risk from exposure in the first trimester still requires further study. Ironically, these agents are being prescribed more frequently to women with diabetes due to their protective effects on kidney function. Exposure to ACE or ARB medications during pregnancy has tripled since the late 1990s.[15] These medications should be replaced when the patient decides to attempt conception. However, at least 50% of pregnancies are unplanned in the United States and lack of adequate access to primary medical care provides further barriers to preconception evaluation. Patients with a history of gestational diabetes will often develop type 2 diabetes. The postpartum examination at the completion of that pregnancy represents the last true opportunity to review the risks and speak with the patient about prevention and planning for the future pregnancies. Patients diagnosed before the second trimester are also at increased risk to develop urinary tract infections and preterm labor. In the early third trimester, insulin resistance peaks. Patients who have been able to maintain good glycemic control until this time may experience frustration as glycemic control deteriorates even under conditions of continued compliance. Deterioration of glycemic control can be dramatic, occasionally requiring hospitalization. Criteria to consider for hospitalization to initiate insulin therapy include the identification of a very early gestation with very poor glycemic control, lack of rapid access to outpatient diabetes care providers, a risk for development of diabetic ketoacidosis, or third trimester fasting blood glucose values in excess of 140 mg/dL.

VII. Addition of Medical Therapy

It is clear from the random blood glucose value of 196 mg/dL and the 3-pound weight gain that Y.L. will not be able to achieve good glycemic control on a program of diet and exercise alone (Figure 1). Although insulin alone has been the mainstay of therapy for gestational diabetes for decades, there is now an expanded array of choices available. Patients with mild-to-moderate degrees of hyperglycemia and in the third trimester of pregnancy are good candidates to achieve glycemic control on oral medications. Because the primary defect causing gestational diabetes is increased insulin resistance, the increased need for insulin during pregnancy can be met in three ways—administration of exogenous insulin, increasing insulin secretion, or improving insulin sensitivity. The sulfonylureas effectively increase insulin secretion and are well tolerated in pregnancy,[16] with the majority of patients being able to maintain good glycemic control. While sulfonylureas do cross the placental barrier, neonates born to women treated with glyburide have not been shown to experience hypoglycemia or other neonatal metabolic complications.[17] It should be noted that if the use of glyburide is extended into populations with more severe forms of hyperglycemia, a significant number of patients will fail to achieve glycemic control.[18] There is also a concern about the long-term consequences of forcing the beta-cell into "overdrive," possibly hastening the process of beta cell apoptosis. Thus, the use of glyburide should be restricted to women who develop a need for additional therapy in the third trimester and whose fasting sugars are consistently below 110–115 mg/dL.

Insulin sensitivity–enhancing medications, such as metformin, act by reversing the pregnancy-induced effects on insulin resistance so that a given amount of insulin secretion is more effective in maintaining euglycemia. This may help to preserve beta cell function over time and may delay the eventual apoptosis. Metformin has found extensive use in the arena of infertility treatment. Its ability to restore ovulatory func-

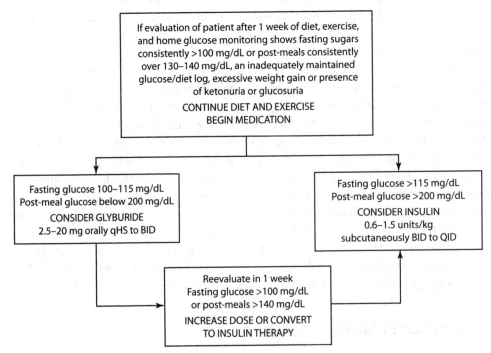

Figure 1. Third Trimester Initiation of Medical Therapy for Patients Unable to Achieve Good Glycemic Control Using Diet and Exercise Alone.

tion in patients with polycystic ovarian disease is due to a reversal of insulin resistance. There are no contemporary large randomized reports of use of metformin for treatment of gestational diabetes. Most reports in the literature focus on the pregnancy outcomes in patients with polycystic ovarian disease who conceived while on metformin therapy.[19,20] One small retrospective study showed an increased risk for the development of preeclampsia and stillbirth in the metformin group compared to groups treated with sulfonylureas or insulin.[21] The use of metformin as a primary agent for treating gestational diabetes during the third trimester should, therefore, await the results of a large prospective trial currently under way.[22] It is appropriate to use metformin as adjunctive therapy for patients who have been unable to achieve adequate glycemic control despite using massive amounts of insulin daily (300–400 units). Insulin therapy can be initiated using both short- and long-acting insulin types to achieve glycemic control rapidly and precisely. With the exception of lispro, which appears to be safe,[23] there is little data available concerning the use of insulin analogs during pregnancy. Inhaled insulin preparations are not recommended for use during pregnancy. The effects of pregnancy on lung permeability and insulin absorption have not been studied. There is additional concern that use of inhaled insulin products may induce the formation of insulin antibodies, which could cross the placenta.[24] For these and other reasons, inhaled insulin has been removed from the U.S. market.

Patients are usually begun on a twice- or three times daily regimen and prepare a customized mix of the two types in order to achieve glycemic control. Prepared concentrations of mixed insulins do not provide the flexibility needed to respond to variations in glycemic control induced during pregnancy. Insulin needs vary widely and increase significantly as the pregnancy progresses. Historically, insulin needs have been calculated in a range of 0.6–0.9 units/kg daily. This total dose is then divided to administer two thirds of the dose before breakfast and one third before dinner. Long-acting insulin forms two thirds of the prebreakfast dose and half of the predinner dose in this standard regimen. However, patients with body mass indexes in the 40–60 range have significantly higher needs for insulin. For these patients, insulin doses at the end of pregnancy may be in the range of 300–400 units a day.

VIII. PATIENT CASE (PART 4): SURVEILLANCE FOR THIRD TRIMESTER COMPLICATIONS

Y.L. is begun on insulin subcutaneously administered twice a day. After 2 weeks of therapy she is noted to have achieved good glycemic control. She continues to receive ongoing support for dietary compliance and is seen frequently to adjust insulin doses. Because of the ongoing risks for stillbirth and the development of preeclampsia, she begins twice-weekly visits at 34 weeks' gestation. Fetal surveillance is performed twice weekly and remains reassuring. At approximately 38 weeks' gestation, the estimated fetal weight is 4000 grams (8 pounds 14 ounces). Her cervical examination is unfavorable for the induction of labor.

IX. Timing and Route of Delivery

Fear of stillbirth, macrosomia, and preeclampsia lie at the heart of discussions concerning route and timing of delivery. Historically, the risk for stillbirth vied with the risk for neonatal death due to premature delivery. Contemporary advances in pregnancy dating, antepartum fetal surveillance, and the use of home glucose monitoring devices have combined to significantly decrease the risk of stillbirth. Antepartum monitoring is generally begun at 32–34 weeks' gestation and proceeds twice weekly until the completion of the pregnancy. There are many protocols that provide adequate surveillance and achieve a risk of stillbirth lower than that in the general population. Whichever protocol is most suited for the local practice pattern is acceptable, as long as there is a clearly defined requirement for immediate contact with the primary care provider for follow-up of abnormal results (Table 4).

The most vexing issue for obstetricians these days concerns the safe delivery of the infant of a diabetic mother. Macrosomic infants are known to have higher risks to experience shoulder dystocia and are prone to develop neonatal complications once delivered. There is little tolerance in the medicolegal arena for the occurrence of a shoulder

Table 4. Protocols to Decrease Risk for Stillbirth in Women with Diabetes: Antepartum Fetal Monitoring Tests

Test Description	Initiate at	Frequency of Testing	Result
Nonstress testing evaluation of fetal heart rate pattern over 20–30 min	32–34 wk for patients on medication or with comorbidities 40 wk for all other patients	Twice weekly	Reactive Reactive with variable or late deceleration* Nonreactive*
Modified biophysical, full biophysical profile	As above	Modified BPP twice weekly Full BPP weekly	Modified BPP: Amniotic fluid volume and NST result
Observation of fetal heart rate, tone, movement, breathing, and amniotic fluid volume	—	—	Full BPP: Scores of 0 or 2 for each of the 5 parameters Abnormal: BPP <8*
Contraction stress test	34 wk for patients on medication; contraindicated in patients with placenta previa or prior classical cesarean section	Weekly; contractions are induced using breast stimulation or Pitocin administration until there are three contractions in a 10-min time period	Reactive Nonreactive* Negative: No decelerations Equivocal: Decelerations with <50% of contractions* Positive: Decelerations with ≥50% of contractions*

BPP = biophysical profile, NST = nonstress test.
*Indicates an immediate need for further evaluation of fetal well-being.

dystocia, even though relatively few of these deliveries result even in temporary birth injury. It has been estimated that even if a policy offered cesarean section only to women with gestational diabetes and estimated fetal weight more than 4500 grams, 443 women would have to undergo cesarean section to prevent one case of permanent brachial plexus palsy.[25] The cohort of women undergoing cesarean section will experience collateral injuries, including infection, incidental damage to bowel or bladder, deep vein thrombosis, and hemorrhage. There is also an increased risk for uterine rupture and hysterectomy in subsequent pregnancies for women who have undergone cesarean delivery. Estimation of birth weight is imprecise and only one of many factors to consider when choosing the route of delivery. Clinical pelvimetry, knowledge of the patient's obstetric history, the presence or absence of comorbidities, and cervical preparedness must also be considered.[26] Shoulder dystocia drills should be practiced routinely and teams prepared to handle the emergency should it occur. A purely elective induction of labor or delivery by cesarean section should never occur before 39 completed weeks of gestation. For every week before 39 completed weeks' gestation that the elective delivery occurs, the neonate experiences increasing risk to need NICU admission and treatment.[27]

Labor and delivery units performing induction of labor for women with insulin-requiring diabetes should have protocols for glycemic management during labor. Because labor is akin to prolonged exercise, many patients will have little need for insulin during the normal processes of labor. Neonatal complication rates are linked closely to glycemic control in labor, however, so adequate surveillance of maternal glycemic values and hydration status during labor must be carried out. Maternal glucose values should be checked at 2–4 hour intervals and ideally kept between 80 and 130 mg/dL.[28] Ketonuria is to be avoided. While most women will go through labor with little or no need for insulin, there will be some who will need either continuous or bolus administration of insulin. Protocols for managing these needs depend on the local level of pharmacy support and nursing skill level.

X. PATIENT CASE [PART 5]: THE POSTPARTUM PERIOD

Y.L. undergoes induction of labor at 39½ weeks' gestation. She delivers a male infant weighing 3700 grams without difficulty. The infant is noted to have hypoglycemia shortly after delivery, which resolves after a day. She is discharged home after 2 days. She is instructed to discontinue insulin and discontinue home glucose monitoring. She is asked to maintain her current diet and exercise regimen. She has established breastfeeding despite the short-term separation from her baby and returns to your office 5 weeks after delivery for further evaluation.

XI. Postpartum Period

Neonatal metabolic complications will occur 10%–15% of the time after delivery, even under circumstances of good third trimester glycemic control. Most are mild, as they were in the case of Y.L.'s son. However, any length of NICU stay disrupts the initiation of breastfeeding. When the average hospital stay after a vaginal delivery is about 48 hours, it can be difficult even for an experienced mother to obtain the support she needs to breastfeed successfully. An additional barrier to breastfeeding exists for type 2 diabetic patients who may wish to discontinue insulin and switch back to oral hypoglycemic agents. Several classes of oral agents have been studied and found to be compatible with breastfeeding.[29] It should be noted that once the placenta is delivered, insulin sensitivity begins to rebound rapidly. Glycemic control should not be excessively "tight" during this time, as the arrival of a newborn will interrupt meal schedules and make the patient prone to develop hypoglycemia. Fasting glucose below 120 mg/dL and postmeals below 180 mg/dL will suffice for the majority of patients in the first week or two after delivery. Patients who began the pregnancy on insulin with good glycemic control can usually revert to their prepregnancy regimen. If that regimen cannot be recalled, then calculate an insulin dose about one third of that used just before delivery. Patients with gestational diabetes should be rescreened at the postpartum visit to determine whether they have reverted to normal glucose tolerance. The counseling at this visit is exceptionally important; it represents perhaps the last opportunity for a physician to counsel the patient concerning her risks to develop type 2 diabetes and the strategies she can employ to prevent the complication from occurring. The information should be presented in a positive context, emphasizing that the patient has already achieved compliance with the recommendations. She has already begun to form new dietary habits and should be encouraged to continue with her new lifestyle. She should be given a sense of empowerment over her medical condition and recognize that she has control over her own medical future. Diet and weight loss should be discussed extensively. If a patient is a candidate for gastric bypass surgery, it should be discussed and recommended. Options for birth control should be explained thoroughly. Patients should hear an emphasis on planning for future pregnancies, not just a plan to avoid pregnancy. Continued future screening for the development of type 2 diabetes should be recommended.[3] When possible, information should be forwarded to the patient's primary care physician so that the dialogue concerning her medical future can continue uninterrupted. Hopefully, when Y.L. returns for her next pregnancy, she will have retained some ability to deal with these issues and be prepared and confident to take control of her own medical issues.

XII. Summary

Gestational diabetes is a condition heralding probable development of type 2 diabetes in later life. As the pregnant population ages and grows more overweight, gestational diabetes occurs more frequently and more severely. Screening strategies should be directed at identifying the patient at high risk to develop gestational diabetes as soon as she presents for prenatal care. Once gestational diabetes has been identified, a diabetes education and treatment team should see the patient promptly. Recommendations should be transmitted expeditiously to the patient's physician, as authorizations for continued care must be coordinated by that office, in most cases. Initial treatment should consist of diet, exercise, and home glucose monitoring. Some patients will be discovered to have very poor glycemic control and require insulin administration or even hospitalization to initiate care. Patients should be seen 1 week after initiating therapy to review the rationale for therapy and to determine whether additional medications are required. Should she require medication, a choice between insulin and glyburide must be made. Due to the increased risks for stillbirth and preeclampsia, the patient who requires medication to achieve glycemic control should start a program of fetal surveillance no later than 34 weeks' gestation. Timing of purely elective delivery should always be after 39 completed weeks' gestation. Postpartum visits should include screening to confirm the resolution of impaired glucose tolerance and an extensive discussion of the future health risks, prevention strategies, and future pregnancy planning.

XIII. Guidelines and/or Position Statements

American Diabetes Association. Gestational Diabetes Mellitus. *Diabetes Care*. 2004; 27(suppl 1):S88–S90.

National Diabetes Data Group. Summary and Recommendations of the Fifth International Workshop-Conference on Gestational Diabetes Mellitus. *Diabetes Care*. 2007;30(suppl 2):S251–S260.

American College of Obstetricians and Gynecologists. Gestational Diabetes. *ACOG Practice Bulletin*. Number 30, September 2001. *Obstet Gynecol*. 2001;98:525–538.

XIV. References

1. Cohen SJ. Border Health Strategic Initiative: overview and introduction to a community-based model for diabetes prevention and control. *Prev Chronic Dis*. 2005;2:A05–A09.

2. Prevalence of diabetes and impaired fasting glucose in adults—United States, 1999–2000. *MMWR Morb Mortal Wkly Rep*. 2003;52:833–837.

3. Metzger BE, Buchanon T, Coustan DR, et al. Summary and recommendations of the Fifth International Workshop-Conference on Gestational Diabetes Mellitus. *Diabetes Care*. 2007;30:S251–S260.

4. Carpenter MW, Coustan DR. Criteria for screening tests for gestational diabetes. *Am J Obstet Gynecol*. 1982;144:768–773.

5. Berger H, Crane J, Farine D, et al. Screening for gestational diabetes mellitus. *J Obstet Gynaecol Can*. 2002;24:894–912.

6. Yogev Y, Ben-Haroush A, Chen R, et al. Diurnal glycemic profile in obese and normal weight non-diabetic pregnant women. *Am Journ Obstet Gynecol*. 2004; 191:949–953.

7. Paretti E, Mecacci F, Papini M, et al. Third trimester maternal glucose levels from diurnal profiles in non-diabetic pregnancies: correlation with sonographic parameters of fetal growth. *Diabetes Care*. 2001;24:1319–1323.

8. De Veciana M, Major CA, Morgan MA, et al. Post-prandial versus pre-prandial blood glucose monitoring in women with gestational diabetes mellitus requiring insulin therapy. *N Engl J Med*. 1995;333:1237–1241.

9. Brody SC, Harris R, Lohr K. Screening for gestational diabetes: a summary of the evidence for the U.S. Preventive Services Task Force. *Obstet Gynecol.* 2003;101:380–392.

10. Crowther CA, Hiller FE, Moss JR, et al, for the Australian Carbohydrate Intolerance Study in Pregnant Women (ACHOIS) Trial Group. Effect of treatment of gestational diabetes mellitus on pregnancy outcomes. *N Engl J Med.* 2005;352:2477–2486.

11. Peled Y, Perri T, Chen R, et al. Gestational diabetes mellitus—implications of different treatment protocols. *J Pediatr Endocrinol Metab.* 2004;17:847–852.

12. Mills JL, Simpson JL, Driscoll SG, et al, for the National Institutes of Child Health and Human Development-Diabetes in Early Pregnancy Study. Incidence of spontaneous abortion among normal and insulin-dependent diabetic women whose pregnancies were identified within 21 days of conception. *N Engl J Med.* 1988;319:1617–1623.

13. Ray JG, O'Brien TE, Chan WS. Preconception care and the risk of congenital anomalies in the offspring of women with diabetes mellitus: a meta-analysis. *QJM.* 2001;94:435–444.

14. Cooper WO, Hernandez-Diaz S, Arbogast PG, et al. Major congenital malformations after first-trimester exposure to ACE inhibitors. *N Engl J Med.* 2006;354:2443–2451.

15. Bowen ME, Ray WA, Arbogast PG, et al. Increasing exposure to angiotensin-converting enzyme inhibitors in pregnancy. *Am J Obstet Gynecol.* 2008;198:291.e1–e5.

16. Langer O, Conway DL, Berkus ME, et al. A comparison of glyburide and insulin in women with gestational diabetes mellitus. *N Engl J Med.* 2000;343:1134–1138.

17. Moretti ME, Rezvani M, Koren G. Safety of glyburide for gestational diabetes: a meta-analysis of pregnancy outcomes. *Ann Pharmacother.* 2008;42:483–490.

18. Moore TR. Glyburide for the treatment of gestational diabetes: a critical appraisal. *Diabetes Care.* 2007;30(suppl 2):S209–S213.

19. Creanga AA, Bradley HM, McCormick C, et al. Use of metformin in polycystic ovary syndrome: a meta-analysis. *Obstet Gynecol.* 2008;111:959–968.

20. Kocak M, Caliskan E, Simsir C, et al. Metformin therapy improves ovulatory rates, cervical scores, and pregnancy rates in clomiphene citrate-resistant women with polycystic ovary syndrome. *Fertil Steril.* 2002;77:101–106.

21. Hellmuth E, Damm P, Molsted-Pedersen L. Oral hypoglycaemic agents in 118 diabetic pregnancies. *Diabet Med.* 2000;17:507–511.

22. Rowan JA et al. Treatment with metformin compared with insulin (the Metformin in Gestational Diabetes [MiG] trial). *Diabetes Care.* 2007;30(suppl 2):S214–S219.

23. Masson EA, Patmore JE, Brash PD, et al. Pregnancy outcome in Type 1 diabetes mellitus treated with insulin lispro (Humalog). *Diabetes Med.* 2003;20:46–50.

24. National Institute for Health and Clinical Excellence (NICE). Inhaled insulin for the treatment of diabetes (types 1 and 2). London (UK): National Institute for Health and Clinical Excellence (NICE); 2006 Dec. 34 p. (Technology appraisal; no. 113).

25. Rouse DJ, Owen J, Goldenberg RL, et al. The effectiveness and costs of elective cesarean delivery for fetal macrosomia diagnosed by ultrasound. *Obstet Gynecol Surv.* 1997;52:337–339.

26. Fetal Macrosomia. ACOG Practice Bulletin Clinical Management Guidelines for Obstetrician-Gynecologists. Number 22, November 2000.

27. Clark S, Belfort M, Saade G, et al. Implementation of a conservative checklist-based protocol for oxytocin administration: maternal and newborn outcomes. *Am J Obstet Gynecol.* 2007;197:480.e1–e5.

28. Andersen O, Hertel J, Schmølker L, et al. Influence of the maternal plasma glucose concentration at delivery on the risk of hypoglycaemia in infants of insulin-dependent diabetic mothers. *Acta Paediatr Scand.* 1985;74:268–273.

29. Briggs G, Freeman R, Yaffe S. *Drugs in Pregnancy and Lactation. A Reference Guide to Fetal and Neonatal Risk.* 8th ed. Philadelphia: Lippincott Williams & Wilkins, 2008.

QUESTIONS AND ANSWERS

1. Which of the following conditions must be present for a woman to be considered at low risk to develop gestational diabetes?

   a. under the age of 25

   b. at or near ideal body weight

   c. no first-degree relatives with diabetes

   d. no glucosuria present

   e. all of the above

2. For women who have undergone gastric bypass, what screening strategy is preferred?

   a. use of the "one-step" method

   b. use of the "two-step" method

   c. no screening indicated due to massive weight loss

   d. use of mixed meal challenge tests or fasting glucose levels

3. Nutritional counseling should be:

   a. completed in a single comprehensive session

   b. culturally appropriate and tailored to include strategies for making healthy choices in many dining situations

   c. offered on a case-by-case basis

   d. discontinued once medical therapy has been initiated

4. Match the test results in the left column to the appropriate intervention in the right column.

a. All fasting glucose <100 mg/dL

b. Poorly maintained glucose log, random blood sugar 160 mg/dL

c. Fasting blood glucose >120 mg/dL

d. Fasting glucose 100–115 mg/ dL at 32 weeks' gestation

1. Begin insulin therapy

2. Continue diet and exercise, consider decreasing frequency of HGM

3. Review therapeutic goals, continue diet and exercise therapy for another week

4. Add glyburide to therapeutic regimen

5. Postpartum counseling should include:

a. discussion of risk for future development of type 2 diabetes and the need for ongoing screening

b. discussion of the effects of unrecognized or uncontrolled diabetes at conception

c. discussion of strategies to delay or prevent development of type 2 diabetes

d. discussion of planning for future pregnancies

e. all of the above

Answers:

1. e; 2. d; 3. b; 4. a-2, b-3, c-1, d-4; 5. e

Epilepsy in Pregnancy and Breastfeeding

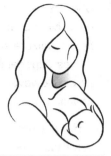

David L. Lourwood and Patricia R. Wigle

LEARNING OBJECTIVES

1. Describe how pregnancy affects seizure disorders.

2. Discuss changes in dosing various anticonvulsants in the pregnant patient.

3. Summarize the potential teratogenic risks associated with the use of various anticonvulsant agents in pregnancy.

I. Introduction

In the United States, it is estimated that almost half of all pregnancies are unplanned.[1] While it is recommended the patient be stabilized on her antiepileptic drug (AED) regimen before conception, this often is not possible with an unexpected pregnancy. This underscores the need to discuss pregnancy planning and epilepsy management with all female patients of child-bearing age who have epilepsy.

The patient with epilepsy experiences pharmacokinetic changes and other pregnancy-related symptomatology that may affect seizure control. Pharmacokinetic changes associated with pregnancy include increases in hepatic metabolism and renal elimination, along with changes in protein binding and increased volume of distribution. These changes can affect many drugs, especially AED therapy.[2,3] Narrow therapeutic index AEDs are particularly sensitive to changes in a pregnant patient's pharmacokinetic parameters. Serum levels for these medications should be monitored, along with seizure frequency. The dosages of AEDs should be adjusted to accommodate both of these factors. Nausea and vomiting, fear of AED adverse events, sleep disturbances, hormonal changes, and stress can also affect the patient's adherence to therapy and seizure frequency.

II. PATIENT CASE (PART 1)

You are working as a clinical pharmacy specialist in a physician group practice. A.G. is a 24-year-old female who presents to the clinic for a family planning visit.

She has been married for 2 years and excitedly wants to discuss the potential of conceiving a child with her husband. Review of her history indicates that she has had a seizure disorder since childhood consisting of grand mal seizures. She denies experiencing an aura or loss of bladder control before or during her seizures. However, she does lose consciousness and is concerned that this may negatively affect her plans for a successful pregnancy.

Her seizure control has been good with only one or two seizures per year; her last seizure occurred 10 months ago. She admits that she was noncompliant with her seizure medicine at that time due to a busy work-related travel schedule. She is currently stabilized on phenytoin, 400 mg PO, at bedtime and denies diplopia, dysarthria, dizziness, sedation, and gingival changes.

Your patient has been reading material on the Internet and is concerned about how pregnancy will affect her seizure control. She is also aware of the fact that several medications can be of concern for the developing fetus and wishes to discuss her medications with you.

III. Epidemiology

Approximately 2.8 million Americans have epilepsy.[3] Of this patient population, almost half are women of child-bearing age. As with other chronic medical conditions, seizures may worsen, improve, or remain the same during pregnancy.[4-6] Most patients with epilepsy will have a normal pregnancy, followed by a healthy delivery.[4] The risk of seizures and AED therapy to both the mother and fetus needs to be weighed carefully. Many factors can contribute to the teratogenic potential of anticonvulsant therapy. These include genetic predisposition, fetal hypoxia and bradycardia due to maternal seizures, cardiovascular function depression, harmful effects of the drugs and their metabolites, and drug interference with folate metabolism.[6,7] Anticonvulsants have been associated with a two- to three-fold increase in major malformations when compared to the general population.[1] Malformations seem to occur more frequently with combination therapy than with monotherapy.[7,8] In addition, the dosage used may affect the teratogenic potential of a given drug, especially valproic acid. Studies have revealed the rate of teratogenic malformation to be 4.6%–15.6% with multidrug regimens, compared to 2.6%–6.5% with the use of a single agent.[9-12] Background risk for harm to the mother and fetus is believed to be 1%–3%.[8,13] Additional risk to the mother is due to postseizure trauma, which can lead to premature rupture of the membranes or vaginal hemorrhage.

Data from one study showed a lower rate of congenital malformations in women taking antiepileptic medication compared to women with epilepsy who were not treated with an AED during pregnancy.[14] However, malformation rates were higher in patients receiving valproate therapy and were not elevated for patients who received carbamazepine, oxcarbazepine, or phenytoin. Information regarding incidence of congenital malformations and pregnancy categories for common AEDs is listed in Table 1.

Table 1. Potential for Human Development Toxicity for Various Anticonvulsant Drugs

Drug	FDA Classification	Potential Teratogenic Risk
Phenytoin	D	FACS, patent ductus arteriosus, renal anomalies, pyloric stenosis
Phenobarbital/ primidone	D	FACS, patent ductus arteriosus, renal anomalies, pyloric stenosis
Carbamazepine	D	Spina bifida, FACS, developmental delay
Valproic acid	D	Appears to be dose related; spina bifida, FACS, bilateral inguinal hernia, cardiac anomalies, developmental delay
Lamotrigine	C	Limited data, cleft lip and/or palate
Topiramate	C	None known
Oxcarbazepine	C	None known
Gabapentin	C	Limited data, delayed ossification (rodent), hypospadias
Zonisamide	C	Limited data, one report of atrial septal defect, one report of anencephaly
Levetiracetam	C	Limited data, three reports of low birth weight

FACS = fetal anticonvulsant syndrome.

It is difficult to determine whether the disease state, the medical treatment, or a combination of both is responsible for the adverse fetal events seen with patients on antiepileptic medications. This has been a controversial point in therapy for a number of years. In one meta-analysis, epilepsy itself was not found to be an independent risk factor for teratogenic risk.[15] Women with epilepsy who took antiepileptic medications had a higher rate of congenital abnormalities compared to those who did not take antiepileptic medications (odds ratio = 3.26, 95% confidence interval 2.15–4.93).[15] However, the type of seizure and frequency of seizures may have been different between the two groups, which complicates the interpretation of the results.

There are several registries that monitor the outcomes of pregnant women exposed to AEDs. These include the North American Pregnancy Registry, the Australian Pregnancy Registry, the Swedish Medical Birth Registry, the Finnish National Medical Birth Registry, the United Kingdom Pregnancy Registry, and the International Lamotrigine Pregnancy Registry. These registries identify a higher frequency of major malformations with valproic acid and with polypharmacy involving multiple AEDs.[6]

Given the limited case and cohort data available, it is difficult to estimate the frequency of adverse events. Confounders such as maternal seizure type and frequency, maternal nutritional status, parental education and IQ, and socioeconomic status should be considered in the evaluation of AED adverse event reports.[16]

IV. Preconception Care and General Management during Pregnancy

In a best-case scenario, a woman with epilepsy who desires to become pregnant would consult with her primary care provider, obstetrician, and neurologist (Table 2). These

Table 2. General Management in Pregnancy Principles

Recommendation	Recommendation Rationale
Preconception	Optimize seizure control on preferably one antiepileptic medication. Educate the patient about medication choices and the impact of a pregnancy on her, her seizure control, and her baby. Begin supplementation with a prenatal vitamin and folic acid.[a] Emphasize medication adherence.
Throughout pregnancy	Avoid medications, if possible, that may precipitate a seizure.
First trimester	11–13 wk: ultrasound. Free AED concentration.[b]
Second trimester	14–16 wk: alpha-fetoprotein concentration. 18–20 wk: ultrasound. Free AED concentration.[b]
Third trimester	36 wk: begin vitamin K, 10 mg/d, to minimize risk of neonatal bleeding for patients on enzyme-inducing anticonvulsants. Free AED concentration.[b]

[a]Folic acid supplementation varies from 0.4 to 5 mg/d. A higher folic acid dose of 4–5 mg/d is warranted in patients who have a history of neural tube effects and those taking anticonvulsant medications.

[b]Concentrations are measured for antiepileptic drugs (AEDs) that have defined therapeutic concentration at the beginning of each trimester. The decision to perform monthly AED concentration versus every trimester is multifactorial and takes into account the patient's prepregnancy seizure control, the frequency of seizures during her pregnancy, and the discretion of the patient and her health care team. Changes in unbound concentrations have been noted for phenobarbital, carbamazepine, phenytoin, and sodium valproate.

From Tomson et al.,[2] ACOG,[3] Yerby MS,[4] and Adab N.[20]

health care professionals would optimize her antiepileptic medication regimen and achieve seizure control before conception. Medication changes and discontinuations, if applicable, would be performed at least 6 months before conception.[2]

Education before conception should include the effect of AEDs on hormonal contraception, the use and risk of these medications during pregnancy, the need for both folic acid and vitamin K supplementation, adherence to medication, and differences in seizure control during pregnancy.[3] The drug interaction between AEDs and hormonal contraception is detailed in the next section. Folate deficiency has been linked to neural tube defects. The data regarding folic acid supplementation in decreasing the risk of neural tube defects in women with epilepsy are positive; however, the optimal dose has not been determined. All pregnant women should receive folic acid supplementation of at least 0.4 mg per day. For patients with a history of a pregnancy with neural tube defects and for those women on AED therapy, a higher folic acid dose of between 4 and 5 mg per day has been recommended.[3]

Phenytoin, carbamazepine, and phenobarbital may be associated with neonatal hemorrhage because of a decrease in vitamin K–dependent clotting factors.[3] Vitamin K supplementation is recommended for patients on AED therapy beginning in the 36th week of gestation.

V. Treatment

A. Goals

The goals of drug therapy in the management of the pregnant patient with epilepsy are to minimize the occurrence of seizures in the mother and to select pharmacotherapy that has the least risk to the fetus from the standpoint of both developmental teratology and long-term learning difficulties. In addition to these issues, consideration must be given to the potential for pregnancy-induced pharmacokinetic alterations to change various anticonvulsants and the increased need for therapeutic drug monitoring.

B. Anticonvulsant Therapy

A woman who wishes to become pregnant and who has been seizure-free for a minimum of 2 years may elect to work with her obstetrician, neurologist, primary care provider, and pharmacist to consider discontinuing her medication.[1,17] This decision should include consideration of the level of risk that the patient is willing to accept. One risk mentioned previously is the potential for a percentage of women to experience a greater frequency of seizures during pregnancy. Another concern is how medication discontinuation may affect other facets of her life, including driving privileges.

If continuing therapy is elected, the most effective drug therapy for the patient's given seizure type should be selected. In this patient case, the use of phenytoin for a grand mal seizure disorder is acceptable. Another consideration in the selection of drug therapy for the pregnant patient with epilepsy is the potential for teratogenicity. Data from the literature have shown that use of the lowest effective dose, preferably as monotherapy, is associated with potential minimization of adverse effects to the fetus.[1,8,17,18] The pharmacokinetics of many anticonvulsants is known to change in pregnancy.[9,18,19] Most important, pregnancy is associated with changes in binding of the drug to plasma proteins, enhancement of drug elimination, and alterations in volume of distribution. These changes must be considered to optimize drug therapy.

Some general pharmacokinetic changes in pregnancy have been noted.[18–20] Up to 85% of women will experience nausea and vomiting during early gestation.[21] This can interfere with drug absorption.[19] Plasma volume increases by 40%–50% as pregnancy progresses, which can result in decreased relative concentrations of albumin.[8,9,18–20] This leads to a decline in both total and bound drug concentrations with a subsequent rise in unbound drug. As a result, drug therapy might best be monitored during pregnancy with the use of the free concentration of the drug. However, free drug concentrations are not always readily available in practice.

Clearance may be altered in pregnancy due to changes in drug metabolism. Alterations in relative concentrations of estrogen and progesterone, seen throughout pregnancy, may have the effect of increasing drug metabolism and clearance of hepatically metabolized drugs (eg, phenytoin, phenobarbital, valproate, carbamazepine, lamotrigine).[9,19,20] In addition, renal function increases as pregnancy progresses, causing serum concentrations of newer drugs, which are predominately excreted unchanged (eg, gabapentin), to be decreased.[19,20,22] As a result of any of these mechanisms, loss of seizure control may occur during pregnancy.

Published guidelines recommend monitoring of anticonvulsant blood concentrations at the beginning of each trimester to ensure continued efficacy.[1,10,20] Further monitoring is suggested if poor seizure control is noted. Monitoring of drug concentrations and corresponding dosage adjustments of any anticonvulsant must take into account seizure frequency as justification for dosage adjustment.[19,20,22]

In addition, each of these gestational alterations in drug handling by the body can rapidly reverse during the puerperium with resultant need for close monitoring and adjustment of drug dosing during the immediate postpartum period to maintain seizure control and minimize drug toxicity.[9,18,19] One guideline recommends that if it has been required to increase the dose of an anticonvulsant during pregnancy, then the dosage should then be gradually reduced to preconception doses within the first few weeks after delivery.[11]

The other area of major concern with the management of the pregnant epileptic patient is the risk for teratogenesis. As previously noted, the occurrence of tonic-clonic seizures has been associated with an increased risk to the mother and fetus by reducing placental blood flow and resultant impairment of fetal oxygenation.[18] Most of the data available to date regarding the risk of drug-induced adverse effects on the developing fetus have related to older agents (eg, phenytoin, phenobarbital, valproate, carbamazepine). Much more limited data, if any, are available for the use of newer agents (eg, gabapentin, topiramate) in pregnancy, with the exception of lamotrigine.

Most malformations occur early in the first trimester, often before the woman is aware of her pregnancy. As a result, planning of the pregnancy, to optimize therapy and minimize risks, as seen with this patient case is highly advisable.[11] Major congenital malformations can occur with most of the anticonvulsants. Malformations that occur with the use of anticonvulsants can be divided into two types—major and minor. *Minor anomalies* are defined as those that occur in less than 4% of the population but that have neither cosmetic nor functional significance to the child. These are not considered a threat to overall health. Minor anomalies account for 6%–20% of all neonatal abnormalities after anticonvulsant exposure. These are usually distinctive and commonly include distal digital and nail hypoplasia and midline craniofacial anomalies, such as ocular hypertelorism, broad nasal bridge, short upturned nose, alterations of the lips, and epicanthal folds. Many of the craniofacial abnormalities are outgrown by the time the child reaches the age of 5 years.[8,23]

Major malformations are defined as those that have cosmetic or functional significance to the child. These malformations are usually noted within the first week of life. Major anomalies commonly associated with antiepileptic drug exposure include congenital heart defects, cleft lip and/or palate, neural tube defects, and urogenital defects.[8,13] Congenital heart defects include atrial septal defect, ventricular septal defect, tetralogy of Fallot, coarctation of the aorta, patent ductus arteriosus, and pulmonary stenosis. Neural tube defects usually consist of spina bifida, but can include hydrocephaly as well as other midline defects. Urogenital anomalies commonly involve glandular hypospadias.

Most of the older anticonvulsants have been associated with an increased risk of teratogenic anomalies. Phenytoin and phenobarbital appear to be the potentially safest agents for use in pregnancy due to a smaller relative risk of adverse fetal

effects. While the majority of abnormalities classified as minor in nature have traditionally been associated with the use of phenytoin and phenobarbital, the abnormalities appear to be more universal in occurrence with other antiepileptic agents.
This cluster of abnormalities is often referred to as the *fetal anticonvulsant syndrome
(FACS)*.[8,12,13,24] The risk of FACS is higher when the mother is exposed to these
drugs during the first trimester.

Differences in incidence of FACS with various antiepileptic medications have
been reported.[8,12,13,24] For example, fetal valproate syndrome is associated with epi-
canthic folds and infraorbital groove, medial deficiencies of the eyebrows, flat nasal
bridge, short nose with anteverted nares, smooth or upturned philtrum, a long thin
upper lip with a thickened lower lip, and a small, downturned mouth. Fetal phenytoin
exposure has been associated with hypertelorism, broad nasal bridge, short nose, and
facial hirsutism. Finally, carbamazepine use during pregnancy is associated with epi-
canthic folds, short nose, long philtrum, and upward slanting palpebral fissures.

Phenytoin is associated with a 6%–11% risk of fetal anomalies.[24,25] Most adverse
effects with the use of the drug relate to previous descriptions for FACS. Data exist
that indicate a mother who has a child with FACS secondary to phenytoin is at greater
risk of having subsequent pregnancies with phenytoin-associated anomalies.[25]

Phenobarbital has also been associated with a relatively smaller number (6.5%) of
serious adverse effects on the fetus, with most focusing on the FACS.[26] Many of these
reports of FACS-related problems have been noted by 5 days of age.[26] There have also
been reports of phenobarbital, primidone, and phenytoin being associated with risk of
long-term neuropsychological effects.[25–28] In a prospective study of 67 children
exposed to these three drugs during pregnancy, a significant lowering of verbal and
performance IQ was noted, with the most significant lowering occurring with poly-
drug therapy using both phenytoin and either phenobarbital or primidone.[27]

None of the older drugs is without teratogenic concerns. Carbamazepine and valproic acid are among those agents for which greatest concern is noted due to risks of
occurrence of spina bifida. This risk is approximately 0.5%–1% for the former and 1%–
3.8% for the latter. This compares with a risk in the general population of 1 in 1300,
resulting in a drug-induced risk of 14-fold over that seen at baseline. Theoretically, the
teratogenic potential of carbamazepine may in part be due to the active metabolite, car-
bamazepine-10,11-epoxide.[7] Other concurrent conditions such as diabetes and excessive prepregnancy weight may increase the risk of spinal malformations.[4]

The relative risk for development of major malformations with fetal exposure to carbamazepine is 4.9 compared to the general population.[8] Of this number, the risk of spina
bifida occurs in 1% of exposed children.[8] The major malformations most reported with
exposure to carbamazepine during pregnancy include neural tube defects, cardiovascular
and urinary tract anomalies, and cleft palate. As with other anticonvulsants, the risk of
anomalies is greatest when carbamazepine is used as part of a polytherapeutic regimen,
with a rate of potential birth defects as high as 18.8%. This is opposed to a risk of 5.2%
when the drug is used alone.[8]

Major and minor physical abnormalities are not the only concern with the use of carbamazepine. The effect of anticonvulsant therapy on learning difficulties in childhood is

controversial. In one study, 249 children older than 6 years of age were administered the Weschler Intelligence Scale.[28] The potential for learning disturbances was noted to be lowest (associated with a reduction of 3 IQ points) in children exposed to monotherapy in utero and higher with combination therapies. When children younger than 6 years of age were examined in the same study, learning deficiencies were observed.[28]

In a separate study of 86 patients exposed to carbamazepine in utero, only minimal changes in the Weschler Intelligence Scale were found in both verbal and nonverbal IQ scores.[29] Conversely, low developmental and IQ scores were noted in a comparable study in the subpopulation of children who had signs of FACS.[23] As a result, it has been theorized that minor anomalies, such as craniofacial abnormalities, may be associated with a greater risk of intelligence abnormalities by the time the child reaches school age.

When comparing the use of valproic acid to carbamazepine, the most striking difference is the risk of malformations. In similar studies of anticonvulsant medications, valproic acid is consistently considered to be most likely (10.7%–17.1%) to induce malformations.[23,30] Whereas risks with valproic acid include those described above for FACS, the greatest concern with this drug is spina bifida.[24,31] In addition, the risk for valproic acid seems to be dose-related, with risk of anomalies being progressively increased with doses above 1000–1400 mg/d.[23,31] This increased risk has been defined as being 3.9- to 6.8-fold higher with elevated doses of valproic acid.[23,32] Risk of malformation with valproic acid seems to be especially increased when the drug is used in polytherapy (rate of malformation, 15.2%).[30] At valproic acid doses of 1000 mg/day or more, the metabolism of the drug changes from fatty acid β-oxidation to glucuronide conjugation.[30,31] Saturation of β-oxidation capacity may result in interference with the metabolism of endogenous branched-chain amino acids. Accumulation of some branched-chain products may play a role in teratogenicity derivation.

Similar to carbamazepine, the use of valproic acid in pregnancy has been associated with an increased risk of delayed psychomotor development in the children of women exposed to valproic acid during gestation. As with carbamazepine, there is some evidence that these neurologic/learning abnormalities may be associated with minor physiologic anomalies that are felt to diminish in severity with time.[31,32] A retrospective study of functional delays in children exposed to valproic acid was conducted by the Mersey Regional Epilepsy Clinic in England. Data were collected for 330 mothers and their 594 children, between the ages of 3 months and 23 years. Of the 400 children attending school, 42 required remedial help. The odds ratio of exposure to valproic acid and additional educational needs was 3.4.[28,33] The evidence concerning learning disabilities for children born to women who took antiepileptic medications during their pregnancies has not been totally convincing. As the authors pointed out, several confounding variables exist, such as differences in epilepsy syndrome, type and severity of seizures, sociodemographic status, mother tongue, parental IQ, and maternal education—each of these not being taken into consideration in the study.[33]

In a second analysis of the data in the Mersey study, more detailed analysis of the mothers and children was obtained.[28] These newer data included assessments of IQ and neuropsychological functioning in the children. Verbal IQ was significantly lower in children exposed to valproic acid, with an odds ratio of 3.5 of the children having a verbal IQ of ≤69. In addition, there may be an association between valproic acid doses of 800 mg/d or more and lower IQ. It is believed that the true impact of valproic acid (and other anticonvulsants) on mental development and functioning will only be able to be truly ascertained from larger, carefully planned, prospective studies.

Effects of older anticonvulsant medications on folate metabolism may explain the mechanism of neural tube adverse effects.[25] Folate is used by the body for several functions, including red and white blood cell development, normal gastrointestinal functioning, neural tube development, and maintenance of integrity of the nervous system. Neural tube defects are malformations caused by abnormal neural tube closure during the third or fourth week of fetal development. Of this number, 40%–50% are accounted for by spina bifida and anencephaly. The greatest risk for neural tube defects, a 10-fold increase, appears to be a previous pregnancy resulting in a neural tube defect. Maternal use of carbamazepine, and to a greater extent, valproic acid, is also associated with an increase in the occurrence of spina bifida.

Phenytoin is metabolized through highly reactive electrophilic intermediaries to form oxidized products. During pregnancy, as described above, the metabolism of phenytoin is elevated, leading to increased formation of these oxidized metabolites. Data indicate that phenytoin and its metabolites alter hepatic distribution and metabolism of folate with resultant symptoms associated with FACS.[25] Phenobarbital and the related drug primidone have also been connected with symptoms associated with FACS, and these symptoms may also be attributable to alterations in folate metabolism. The mechanism of this interaction is not well understood, but is hypothesized to be similar to the mechanism described for phenytoin.[25] Carbamazepine also affects folate metabolism with resultant symptoms associated with FACS and spina bifida. In the case of this drug, it is believed carbamazepine's increased metabolism in the gravid patient is associated with formation of epoxide intermediates similar to those formed with use of phenytoin. In addition, these carbamazepine-induced epoxide metabolites may be associated with covalent binding to DNA and proteins with resultant soft tissue and skeletal malformations.[25]

Teratogenic concentrations of valproic acid have been associated with alterations in folate metabolism resulting in adverse fetal effects.[25] It appears valproic acid's effects on folic acid are a dose-related phenomenon, with risks of anomalies being much less with doses less than 1000–1400 mg/d. This dose-related phenomenon appears to be related to saturation of plasma protein binding at higher concentrations of valproic acid. This results in an increase in unbound drug available for placental transfer and accumulation of the drug in the fetus.

Of the newer anticonvulsants, the most is known regarding the use of lamotrigine in pregnancy. The International Lamotrigine Pregnancy Registry was created to gather data related to the use of the drug in pregnancy. One of the first reports from the lamotrigine registry was that of a group of 414 first-trimester exposures to the drug. In this group, 12 outcomes (2.9%) with major birth defects occurred.[34] Adverse outcomes included problems such as esophageal malformation, cleft palate, club foot, ventricular septal defect, and hydronephrosis. This rate of malformation is not statistically different from that seen in the general population.

When lamotrigine was given as polytherapy with other anticonvulsants, there was no greater risk of malformation, except in patients exposed to the combination of lamotrigine and valproic acid (12.5%).[34] This registry report contained no adverse fetal effects from exposure to lamotrigine in the second or third trimesters.

In September 2006, the U.S. Food and Drug Administration (FDA) issued an alert regarding preliminary data from the North American Antiepileptic Drug Pregnancy Registry describing a possible association between lamotrigine monotherapy during the first trimester of pregnancy and cleft lip and/or palate. The number of occurrences were few and not associated with other birth defects. The rate of malformation was 0.89% (5 cases in 564 pregnancies). This compares with a risk from European and Australian reports of 0.05–0.22%.[35] A second report from the North American Antiepileptic Drug Pregnancy Registry found an incidence of major malformations in 16 of 684 (2.3%) infants exposed to lamotrigine in utero. Of note, five of the infants (7.3/1000) had oral clefts.[36]

As with other anticonvulsants, lamotrigine metabolism is altered in pregnancy. The increased rate of clearance of lamotrigine in pregnancy is greater than that seen for other AEDs. A significant decrease in serum concentrations of the drug, which is related to increased hepatic metabolism of the drug, has been seen in pregnant patients. This increased metabolism resolves within the 6-week puerperium, indicating a need to follow therapy closely after delivery to adjust drug dosage to maintain efficacy.[12,20,37] Topiramate is a new anticonvulsant that has potential for teratogenicity.[38] Studies in rats and rabbits have noted ossification-related malformations. Few human studies in pregnancy are available. In a review of 28 cases given polytherapy, which included topiramate, three cases of birth defects were reported. Postmarketing surveillance reported 139 cases of topiramate exposure with 87 live births and five cases of hypospadias.[4]

Oxcarbazepine is the 10-keto analog of carbamazepine. Its metabolism differs from that of carbamazepine. Oxcarbazepine is rapidly metabolized to 10-hydroxycarbamazepine, which has anticonvulsant activity, and does not interfere with folate metabolism. It forms an epoxide intermediate and is independent of the cytochrome P-450 system.[12,38] Limited animal and human reports suggest that oxcarbazepine may not be a teratogen.[12,38]

Animal data associated with gabapentin use in pregnancy have shown that the drug may cause delayed bone ossification in rodent fetuses.[38] The Gabapentin Pregnancy Registry monitors the use of this drug in pregnancy.[39] In a report of 44 live births exposed to the drug in pregnancy, major malformations were noted in two patients and minor malformations in a third child. The major malformations were hypospadias in a child exposed to gabapentin with phenobarbital and an absent kidney in a child exposed to gabapentin along with valproic acid. Eleven children exposed to gabapentin alone did not demonstrate birth defects.

Zonisamide has also been used only rarely in the treatment of epilepsy in the gravid patient. In a preliminary report of 26 offspring exposed to the drug in utero (four monotherapy and 22 polytherapy), malformations were noted in two of the polytherapy-exposed offspring—one was an anencephalic child diagnosed at 16 weeks' gestation, the other had an atrial septal defect.[40] In both cases, the serum concentrations of zonisamide were below the therapeutic range reported for the drug.

Although levetiracetam has been associated with growth retardation and skeletal abnormalities in rodents, there are only limited data in human patients.[41] In a study involving rat pups, levetiracetam monotherapy and in combination with carbamazepine did not induce cell death.[42] A small study of 11 patients did not show an increased risk of malformations.[41] Levetiracetam concentrations also decrease during pregnancy. The decline in serum concentrations during gestation may be as high as 50%, which can be due to increased renal clearance, enhanced enzymatic hydrolysis, or a combination of these factors.[43]

C. Adjunctive Drug Therapy

1. Folic Acid

As previously mentioned for many anticonvulsants, especially older agents, drug-induced folate deficiency may explain some of the risks of teratogenicity in the children of women exposed to these drugs during pregnancy.[4,25] As a result, folic acid supplementation may reduce the risk of neural tube defects. Unfortunately, no definitive data exist to demonstrate the clear benefit of folic acid supplementation in preventing birth defects in women receiving anticonvulsant therapy. However, due to the increased risk in this group of patients, folic acid supplementation is recommended. Folic acid supplementation is usually administered in a dose of 4–5 mg/d and should be begun prior to conception and continuing at least throughout the first trimester of pregnancy to achieve potentially effective serum concentrations before fetal neural tube closure.[1,18]

2. Vitamin K

Anticonvulsant drugs that induce hepatic enzymes can accelerate the metabolism of vitamin K with a resultant deficiency of the vitamin in neonates. This can result in increased concentrations of nonfunctional procoagulants that are decarboxylated forms of vitamin K–dependent clotting factors in the cord blood of infants exposed to AEDs in utero. These factors have been associated with an increased risk of intracranial bleeds in the neonate.[18,22]

To reduce this risk, some have recommended that vitamin K, 10 mg PO daily, be administered to the mother during the last month of the pregnancy.[1,18] As with folate supplementation, no definitive data exist to prove that this intervention actually reduces the risk of neonatal intracranial hemorrhage. To avoid coagulation defects, it is also recommended that all newborns receive 1 mg of vitamin K IM postpartum.

VI. Drug Interactions

Two important considerations for the management of a female patient with epilepsy are how the AEDs might affect both her pregnancy and medications for the prevention of pregnancy. AEDs can interact with multiple medications and with each other (Tables 3 and 4). Phenytoin, carbamazepine, phenobarbital, and primidone are

Table 3. Antiepileptic Drug [AED] and Antiepileptic Drug Interactions

	CBZ	LTG	OXC	PB	PHT	TOP	VA	LEV
CBZ	—	↓LTG	↓OXC ↓CBZ	↓CBZ	↓CBZ ↓/↑PHT	↓TOP	↓VA ↑CBZ	↑CBZ
LTG	↓LTG	—		↓LTG	↓LTG	↑TOP	↑LTG	
OXC	↓OXC ↓CBZ		—	↑PB ↓OXC	↑PHT ↓OXC		↓VA ↓OXC	
PB	↓CBZ	↓LTG	↓OXC ↑PB	—	↑PB ↓/↑PHT		↑PB	
PHT	↓CBZ ↓/↑PHT	↓LTG	↓OXC ↑PHT	↑PB ↓/↑PHT	—	↓TOP ↑PHT	↑free VA	
TOP	↓TOP	↑TOP			↓TOP ↑PHT	—	↓TOP ↓VA	
VA	↑CBZ ↓VA	↑LTG	↓OXC ↓VA	↑PB	↑free VA	↓TOP ↓VA	—	
LEV	↑CBZ							—

CBZ = carbamazepine, LEV = levetiracetam, LTG = lamotrigine, OXC = oxcarbazepine, PB = phenobarbital, PHT = phenytoin, TOP = topiramate, VA = valproic acid, ↓ = decreased, ↑ = increased.
From Perucca E,[45] Sandson et al.,[46] and Patsalos PN and Perucca E.[47]

Table 4. Antiepileptic Drug [AED] Interactions with Non-AED Interactions

	CBZ	PB	PHT	VA
Antineoplastic[a]	↓[a]		↑/↓[a]	↓[a]
Benzodiazepines	↓bnz	↓bnz	↑PHT ↓bnz	↑bnz
Carbapenems				↓VA
Cimetidine	↑CBZ		↑PHT	↑VA
Cyclosporine	↓cyclosporine	↓cyclosporine	↓cyclosporine	
Diltiazem	↑CBZ		↑PHT	
Erythromycin	↑CBZ			
Fluconazole	↑CBZ		↑PHT	
Fluoxetine	↑CBZ		↑PHT	
Folic acid	↓folic acid	↓folic acid	↓folic acid	↓folic acid
Isoniazid	↑CBZ		↑PHT	↑VA
Methadone	↓methadone	↓methadone	↓methadone	
NSAIDs	↓NSAID	↓NSAID	↓NSAID	
Quetiapine[b]	↓quetiapine	↓quetiapine	↓quetiapine	
Rifampin	↓CBZ		↓PHT	↓VA
Salicylates				↑free VA
Sulfonamides			↑PHT	
Warfarin	↓warfarin	↓warfarin	↓warfarin	

bnz = benzodiazepine, CBZ = carbamazepine, LTG = lamotrigine, NSAID = nonsteroidal anti-inflammatory drug, OXC = oxcarbazepine, PB = phenobarbital, PHT = phenytoin, TOP = topiramate, VA = valproic acid, ↓ = decreased, ↑ = increased.
[a]Cisplatin and other antineoplastics can have varying effects on antiepileptic medications.
[b]Effect of risperidone and ziprasidone is reduced with CBZ, PB, and PHT.
From Report of the Quality Standards Subcommittee of the American Academy of Neurology,[1] Perucca E,[45] Sandson et al,[46] and Patsalos PN and Perucca E.[47]

enzyme-inducing antiepileptic medications and can lower the concentrations of drugs metabolized by cytochrome P-450 1A2, 2C9, 2C19, and 3A4.[28] These antiepileptic medications, along with topiramate at doses ≥200 mg/d, can decrease combined oral contraceptive levels and effectiveness.[44–47]

If a patient is taking an enzyme-inducing anticonvulsant medication, there is an older recommendation for the patient to take a combined oral contraceptive pill containing 50 µg ethinyl estradiol.[1] Newer recommendations include continuous combined oral contraceptives, progestin products at doses high enough to inhibit ovulation as monotherapy without estrogen (ie, levonorgestrel 0.06 mg/d), and intrauterine devices.[47] Because the progestin-only contraceptive tablets do not contain high enough amounts of progestin activity to inhibit ovulation as their primary mechanism, these products are not recommended for contraceptive purposes for patients on enzyme-inducing anticonvulsants.[47] A back-up contraceptive method or a change in anticonvulsant are two additional options to minimize these interactions. There does not appear to be an interaction with combined oral contraceptive pills and gabapentin, levetiracetam, pregabalin, tiagabine, valproate, or zonisamide.[44–47]

Unlike the antiepileptic medications that are enzyme-inducing, valproic acid can have inhibitory effects on the cytochrome P-450 enzyme system.[44–47] In addition to cytochrome P-450 enzyme and protein binding drug interactions, there is also the potential for additive toxicity. For example, the combination of cyclosporine and valproic acid may increase the patient's risk of hepatotoxicity.

VII. Considerations in Breastfeeding

Several anticonvulsants are excreted in breast milk. The risk of use of a given drug in the lactating mother–child pair is related to the amount of drug excreted into the mother's milk. In a few cases, specific effects of the drug on the nursing infant have been noted.

For example, the pharmacokinetics of phenytoin and phenobarbital in lactation have been reviewed. Little risk exists for the nursing infant if maternal drug levels are maintained in the therapeutic range.[48] Reports have noted methemoglobinemia, drowsiness, and decreased sucking ability in one infant.[49] In the case of the use of phenobarbital, drug-induced sedation has been noted due to amounts of the drug accumulating in the infant secondary to the child's slower metabolism.[48]

Carbamazepine is also noted to be excreted in small amounts in the mother's milk.[48] The occurrence of seizurelike activity has been noted in a child receiving carbamazepine, fluoxetine, and buspirone from nursing.[50] Valproic acid passes into breast milk to produce infant serum levels that are less than 15% of that seen in the mother.[51] A single report of an adverse event in a nursing child was thought to be attributable to valproic acid. Thrombocytopenia purpura, anemia, and reticulocytosis were noted in the 3-month-old breastfed infant.[52]

Little is known regarding the newer anticonvulsants. Lamotrigine is excreted into breast milk in concentrations 30%–60% of that seen in the maternal blood.[53] No adverse effects have been reported in infants exposed to the drug in breast milk. Likewise, zonisamide and topiramate have also been reported in breast milk in levels 60%–90% of that seen in maternal serum.[38,54] While no adverse effects in nursing infants have been reported with zonisamide use, topiramate has been associated with reports of changes in neonatal alertness, behavior, and feeding habits.[38]

No data exist for breastfeeding with maternal use of levetiracetam, gabapentin, and oxcarbazepine. With the exception of phenobarbital, the American Academy of Pediatrics has found all anticonvulsants to be compatible with breastfeeding.[55]

VIII. PATIENT CASE [PART 2]

After discussing these questions with A.G., her husband, and her physicians, the decision is made to continue phenytoin therapy during this gestation. You follow therapy throughout the pregnancy and check concentrations periodically, making adjustments to her phenytoin dosage as required. At 39 weeks, she delivers a healthy baby boy who has only slight facial anomalies. You reassure her that her son should "grow out" of these problems in the first few years of life.

IX. Clinical/Practice Pearls

- Prior to conception, optimize AED therapy. Modification and/or discontinuation of AED therapy should occur at least 6 months prior to conception.
- The best AED is the one, at the lowest effective dose, that controls the patient's seizures.
- When possible, avoid polypharmacy with multiple AEDs, especially with valproic acid.

X. Summary

The management of the pregnant patient with epilepsy presents unique challenges to her health care team. Each of the available anticonvulsants has the potential for fetal adverse effects. Many of the newer agents lack the clinical experience to determine their safe use in the pregnant patient. Seizure frequency is noted to increase, decrease, or remain similar to that seen before conception. An increase in seizure frequency can be due to many reasons, including alterations in drug pharmacokinetic parameters. As such, drug concentrations should be monitored throughout pregnancy and dosage adjustments made based on both drug levels and seizure frequency.

The use of one antiepileptic medication, when possible, is preferable for the management of this patient population. Monotherapy has been associated with less potential for drug–drug interactions, alterations in drug handling, and adverse effects on the fetus. Of the available anticonvulsants, phenytoin and phenobarbital have the best safety record for use. Valproic acid and carbamazepine have been associated with spina bifida and other disorders of the developing neural tract and should be avoided, if possible. Among newer agents, the most human experience is available for lamotrigine. Yet, it too has been associated with the risk of adverse fetal effects. Supplementation with folic acid has been recommended during pregnancy to attempt to minimize the risk of neural tube defects. Doses of 4–5 mg/d are used. Vitamin K supplementation is also proposed to reduce the risk of drug-induced bleeding difficulties in the neonate.

XI. References

1. Report of the Quality Standards Subcommittee of the American Academy of Neurology. Practice parameter: management issues for women with epilepsy (summary statement). *Neurology*. 1998;51:944–948.

2. Tomson T, Hiilesmaa V. Epilepsy in pregnancy. *BMJ*. 2007;335:769–773.

3. ACOG Education Bulletin. Seizure disorders in pregnancy. *Int J Gyn Obstet*. 1997;56:279–286.

4. Yerby MS. Clinical care of pregnant women with epilepsy: neural tube defects and folic acid supplementation. *Epilepsia*. 2003;44(suppl 3):33–40.

5. Crawford P, Appleton R, Betts T, et al, for the Women with Epilepsy Guidelines Development Group. Best practice guidelines for the management of women with epilepsy. *Seizure*. 1999;8:201–217.

6. Meador KJ, Brandel JP, Preese M, et al. In utero antiepileptic drug exposure: fetal death and malformations. *Neurology*. 2006;67:407–412.

7. Kaneko S, Otani K, Fukushima Y, et al. Teratogenicity of antiepileptic drugs: analysis of possible risk factors. *Epilepsia*. 1988;29:359–367.

8. Pennell PB. The importance of monotherapy in pregnancy. *Neurology*. 2003;60(suppl 4):S31–S38.

9. Perucca E, Crema A. Plasma protein binding of drugs in pregnancy. *Clin Pharmacokinet*. 1982;7:336–352.

10. Tomson T, Perucca E, Battino D. Navigating toward fetal and maternal health: the challenge of treating epilepsy in pregnancy. *Epilepsia*. 2004;45:1171–1175.

11. Crawford P. Best practice guidelines for the management of women with epilepsy. *Epilepsia*. 2005;46(suppl 9):117–124.

12. Pennel PB. Antiepileptic drug pharmacokinetics during pregnancy and lactation. *Neurology*. 2003;61(suppl 2):S35–S42.

13. Moore SJ, Turnpenny P, Quinn A, et al. A clinical study of 57 children with fetal anticonvulsant syndromes. *J Med Genet*. 2000;37:489–497.

14. Artama M, Auvinen A, Ravdaskoski T, et al. Antiepileptic drug use of women with epilepsy and congenital malformations in offspring. *Neurology*. 2005;64:1874–1878.

15. Fried S, Kozer E, Nulman I, et al. Malformation rates in children of women with untreated epilepsy: a meta-analysis. *Drug Safety*. 2004;27:197–202.

16. Adab N, Tudur Smith C, Vinten J, et al. Common antiepileptic drugs in pregnancy in women with epilepsy. *Cochrane Database Syst Rev.* 2004;(3): CD004848.

17. Kalviainen R, Tomson T. Optimizing treatment of epilepsy during pregnancy. *Neurology.* 2006;67(suppl 4):S59–S63.

18. Tettenborn B. Management of epilepsy in women of childbearing age: practical recommendations. *CNS Drugs.* 2006;20:373–387.

19. McAuley JW, Anderson GD. Treatment of epilepsy in women of reproductive age: pharmacokinetic considerations. *Clin Pharmacokinet.* 2002;41:559–579.

20. Adab N. Therapeutic monitoring of antiepileptic drugs during pregnancy and in the postpartum period: is it useful? *CNS Drugs.* 2006;20:791–800.

21. American College of Obstetricians and Gynecologists. Nausea and vomiting of pregnancy. *ACOG Practice Bulletin.* Number 52, April 2004. *Obstet Gynecol.* 2004;103:803–815.

22. Nulman I, Laslo D, Koren G. Treatment of epilepsy in pregnancy. *Drugs.* 1999;57:535–544.

23. Kini U, Adab N, Fryer A, et al. Dysmorphic features: an important clue to the diagnosis and severity of fetal anticonvulsant syndromes. *Arch Dis Child Fetal Neonatal Ed.* 2006;91:F90–F95.

24. Holmes LB, Harvey EA, Coull BA, et al. The teratogenicity of anticonvulsant drugs. *N Engl J Med.* 2001;344:1132–1138.

25. Lewis DP, vanDyke DC, Stumbo PJ, et al. Drug and environmental factors associated with adverse pregnancy outcomes: part I: antiepileptic drugs, contraceptives, smoking, and folate. *Ann Pharmacother.* 1998;32:802–817.

26. Holmes LB, Wyszynski DF, Lieberman E, et al. The AED (antiepileptic drug) pregnancy registry: a 6-year experience. *Arch Neurol.* 2004;61:673–678.

27. Koch S, Titze K, Zimmerman RB. Long-term neuropsychological consequences of maternal epilepsy and anticonvulsant treatment during pregnancy for school-aged children and adolescents. *Epilepsia.* 1999;40:1237–1243.

28. Adab N, Kini U, Ayres G, et al. The longer-term outcome of children born to mothers with epilepsy. *J Neurol Neurosurg Psychiatry.* 2004;75:1575–1582.

29. Gaily E, Kantola-Sorsa E, Hiilesmaa V, et al. Normal intelligence in children with prenatal exposure to carbamazepine. *Neurology.* 2004;62:28–32.

30. Vajda FJE, Eadie MJ. Maternal valproate dosage and foetal malformations. *Acta Neurol Scand.* 2005;112:137–143.

31. Genton P, Semah F, Trinka E. Valproic acid in epilepsy: pregnancy-related issues. *Drug Safety.* 2006;29:1–21.

32. Mawer G, Clayton-Smith J, Coyle H, Kini U. Outcome of pregnancy in women attending an outpatient epilepsy clinic: adverse features associated with higher doses of sodium valproate. *Seizure.* 2002;11:512–518.

33. Adab N, Jacoby A, Smith D, et al. Additional educational needs in children born to mothers with epilepsy. *J Neurol Neurosurg Psychiatr.* 2001;70:15–21.

34. Cunnington M, Tennis P. Lamotrigine and the risk of malformations in pregnancy. *Neurology.* 2005;64:955–960.

35. U.S. Food and Drug Administration. Information for healthcare professionals: lamotrigine (marketed as Lamicital®). www.fda.gov/cder/drug/InfoSheets/HCP/lamotrigineHCP.htm. Issued September 2006. Updated January 2008. Accessed March 25, 2008.

36. Holmes LB, Baldwin EI, Smith CR, et al. Increased frequency of isolated cleft palate in infants exposed to lamotrigine in pregnancy. *Neurology.* 2008;70:2152–2158.

37. Ohman I, Vitols S, Tomson T. Lamotrigine in pregnancy: pharmacokinetics during delivery, in the neonate, and during lactation. *Epilepsia.* 2000;41:709–713.

38. Palmieri C. Teratogenic potential of the newer antiepileptic drugs: what is known and how should this influence prescribing? *CNS Drugs.* 2002;16:755–764.

39. Montouris G. Gabapentin exposure in human pregnancy: results from the Gabapentin Pregnancy Registry. *Epilepsy Behav.* 2003;4:310–317.

40. Kondo T, Kaneko S, Amano Y, et al. Preliminary reports on teratogenic effects of zonisamide in the offspring of treated women with epilepsy. *Epilepsia.* 1996;37:1242–1244.

41. Berg KT, Samren EB, Oppen CV, et al. Levetiracetam use and pregnancy outcome. *Reproductive Toxicology.* 2005;20:175–178.

42. Kim J, Kondratyev A, Gale K. Antiepileptic drug-induced neuronal cell death in the immature brain: effects of carbamazepine, topiramate and levetiracetam as monotherapy versus polytherapy. *J Pharmacol Exp Ther.* 2007;323:165–173.

43. Tomson T, Battino D. Pharmacokinetics and therapeutic drug monitoring of newer antiepileptic drugs during pregnancy and the puerperium. *Clin Pharmacokinet.* 2007;46:209–219.

44. Perucca E. Clinically relevant drug interactions with antiepileptic drugs. *Br J Clin Pharmacol.* 2005;61:246–255.

45. Sandson NB, Marcucci C, Bourke DL, et al. An interaction between aspirin and valproate: the relevance of plasma protein displacement drug-drug interactions. *Am J Psychiatry.* 2006;163:1891–1896.

46. Patsalos PN, Perucca E. Clinically important drug interactions in epilepsy: interactions between antiepileptic drugs and other drugs. *Lancet Neurol.* 2003;2:473–481.

47. Schwenkhagen AM, Stodieck SRG. Which contraception for women with epilepsy. *Seizure.* 2008;17:145–150.

48. Nau H, Kuhnz W, Egger HJ. Anticonvulsants during pregnancy and lactation: transplacental, maternal, and neonatal pharmacokinetics. *Clin Pharmacokinet.* 1982;7:508–543.

49. Finch E, Lorber J. Methaemoglobinaemia in the newborn: probably due to phenytoin excreted in the milk. *J Obstet Gynaecol Br Emp.* 1954;61:833.

50. Brent NB, Wisner KL. Fluoxetine and carbamazepine concentrations in a nursing mother/infant pair. *Clin Pediatr.* 1998;37:41–44.

51. Wisner KL, Perel JM. Serum levels of valproate and carbamazepine in breastfeeding mother-infant pairs. *J Clin Psychopharmacol.* 1998;18:167–169.

52. Stahl MMS, Neiderud J, Vinge E. Thrombocytopenic purpura and anemia in a breast-fed infant whose mother was treated with valproic acid. *J Pediatr.* 1997;130:1001–1003.

53. Tomson T, Ohman I, Vitols S. Lamotrigine in pregnancy and lactation: a case report. *Epilepsia.* 1997;38:1039–1041.

54. Shimoyama R, Ohkubo T, Sugawara K. Monitoring of zonisamide in human breast milk and maternal plasma by solid-phase extraction HPLC method. *Biomed Chromatogr.* 1999;13:370–372.

55. Committee on Drugs. American Academy of Pediatrics. The transfer of drugs and other chemicals into breast milk. *Pediatrics.* 2001;108:776–789.

QUESTIONS AND ANSWERS

1. Among the available anticonvulsants, which is the safest for use in pregnancy?

2. A patient who is 20 weeks pregnant presents with a serum phenytoin level of 6.5 µg/mL. She has been seizure-free to this point in her pregnancy. Should her dose be adjusted?

3. A 22-year-old female patient with epilepsy presents to clinic for a routine follow-up visit. She recently delivered a healthy baby boy and wants to know whether she can breastfeed while on carbamazepine therapy.

4. Eight weeks after delivery, a patient presents to your pharmacy with a prescription for the NuvaRing. She is currently taking phenytoin for epilepsy and has not had a seizure for 8 months. Her last seizure was due to noncompliance with therapy. What do you recommend?

Answers

1. Only limited data are available for most of the newer agents such as gabapentin and topiramate. In the nonpregnant patient, valproic acid is the drug of choice for most seizure types. Yet, due to the potential for causing neural tube defects, the use of valproic acid and carbamazepine should be avoided, when possible. Phenytoin and phenobarbital are not free of adverse effects on the developing fetus, with fetal anticonvulsant syndrome being most frequently reported. Based on relative safety, the use of one of these two latter agents is usually chosen for use in pregnancy. In addition, studies have shown that monotherapy for seizure control is less likely to be associated with teratogenic risk.

2. This has been a controversial area. The consensus is that since albumin is decreased and biopharmaceutic parameters of phenytoin usage are altered in pregnancy that a free phenytoin level, when available, should be followed during therapy. Since this woman is seizure-free, no adjustment in therapy is required. It would be reasonable to recheck her free phenytoin level in 1 month.

3. Similar to concerns about use of antiepileptic medications during pregnancy, risks versus benefits must be weighed for nursing mothers and their babies. Carbamazepine and its metabolite are both transferred into breast milk. However, the American Academy of Pediatrics considers carbamazepine generally compatible with breastfeeding. The newborn should be monitored for excessive sedation.

4. Her last seizure was due to noncompliance with therapy. The NuvaRing contains a low dose of ethinyl estradiol (15 μg/d) and is not an appropriate option for this patient who is on an enzyme-inducing antiepileptic medication. Three options exist: (i) since she has been controlled on phenytoin, a change to a nonenzyme inducing antiepileptic medication can be made; (ii) the NuvaRing prescription can be changed to a combined oral contraceptive pill containing 50 μg ethinyl estradiol per day, continuous oral contraceptive pill therapy, or a progestin product at doses effective for ovulation inhibition; or (iii) elect to use nonhormonal forms of contraception. The first option is unattractive because she has been controlled on therapy. The second option is a better option, but the patient must be monitored for both signs and symptoms of too much estrogen exposure and breakthrough bleeding, which may indicate lowered estrogen levels or decreased efficacy. The third option is not appropriate due to the higher rates of perfect and typical use failure with this contraceptive choice, but it can be used as a second form of contraception. It should be noted lamotrigine's concentrations can be affected by ethinyl estradiol in combined contraceptive methods.

Chronic Hypertension in Pregnancy

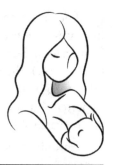

Kimey Ung and Elizabeth Yi

CHAPTER

22

LEARNING OBJECTIVES

1. Compare the criteria for diagnosis of both mild and severe chronic hypertension in pregnancy.

2. Identify the common maternal and fetal complications of chronic hypertension in pregnancy.

3. Describe the treatment options for management of mild chronic hypertension in pregnancy.

4. Summarize the treatment options for management of severe chronic hypertension in pregnancy.

I. Introduction

According to the Joint National Committee for Prevention, Detection, Evaluation, and Treatment of High Blood Pressure, chronic hypertension is defined as sustained elevation in systolic blood pressure ≥140 mmHg and diastolic blood pressure ≥90 mmHg.[1] In pregnancy, the diagnosis of chronic hypertension is made in the presence of hypertension before pregnancy or presence of hypertension before the 20th week of gestation. For those women diagnosed as having hypertension for the first time after 20 weeks' gestation, chronic hypertension becomes a diagnosis of exclusion and is given when the elevated blood pressure persists longer than the postpartum period (12 weeks postdelivery).[2,3]

Pregnancy complicated by chronic hypertension is associated with significant adverse maternal and fetal outcome. Expectant mothers with chronic hypertension face a three-fold increase in risk of perinatal mortality and approximately a two-fold increase in risk of placental abruption.[4] Increased rates of both fetal and maternal adverse outcomes, such as fetal growth restriction, small for gestational age (SGA) infants, premature birth, superimposed preeclampsia, and rate for cesarean section have all been reported.[2-4] Higher frequencies of these complications are seen in women with severe hypertension, those who develop superimposed preeclampsia, and/or those with long-standing hypertension with preexisting cardiovascular and renal disease.[4]

The prevalence of chronic hypertension among women of childbearing age increases significantly with age. According to the National Health and Nutrition Examination Survey data conducted by the National Center for Health Statistics (1988–1991), the prevalence of chronic hypertension was 0.6%–2.0% in women 19–29 years old and 4.6%–22.3% in women 30–39 years old.[5] The average prevalence of hypertension at that time was 5.1% in women 18–39 years of age. However, the average prevalence has increased to 6.1% in 1991–1994 and 7.2% in 1999–2000.[6]

Chronic hypertension has been reported to occur in approximately 5% of pregnancies.[4] Given the recent increase in the overall prevalence rate of chronic hypertension and the current demographic trend of childbearing at older age,[7] the incidence is expected to rise, further contributing to the economic burden of caring for the sick mothers and neonates.[4,5]

II. PATIENT CASE [PART 1]

G.G. is a 33-year-old gravida 3 para 2 who presents at her first obstetric appointment at 12 weeks' gestation. She was diagnosed with chronic hypertension 1 year ago when her blood pressures were consistently elevated above 140/100 mmHg. An angiotensin-converting-enzyme (ACE) inhibitor, benazepril (Lotensin) 10 mg/d, was started at that time by her physician. Her blood pressure values have been controlled since starting benazepril. Three years ago she was diagnosed with type 2 diabetes mellitus that is controlled by diet and exercise. Her family history is positive for type 2 diabetes, hypertension, and dyslipidemia. She denies use of alcohol and tobacco. Other than benazepril, she is taking no other medications. She has no allergies to drugs or food. Her current blood pressure is 120/74 mmHg, heart rate is 70 beats/min, and her respiratory rate is 13 breaths/min. Her electrolytes, a complete blood count, and renal function (serum creatinine 0.5 mg/dL) are within normal limits, and her urine is negative for ketones, glucose, and protein. She denies any symptoms of headaches, visual changes, abdominal pain, or edema. Clinically, there is no evidence of end-organ disease.

III. Clinical Presentation

Patients with chronic hypertension are usually asymptomatic with elevated blood pressure measurement as the only demonstrable finding. When hypertension is severe, patients may exhibit signs and symptoms signifying an acute insult to the vasculature of the target organs such as the eye, brain, heart, kidney and the peripheral arteries. Patients with comorbid diseases and/or those with end organ damage may also present with symptoms. However, the presence of end-organ damage represents a long-term complication of chronic hypertension and is not commonly associated with young women.

Patients may complain of visual disturbances, headaches, dizziness, and feelings of malaise. Fundoscopic examinations of patients with visual disturbances may reveal evidence of retinopathy characterized by the narrowing of the arterial diameter (Grade 1), arteriovenous nicking (Grade 2), cotton wool exudates and flame hemorrhages (Grade 3), or papilledema (Grade 4) in severe cases. Elevations in serum creatinine and microalbuminuria and/or proteinuria are seen in patients with acute or chronic compromise to the kidney function. Abnormal baseline electrocardiographic findings may reveal the presence of left ventricular hypertrophy. Patients with a history of cerebrovascular accident or transient ischemic attacks may complain of transient or residual functional deficits evident in neurologic examination. Frequent complaints of infections or presence of necrotic extremities may indicate presence of peripheral arterial disease.

Other objective and subjective findings, such as the presence of unexplained hypokalemia (primary aldosteronism), hypercalcemia (hyperparathyroidism), labile, paroxysysmal hypertension with headache, palpitation, pallor and perspiration (pheochromocytoma), and delayed or absent femoral arterial pulses (aortic coarctation), represent symptoms associated with hypertension with underlying disease.[1]

IV. Etiology and Classification

The reported incidence of fetal and maternal complications associated with chronic hypertension, along with degree of complications, is dependent on the etiology, severity of hypertension, and the degree of target organ damage.[3,5] Identification of etiology as well as classification of hypertension serve an important role in consideration of therapeutic interventions in the management of pregnant women with chronic hypertension.[5]

Chronic hypertension is subdivided as primary (essential or idiopathic) and secondary hypertension. Primary hypertension is, by far, the most common cause of chronic hypertension in pregnancy and is responsible for 90% of the cases.[1,5] The pathophysiologic feature of essential hypertension is vasoconstriction. Although various abnormalities in peripheral and central adrenergic, renal, hormonal, and vascular systems have been described, the exact mechanism contributing to the pathophysiology leading to vasoconstriction remains largely unknown.[8] Therefore, treatment is geared toward symptomatic management in attempts to prevent cardiovascular complications, primarily by using pharmacologic agents to decrease blood pressure by regulating fluid balance and vascular muscle tone.

Chronic hypertension can be secondary to one or more of the underlying disorders, such as renal disease (glomerulonephritis, interstitial nephritis, polycystic kidneys, renal artery stenosis), collagen vascular disease (lupus, scleroderma), endocrine disorders (diabetes with vascular involvement, pheochromocytoma, thyrotoxicosis, Cushing's disease, hyperaldosteronism), and vascular disease (coarctation of aorta).[2,3,5] Secondary hypertension accounts for approximately 10% of the cases in the general population with a higher prevalence rate in young women. Management of secondary hypertension is focused on treating the underlying disorder, in addition to symptomatic management of elevated blood pressure.

In pregnancy, chronic hypertension is further classified as mild or severe, depending on the blood pressure measurement.[3] Mild hypertension is defined as systolic or diastolic blood pressures of ≥140 or 90 mmHg, respectively. Severe hypertension is defined as systolic or diastolic blood pressures of ≥180 or 110 mmHg, respectively.

V. Maternal and Perinatal Complications

Chronic hypertension complicates pregnancy and increases the risk for adverse maternal and perinatal outcome. Complications include abruptio placentae, superimposed preeclampsia, premature birth, intrauterine growth restriction (IUGR), cesarean birth, and fetal demise.[2,3,9–13]

Abruptio placentae is the separation of the placenta from its site of implantation before birth and is a significant contributor of stillbirth (see Chapter 12, Abruptio Placentae). The fetal mortality is especially high when abruptio placentae is associated with preterm birth, but, even in those infants born at term, the perinatal mortality is reported to be 25-fold higher.[6] In expectant mothers with chronic hypertension, the risk for abruption is doubled,[4,14] with reported incidence as high as 10% in those with severe hypertension.[11,13] In patients with mild hypertension, the reported incidence ranges from 0.7% to 2.3%,[9,11,12,15] The presence of superimposed preeclampsia or history of abruptio placentae further increases the risk,[11,12,16] and rates as high as 12% have been reported in the setting of superimposed preeclampsia.[10]

Development of superimposed preeclampsia is a relatively common occurrence in chronic hypertension.[3] Clinically, hypertensive women have almost a four-fold risk of developing preeclampsia.[14] In patients with mild disease, superimposed preeclampsia occurs in approximately 10%–25% of all pregnancies.[11,12,15] In patients with severe hypertension, approximately half of the women have been found to develop superimposed preeclampsia with reported rates between 46% and 52%.[10,12,13] A multicenter randomized trial carried out by the Network of Maternal-Fetal Medicine Units of the National Institute of Child Health and Human Development evaluated 774 women with chronic hypertension. The overall rate of superimposed preeclampsia was reported to be 25%. This incidence was increased in those women who had chronic hypertension for more than 4 years (p = .007), those with history of preeclampsia (p = .02), and those with severe hypertension with diastolic blood pressure ≥110 mmHg when compared to those with diastolic blood pressure <100 mmHg (p = .01).[12]

Chronic hypertension triples the risk of perinatal mortality.[4] In a study of 337 pregnancies in 298 women with chronic hypertension, the rate of perinatal mortality was 45 in 1000 compared with 12 in 1000 in the general population (p <.001).[9]

There is an increased rate of premature birth and SGA infants in women with chronic hypertension.[9,10,17] The rate for premature birth is between 24% and 35%[9,10,12], with reported rates as low as 12% in patients with mild disease[9,10,12] and as high as 62%–70% in severe cases.[5,12,16] The incidence rate for SGA infants is 11%–15.5%,[9,10,12], with rates as low as 8% in patients with mild disease and as high as 31%–40% in severe cases.[5,10,13]

Development of superimposed preeclampsia is associated with the greatest perinatal morbidity, and most adverse perinatal outcomes related to chronic hypertension are seen in those who develop superimposed preeclampsia and in those with severe hypertension early in pregnancy.[10,12] Patients with superimposed preeclampsia are four times as likely to have preterm delivery (p <.001), twice as likely to experience perinatal death (p = .02), and four to five times as likely to have an infant with ventricular hemorrhage (p <.01) compared with those patients without superimposed preeclampsia.[12] In addition, those women with superimposed preeclampsia have increased risk of having SGA infants (odds ratio 2.3; 95% confidence interval 1.85–2.84)[18] and are more likely to deliver earlier than 32 weeks than women without superimposed preeclampsia.[10] In a study of 44 pregnant women with severe hypertension in the first trimester, a subgroup analysis of patients who developed superimposed preeclampsia revealed significantly higher rates of perinatal morbidity and mortality in comparison with those with just severe hypertension.[13] The trial was not designed to study this subset of patients and the power of the study was too small to make any generalizations, but a definite trend of worsening fetal outcome was observed. In comparisons of patients with and without superimposed preeclampsia, the rate of prematurity and SGA infants was 100% versus 38% and 78% versus 15%, respectively. All perinatal mortality was seen in the setting of superimposed preeclampsia (48%).

Although it is true that, given the short time frame of pregnancy, the risk for developing cardiovascular complications such as myocardial infarct, heart failure, stroke, and kidney disease is low, the natural physiologic changes that accompany pregnancy can become pathogenic in women with chronic hypertension, increasing the risk for maternal cardiovascular complications. This is especially true in those women with severe hypertension and those with preexisting comorbid disease or end organ damage, such as renal insufficiency, diabetes with vascular compromise, and left ventricular dysfunction.[2,5] Physiologic changes such as an increase in blood volume and decrease in vascular tone with a resulting decrease in colloid oncotic pressure are a natural occurrence in pregnancy necessary to accommodate the growing fetus in the womb.[3] In expectant mothers with chronic hypertension, such changes can burden the already compromised cardiovascular system affected by hypertensive disease and can exacerbate preexisting vascular conditions.[3] These mothers are predisposed to developing complications such as congestive heart failure, worsening renal function leading to acute renal failure, retinopathy, pulmonary edema, and cerebral hemorrhage.[2,3] In patients with moderate to severe renal insufficiency at conception (serum creatinine >1.4 mg/dL), hypertensive disease can lead to acceleration of maternal renal disease with potential need for dialysis along with increased risk for fetal loss.[3,16] In the presence of uncontrolled blood pressure, the relative risk of fetal loss is increased 10-fold in patients with renal insufficiency compared to those with well-controlled hypertension or pregnancy without hypertension.[3,16]

VI. Screening and Diagnosis

The diagnosis of hypertension is based on the blood pressure at the initial visit, whether the patients are on antihypertensive medications or not.[5] Patients are classified as having mild hypertension if they have systolic or diastolic blood pressures ≥140 mmHg or 90 mmHg, respectively, and severe hypertension if their systolic or diastolic blood pressures are ≥180 mmHg or 110 mmHg, respectively.[3]

An in-depth history, including the duration of hypertension, use of antihypertensive medications, types of and response to drug therapy, along with a medical, family, and obstetric history, is obtained to assess the risk and severity of the disease.[5] The obstetric history should identify maternal and neonatal outcomes, especially with regard to superimposed preeclampsia, abruptio placentae, preterm delivery, SGA infants, and intrauterine fetal demise.

Baseline laboratory tests and physical examinations are focused on the organ systems likely to be affected by chronic hypertension or likely to deteriorate during pregnancy. Laboratory tests include serum creatinine, blood urea nitrogen, urinalysis, urine protein/creatinine ratio to screen for proteinuria, electrolytes, and a complete blood count.[2,3,5]

Although the random urine protein/creatinine ratio in a nonpregnant patient population is a reliable estimator of 24-hour urine protein excretion levels, this has not been proven to be true in pregnancy. Therefore, to obtain a reliable estimate of total protein excretion, a 24-hour urine collection is recommended, especially in those patients suspected of having significant proteinuria or in the setting of superimposed preeclampsia.[19,20] Physical examination includes optic fundus examination; auscultation of carotid, abdominal, and femoral bruits; palpation of thyroid gland; examination of heart and lung; abdominal examination for enlarged kidney, masses, or abnormal aortic pulsation; palpation of lower extremity for edema and pulses; and neurologic assessment.[1]

In patients with poor blood pressure control, significant proteinuria, or long-standing hypertension, additional tests, such as chest x-ray, electrocardiography, echocardiography, ophthalmologic examination, and renal ultrasonography, might be required to evaluate for the presence of target organ damage involving the heart (left ventricular hypertrophy, angina, history of myocardial infarct, prior coronary revascularization, congestive heart failure), brain (history of stroke or transient ischemic attack), kidney (nephrosclerosis, chronic kidney disease), peripheral arterial vasculature, and the eye (retinopathy).[2,3] Abdominal protection is needed to prevent radiation exposure to the fetus if chest x-rays are performed.[21]

Young women with hypertension are more likely to have secondary hypertension.[2,3] Therefore, secondary causes should be excluded, especially if the patient presents with severe hypertension early in pregnancy, or if she has symptoms. The presence of pheochromocytoma in particular should be excluded as this disease is associated with high morbidity and mortality.[3] Patients with pheochromocytoma can present with paroxysmal severe hypertension with headaches, hyperglycemia, sweating, frequent hypertensive crisis, seizure disorders, and anxiety attacks.

In pregnancy, a physiologic decrease in blood pressure usually begins at the end of the first trimester and returns to its prepregnancy state in the third trimester.[3,4] In women with chronic hypertension, this effect may be exaggerated and the diagnosis of chronic hypertension may be masked during this period. As many as 50% of patients with mild hypertension will have normal blood pressure during weeks 20–26 of gestation.[11] Therefore, chronic hypertension may be difficult to detect in women with previously undiagnosed disease who begin prenatal care after 20 weeks' gestation. Moreover, it also will be difficult to differentiate worsening chronic hypertension from the development of preeclampsia or superimposed preeclampsia.

The diagnosis becomes more challenging in the presence of proteinuria along with elevated blood pressure findings. Worsening of undiagnosed renal impairment cannot be easily differentiated from new onset proteinuria that may be suggestive of superimposed preeclampsia or preeclampsia. In these patients, baseline laboratory values should include uric acid level, platelet count, liver function tests, serum creatinine, complete blood count, and a 24-hour urine collection to screen for superimposed preeclampsia and preeclampsia. These laboratory values may also be useful for diagnosing the HELLP (*hemolysis, elevated liver enzymes, and low platelets*) syndrome (see Chapter 11, Gestational Hypertension, Preeclampsia, and Eclampsia).[3]

Most adverse maternal and perinatal outcomes in chronic hypertension are often observed with the development of superimposed preeclampsia. It is important to distinguish superimposed preeclampsia from worsening chronic hypertension, as severe superimposed preeclampsia may warrant immediate hospitalization requiring IV administration of antihypertensive agents to control blood pressure and continuous fetal monitoring. Severe superimposed preeclampsia may be an indication for delivery in patients with gestational age >28 weeks.[9]

Onset of superimposed preeclampsia should be suspected in expectant mothers with chronic hypertension who have worsening blood pressure, especially if they present with clinical symptoms such as severe headache, visual disturbances, generalized edema, pulmonary edema, and oliguria.[3] In general, the diagnosis of superimposed preeclampsia is likely if there is new onset of proteinuria (300 mg/24 hours) in women diagnosed with hypertension early in pregnancy (<20 weeks) without baseline proteinuria.[2,5] In women with baseline proteinuria, this diagnosis is given for a sudden increase in proteinuria, development of thrombocytopenia (platelets <100,000 cells/mm^3), and/or presence of elevated alanine aminotransferases or aspartate aminotransferases to abnormal levels.[2] Diagnosis also is suspected in patients with an exacerbated increase in hypertension to the severe range (systolic ≥180 mmHg or diastolic ≥110 mmHg) when their blood pressure was previously well controlled on antihypertensive agents, and for symptomatic patients with exacerbated hypertension with or without a significant increase in liver enzymes (unrelated to methyldopa) or thrombocytopenia.[2] Although uric acid levels are nonspecific to superimposed preeclampsia and are increased in patients with renal dysfunction, elevated uric acid levels of ≥5.5 mg/dL may be helpful in confirming the diagnosis of superimposed preeclampsia.[3]

VII. Guidelines

American College of Obstetricians and Gynecologists summary of recommendations[3]:

1. "ACE Inhibitors are contraindicated in pregnancy and are associated with fetal and neonatal renal failure and death. (Level A)"

2. "Antihypertensive therapy should be used for pregnant women with severe hypertension for maternal benefit. (Level B)"

3. "Methyldopa and labetalol are appropriate first-line antihypertensive therapies. (Level B)"

4. "Treatment of women with uncomplicated mild chronic hypertension is not beneficial because it does not improve perinatal outcome. (Level B)"

5. "The beta-blocker atenolol may be associated with growth restriction and is not recommended for use in pregnancy. (Level B)"

6. "Women with chronic hypertension should be evaluated for potentially reversible etiologies, preferably prior to pregnancy. (Level C)"

7. "Women with long-standing hypertension should be evaluated for end-organ disease, including cardiomegaly, renal insufficiency, and retinopathy, preferably prior to pregnancy. (Level C)"

8. "When chronic hypertension is complicated by IUGR or preeclampsia, fetal surveillance is warranted. (Level C)"

Definitions:

Level A: recommendations based on good and consistent scientific evidence

Level B: recommendations based on limited or inconsistent scientific evidence

Level C: recommendations based on consensus and expert opinion

VIII. Treatment

A. Goals and Management

Chronic hypertension in pregnancy is associated with both maternal and perinatal morbidity and mortality. The goal of treatment is to reduce maternal cardiovascular risks and optimize fetal and neonatal outcomes.

The blood pressure goal and approach to therapeutic management of chronic hypertension is different in pregnancy than in nongravid patients. In the general population, the treatment is aimed at preventing cardiovascular events while minimizing potential adverse side effects of antihypertensive agents. In pregnancy, the duration of treatment is very short and the exposure of the fetus to hypertensive medication is unavoidable, raising additional concerns for safety and effectiveness of therapeutic intervention.

The target blood pressure goal in pregnancy is higher than in the general population. Although severe vasoconstriction from hypertension itself can lead to decreased uteroplacental perfusion that contributes to SGA infants,[10] there is a theoretical concern that lowering blood pressure to normal physiologic levels using therapeutic agents might also cause decreased placental perfusion that compromises fetal growth.[2,3,22] Pregnant women with chronic hypertension may require higher sustained blood pressure to maintain adequate uteroplacental blood flow than normotensive obstetric patients.[22] As a result, the target blood pressure goals in chronic hypertension in pregnancy are relatively higher in comparison with the general public; the desired blood pressures are systolic 140–150 mmHg and diastolic 90–100 mmHg

(Table 1). Patients with end-organ damage or comorbid disease states have a more stringent target goal range. Despite the lack of scientific data examining patients with comorbid diseases, these patients are treated aggressively, targeting a goal of ≤140/90 mmHg because they are at higher risk for adverse maternal and perinatal outcomes.[5]

There are various guidelines on how to treat pregnant patients with preexisting hypertension. Due to lack of randomized trials in this area, most of the recommendations are based on consensus and expert opinion. There is quite a discord among clinicians about when to initiate antihypertensive medications, what the optimal blood pressure goals should be, and which antihypertensive medications should be used during pregnancy. The current practices and recommendations are based on consensus statements and expert opinions (see Table 1).

An initial evaluation of patients with chronic hypertension should be done at preconception or at least before 20 weeks' gestation. The risk assessment is conducted to ascertain the severity of hypertension, etiology of the disease, and presence of comorbid disease and/or end-organ damage.[2,3,5] Ideally, women with long-standing hypertension or severe hypertension should begin management before conception. Antihypertensive medication also should be reviewed to prevent drug-induced embryo-fetal toxicity and, if necessary, changed to agents known to be low risk in pregnancy.[2] Agents such as ACE inhibitors and angiotensin receptor blockers (ARBs) should be avoided in pregnancy because they are known to cause fetal renal toxicity, leading to oligohydramnios, anuria, pulmonary hypoplasia, and growth retardation.[4] Therapeutic intervention for patients with severe and uncontrolled hypertension, who are at highest risk for poor maternal and fetal outcomes, should be optimized before conception.

Table 1. Treatment Management

Low Risk: Mild Hypertension
- Implement nonpharmacologic intervention
- In newly diagnosed patients, consider delay in initiation of pharmacologic therapy
- In patients already on antihypertensive medications, consider discontinuation or reduction in dose of antihypertensive mediation in the absence of target organ damage
- In all cases, therapy should be reinstituted or started if blood pressures exceed 150–160 mmHg systolic, and/or 100–110 mmHg diastolic
- Natural physiologic decline in blood pressures usually occurs during second trimester
- Blood pressures should be monitored closely at each prenatal visit, especially during third trimester when blood pressures will start to rise back to prepregnancy levels

High Risk: Severe Hypertension
Goals: SBP 140–150 mmHg, DBP 90–100 mmHg
- Initiate pharmacologic therapy and encourage lifestyle modifications in diet and level of activity
- If currently on medication, evaluate medication for safety in pregnancy and change if necessary
- Optimize dose to control blood pressure, may require hospitalization
- Assess for target organ damage

Target organ damage
- Goals: SBP <140 mmHg, DBP <90 mmHg
- Hypertension may exacerbate target organ damage during pregnancy in women with renal disease, diabetes with vascular disease, those with left ventricular failure

DBP = diastolic blood pressure, SBP = systolic blood pressure.
From National High Blood Pressure Education Program,[2] ACOG,[3] and Sibai BM.[5]

Classification of chronic hypertension is markedly different in pregnancy than in nonpregnant individuals. Patients are stratified according to blood pressure control and presence of end-organ target damage as either *low risk* or *high risk* for management and counseling purposes.

B. Risk Assessment

1. Low Risk

The majority of women with chronic hypertension have mild to moderate, uncomplicated disease. In the absence of target end-organ damage, these women are at low risk for adverse outcomes. Pregnancy outcomes are similar in low-risk women who do not go on to develop superimposed preeclampsia when compared with the general obstetric population.[11,15,23,24] Most women with mild hypertension have good outcomes, as the risk for complications related to chronic hypertension are mostly associated with the presence of severe hypertension or the development of preeclampsia.[2,11,13]

Several studies have shown that discontinuation of antihypertensive therapy during the first trimester does not further predispose these patients to preeclampsia, abruptio placentae, preterm delivery, or perinatal death when compared to treated patients.[11,15,24] The use of antihypertensive medications has led to a reduction in the rate of exacerbation of hypertension, but this benefit was not translated into improved perinatal outcome.[15] Sibai et al conducted a randomized controlled trial consisting of 263 pregnant patients with mild hypertension who were randomized at 6–13 weeks' gestation to methyldopa, labetalol, or no treatment. The treatment group had significantly lower systolic and diastolic blood pressure, but this finding did not translate into improved perinatal outcome. There was no statistical difference in the incidence of superimposed preeclampsia (18.4%, 16.3%, 15.6%, respectively), abruptio placentae (1.1%, 2.3%, 2.2%, respectively), preterm delivery (23.5%, 11.6%, 10%, respectively), IUGR, or perinatal mortality. In another study, 145 pregnant women with mild hypertension were randomized to receive either no treatment or nifedipine.[24] There was no difference in the incidences of SGA infants, preterm delivery, cesarean section, and mean birthweight between the two groups. The investigators recommended delaying treatment until hypertension became more severe.

However, treatment may not be necessary because there is a natural physiologic decline in blood pressure that usually begins during the second trimester.[2] A study examining 211 pregnant patients with mild chronic hypertension found that up to 50% of patients reported a decrease in blood pressure during the second trimester and 66% had increased their blood pressure during the third trimester back to their baseline.[11] Thus, close monitoring of blood pressure is still required because it will eventually start to rise in the third trimester.

For the most part, studies conducted to determine benefits of antihypertensive agents in this low-risk group on perinatal outcome have been inconclusive. There is no proven evidence that short-term pharmacologic treatment results in improved perinatal outcome.[4,15,24] The Agency for Healthcare Research and Quality conducted a review of the published literature from 1947 to February 1999 for data on the management of mild-to-moderate hypertension.[4] The study concluded that "the evidence base regarding pharmacologic management of chronic hypertension during pregnancy is too small to either prove or disprove moderate to large benefit (>20% improvement) of antihypertensive therapy."[4]

The current recommendation for management of mild chronic hypertension is to delay initiation of pharmacologic therapy in those patients currently not on antihypertensive medication or, if the patient is receiving therapy, to decrease the dose or stop the drug therapy. The basis for initiating antihypertensive therapy is an attempt to lower the risk of progression to severe hypertension. Medication therapy should be initiated or reinstituted if blood pressures are elevated to 150–160 mmHg/90–100 mmHg or there is a presence of target organ damage.[2] Monitoring for early signs of preeclampsia and fetal growth restriction is necessary with serial ultrasound examinations.

2. High Risk

Women with severe chronic hypertension are markedly more susceptible to maternal and neonatal complications. This high-risk group includes patients who have systolic blood pressures of ≥180 mmHg or diastolic pressures ≥110 mmHg, have target organ damage, or secondary hypertension.[5]

Preexisting diseases, such as renal insufficiency (serum creatinine >1.4 mg/dL), diabetes with vascular involvement, severe collagen vascular disease, cardiomyopathy, coarctation of aorta, or history of cerebrovascular accident or myocardial infarct, are associated with both poor maternal and perinatal outcomes and, in some instances, pregnancy may be contraindicated.[5] In patients with preexisting vascular disease, appropriate counseling regarding the potential risk of adverse outcome should be provided to assist in planning for the pregnancy. Pregnancy can exacerbate these vascular conditions and can lead to congestive heart failure, acute renal failure requiring dialysis, and possibly death.[5] Women with compromised renal function before conception are generally encouraged to complete childbearing while their renal function is still well preserved, because an increase in hypertension, high-grade proteinuria, and rapid progression to end-stage renal failure can occur.[25] The risk of acceleration to end-stage renal failure and possible need for hemodialysis is greatest in women whose serum creatinine is >2 mg/dL in the first trimester. Rates of maternal complications are dramatically increased for pregnant women with moderate-to-severe renal insufficiency, but fetal survival was reported to be as high as 93% in one small study.[25]

Severe hypertension also is associated with increased cardiovascular morbidity and mortality. Death from ischemic heart disease and stroke increases linearly and progressively, with elevated blood pressure from measurements as low as 115/75 mmHg. Mortality for both ischemic heart disease and stroke doubles for every 20 mmHg systolic or 10 mmHg diastolic rise in blood pressure.[2] In pregnancy, the risk of adverse outcome is greatest in women with severe hypertension, especially early in pregnancy.[10,13]

The incidence of superimposed preeclampsia and abruptio placentae is dramatically increased in severe hypertension with reported rates as high as 50% and 12%, respectively.[5,10,11,13] In one study of 44 pregnant patients with severe hypertension in the first trimester, the prevalence rate of prematurity, SGA infants, and perinatal mortality was reported to be 70%, 43%, and 25%, respectively, with the highest incidence in those patients who developed superimposed preeclampsia.[13] Pregnant women with uncontrolled severe hypertension also are at risk for complications, such as pulmonary edema, hypertensive encephalopathy, retinopathy, cerebral hemorrhage, retinopathy, and acute renal failure.[2,3,5]

There are no controlled studies examining the benefits of treatment in women with severe hypertension because of the potential risk to the mother and fetus. Given the acute risk of untreated severe hypertension, pharmacologic therapy is initiated for systolic blood pressures ≥180 mmHg and diastolic pressures ≥110 mmHg.

C. Nonpharmacologic Therapy

In the general population, lifestyle modifications have been shown to reduce blood pressure, prevent or delay the incidence of hypertension, enhance efficacy of antihypertensive agents, and decrease cardiovascular risk factors.[1] In pregnancy, however, there is a lack of clinical trials examining the efficacy of nonpharmacologic therapy affecting outcome in patients with chronic hypertension.[4] Nonetheless, many nonpharmacologic interventions, such as bed rest, limited activity, diet modification (eg, salt and protein intake restriction), stress reduction, and cessation of smoking and alcohol use, are recommended by many experts, although bed rest is not routinely recommended for women with chronic hypertension in the absence of complications.[2–5,7,14]

Use of tobacco and alcohol is strongly discouraged in pregnancy. Cigarette smoking has been associated with an increased risk for placental abruption and IUGR. Excessive alcohol consumption, in addition to its well-known embryo-fetal toxicity, can aggravate maternal hypertension, increasing the risk for adverse outcome.[2] (See Chapter 2, Developmental Toxicity and Drugs, for the entire range of embryo-fetal toxicities from cigarette smoking and alcohol.)

A nutritionist should be consulted regarding weight gain and sodium intake. Although data on pregnant women are scarce, patients are advised to restrict their sodium intake to 2.4 g/d. Patients are encouraged to follow a diet rich in fruits, vegetables, low-fat dairy products with reduced cholesterol as well as saturated and total fat, and rich in potassium and calcium.[2]

Although regular exercise is beneficial in management of hypertension in nongravid women, there are no data on its safety in pregnancy. In view of the theoretical concerns to maintain adequate placental blood flow in pregnant women already at risk for preeclampsia, patients should be advised to refrain from aerobic exercise or any vigorous activity and to restrict activity at work and home.[2]

Obesity predisposes patients to develop chronic hypertension, and it may be a risk factor for the development of superimposed preeclampsia. However, there is no evidence that limiting weight gain leads to decreased occurrence of superimposed preeclampsia. Therefore, weight reduction, even in obese pregnant women, should not be recommended during pregnancy.[2]

D. Pharmacologic Therapy

Before initiation of pharmacologic therapy, clinicians must weigh the potential benefits to the mother and possible harm to the fetus. Antihypertensive therapy should be initiated based on maternal and fetal risk assessment. The severity of blood pressures, presence of target organ damage, potential for drug-induced developmental toxicity, and gestational age must be considered before initiation of therapy.

There are limited data in the literature examining the potential for developmental toxicity of antihypertensives. Most of the evidence to date relies solely on case reports and state medical registries data.[28] Although there is a lack of randomized clinical trials comparing antihypertensives in pregnancy, large clinical experiences and expert opinions guide therapeutic recommendations on the treatment of chronic hypertension during pregnancy.[2,3,5]

In the management of women with mild chronic hypertension, antihypertensives should be discontinued or the dose decreased, based on expert opinion.[5] Studies have shown that women with mild chronic hypertension who do not develop superimposed preeclampsia will have outcomes similar to the general obstetric population.[9,11,15] It is prudent to discontinue these medications and limit the exposure of the embryo-fetus to potentially toxic agents if there are no proven benefits. Discontinuation of antihypertensives in this low-risk population does not affect the rates of preeclampsia, abruptio placentae, or preterm delivery.[11,15] However, if blood pressures become elevated above 150–160 mmHg systolic or 100–110 mmHg diastolic, antihypertensive medications should be initiated because the patient is now at risk for developing severe hypertension.[2,3,5]

In severe hypertension, antihypertensive medications are essential because of the acute risk of stroke, congestive heart failure, or renal failure.[2,3] Gravid patients with uncontrolled mild-to-moderate hypertension with target organ damage are also vulnerable to similar adverse outcomes if blood pressures are not controlled adequately.[25] For initial therapy, hospitalization may be necessary to control critically high blood pressures (systolic blood pressures >180 mmHg and/or diastolic blood pressure >110 mmHg) with IV medications, such as hydralazine and labetalol (see Table 2). Once blood pressures have been adequately controlled, an oral antihypertensive drug can be started. For maintenance regimens, the oral antihypertensive therapies most commonly used are methyldopa, labetalol, or extended release nifedipine (Table 2). A summary of other antihypertensive drugs used during pregnancy is listed in Table 3.

1. Methyldopa

Methyldopa (Aldomet) is a centrally acting α-adrenergic agent that acts by decreasing sympathetic outflow to decrease blood pressure.[26] It is one of most common antihypertensive agents used in pregnancy because of its long record of use and safety pro-

Table 2. Recommended Drugs Used to Treat Chronic Hypertension in Pregnancy

Drug Therapy	Starting Dosages	Maximum Dosages
Acute therapy		
Hydralazine	5–10 mg IV every 20 min	30 mg
Labetalol	20–40 mg IV every 10–15 min	300 mg
Maintenance therapy		
Methyldopa	250 mg two to three times daily	2 grams daily
Labetalol	100–200 mg twice daily	2400 mg daily
Nifedipine	30 mg once daily	120 mg daily

From Sibai BM,[5] and Wickersham RM and Novak KK.[26]

Table 3. Risk Assessment of Antihypertensive Drugs Used during Pregnancy

Pharmacologic Agent	Risk Assessment

Calcium channel blockers
  Amlodipine (Norvasc)
  Diltiazem (Cardizem)
  Felodipine (Plendil)
  Isradipine (DynaCirc)
  Nicardipine (Cardene)
  Nifedipine (Adalat, Procardia)
  Nisoldipine (Sular)
  Verapamil (Calan)
	Animals: embryo and fetal toxicity
	Humans: no evidence of teratogenicity, limited first trimester data; do not appear to cause developmental toxicity when used in the second and third trimester; broad clinical experience with nifedipine XR use for severe hypertension and nifedipine IR for tocolysis; appear to be relatively safe

Peripheral vasodilators
  Hydralazine (Apresoline)
  Minoxidil (Loniten)
	Animals: no data with hydralazine, but minoxidil is teratogenic at high doses
	Humans: limited first trimester data prevent assessment; hydralazine in the second and third trimesters is relatively safe, but neonatal thrombocytopenia is a risk with chronic use; maternal hypotension and neonatal hypertrichosis are a concern with minoxidil

β-Adrenergic blocking agents
  Acebutolol (Sectral)[a]
  Atenolol (Tenormin)
  Betaxolol (Kerlone)
  Bisoprolol (Zebeta)
  Carteolol (Cartrol)[a]
  Metoprolol (Lopressor/Toprol)
  Nadolol (Corgard)
  Penbutolol (Levatol)[a]
  Pindolol (Visken)[a]
  Propranolol (Inderal)
  Timolol (Blocadren)
	Animals: dose-related embryo and fetal toxicity; no evidence of teratogenicity
	Humans: no evidence of teratogenicity; agents without ISA associated with reduced placental weight and IUGR; most pronounced with atenolol; effect is dose and time related with greatest reductions occurring when agents are used in the second and third trimesters; β-blockade in newborn is a risk when used close to delivery

Dual α/β-adrenergic blocking agents
  Carvedilol (Coreg)
  Labetalol (Normodyne/
    Trandate)
	Animals: embryo and fetal toxicity, but no evidence of teratogenicity
	Humans: no first trimester experience with carvedilol, and limited data for labetalol prevents assessment of risk; IUGR is potential concern in second and third trimesters but less than β-blockers without ISA; β-blockade in newborn is a risk when used close to delivery

Antiadrenergic agents: centrally acting
  Clonidine (Catapres)
  Guanabenz (Wytensin)
  Guanfacine (Tenex)
  Methyldopa (Aldomet)
	Animals: embryo and fetal toxicity documented, but not with methyldopa
	Humans: no evidence of human teratogenicity, but only methyldopa has first trimester experience; methyldopa has most data in second and third trimesters; limited data for other agents

α_1-Adrenergic blocking agents: peripherally acting
  Doxazosin (Cardura)
  Prazosin (Minipres)
  Terazosin (Hytrin)
  Tolazoline (Priscoline)
	Animals: fetal toxicity, but no teratogenicity
	Humans: limited data, no assessment of risk is possible

(continued)

Table 3. Risk Assessment of Antihypertensive Drugs Used during Pregnancy (Continued)

Pharmacologic Agent	Risk Assessment
Angiotensin-converting enzyme inhibitors Benazepril (Lotensin) Captopril (Capoten) Enalapril (Vasotec) Fosinopril (Monopril) Lisinopril (Prinivil, Zestril) Moexipril (Univasc) Perindopril (Aceon) Quinapril (Accupril) Ramipril (Altace) Trandolapril (Mavik)	**Animals:** embryo and fetal toxicity, but no teratogenicity **Humans:** possible increased risk of major defects, including cardiovascular and central nervous system defects when used during first trimester, confirmation required; use in second and third trimesters is associated with renal failure and anuria with resulting oligohydramnios and fetal hypotension associated with hypocalvaria and pulmonary hypoplasia (limb contractures, persistent patent ductus arteriosus, craniofacial deformation, neonatal death); neonatal anuria and hypotension resistant to volume expansion and pressor agents may occur; exchange transfusion and dialysis may be required
Angiotensin II receptor blocking agents Candesartan (Atacand) Eprosartan (Teveten) Irbesartan (Avapro) Olmesartan (Benicar) Telmisartan (Micardis) Valsartan (Diovan)	**Animals:** embryo and fetal toxicity, but no teratogenicity **Humans:** toxicity identical to that observed with ACE inhibitors in the second and third trimesters
Diuretics Bumetanide (Bumex) Ethacrynic acid (Edecrin) Furosemide (Lasix) Hydrochlorothiazide (Microzide, HydroDiuril) Spironolactone (Aldactone) Torsemide (Demadex) Triamterene (Dyrenium)	**Animals:** embryo and fetal toxicity, but no teratogenicity **Humans:** decreases plasma volume; may exacerbate hypovolemic state in superimposed preeclampsia; discontinue immediately if superimposed preeclampsia develops or if there is a suspicion of IUGR; avoid in gestational hypertension; risks to the newborn include possible hypoglycemia, thrombocytopenia, hyponatremia, or hypokalemia

ACE = angiotensin-converting enzyme, ISA = intrinsic sympathomimetic activity, IUGR = intrauterine growth restriction.
[a]Denotes β-adrenergic receptor blockers with ISA activity.
From Wickersham RM and Novak KK,[26] and Briggs GG, et al.[28]

file. Stable uteroplacental blood flow and fetal hemodynamics have been documented in several reports.[27,28] There have been only a few reports of adverse neonatal effects from maternal use of methyldopa and no association of any congenital malformations.[28] Despite its common use, methyldopa has its drawbacks. Methyldopa is often used in patients with mild chronic hypertension, but it can be ineffective in severe hypertension. It has low potency, dosed multiple times daily, and possibly can increase liver function tests. Adverse side effects include dizziness and sedation, which usually begin at the start of therapy and will eventually subside, but may return at increasing doses.[26] Many patients may be intolerant of these side effects and may need to be switched to another agent, such as labetalol. The starting doses of methyldopa are 250 mg orally 2–3 times daily, and dosage is increased to a maximum of 2 grams daily.[26]

2. Labetalol

Labetalol (Trandate) is an α/β-adrenergic blocking agent commonly used to treat severe hypertension during pregnancy.[26] Intravenous labetalol is used to lower blood pressures acutely and can be started at 20 mg, then incrementally increased to 40 mg then 80 mg IV every 10–15 minutes to a cumulative dose of 300 mg. The maximum effect usually occurs in 5 minutes and the duration of action can last from 45 minutes to 6 hours.[26] Intravenous labetalol was found to be as effective as IV hydralazine in lowering blood pressures in late-onset hypertension in pregnancy and found to be associated with less maternal hypotension, fewer cesarean deliveries, and no increase in perinatal mortality.[29] Oral labetalol is also used as maintenance therapy to treat severe hypertension during pregnancy.[3,5,28] Doses start at 100 mg twice daily and can be incrementally increased to a maximum daily dose of 2400 mg. Peak plasma levels occur in approximately 1–2 hours, and steady state is achieved after 3 days of repetitive dosing. The duration of effect depends largely on the dose but usually lasts 8–12 hours.[26]

Labetalol is moderately lipid-soluble, crosses the placenta, and produces cord serum concentrations approximately 40%–80% of maternal serum levels.[28] No teratogenicity has been documented in animal studies at oral doses 4–6 times the maximum recommended human dose; however, studies are lacking with first trimester use in humans. Reduced placental weight and IUGR can occur with use of labetalol, as well as with other β-blockers when used in the second and third trimesters. However, the benefit of labetalol therapy is far greater than the risk of severe hypertension on the developing fetus. Uteroplacental blood flow does not seem to be compromised with the decrease in maternal blood pressures. Labetalol should be used with caution in women with asthma and heart failure. If labetalol is used close to term or delivery, newborns should be monitored for 24–48 hours for signs and symptoms of β-blockade, such as bradycardia and hypotension.[28]

3. Hydralazine

Hydralazine (Apresoline) is a peripheral vasodilator that works directly on arterial smooth muscle causing reflex tachycardia which increases heart rate and cardiac output, eventually lowering blood pressures without compromising uterine blood flow.[26,28] It is the drug of choice for acute treatment of severe hypertension in pregnancy. Intravenous hydralazine can be given in doses of 5–10 mg every 20–30 minutes for a cumulative dose of 20 mg. The onset of action ranges from 10 to 20 minutes and lasts for approximately 3–6 hours. Repeat doses need to be separated by intervals of at least 20–30 minutes to avoid drug accumulation.[26] If desired blood pressures have not been reached with maximum dosages of hydralazine, IV labetalol may be used.

Although hydralazine readily crosses the placenta, causing fetal serum concentrations to be equal or greater than maternal levels, several reports have found it to be relatively safe in pregnancy.[28] The Collaborative Perinatal Project monitored 136 cases of maternal exposure to hydralazine during pregnancy, which found no defects with first trimester use. Adverse side effects include nausea, vomiting, tachycardia, flushing, headache, and tremors.[26] These adverse side effects could potentially mimic the signs and symptoms of preeclampsia.

4. Nifedipine

Nifedipine (Procardia, Adalat) is an oral dihydropyridine calcium channel blocker used during pregnancy for treatment of severe hypertension.[26] On occasion, immediate-release nifedipine can be used acutely to treat hypertension with oral doses of 10–20 mg every 30 minutes to a maximum dose of 50 mg.[5] The immediate-release formulation is no longer recommended by the U.S. Food and Drug Administration for treatment of acute hypertensive urgencies because of the risk of stroke or myocardial infarction in the general population.[26] However, it continues to be used in pregnancy for acute treatment of severe hypertension because the risk of an ischemic event secondary to atherosclerotic disease is unlikely in this patient population. Immediate-release nifedipine is commonly also used as a tocolytic agent for preterm labor. The extended-release formulation of nifedipine is used for maintenance therapy for severe hypertension with starting doses at 30 mg once daily to a maximum of 120 mg per day. Doses should be titrated every 7–14 days, and possibly earlier if blood pressures are closely monitored.[26] Hypotension and neuromuscular blockade can occur if nifedipine is used concurrently with magnesium sulfate because of the synergistic effect between these two drugs.[28]

Use of nifedipine during early pregnancy is controversial because animal studies in rats and rabbits noted teratogenic effects which include stunted fetuses, rib anomalies, cleft palate, and embryo and fetal deaths when these animals were exposed to doses 3.5–42 times the maximum recommended human dose.[28] However, a prospective multi-centered cohort study of 78 women with exposure to calcium channel blockers failed to find an increase rate of congenital malformations when compared with controls. Forty-four percent of these women used nifedipine during this study.[30] Although there are limited data on the safety of nifedipine during pregnancy, it does not appear to be a major teratogen in humans.[28]

5. Diuretics

Diuretics are common first-line agents to treat hypertension in the general population.[2] However, their use is controversial in pregnancy because diuretics can prevent normal plasma expansion. This reduction in plasma volume was not associated with any adverse effects on fetal outcome, but it can exacerbate the hypovolemic state of chronic hypertensive women who develop superimposed preeclampsia.[31] IUGR can occur because uteroplacental blood flow is compromised from the decrease in intravascular plasma volume. Animal studies have revealed no correlation between diuretics and congenital malformations.[28] The Collaborative Perinatal Project evaluated 233 women who had cardiovascular disorders with first trimester exposure to a thiazide or related diuretic and found an increase incidence of defects. However, the significance of these results is unknown because a causal relationship cannot be inferred.[28] In the Michigan Medicaid recipient surveillance study, 635 newborns were exposed during the first trimester to chlorothiazide (Diuril), chlorthalidone (Hygroton), or hydrochlorothiazide (HydroDiuril). There was no association between these diuretics and incidence of congenital defects.[28] Diuretics may be used during pregnancy in patients with excessive salt retention as a single agent or in combination with other agents. When used in combination with other agents, diuretics can potentiate the response to other antihypertensives. Cessation of diuretic therapy should occur immediately if superimposed preeclampsia develops or if there is a suspicion of fetal growth restriction.[5] Risks to the newborn include possible hypoglycemia, thrombocytopenia, hyponatremia, or hypokalemia.[28]

6. Angiotensin-Converting Enzyme Inhibitors and Angiotensin Receptor Blockers

ACE inhibitors block the conversion from angiotensin I to angiotensin II, whereas ARBs selectively block the binding of angiotensin II to AT_1 receptors.[26] Both classes of drugs are contraindicated during pregnancy because of their deleterious effects on the fetal and neonatal kidneys when used in the second and third trimesters.[28] High levels of angiotensin II are thought to be necessary to maintain glomerular filtration at low perfusion pressures. Without adequate perfusion, fetal hypotension and decreased renal blood flow occur, which can cause fetal anuria and oligohydramnios. Low levels of amniotic fluid can lead to pulmonary hypoplasia, hypocalvaria, limb contractures, persistent patent ductus arteriosus, craniofacial deformation, and possibly neonatal death.[32]

No teratogenic effects were seen in experimental animals exposed to ACE inhibitors at doses 9–60 times the maximum recommended human dose (MRHD).[28] Animal studies with ARBs at doses <10 times the MRHD revealed no teratogenicity, but exposure late in gestation was associated with severe fetal and newborn toxicity. Before 2006, there was no evidence that first trimester exposure to ACE inhibitors caused structural anomalies but, in that year, a retrospective study from the Tennessee Medicaid program using pharmacy-based data observed an increased risk of major defects (cardiovascular and central nervous system defects) when these agents were used early in pregnancy. The investigators concluded that it was best to avoid ACE inhibitors during all portions of pregnancy.[33] However, this type of study can only raise hypotheses and, because of the absence of supporting animal and human data, the findings are controversial and require confirmation.[28] The human pregnancy experience with ARBs is too limited to draw any conclusions. Nevertheless, women who have been exposed to ACE inhibitors or ARBs during the first trimester should be counseled as to the potential for structural defects.

7. β-Blockers

Some β-adrenergic receptor antagonists, including metoprolol (Lopressor) and atenolol (Tenormin), which lack intrinsic sympathomimetic activity, can cause IUGR and reduced placental weight.[28] The duration of therapy and the gestational age at which therapy was initiated determine the severity of growth restriction. Treatment that begins in the second trimester is associated with the greatest decrease in fetal and placental weight. Treatment beginning in the third trimester is associated with only a decrease in placental weight. Vascular resistance is increased in both the mother and fetus, which may contribute to the growth restriction.[28] Several other β-blockers, such as pindolol (Visken), acebutolol (Sectral), and the α/β-blocker labetalol, have more favorable effects on birth weight. In general, these agents should be reserved in women where the benefits outweigh the risk of growth restriction (eg, cardiomyopathy or arrhythmias). Newborns should be observed closely for signs and symptoms of β-blockade, such as bradycardia and hypotension, during the first 24–48 hours after birth.

IX. PATIENT CASE [PART 2]

The patient's blood pressure is well controlled on benazepril at 120/74 mmHg at her first trimester prenatal visit. She is considered to have low-risk chronic hypertension during pregnancy because her blood pressures are well below 180/110 mmHg, there is no history of prenatal loss, and she has no evidence of end-organ disease. G.G. will be educated about nutritional requirements, appropriate weight gain during pregnancy, and the need to restrict sodium in her diet to a maximum of 2.4 grams per day. She also will be advised to avoid tobacco and alcohol, which not only will cause detrimental effects on the functional and developmental growth of the fetus, but also can aggravate maternal hypertension. Benazepril should be discontinued at this time because of the possible adverse effects on the embryo-fetus. However, G.G. should be counseled on the potential risk because her embryo was exposed during the first trimester. She may not need any antihypertensive medications during the first and second trimesters because of the normal physiologic decline of blood pressure during these periods of pregnancy.

Early signs of preeclampsia and fetal growth restriction will be monitored at each subsequent prenatal visit, as well as monitoring her blood pressure. If possible, she also should monitor her blood pressures at home. If her blood pressures start to rise above systolic pressures of 150–160 mmHg and/or diastolic pressures above 100–110 mmHg, she may need to be restarted on an oral antihypertensive agent, such as methyldopa or labetalol, and be evaluated for possible preeclampsia if she develops symptoms.

G.G. should be educated about the signs and symptoms of preeclampsia. Preconception counseling should be emphasized because she has chronic hypertension and diabetes that should be in tight control before she tries to conceive again.

X. Summary

Chronic hypertension during pregnancy poses a great risk for maternal and neonatal morbidity and mortality. There is an increased risk for development of preeclampsia and abruptio placentae, which, in turn, can detrimentally affect the growth and well-being of the fetus. Adverse outcomes associated with chronic hypertension include IUGR, low birth weight, preterm birth, and possible perinatal death. The primary objective in treatment of chronic hypertension during pregnancy is to reduce maternal cardiovascular risks and optimize fetal and neonatal outcomes. These outcomes can be achieved through preconception counseling, early prenatal care, frequent blood pressure monitoring, intensive antepartum monitoring of the fetus, and appropriate therapeutic intervention.

XI. References

1. Chobanuab AV, Bakris GL, Black HR, et al. The seventh report of the Joint National Committee on Prevention, Detection, Evaluation, and Treatment of High Blood Pressure. *JAMA*. 2003;289:2560–2572.

2. National High Blood Pressure Education Program. Report of the National High Blood Pressure Education Program Working Group on High Blood Pressure in Pregnancy. *Am J Obstet Gynecol*. 2000;183(suppl):S1–S22.

3. American College of Obstetrician and Gynecologists. Chronic hypertension in pregnancy. *ACOG Practice Bulletin*. Number 29. July 2000. *Obstet Gynecol*. 2001;98: 177–185.

4. Agency for Healthcare Research and Quality. Management of chronic hypertension during pregnancy. Evidence report/technology assessment no.14. *AHRQ Publication No. 00-E011*. Rockville, MD: AHRQ, 2000.

5. Sibai BM. Chronic hypertension in pregnancy. *Obstet Gynecol*. 2002;100:369–377.

6. Cunningham FG, MacDonald PC, Gant NF, et al, eds. *Williams Obstetrics*. 22nd ed. New York: McGraw-Hill, 2005.

7. Ventura SJ, Abma JC, Mosher WD, et al. Estimated pregnancy rates by outcome for the United States, 1990–2004. *National Vital Statistics Reports*. Vol 56, Number 15. Hyattsville, MD: National Center for Health Statistics, 2008.

8. Beevers G, Lip G, O'Brien E. ABC of hypertension: the pathophysiology of hypertension. *BMJ*. 2001;322;912–916.

9. Rey E, Couturier A. The prognosis in pregnancy in women with chronic hypertension. *Am J Obstet Gynecol*. 1994;171:410–416.

10. McGown LM, Buist RG, North RA, et al. Perinatal morbidity in chronic hypertension. *Br J Obstet Gynaecol*. 1996;103:123–129.

11. Sibai BM, Abdella TN, Anderson GD. Pregnancy outcome in 211 patients with mild chronic hypertension. *Obstet Gynecol*. 1983;61:572–576.

12. Sibai BM, Lindheimer M, Hauth J, et al. Risk factors for preeclampsia, abruption placentae, and adverse neonatal outcomes among women with chronic hypertension. National Institute of Child Health and Human Development Network of Maternal-Fetal Medicine Units. *N Engl J Med*. 1998;339:667–671.

13. Sibai BM, Anderson GD. Pregnancy outcome of intensive therapy in severe hypertension in first trimester. *Obstet Gynecol*. 1986;67:517–522.

14. Zetterstrom K, Lindeberg SN, Haglund B, et al. Maternal complications in women with chronic hypertension: a population-based cohort study. *Acta Obstet Gynecol Scand*. 2005;84:419–424.

15. Sibai BM, Mabie WC, Shamsa F, et al. A comparison of no medication versus methyldopa or labetalol in chronic hypertension during pregnancy. *Am J Obstet Gynecol*. 1990;162:960–967.

16. Sibai BM. Diagnosis and management of chronic hypertension in pregnancy. *Obstet Gynecol*. 1991;74:451–461.

17. Catov JM, Nohr EA, Olsen J, et al. Chronic hypertension related to risk for preterm and term small for gestational age births. *Obstet Gynecol*. 2008;112:290–296.

18. Chappell LC, Enye S, Seed P, et al. Adverse perinatal outcomes and risk factors for preeclampsia in women with chronic hypertension: a prospective study. *Hypertension.* 2008;51:1002–1009.

19. Dumwald C, Merce B. A prospective comparison of total protein/creatinine ratio versus 24-hour urine protein in women with suspected preeclampsia. *Am J Obstet Gynecol.* 2003;189:848–852.

20. Papanna R, Mann LK, Kouides RW, et al. Protein/creatinine ratios in pre-eclampsia: a systemic review. *Obstet Gynecol.* 2008;112:135–144.

21. American College of Obstetricians and Gynecologists. Guidelines for diagnostic imaging during pregnancy. *ACOG Committee Opinion.* No. 299. *Obstet Gynecol.* 2004; 104:647–651.

22. Von Dadelszen P, Ornstein MP, Bull SB, et al. Fall in mean arterial pressure and fetal growth restriction in pregnancy hypertension: a meta-analysis. *Lancet* 2000;355:1332–1336.

23. Giannubilo SR, Dell'Uomo B, Tranquilli AL. Perinatal outcomes, blood pressure patterns and risk assessment of superimposed preeclampsia in mild chronic hypertensive pregnancy. *Eur J Obstet Gynecol Reprod Bio.* 2006;126:63–67.

24. Gruppo di Studio Ipertensione in Gravidanza. Nifedipine versus expectant management in mild to moderate hypertension in pregnancy. *Br J Obstet Gynaecol.* 1998;105:718–722.

25. Jones DC, Hayslett JP. Outcome of pregnancy in women with moderate or severe renal insufficiency. *N Engl J Med.* 1996;335:226–232.

26. Wickersham RM, Novak KK, eds. *Drug Facts and Comparisons.* St. Louis, MO: Wolters Kluwer Health, Inc., 2008.

27. Rosenthal T, Oparil S. The effect of antihypertensive drugs on the fetus. *J Hum Hypertens.* 2002;16:293–298.

28. Briggs GG, Freeman RK, Yaffe SJ. *Drugs in Pregnancy and Lactation: A Reference Guide to Fetal and Neonatal Risk.* 8th ed. Baltimore: Lippincott Williams & Wilkins, 2008.

29. Magee LA, Elran E, Bull SB, et al. Risks and benefits of beta receptor blockers for pregnancy hypertension: overview of the randomized trials. *Eur J Obstet Gynecol Reprod Biol.* 2000;88:15–26.

30. Magee LA, Schick B, Donnenfeld AE, et al. The safety of calcium channel blockers in human pregnancy: a prospective, multicenter cohort study. *Am J Obstet Gynecol.* 1996;174:823–828.

31. Sibai BM, Grossman RA, Grossman HG. Effects of diuretics on plasma volume in pregnancies with long-term hypertension. *Am J Obstet Gynecol.* 1984;150:831–835.

32. Shotan A, Widerhorn J, Hurst A, et al. Risks of angiotensin-converting enzyme inhibition during pregnancy: experience and clinical evidence, potential mechanisms, and recommendations for use. *Am J Med.* 1994;96:451–456.

33. Cooper WO, Hernandez-Diaz S, Arbogast PG, et al. Major congenital malformations after first-trimester exposure to ACE inhibitors. *N Engl J Med.* 2006;354:2443–2451.

QUESTIONS AND ANSWERS

1. How is chronic hypertension diagnosed during pregnancy?

2. How is mild chronic hypertension defined in pregnancy?

3. What are the maternal and fetal risks for patients with mild chronic hypertension diagnosed during pregnancy?

4. What are the treatment recommendations for patients with mild chronic hypertension during pregnancy?

5. What are the maternal and fetal risks for patients with severe chronic hypertension during pregnancy?

Answers

1. During pregnancy, chronic hypertension is diagnosed before 20 weeks' gestation with sustained blood pressures >140 mmHg systolic and/or >90 mmHg diastolic on two occasions at least 4 hours apart.

2. Women with mild chronic hypertension usually have systolic blood pressures of at least 140 mmHg and diastolic blood pressures of 90 mmHg and usually have no evidence of target end organ damage.

3. In the absence of target end organ damage, these women are at low risk for adverse outcomes. Pregnancy outcomes are similar in these low-risk women who do not go on to develop superimposed preeclampsia when compared to the general obstetric population. Most women with mild hypertension have good outcomes as the risk for complications related to chronic hypertension are mostly associated with the presence of severe hypertension or the development of preeclampsia.

4. Based on expert opinion, antihypertensives should be discontinued or tapered down. Studies have shown that women with mild chronic hypertension who do not go on to develop superimposed preeclampsia will have similar outcomes to the general obstetric population. It is prudent to discontinue these medications and limit the exposure of possible teratogens to the fetus, especially if there are no fetal and neonatal benefits. Discontinuation of antihypertensives in this low-risk population did not affect the rates of preeclampsia, abruptio placentae, or preterm delivery. Once blood pressure becomes elevated (≥180 mmHg systolic and/or ≥110 mmHg diastolic), antihypertensive medications, such as methyldopa or labetalol, should be initiated because the patient has now developed severe hypertension.

5. Expectant mothers with severe chronic hypertension face a three-fold increase in risk of perinatal mortality and approximately a two-fold increase in risk of placental abruption. Increased rates of both fetal and maternal adverse outcomes, such as IUGR, SGA infants, premature birth, superimposed

preeclampsia, and increased rates for cesarean section have all been reported. Higher frequencies of these complications are seen in women with severe hypertension, those who develop superimposed preeclampsia, and/or those with long-standing hypertension with preexisting cardiovascular and renal disease.

Infectious Disease

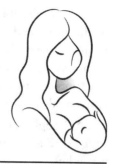

Stephanie R. Chao

LEARNING OBJECTIVES

1. Summarize the standards for routine antenatal screening for infectious diseases during pregnancy.

2. Describe recommendations for immunization of pregnant women, and the risks and benefits for a developing fetus from vaccination of the mother.

3. Select the appropriate antibiotic agent(s) for use during pregnancy based on the indication for use and available information on maternal and fetal safety.

4. Identify three common infections during pregnancy (urinary tract infections, chorioamnionitis, and endometritis) and be able to discuss their basic clinical presentation, pathophysiology, diagnoses, and prevention and treatment options.

5. Describe guidelines for prevention of certain perinatal infectious diseases (neonatal Group B streptococcal disease and postpartum wound infection).

I. Introduction

A discussion on infectious diseases during pregnancy involves the diagnosis and management, as well as the prevention, of certain conditions that may be present in nonpregnant women or which are unique to pregnancy. Because of certain proposed physiologic changes in cell-mediated immunity that occur normally in pregnancy, it is theorized that pregnancy can enhance the susceptibility to infection caused by certain microorganisms and increase the virulence of others. Such proposed alterations include a decrease in the absolute number of lymphocytes, a decline in helper T-cell numbers, and changes in the production of lymphokines such as interleukins and interferons. Further, anatomic variations that occur as a result of hormonal fluctuations or a growing gravid uterus may predispose a pregnant woman to higher rates of certain infections, such as urinary tract infections.

The management of certain infectious diseases during pregnancy may differ from management in the nonpregnant state. Antibiotic selection during pregnancy requires not only knowledge about the general principles of antimicrobial therapy, but also of the altered physiology of pregnancy and how this may alter the pharmacokinetics of medications, and the potential effects of any drug on the fetus. Further, consideration of how a particular condition may result in maternal and fetal complications is paramount as well. Untreated disease or failure to provide adequate prophylaxis for specific infections can lead to adverse fetal or neonatal complications, including congenital anomalies, cerebral palsy, or neonatal infection and septicemia.

Although a comprehensive review of all infectious diseases that may occur during pregnancy is beyond the scope of this chapter, the most common infections due to ascending contamination of the uterine cavity by normal vaginal or rectal flora are discussed. Additionally, early pregnancy screening for infectious diseases, immunization, and the prevention of such infections as neonatal Group B streptococcal disease and postpartum wound infection are reviewed.

II. PATIENT CASE [PART 1]

S.K., a 22-year-old nulliparous female, presents to her obstetrician at 8 weeks' gestation for a scheduled follow-up prenatal visit. Today she has no major complaints, except for some mild nausea in the evening controlled with promethazine, 25-mg suppositories. She reports generally feeling well. Vital signs are stable and she is afebrile. Physical and pelvic examinations are within normal limits, and personal and family history are noncontributory. She is 5'4", 140 pounds (63.6 kilograms) current weight, and 135 pounds (61.4 kilograms) pregravid weight, with no known drug allergies. Blood work and laboratories obtained before today's visit show a complete blood count (CBC) within normal limits, a negative endocervical culture for gonorrhea and chlamydia, nonreactive rapid plasma reagin (RPR), negative hepatitis B surface antigen, blood type O, Rh-positive status, and rubella antibody positive test results. She "opts-out" of HIV testing and provides documentation that she is up-to-date on her vaccinations, except for her annual flu shot.

III. Early Pregnancy Screening for Infectious Diseases

Question 1: What antenatal tests are considered routine for screening of certain infectious diseases early in pregnancy?

A. Routine Prenatal Screening

Routine tests performed early in pregnancy assist the clinician in detecting certain infectious diseases that can be detrimental to the health of the fetus or newborn. In asymptomatic women or those with a negative history, routine antepartum surveillance includes a pelvic examination during the initial prenatal visit, during which the cervix is inspected for genital herpes, venereal warts, trichomonas, or candidal infection. A Pap smear is performed, and cultures for gonorrhea and chlamydia may be obtained for high-risk patients. Guidelines from the Centers for Disease Control and Prevention (CDC) recommend chlamydia screening in all pregnant women,[1] whereas the American College of Obstetricians and Gynecologists (ACOG) and the U.S. Preventive Services Task Force (USPSTF) recommend testing only in women at high risk.[2,3] The high-risk patient is defined as any individual living in a geographic area in which Neisseria gonorrhoeae is highly-prevalent, and in those patients who are younger than 25 years of age with a history or current evidence of any sexually transmitted infection (STI), a new sexual partner within the preceding 3 months, or multiple sexual partners.[4]

Additional laboratory tests routinely performed at the first prenatal visit to screen for infectious diseases include a CBC to evaluate white blood cell count (WBC), urinalysis with microscopic examination and culture testing to detect asymptomatic bacteriuria, a serologic test for syphilis (RPR or venereal disease research laboratory), determination of immunity to rubella virus, and a hepatitis B surface antigen.[2] Other tests that may be performed in at-risk individuals are available, but not routinely recommended in all pregnant women. Assessment and testing for toxoplasmosis, tuberculosis, cytomegalovirus, herpes simplex virus, and varicella immunity may be obtained if indicated based on the patient's history, physical examination, geographic location, parental desire, or in response to public health guidelines. Screening for bacterial vaginosis (BV) is also available, although this remains controversial and is not considered routine.

B. Bacterial Vaginosis

BV is a common vaginal infection in women and results from an overgrowth of normal anaerobic bacteria in the vagina. In the United States, the prevalence of BV is estimated to be approximately 29% in women aged 14–49 years.[5] Symptomatic BV may cause a malodorous vaginal discharge and is diagnosed using Gram stain. Women may also have BV and be asymptomatic. In pregnancy, BV has been associated with increased rates of preterm birth, low birth weight, and premature rupture of membranes.[6] However, studies in general obstetric populations have not found that treatment of asymptomatic infection reduces the incidence of preterm labor or birth, despite using antibiotic therapies that are effective in eradicating BV.[7] Therefore, ACOG does not recommend routine screening and treatment for BV in asymptomatic U.S. populations.[8] Consideration may be given to screening for and treating BV in high-risk women, particularly those with prior preterm births; however, studies have shown conflicting results in this population as well.[6] For those women with symptomatic BV or who receive testing for BV and are found positive, standard antibiotic therapy with oral metronidazole (500 mg orally twice daily for 7 days) or clindamycin (300 mg orally twice daily for 7 days) is effective in eradicating BV in pregnant women. Some clinicians advise against the use of intravaginal or topical therapy for BV (eg, clindamycin 2% cream or metronidazole 0.75% gel), due to the rationale that they may be less effective against potential systemic, subclinical upper genital tract infection. Additionally, other clinicians recommend against using metronidazole in the first trimester due to data showing mutagenicity in bacteria and carcinogenicity in mice.[9] However, in human reports, no relationship between first-trimester exposure to metronidazole and harmful fetal effects has been found, including carcinogenic, mutagenic, or teratogenic effects. A suggested management plan may be to use oral clindamycin if treatment is desired in the first trimester, or to wait until the second trimester to use either of the two oral agents for eradication of BV.

C. Human Immunodeficiency Virus

Human immunodeficiency virus (HIV) antibody testing should be performed on all pregnant women with patient notification as part of the routine battery of prenatal blood tests, unless the patient declines. Refusals are documented in the prenatal records. It is also important for obstetricians to be aware of their own states' prenatal HIV screening guidelines and local laws regarding signed consent forms indicating permission for HIV testing. Routine testing for HIV (unless the patient refuses) is referred to as the "opt-out" approach recommended by ACOG to achieve higher rates of testing and hopefully provide the advantages of informed decision-making, appropriate medical management during pregnancy, and prevention of perinatal HIV-1 transmission to the fetus.[10] With appropriate antiretroviral management of HIV during pregnancy, the perinatal transmission rate can be decreased by nearly 70%, as demonstrated by the Pediatric AIDS Clinical Trials Group (PACTG) Protocol 076 (Table 1).[11] Although use of the intrapartum and postnatal components of the PACTG 076 zidovudine regimen is recommended for all HIV-1 infected pregnant women in the United States, regardless of their therapy throughout pregnancy, other regimens exist and may be considered based on patient population and risk factors. Readers interested in additional details are encouraged to seek the most recent recommendations from the CDC.

Table 1. Pediatric AIDS Clinical Trials Group 076 Zidovudine (ZDV) Regimen

Time of ZDV Administration	Regimen
Antepartum	Oral administration of 100 mg ZDV five times daily,[a] initiated at 14–34 wks' gestation and continued throughout the pregnancy.
Intrapartum	During labor, IV administration of ZDV in a 1-h initial dose of 2 mg/kg body weight, followed by a continuous infusion of 1 mg/kg body weight/h until delivery.
Postpartum	Oral administration of ZDV to the newborn (ZDV syrup at 2 mg/kg body weight/dose every 6 h) for the first 6 wk of life, beginning 8–12 h after birth.[b]

[a]Oral ZDV, administered as 200 mg three times daily or 300 mg twice daily, is used in general clinical practice and is an acceptable alternative regimen to 100 mg orally five times daily.
[b]Intravenous dosage for infants who cannot tolerate oral intake is 1.5 mg/kg body weight intravenously every 6 h.
From Centers for Disease Control and Prevention.[11]

ACOG also recommends repeat screening for chlamydia during the third trimester (ideally before 36 weeks of gestation) for women younger than 25 years, along with repeat testing for gonorrhea, syphilis, hepatitis B virus, and HIV. Repeat testing for these STIs may be considered in high-risk patients, as defined above, or in those who use illicit drugs, engage in high-risk sexual activity, or who exhibit signs and symptoms suggestive of acute STIs.[1]

IV. Immunization during Pregnancy

Question 2: What are the recommendations for immunization of pregnant women?

Immunization of pregnant women to prevent disease in the offspring is ideally done in the preconception period. If this is not feasible and immunizations are indicated during pregnancy, the benefits of immunization generally outweigh the theoretical risks of adverse effects to the fetus. Further, no evidence of risk exists with the vaccination of pregnant women with inactivated virus or bacterial vaccines or toxoids.[12] However, immunizations using vaccines containing live attenuated viruses are relatively contraindicated in pregnancy, because of the theoretical risk of transmission of the vaccine virus to the fetus. These include measles, mumps, rubella, yellow fever, and vaccinia. Certain vaccines are also generally not recommended for use in pregnancy because they are live attenuated vaccines or their safety has not been established; these include vaccines for human papillomavirus, poliomyelitis, varicella, bacille Calmette-Guérin, Japanese encephalitis, and zoster. Other vaccines not mentioned (eg, pneumococcal polysaccharide, hepatitis B virus, or meningococcal conjugate) may be given if indicated. It is important for the clinician to consider in susceptible patients the benefits of an efficacious vaccine, especially if the potential deleterious effects of the disease on the pregnancy outweigh the risks of exposure to the fetus. The most current recommendations and updates on immunization during pregnancy are obtained from the CDC (http://www.cdc.gov/vaccines/).

Vaccination with inactivated influenza vaccine is recommended for all pregnant women in any trimester, especially those who will be pregnant in the second and third trimesters during the influenza season (October–March), and to women at high risk for pulmonary complications regardless of their gestational age.[13] No adverse fetal effects have been demonstrated in those exposed to inactivated influenza immunization. However, FluMist®, the nasal-spray flu vaccine, is a live attenuated influenza vaccine, and is contraindicated in pregnancy.

For measles, mumps, and rubella, vaccination of susceptible women should be part of preconception or postpartum care. The risks of these diseases to the fetus or neonate may be significant; measles has been associated with a significant increase in spontaneous abortions and may cause malformations, mumps may increase first trimester spontaneous abortions, and rubella has been associated with high spontaneous abortions as well as congenital rubella syndrome.[13]

If a woman becomes pregnant within 4 weeks of immunization with a live attenuated vaccine, or if it is inadvertently given to a pregnant woman, she should be counseled about the potential effects on the fetus and the theoretical basis of this concern;

however, vaccination with these live-virus vaccines should not be regarded as a reason to terminate pregnancy.[12] The CDC, along with some manufacturers, have established a vaccine in pregnancy registry to monitor outcomes of women who receive certain vaccines 3 months before or any time during pregnancy; eligible patients and clinicians are encouraged to call (800) 986-8999.

V. Antibiotic Selection in Pregnancy

A. General Considerations

The goals of antimicrobial therapy during pregnancy are to reach or exceed desired minimum inhibitory concentrations in the affected tissue without incurring toxicity to the mother or her fetus. Such therapy is administered during pregnancy to treat maternal infection and to prevent neonatal disease. Antibiotic courses are usually short, but may be prolonged as well—as in the case of suppression therapy provided to prevent recurrent pyelonephritis in pregnancy. The selection of the appropriate agent requires careful consideration of several factors, including the potential pathogens and the emergence of resistant organisms (especially in the setting of empiric selection), as well as maternal considerations, such as risk of adverse reaction, history of anaphylaxis and allergies, and likelihood of compliance to the prescribed regimen. Additionally, proper antibiotic dosage selection requires knowledge of the physiologic changes that occur during pregnancy, and how that may alter the absorption, distribution, metabolism, and elimination of the drug. Finally, evaluation of the risks associated with drug exposure to the fetus is also paramount.

B. Potential Pathogens

Most infections encountered during pregnancy result from ascending contamination of the lower genital tract flora, most commonly by aerobic and anaerobic organisms. Common bacterial pathogens of this nature include gram-negative aerobes (*Escherichia coli*, *Klebsiella* species, *Proteus mirabilis*, *Enterobacter*, *Morganella morganii*, and *Gardnerella vaginalis*), gram-positive aerobes (Groups A, B, and D streptococci, *Streptococcus viridans*, enterococci, and *Staphylococcus aureus*), gram-negative anaerobes (*Bacteroides fragilis*, *Prevotella* species, *Fusobacterium* species, *Mycoplasma hominis*, *Ureaplasma urealyticum*, and *Mobiluncus* species), and gram-positive anaerobes (*Peptostreptococcus* species and *Clostridium perfringens*).[14]

Most antepartum infections require prompt treatment upon discovery, making the correct empiric selection of antibiotics prudent before the offending pathogen is identified or until the treatment goals are attained. This requires knowledge of the most common offending organisms and local resistance patterns. For instance, monotherapy with ampicillin or sulfonamides for urinary tract infections has become problematic in most geographic areas, and traditionally dosed penicillin has also become less effective for treating most pulmonary infections. Treatment or prevention of Group B streptococcal (GBS) disease in penicillin-allergic patients has also been complicated by increasing resistance to clindamycin and/or erythromycin.[15] This emphasizes the importance of requesting sensitivities for this organism in penicillin-allergic patients.

When antibiotics are administered late in gestation, such as during labor and childbirth, issues related to increasing resistant organisms in the neonate have become a concern as well. In a study of 5447 very-low-birth-weight (VLBW) infants born between 1998 and 2000, a marked decrease in neonatal GBS sepsis was found when compared to VLBW infants born between 1991 and 1993; however, there was also an increase in neonatal *E. coli* sepsis resistant to ampicillin.[16]

The use of broad-spectrum agents or multiantibiotic regimens may be required initially, especially when polymicrobial infections are suspected. After culture and sensitivity results are available, a narrower-spectrum or more cost-effective single agent may be substituted.

C. Pharmacokinetics of Antibiotics during Pregnancy

Like all medications, pregnancy can affect the pharmacokinetics and pharmacodynamics of both oral and parenteral antibiotics through a variety of mechanisms (see Chapter 4, Clinical Pharmacokinetics in the Pregnant Patient). Gradual increases in intravascular fluid volume and cardiac output ultimately lead to increased volume of distribution and dramatically improved clearance of drugs, especially those cleared by the kidneys. Combined with greater volume of distribution, increased hepatic metabolism, and sequestration of drugs into the fetal compartment, maternal drug levels of antibiotics in serum and tissue are approximately 10%–50% lower in late pregnancy and in the immediate postpartum period when compared to nonpregnant women.[17] Antibiotics that may be affected by this include penicillins, cephalosporins, aminoglycosides, and erythromycin. Most of these pharmacokinetic effects have not been extensively studied, and it is unclear what the clinical significance of these decreased drug levels in pregnancy may be. Monitoring serum drug concentrations may be necessary to ensure adequate treatment for some medications; however, measuring antibiotic serum levels may not provide additive benefit. Monitoring clinical improvement of symptoms is more important and more cost-effective; serum levels may be reserved for patients with renal or hepatic insufficiency, for medications with narrow therapeutic windows, or in cases of suspected toxicity or inefficacy. In a study of 56 immediately postpartum women with endometritis, women receiving pharmacokinetically dosed gentamicin were randomized into two groups: serum gentamicin levels determined after the third dose (control group), and serum levels determined only if renal dysfunction was evident or if the patient did not respond to therapy (study group).[18] There were no differences between the two groups with regard to length of hospital stay, duration of treatment, total cost of antibiotics, or readmission rate. However, the anticipated annual cost-savings of determining drug levels only in selected patients was $24,450. The conclusion from this study was that routine monitoring of gentamicin serum levels in otherwise healthy women with endometritis and normal renal function is not required.

D. Fetal Safety Concerns

All antibiotics are able to cross the placenta and enter the fetal circulation to some degree. Like any medication, antibiotics should only be given when the benefits to the mother or fetus outweigh the risks. In general, relatively few antibiotics are contraindicated in pregnancy, and most are considered compatible or have low risk of adverse fetal effects. Most of the commonly used antibiotics for infectious diseases are compatible with pregnancy, including penicillins, cephalosporins, clindamycin, vancomycin, and erythromycin (base, stearate, or ethylsuccinate).[9] Short courses of aminoglycosides at standard doses (eg, gentamicin, 1.5–2 mg/kg, given every 8 hours) are also compatible, but peak maternal serum concentrations should not exceed normal therapeutic levels. Since maternal drug concentrations are a major determinant of fetal concentrations, standard dosing may be preferred over extended-interval dosing because the latter regimen can result in supratherapeutic peak maternal serum aminoglycoside levels. Additionally, extended-interval dosing is typically only indicated in those patients with predictable volumes of distribution and drug clearance, conditions that can vary greatly during pregnancy.

A few antibiotics are either contraindicated or to be used with caution during pregnancy (Table 2); however, the gestational age of fetal exposure to the drug is an important consideration. Trimethoprim (as a single agent or in combination with sulfamethoxazole [Septra® or Bactrim®]) is a folate antagonist and should be avoided in the first trimester due to fear of fetal abnormalities. Sulfonamides should be avoided near term because of the potential for jaundice and hemolytic anemia in the newborn. Human data on nitrofurantoin exposure in the third trimester also suggest risk, and it should be avoided near term (ie, after 36 weeks' gestation) or if delivery is imminent secondary to induction of hemolytic anemia in glucose-6-phosphate dehydrogenase–deficient newborns and in newborns whose red blood cells are deficient in glutathione. This is a concern in newborns secondary to their glutathione instability. Tetracyclines are not recommended for use in the second and third trimesters (unless no other alternative exists) secondary to adverse effects on fetal teeth and bones. The use of fluoroquinolones during pregnancy is generally not recommended because of reports of arthropathy in immature animals after fluoroquinolone administration. Although no reports have confirmed this association in humans after in utero exposure, it is still advisable to avoid the use of fluoroquinolones in pregnancy, unless there are no acceptable alternatives. Even then, fluoroquinolones should be avoided in the first trimester. Dose-related toxicities with streptomycin and kanamycin have been reported, specifically eighth-cranial nerve and kidney damage in the mother and neonate; the prolonged use of these agents should be avoided throughout pregnancy.[9]

Antibiotics not mentioned in this chapter, especially those recently introduced to the market, are those not commonly used in pregnancy. Risk factors assigned to these agents by the U.S. Food and Drug Administration are typically category C (see Table 2 for definitions of risk categories). In situations in which the most commonly used antibiotics with fetal safety data are not indicated or not available for use, alternative antibiotic agents may be considered if the benefits of their administration outweigh any potential or unknown risks.

VI. PATIENT CASE [PART 2]

During S.K.'s prenatal visit, a urine specimen is collected by midstream clean-catch. She denies any urinary symptoms; however, dipstick analysis shows 1+

Table 2. Fetal Safety Concerns for Selected Antibiotics

Antibiotic	Recommendation Based on Human Data	Risk Category[a]	Fetal Effects/Comments
Aminoglycosides			
Amikacin	Low risk	C	None found
Gentamicin	Low risk	C	None found
Kanamycin	Risk is suggested	D	Eighth cranial nerve damage
Streptomycin	Risk is suggested	D	Eighth cranial nerve damage
Tobramycin	Low risk	C	None found
Azithromycin	Low risk; data are limited	B	None found
Aztreonam	No human data; animal data suggest low risk	B	None found
Cephalosporins[b]	Compatible	B	None found
Clindamycin	Compatible	B	None found
Erythromycin	Compatible	B	None found; excludes estolate salt, which is associated with maternal hepatotoxicity
Fluoroquinolones	Low risk; animal data suggest risk	C	Controversial use due to reports of arthropathy in immature animals; avoid use (especially in first trimester) unless there are no acceptable alternatives
Imipenem-cilastatin sodium	Low risk; data are limited	C	None found
Metronidazole	Low risk	B	None found; controversial use due to reports of mutagenicity in bacteria and carcinogenicity in rodents
Nitrofurantoin	Risk suggested in third trimester	B	Potential induction of hemolytic anemia in G6PD-deficient newborns
Penicillins[c]	Compatible	B	None found
Sulfonamides	Risk suggested in third trimester	C	Category D when used near term due to theoretical risk of kernicterus in newborns
Tetracyclines	Contraindicated	D	In second and third trimesters, adverse effects on fetal teeth and bones, and other congenital defects; associated with maternal hepatotoxicity
Trimethoprim	Risk is suggested; avoid in first trimester	C	Folate antagonist; may lead to possible teratogenic effects
Vancomycin	Compatible	B	None found

G6PD = glucose-6-phosphate dehydrogenase.

[a]FDA Risk Category definitions: A = controlled studies in women show no risk, B = either animal studies show no risk but there are no controlled studies in women, or animal studies showed risk that was not confirmed in women, C = either animal studies show risk but there are no controlled studies in women, or no available studies in women and animals, D = positive evidence of human risk, but benefits from use may be acceptable despite the risk, X = contraindicated in pregnancy.

[b]First, second, third, fourth generations.

[c]Natural, aminopenicillins, antistaphylococcal, antipseudomonal, extended-spectrum.

From Briggs GG, et al.[9]

glucose, negative blood, negative protein, 1+ nitrites, positive leukocyte esterase, negative red blood cell count (RBC), and negative WBC. Laboratory analysis of this second consecutive urine specimen revealed 50,000 colony-forming units (CFUs) per mL of *Escherichia coli*.

VII. Urinary Tract Infections

A. General Overview

Urinary tract infections (UTIs) are the most common medical complications of pregnancy and the most common bacterial infections in pregnancy, occurring in approximately 8%–10% of pregnancies and accounting for 10% of office visits by women.[19] They may be asymptomatic (asymptomatic bacteriuria) or symptomatic (acute cystitis or acute pyelonephritis) in nature, and may place the fetus at increased risk for such complications as preterm birth and low birth weight.

Females are at increased risk over males for development of UTIs, likely due to a shorter urethra in the female, ascending contamination of the external portion of the urethra by pathogenic bacteria from the vagina and rectum, entry of bacteria into the bladder during intercourse, and possible incomplete bladder emptying. During pregnancy, normal physiologic changes occur that further predispose the female to asymptomatic and symptomatic UTIs. Increases in plasma volume decrease urine concentration. Glycosuria has a higher incidence in pregnancy; this encourages bacterial growth in the urine. Hormonal effects caused by increased progestin and estrogen produce uterine atony, and a growing gravid uterus can obstruct the ureters. Beginning in the first trimester and peaking during weeks 22–24, approximately 90% of pregnant women develop ureteral dilatation or hydronephrosis of pregnancy. This may lead to increased bladder volume, decreased bladder tone, and decreased ureteral tone. Urinary stasis and uterovesical reflux occur, in addition to the aforementioned physiologic changes. These factors all contribute to a higher incidence of UTIs in pregnancy.[19]

The causative bacterial organisms for UTIs in pregnancy are the same as those found in nonpregnant women. They include gram-negative rods like *E. coli* (most commonly), *Proteus mirabilis*, *Klebsiella pneumoniae*, and *Pseudomonas aeruginosa*. Other organisms, which are less common, include GBS, *Enterococcus* species, *Staphylococcus saprophyticus*, *Gardnerella vaginalis*, and *Ureaplasma ureolyticum*.

B. Asymptomatic Bacteriuria

Asymptomatic bacteriuria (ASB) is the presence of bacteria in the urine of an asymptomatic patient. In women, it is defined as at least 10^5 CFUs of bacteria per milliliter of midstream clean-catch urine in two consecutive specimens obtained on separate occasions. The Infectious Diseases Society of America (IDSA) additionally defines ASB as a single catheterized urine specimen with at least 10^2 CFUs/mL of one bacterial species.[20] ASB occurs in approximately 4%–7% of pregnancies, and the frequency of bacteriuria increases with age, sexual activity, parity, the presence of genitourinary abnormalities, socioeconomic status, and comorbidities, such as diabetes and sickle cell trait.

Current recommendations from ACOG, IDSA, and the USPSTF state that pregnant women should be routinely screened for bacteriuria by urine culture at least once in early pregnancy[2]; this is typically done at the initial prenatal visit. Leukocyte esterase dipstick, nitrite dipstick, urinalysis, and urine Gram staining may be used for faster and less expensive screening; however, the increased number of false negatives and the poor predictive value of a positive test make these methods less effective. The urine culture is considered gold standard for detection of bacteriuria. Urine cultures that initially yield positive results should be repeated, because almost half of those women will not have significant bacteria on a second clean-catch midstream specimen. For women with persistent ASB, a repeat urine culture should be obtained during the third trimester, for confirmation or follow-up of bacterial eradication.

Subsequent development of symptomatic infection or pyelonephritis and higher rates of delivering premature or low-birth-weight infants have been reported in women with untreated ASB during pregnancy. In a Cochrane Database systematic review done in 2001, it was reported that treatment of ASB during pregnancy decreases the risk of subsequent pyelonephritis from 20%–35% to 1%–4%, when compared with no treatment or placebo.[21] Additionally, antimicrobial treatment for ASB decreases the frequency of low-birth-weight infants and preterm birth.

Based on the asymptomatic nature of the clinical presentation of ASB, it is not necessarily imperative to immediately treat; therefore, pregnant women identified with ASB should be treated with antibiotics based on the pathogen reported and sensitivity testing results. Resistance of common gram-negative rod bacteria found in urine to amoxicillin and sulfonamide preparations in many geographic areas has become a problem; therefore, oral therapy with cephalosporins (eg, cephalexin, 250–500 mg, two to four times daily), the combination agent amoxicillin-clavulanate (250 mg four times daily), or nitrofurantoin (50–100 mg four times daily) may be successful. These agents reach high enough concentrations in the urine. Additionally, consideration of the risks associated with drug exposure to the fetus at specific gestational ages is important (see Section V. Antibiotic Selection in Pregnancy, above).

The optimal duration of treatment for ASB in pregnancy has not been established, and data exist on single-dose, short-course (3–5 days), longer-course (7–10 days or 14 days), as well as continuous (given until term) regimens. Differences in study design and population enrollment make comparisons of these regimens difficult. Adverse effects on the mother and poor compliance make continuous regimens unpopular, coupled with no differences in efficacy found with shorter-course therapies. Therapy with 7–10 days of antibiotics followed by a urine culture 1 week later to monitor for recurrence has become standard and recommended by most experts.

Question 3: What interventions, if any, should be considered for S.K.?

S.K. has ASB, which increases her subsequent risk of acute cystitis or pyelonephritis during pregnancy. She should be offered a 7- to 10-day course of oral antibiotic treatment to eradicate the infecting organism. Selection of the appropriate antibiotic should be based on culture and sensitivity reports, as well as consideration of the risks associated with drug exposure to the fetus.

C. Acute Cystitis

Acute cystitis is distinguished from ASB by the presence of lower urinary tract symptoms such as frequency, urgency, dysuria, and suprapubic pain in afebrile patients with no evidence of systemic illness. While treatment of ASB has been shown to reduce the incidence of pyelonephritis, the incidence of acute cystitis has remained relatively constant. Those with cystitis often have not had preceding ASB; however, up to 30% of patients with untreated ASB may develop symptomatic cystitis.[22] Mechanisms behind the development of cystitis, as well as the causative organisms, are identical to those that cause asymptomatic bacteriuria. In pregnant women presenting with lower urinary tract symptoms, urinalysis and urine culture should be performed.

Although the treatment of ASB should begin after sensitivity results are obtained, the treatment of acute cystitis is generally initiated empirically before culture results are available. The choice of antibiotic is generally based on coverage of common pathogens and local resistance patterns. Similar to ASB and the growing problem of resistance of Enterobacteriaceae to monotherapy with ampicillin or sulfonamides, initial therapy for acute cystitis may include a cephalosporin or amoxicillin-clavulanate. If necessary, the antibiotic may be changed after the culture and sensitivities are reported. While the duration of therapy for cystitis is debated as well, most experts recommend an antibiotic course of at least 7–10 days, to decrease the probability of recurrence. In nonpregnant females, a 3-day course has similar eradication rates compared to a 7- to 10-day course; however, this has not been confirmed in pregnant women.[19] Pregnant women being treated for acute cystitis should be counseled on the importance of compliance with their medication and appropriate follow-up. As in the treatment of ASB, a repeat urine culture should be obtained after therapy is complete to test for eradication. If the same organism is persistent in the urine, prolonged (ie, at least 6 weeks) or suppressive therapy should be considered.

D. Acute Pyelonephritis

Acute pyelonephritis in pregnancy is a serious systemic illness that occurs in 1%–2% of pregnant women, with recurrence reported in 10%–18% of these patients in the same pregnancy.[23] Preceding asymptomatic bacteriuria is a risk factor for pyelonephritis; however, timely identification of ASB and eradication with antibiotics have been shown to reduce the incidence of pyelonephritis by approximately 10-fold. The pathophysiology and causative microbiology are the same as for ASB and acute cystitis, with its occurrence more common in the second and third trimesters due to increasing urinary tract obstruction with stasis caused by the gravid uterus. It is well documented that pyelonephritis can progress to maternal sepsis, preterm labor, and premature birth.[23] Adult respiratory distress syndrome (ARDS) is a rare complication of antepartum pyelonephritis, usually occurring in the third trimester, and may have severe maternal and fetal consequences. Towers and colleagues identified several risk factors for ARDS in antepartum pyelonephritis: heart rate greater than 110 beats per minute, temperature of 103°F (39.4°C) in the first 24 hours, gestational age greater than 20 weeks, tocolytic use, monotherapy with ampicillin, and fluid overload.[24] Endotoxin-mediated tissue damage is thought to be the culprit for the adverse effects of pyelonephritis in pregnant women.

The diagnosis of pyelonephritis is made when presence of bacteria is accompanied by systemic symptoms suggesting upper UTI, such as fever, chills, flank pain, nausea/vomiting, or costovertebral angle tenderness. Symptoms that are suggestive of cystitis also may be present. Most cases will be right-sided, because ureteral atony produced by a gravid uterus produces more dilatation in the right ureter than the left. Left-sided symptoms may warrant further work-up. Differential diagnosis includes pelvic inflammatory disease, appendicitis, cholecystitis, and lower lobe pneumonia, to name a few. Laboratory analysis in acute pyelonephritis may show such hematologic and hemodynamic dysfunctions as thrombocytopenia and hypotension, and urinalysis and urine culture confirm the diagnosis of acute pyelonephritis. The IDSA defines quantitative bacteriology for pyelonephritis similar to criteria for ASB: the presence of 10^5 or more CFUs per milliliter of midstream clean-catch urine—although lower counts may be of concern in pregnancy.

Aggressive treatment is important in preventing complications from pyelonephritis. Uncomplicated pyelonephritis in nonpregnant females may be successfully treated with outpatient oral antibiotics, and some authors have evaluated various outpatient regimens for pyelonephritis during pregnancy. Angel and colleagues studied oral cephalexin (500 mg every 6 hours) compared with another first-generation cephalosporin given IV (cephalothin, 1 gram every 6 hours) in antepartum pyelonephritis patients and concluded that no difference was found between the two groups in terms of successful therapy.[25] However, this small study of 77 patients did not evaluate those who were bacteremic, and both study groups were evaluated in a hospital setting. Millar and colleagues also proposed an outpatient treatment regimen for acute pyelonephritis in pregnancy, comparing two doses of IM ceftriaxone, 1 gram, given 18–36 hours apart, to IV cefazolin, given 1 gram every 8 hours for 48 hours.[26] They concluded that both regimens were effective in their select population. In this study, only women less than 24 weeks' gestation were included, and observation in the emergency room for up to 24 hours to verify patient stability and oral tolerability was performed. In a later study, the same author (Millar) stated close follow-up and patient compliance were important for successful outpatient management.

Most experts and obstetric textbooks still recommend that women with acute pyelonephritis at any gestational age be hospitalized and treated with IV antibiotics, IV hydration, and close monitoring for maternal complications and fetal well-being.[23] During their hospitalization, patients with antepartum pyelonephritis should have their vital signs (including oxygen saturation) evaluated frequently, as well as be monitored for symptoms such as worsening fever or chills, shortness of breath, increased costovertebral angle (CVA) tenderness or pain, uterine contractions, vaginal bleeding or discharge, and increasing positive fluid balance. Fetal heart rate should also be assessed. Laboratory analysis to evaluate renal function and white blood cell count is also important.

Empiric choice of antibiotic should be based on the common causative organisms, local resistance patterns, cost-effectiveness of various regimens, and maternal/fetal safety concerns. Adjustment of antibiotics may be done once susceptibilities are obtained. A different antibiotic may be warranted for patients with recurrent bacterial colonization with the same organism, or those who have been exposed to antibiotics during the same pregnancy (as in S.K.'s case). Some suggested treatment regimens for initial empiric therapy include IV cefazolin (1 gram every 8 hours) with or without an aminoglycoside (eg, gentamicin dosed as per pharmacokinetic guidelines or approximately 1.5–2 mg/kg every 8 hours), or an IV third-generation cephalosporin (eg, cefotaxime, 1–2 grams every 8–12 hours), also with or without an aminoglycoside. Dual antibiotic therapy may be warranted for patients with recurrent disease, septic symptoms, or in those patients with multiple risk factors for severe complications, like ARDS, as mentioned above. Aminoglycosides are a good option for empiric therapy due to their acceptable coverage of offending organisms; however, consideration of the patient's renal function and clearance of the drug is important. Once patients are stable and afebrile for 24–48 hours, they may be discharged on oral antibiotics to complete a 14-day course. Oral antibiotics are selected based on culture and sensitivity results; cephalexin, 500 mg orally four times daily, is a common regimen. Suppression therapy should then be provided until close to childbirth. Suppression is important because the recurrence rate of pyelonephritis in the same pregnancy is significant. A study by Harris and Gilstrap demonstrated a recurrence rate of 2.7% in those patients who received suppressive therapy for the duration of the pregnancy, versus 60% in those patients who did not receive suppressive therapy.[27] Suppression therapy may be accomplished with nitrofurantoin, 100 mg orally every night at bedtime, starting after her 14 days of therapeutic antibiotics are complete, and continuing until 36 weeks' gestation. As stated earlier in the chapter, nitrofurantoin should not be continued in pregnant women beyond 36 weeks or if delivery is imminent.[9] Repeat cultures may be considered for patients not receiving suppression or who may be noncompliant. In addition to reinforcing compliance and follow-up with her treatment plan, additional patient education includes identification of the signs and symptoms of lower and upper UTIs, voiding before and after intercourse, emptying her bladder every 3 hours while awake, adequate hydration with 8–10 ounces of fluids (ie, water, cranberry juice, or milk) each day, and wiping her perineum from front to back for correct hygiene.

VIII. PATIENT CASE [PART 3]

S.K. presents to the emergency room several weeks later, at 14 weeks' gestation, with complaints of fever/chills, fatigue, right-sided flank pain, and CVA tenderness. She also reports mildly painful urination and persistent vomiting unrelieved with her promethazine suppositories. No vaginal discharge is noted. S.K. states these symptoms have persisted for the last 2 days, and admits she never finished her course of antibiotics (cephalexin, 500 mg four times daily, for 7 days) prescribed for asymptomatic bacteriuria. Vital signs on admission: temperature 101.4°F (39°C), heart rate 98, blood pressure 101/66, respiratory rate 22, and peripheral oxygen saturation (SpO$_2$) 98%. A Gram stain of S.K.'s urine reveals gram-negative rods, and dipstick urinalysis demonstrates a straw-colored appearance, specific gravity 1.032, pH 8.0, ketonuria 3+, glucosuria, macroscopic hematuria, WBCs 20–25 cells/mm^3, numerous bacteria, and RBCs 0-1 cells/mm^3. Pelvic examination is negative for pelvic inflammatory disease. Blood and urine samples are obtained from S.K. for laboratory analysis.

Question 4: What is S.K.'s suspected diagnosis and proposed treatment plan?

S.K. has a suspected diagnosis of acute bacterial pyelonephritis. Empiric intravenous antibiotic therapy and hydration support should be initiated in the hospital and continued until she is afebrile and no longer exhibiting signs of dehydration or systemic disease for at least 24–48 hours. Vital signs, along with oxygen saturation by pulse oximetry, are closely monitored and the antibiotics should be changed if culture and sensitivity reporting warrant it. Oral antibiotics are continued for a total of 14 days, followed by suppressive therapy until close to childbirth. Close follow-up of S.K. with repeat cultures and compliance reporting is paramount to prevent recurrent disease and complications related to pyelonephritis in pregnancy.

IX. PATIENT CASE (PART 4)

S.K. is seen in labor and delivery triage at 38 3/7 weeks for the possible onset of labor. She arrives with intact membranes, but is reporting uterine contractions every 6–10 minutes and increasing back ache for the last week. She feels that her baby has "dropped" lower into her pelvis. Vital signs are stable. Two weeks ago she was screened per universal guidelines for GBS colonization from a vaginal culture swab. The results were positive for colonization, and this is noted on her chart. On cervical examination, she is 2 centimeters dilated and 30% effaced. She is admitted to the hospital.

X. Group B Streptococcus Prophylaxis

Maternal and fetal infections caused by GBS (also known as *Streptococcus agalactiae*) range from asymptomatic colonization to sepsis. Women carry GBS as part of the normal fecal and vaginal flora, and between 10% and 30% of pregnant women are colonized with GBS.[28] Vaginal colonization may be transient (more common) or chronic throughout pregnancy, and women who were colonized in a previous pregnancy are not necessarily colonized in a subsequent pregnancy. Although there are differences in culture technique used and the number of samples collected in demographic studies, risk factors for colonization include use of an intrauterine device, African American or Hispanic ethnicity, sexual intercourse, and age younger than 20 years.[28]

GBS infection is recognized as an important cause of maternal uterine infection and septicemia, associated with urinary tract infection, chorioamnionitis when heavy colonization is present in the second trimester, and with postpartum endometritis. It is also a significant cause of neonatal infection and the major cause of sepsis in newborns. When maternal colonization is present, vertical transmission of GBS to the neonate during labor and childbirth occurs approximately 60% of the time, and may result in early-onset neonatal GBS invasive disease in approximately 1%–2% of the cases. Invasive GBS disease in the newborn may be manifested as sepsis, pneumonia, or meningitis. Early-onset neonatal disease is defined as infection within the first 6 days after birth, and accounts for most GBS infection in neonates. It usually reflects exposure to the organism in utero or through maternal vertical transmission. Other risk factors for early-onset neonatal GBS infection include prematurity and low birth weight, along with maternal factors such as premature rupture of membranes (PROM), prolonged labor, chorioamnionitis, multiple gestation, high bacterial concentration of genital GBS, and GBS bacteremia during pregnancy. Late-onset disease occurs 7 days to 3 months after birth. It has a much lower incidence than early-onset disease, but carries a mortality rate of approximately 10%. The route of transmission to the neonate is less clear, but may be secondary to nosocomial, environmental, or maternal causes.[29]

ACOG, along with the CDC and American Academy of Pediatrics, have collaboratively endorsed guidelines on a culture-based approach for screening of GBS and for the prevention of early-onset GBS disease in the newborn. Vaginal or rectal culture–based methods are recommended as universal prenatal screening for GBS colonization in women at 35–37 weeks' gestation. Women who are positive for GBS colonization should receive intrapartum antibiotic prophylaxis for perinatal GBS disease prevention. Other women who should receive intrapartum prophylaxis (Figure 1) include those with a previous infant with invasive GBS disease, GBS bacteriuria during current pregnancy, or unknown GBS status at time of childbirth with any of the following risk factors: less than 37 weeks' gestation, amniotic membrane rupture 18 hours or more,

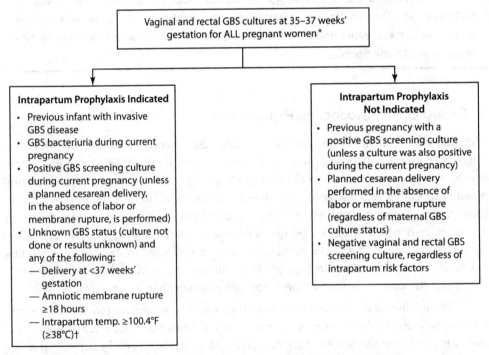

Figure 1. Indications for intrapartum antibiotic prophylaxis to prevent perinatal Group B streptococcal (GBS) disease. *GBS screening is performed in all pregnant women, unless she had GBS bacteriuria during the current pregnancy or a previous infant with invasive GBS disease. †If amnionitis is suspected, broad-spectrum antibiotic therapy that includes an agent (or agents) known to be active against GBS should replace GBS prophylaxis. From Centers for Disease Control and Prevention.[28]

or intrapartum temperature 100.4°F (38.0°C) or above.[28] For women undergoing elective cesarean section in the absence of labor or ruptured membranes, intrapartum prophylaxis is not recommended, regardless of GBS colonization status. Retrospective data and a review of CDC surveillance data revealed that the risk of vertical transmission of GBS in this setting (during a prelabor cesarean section with intact membranes) is low.[30] However, women who are scheduled for an elective cesarean section should still be screened for GBS colonization at 35–37 weeks' gestation, in case the onset of labor or rupture of membranes occurs before the planned cesarean section date.

Penicillin is the antibiotic of choice for intrapartum prophylaxis (Table 3).[28] Ampicillin is an acceptable alternative; however, increasing ampicillin-resistant *E. coli* in neonates is a concern.[16] Antibiotics are most effective when initiated at least 4 hours before childbirth. Cefazolin is recommended for patients who are allergic to penicillin and not at high risk for anaphylaxis. For patients who are allergic to penicillin and at high risk for anaphylaxis, clindamycin or erythromycin may be administered, as long as susceptibility testing performed on GBS isolates confirm sensitivity. Increasing resistance of GBS isolates to clindamycin and erythromycin has been reported,[15] making it necessary to obtain susceptibility reports before using these agents for intrapartum prophylaxis of GBS. Additionally, erythromycin does not cross the placenta; therefore, clindamycin may be the preferred choice over erythromycin to achieve adequate concentrations in the fetal circulation. In the event of GBS iso-

Table 3. Recommended Regimens for Intrapartum Antimicrobial Prophylaxis for Perinatal Group B Streptococcal (GBS) Disease Prevention

Recommended	Penicillin G, 5 million units IV initial dose, then 2.5 million units IV every 4 h until delivery
Alternative	Ampicillin, 2 g IV initial dose, then 1 g IV every 4 h until delivery
If penicillin allergic	
Patients not at high risk for anaphylaxis	Cefazolin, 2 g IV initial dose, then 1 g IV every 8 h until delivery
Patients at high risk for anaphylaxis[a] GBS susceptible to clindamycin and erythromycin[b]	Clindamycin, 900 mg IV every 8 h until delivery *or* Erythromycin, 500 mg IV every 6 h until delivery
GBS resistant to clindamycin or erythromycin or susceptibility unknown	Vancomycin,[c] 1 g IV every 12 h until delivery

[a]Clindamycin and erythromycin susceptibility testing should be performed on prenatal GBS isolates from penicillin-allergic women at high risk for anaphylaxis.
[b]Resistance to erythromycin is often but not always associated with clindamycin resistance. If a strain is resistant to erythromycin but appears susceptible to clindamycin, it may still have inducible resistance to clindamycin.
[c]Cefazolin is preferred over vancomycin for women with a history of penicillin allergy other than immediate hypersensitivity reactions. Vancomycin should be reserved for penicillin-allergic women at high risk for anaphylaxis.
From Centers for Disease Control and Prevention.[28]

lates resistant to clindamycin or erythromycin, or if the susceptibility is not determined, vancomycin must be used.

Question 5: What is recommended for intrapartum administration of antibiotics for S.K.'s positive GBS colonization status?

S.K. should be initiated on Penicillin G, 5 million units IV, then 2.5 million units IV every 4 hours until childbirth.

XI. Chorioamnionitis

Chorioamnionitis is infection of the outer membrane (chorion) and the fluid-filled sac (amnion) that encloses the embryo. It is also sometimes referred to as *intra-amniotic infection, amnionitis, amniotic fluid infection*, or *intrapartum fever*. Chorioamnionitis occurs in approximately 0.5%–10% of all pregnancies, with a higher occurrence rate in patients with preterm births.[23] Chorioamnionitis may be identified before, during, or immediately (within 24 hours) after birth. It is associated with maternal bacteremia and post-cesarean wound infection, neonatal sepsis, pneumonia, meningitis, and complications related to premature birth, such as cerebral palsy, intraventricular hemorrhage, and respiratory distress syndrome.

Chorioamnionitis most likely results from ascending contamination of the lower genital tract flora into the intra-amniotic cavity with such organisms as *E. coli*, GBS, *Bacteroides*, or *Clostridium*. Polymicrobial infection with aerobic and anaerobic organisms is probable as well. Chorioamnionitis may also occur when the amniotic sac membranes are ruptured for a prolonged period of time (greater than 12 hours), because this allows vaginal organisms to move upward into the uterus. Other risk factors include the number of vaginal examinations performed, preterm labor, rupture of membranes before the onset of labor, and maternal chronic autoimmune disease.

Diagnosis of chorioamnionitis is typically made by clinical findings alone and in the absence of other etiologies of infection (ie, a disease of "rule out"). It requires a high index of suspicion because clinical signs and symptoms are not always sensitive or specific. Symptoms may include maternal temperature, maternal and/or fetal tachycardia, uterine tenderness, or malodorous amniotic fluid. Chorioamnionitis should be considered in any febrile pregnant woman, especially if rupture of membranes has occurred. In many cases, elevated maternal temperature may be the only presenting symptom. Fetal heart rate changes (specifically tachycardia or variable decelerations) may also accompany the diagnosis of chorioamnionitis. Although it is a nonspecific finding, in the setting of chorioamnionitis, fetal heart variability can reflect an adverse fetal response to an infectious environment. Direct laboratory confirmation of chorioamnionitis (via Gram staining and culturing of amniotic fluid by amniocentesis) may be useful in the setting of nonruptured membranes, especially if chorioamnionitis is suspected at a gestational age remote from term. However, waiting for the results of laboratory examination can delay initiation of treatment, which should be prompt secondary to potentially adverse maternal and fetal complications. Once chorioamnionitis is suspected, expeditious delivery, along with empiric antibiotic administration, is the treatment of choice. Some experts define expeditious delivery as within 12 hours of diagnosis.[31]

Choice of intrapartum antibiotics is empiric in the setting of chorioamnionitis. Although there are few controlled clinical trials to guide the choice of antibiotics, parenteral antibiotic treatment is aimed primarily toward the most common pathogens involved in chorioamnionitis: *E. coli* and GBS. Ampicillin (2 g IV every 6 hours) plus gentamicin (1.5–2 mg/kg IV every 8 hours or as per institution-specific pharmacokinetic dosing guidelines) is a common treatment regimen. The addition of clindamycin (900 mg IV every 8 hours) to this regimen is advocated by some authors to provide additional anaerobic coverage in the setting of cesarean section, especially due to the importance of resistant *Bacteroides* species and the high failure rate of ampicillin-gentamicin alone in postcesarean endometritis.[31] In penicillin-allergic patients, use of gentamicin-clindamycin or replacing ampicillin with vancomycin (1 gram IV every 12 hours or as per institution-specific pharmacokinetic dosing guidelines) may be done. There are very few reports or recommendations on the use of third-generation cephalosporins, extended-spectrum penicillins, or combination β-lactam/β-lactamase inhibitors in the treatment of chorioamnionitis. Although their spectrum of activity may be suitable for the common pathogens involved, the efficacy of these agents for chorioamnionitis is largely unknown, and they are more expensive and not shown to be superior to the above-noted regimens.

The duration of antibiotic therapy for chorioamnionitis is largely based on clinical resolution of symptoms. Therapy should continue until the patient is afebrile and asymptomatic for at least 24–48 hours postoperatively. After vaginal birth, antibiotics are usually discontinued shortly after childbirth or within 24 hours of being afebrile. In a study of 292 patients with chorioamnionitis receiving antibiotics (ampicillin and gentamicin, plus clindamycin if delivered by cesarean section), no difference was found in the primary outcome of postpartum maternal temperature between women who received antibiotics until 24 hours afebrile and women who received just one additional dose of each after childbirth.[32] Some clinicians will also discontinue antibiotic therapy once the baby is born. Outpatient or oral antibiotics after treatment of chorioamnionitis or postpartum endometritis are rarely indicated. If fever persists after 24 hours of starting the antibiotics, addition of a third agent (ie, clindamycin or metronidazole if not already added), or substitution of an agent if resistance is suspected (eg, metronidazole for clindamycin in resistant *Bacteroides* species or vancomycin for ampicillin), should be considered. If the patient continues to be febrile, other sources of infection must be included in the differential diagnosis. Septic pelvic thrombosis, abscesses, wound infection, retained parts of conception, urinary tract infection, and vaginitis are examples of other sources to be ruled out.

XII. PATIENT CASE (PART 5)

After laboring for 14 hours, S.K. has stalled in the active phase of labor. Her physician has already manually ruptured her membranes. She is afebrile and vital signs are stable. Fetal heart rate decelerations are detected on the fetal monitor. The decision is made to proceed with cesarean section, for which patient consent has been obtained.

XIII. Antibiotic Prophylaxis for Postcesarean Infection

Postpartum maternal infection consists primarily of cesarean wound infection and endometritis. Cesarean section, therefore, is a significant risk factor for the development of infectious morbidity postpartum, with the highest risk occurring in those patients whose cesarean birth is performed in the setting of ruptured membranes or during labor. Other risk factors that predispose a mother to postcesarean infection include emergency procedures performed without adequate preoperative cleansing, surgeries lasting longer than 1 hour, and high blood loss during the operation. In studies evaluating the rate of postcesarean infection in high-risk patients such as these, antibiotic prophylaxis was found to reduce the incidence of postpartum infection by about two thirds.[33] ACOG recommends routine prophylactic antibiotics in this setting.[34]

The decision to administer perioperative antibiotics in the setting of lower-risk patients (ie, those women undergoing elective cesarean sections, or cesarean deliveries performed in the setting of nonruptured membranes and no labor) is more controversial. ACOG notes that the benefit of such therapy in lower-risk patients is "less clear," citing conflicting results from studies evaluating antibiotic prophylaxis in patients undergoing elective cesarean section. However, meta-analysis of nine prior studies in this setting show that antibiotic prophylaxis can reduce the incidence of postcesarean infection by as much as 75%.[35] Most experts and consensus opinions agree that antibiotic prophylaxis is appropriate in high- and low-risk patients because postpartum endometritis and wound infection can lead to more serious morbidities, such as increased pain and poor recovery, need for further interventions such as surgery or drain placement, and extended hospital stays and treatment costs. Therefore, current publications recommend the use of prophylactic antibiotics in both planned and emergent cesareans.

First-generation cephalosporins are the most commonly used antibiotics in this setting. Single-dose clindamycin plus gentamicin is an alternate regimen for women with cephalosporin allergy or penicillin allergy at high risk for anaphylaxis. While a number of antibiotics have been studied and deemed efficacious for prophylaxis, including cefazolin, broader-spectrum second-, third-, and fourth-generation cephalosporins, ampicillin, piperacillin, and ampicillin-sulbactam, none of these studies has demonstrated greater efficacy in choosing one agent over another. Two separate comparative studies evaluating cefazolin versus cefoxitin[36] or cefotetan[37] showed no significant differences in outcome; however, cefazolin costs substantially less than the other two agents. Ampicillin is not routinely used any more because of the increasing prevalence of ampicillin-resistant *E. coli* in the mother and the neonate. Cefazolin, 1–2 grams IV, is the preferred agent due to its longer half-life and lower allergic and anaphylactic risk.

Historically, administration of antibiotic prophylaxis at cord-clamping has been recommended for both elective and nonelective cesarean sections to minimize antibiotic exposure to the fetus.[33–34] This concept is based on pharmacokinetic studies demonstrating bactericidal and minimum inhibitory concentrations in cord or fetal blood within 5–30 minutes of administration of antibiotics administered to the mother for GBS prophylaxis.[38,39] However, in a recent randomized, double-blinded, placebo-controlled trial of 357 women requiring cesarean sections (excluding emergent cesareans) comparing the administration of prophylactic antibiotics 15–60 minutes before skin incision with administration at cord-clamping, there were significant decreases in the incidence of endometritis and total infectious postpartum morbidity in the group receiving prophylaxis before skin incision.[40] There were also trends toward decreased neonatal intensive care unit admissions and length of stay in the preoperative group, perhaps indicating no additional neonatal harm in terms of sepsis or selection of resistant organisms. Further, a meta-analysis of five randomized controlled trials comparing the timing of single antibiotic prophylaxis (preoperative vs at cord-clamping) before cesarean section demonstrated that when the antibiotic was given before skin incision, there were significant decreases in the incidence of postpartum endometritis and total infectious morbidity, without any differences in neonatal outcomes.[41] It is noted that in general, patients with chorioamnionitis or need for emergency cesarean section due to infectious morbidity were excluded in these studies, while the meta-analysis did include laboring and nonlaboring patients. Despite these recent studies, debate still exists on the appropriate timing of administration of antibiotic prophylaxis for cesarean section. Individual institutions should address this issue with respect to information provided from their own infection control committees and neonatology departments. A reasonable approach may be to provide antibiotic prophylaxis 15–60 minutes before skin incision for nonemergent cesareans only.

Question 6: What, if any, antibiotics should be administered for postoperative wound infection prophylaxis in S.K.?

S.K. should receive routine perioperative antibiotic prophylaxis per institution-specific guidelines for the prevention of postcesarean infection. A single dose of a parenteral first-generation cephalosporin, such as cefazolin 1 gram, may be given.

XIV. PATIENT CASE [PART 6]

On postoperative day 2, S.K. spikes a temperature to 100.8°F (38.2°C). Other vital signs: heart rate 98, blood pressure 111/72, and respiratory rate 20. WBC count is 13.1 cells/mm³. Her fundus is slightly tender to palpation; otherwise, she has no other complaints. There is no lochia and no abdominal pain. Her cesarean section wound is clean, dry, and intact, with no obvious signs of infection. She has been attempting to breastfeed, with assistance from a lactation consultant, and her breasts are not tender or engorged.

XV. Endometritis

Endometritis is an infection of the endometrium or decidua, with extension into the myometrium and parametrial tissues, occurring after the first 24 hours following childbirth. Maternal fever detected within the first 24 hours after childbirth, especially after a vaginal birth, is sometimes considered chorioamnionitis, and additional antibiotic treatment after childbirth may not be required. In the setting of cesarean section, further management is usually considered and treated as endometritis. Endometritis is the most common infectious complication in the postpartum period. It occurs in approximately 1%–3% of women who deliver vaginally and in approximately 20% of those who deliver by cesarean section.[23] The rate of postpartum endometritis has also been reported in some studies to be up to 50%–60% higher in women who do not receive antibiotic prophylaxis before cesarean section, when compared to women who do receive antibiotic prophylaxis.[23] Although most patients with endometritis respond well to prompt IV antibiotic therapy, rare but potentially serious complications of endometritis include sepsis, wound infection, necrotizing fasciitis, septic thrombophlebitis, and abscess formation.

Most cases of endometritis are polymicrobial, caused by ascending infection with contamination of the uterine cavity by organisms present in the vagina. The common microorganisms are similar to those mentioned in earlier sections of this chapter: *E. coli*, *Klebsiella* species, GBS, enterococci, *Gardnerella vaginalis*, *Peptostreptococci*, *Bacteroides* species, *Clostridium* species, and *Fusobacterium* species. Endometritis may occur as a result of subclinical or clinical infection before childbirth (ie, chorioamnionitis), or may occur as a corollary to parturition. In addition to cesarean section, other risk factors for endometritis include operative technique, length of operation, presence of and duration of labor, preterm birth, PROM, bacterial vaginosis, colonization with GBS, high colony counts of bacteria in the amniotic fluid, tissue trauma, and retained parts of conception.[31]

Endometritis most commonly presents with fever. Persistent temperature at or above 100.4°F (38.0°C) is a hallmark of endometritis. Much like chorioamnionitis, it is a disease of "rule out"; endometritis should be considered the cause of postpartum maternal temperature unless other sources such as wound infection, urinary tract infection, atelectasis, or episiotomy infection are diagnosed. Other signs and symptoms of endometritis include uterine tenderness, lower abdominal pain, malodorous or purulent lochia, or leukocytosis. WBC might be normally slightly elevated during pregnancy and in the postpartum state; therefore, leukocytosis as a singular clinical sign is not always specific for endometritis or other pregnancy-related infections. Similar to chorioamnionitis, low-grade maternal fever may be the only presenting sign of endometritis. Virulent organisms associated with endometritis, such as β-hemolytic streptococci, *S. aureus*, or *Clostridium perfringens*, have been reported to cause such symptoms as chills, high fever, severe pain, abdominal distention, and serosanguineous discharge.[31]

Debate exists on the utility of blood cultures in the management of endometritis. Once endometritis is diagnosed, most authors advocate prompt empiric treatment with close observation for resolution of fever and other symptoms, without the need for routine cultures. Others advocate obtaining cultures before antibiotic initiation in the event that prolonged treatment is needed for bacteremia or if resistant organisms are present. The decision to draw cultures or not may be reasonably made based on the severity of fever or other symptoms. In a study of 168 patients with postpartum pyrexia, those women with a temperature higher than 101.8°F (38.8°C) were more likely to have documented bacteremia than those with a temperature lower than 101.8°F (38.8°C) (21.4% vs 0.8%, *p* <.001).[42] Noninsidious and rapid progression of clinical symptoms, such as those reported with virulent organisms, may be a consideration for obtaining blood cultures before antibiotic therapy as well. Regardless of whether cultures are obtained or not, treatment of endometritis with IV antibiotics should be started promptly and empirically based on common pathogens, and continuing until the patient is afebrile and asymptomatic for a minimum of 36–48 hours. Long-term or outpatient antibiotics are indicated only in those patients in whom bacteremia is documented. In those cases, antibiotic treatment for a total of 14 days is necessary for most isolated organisms.

Standard antibiotic therapy for endometritis consists of clindamycin (900 mg IV every 8 hours) plus gentamicin (1.5–2 mg/kg IV every 8 hours or as per institution-specific pharmacokinetic dosing guidelines).[43] As previously discussed, routine gentamicin levels are not recommended in this setting, unless the patient has preexisting renal disease or if failed therapy is suspected. Ampicillin (2 grams IV every 6 hours) may be added, either initially or within the first 48 hours if there is no response. Broader-spectrum agents, such as aztreonam, extended-spectrum penicillins, extended-spectrum cephalosporins, and imipenem-cilastatin, have been evaluated for use in endometritis; however, these agents have not been proven to be any more effective than the standard regimen and are more expensive.

Patients who remain febrile 48–72 hours after appropriate antibiotics have been initiated warrant evaluation for other sources or bacterial causes of infection. Adding a third antibiotic agent if not already done (eg, ampicillin to clindamycin-gentamicin), or switching antibiotic agents may be considered for treatment-resistant organisms. Some examples include vancomycin for ampicillin in isolated enterococci, or metronidazole for clindamycin in clindamycin-resistant *Bacteroides*. Assessing the cesarean section incision site, if applicable, for wound infection may be necessary. Other diagnostic tools include pelvic ultrasonography, computed tomography, or magnetic resonance imaging. These tools may aid in the detection of parametrial abscess or uterine gas formation. Examples of other infections to rule out in the event of persistent fever include mastitis, septic pelvic thrombophlebitis, retained products of conception, urinary tract infection, and vaginitis. Wide fluctuations in maternal temperature, from febrile to afebrile every few hours, accompanied by clinical response to therapeutic anticoagulation, may be characteristic of septic pelvic thrombophlebitis (SPT). The utility of anticoagulation with heparin in the setting of SPT is controversial,[44] but may be considered for patients with persistent fever and no other sources of infection.

Question 7: What interventions, if any, should be considered for S.K.?

S.K. is suspected to have endometritis. Broad-spectrum antibiotic coverage should be begun and continued until she is afebrile for 36–48 hours. Standard therapy consists of clindamycin plus gentamicin, with or without ampicillin. S.K. should also be counseled that these medications are compatible with breastfeeding.

XVI. Summary

An understanding of infectious disease in pregnancy involves not only the identification and timely management of women who are symptomatic for disease, but also those who may be asymptomatic. Asymptomatic infections in pregnancy, such as

asymptomatic bacteriuria, GBS colonization, or bacterial vaginosis, can have adverse maternal and fetal complications if untreated or undetected. Other infectious or sexually transmitted infections may be screened for in pregnancy, either as part of a routine battery of prenatal tests or offered to at-risk women. Timely identification of risks for particular diseases and diagnoses of infectious conditions can assist in the appropriate management of the pregnancy, by offering intervention to the pregnant women for vaccination, eradication of the disease, or treatment to reduce both maternal and fetal complications.

Acute pyelonephritis in pregnancy and puerperal infections that occur around the time of childbirth, including chorioamnionitis, endometritis, or postpartum wound infection, have standard regimens that are successful in managing maternal temperature and decreasing the risk of further complications. It is important for the obstetrician and pharmacist to be aware of these standard regimens and how geographic resistance or other practice patterns may influence treatment. Additionally, management of these infectious diseases can be particularly unique in pregnancy, due to the fact that any intervention—or lack thereof—in the mother will invariably affect the fetus or neonate. Knowledge of the consequences of untreated disease, as well as principles behind appropriate antibiotic selection during pregnancy, are paramount for any clinician involved in the management of pregnant women.

XVII. References

1. Centers for Disease Control and Prevention. Sexually transmitted diseases treatment guidelines, 2006. *MMWR Recomm Rep.* 2006;55(RR-11):1–94.

2. American Academy of Pediatrics, American College of Obstetricians and Gynecologists. *Guidelines for Perinatal Care.* 5th ed. Elk Grove Village, IL: AAP; Washington, DC: ACOG, 2002.

3. U.S. Preventive Services Task Force. Screening for chlamydial infection, June 2007. Available at: http://www.ahrq.gov/clinic/uspstf/uspschlm.htm. Accessed March 8, 2008.

4. Katz VL. Prenatal care. In Scott JR, Gibbs RS, Karlan BY, et al., eds. *Danforth's Obstetrics and Gynecology.* 9th ed. Philadelphia: Lippincott Williams & Wilkins, 2003:6.

5. Allsworth JE, Peipert JF. Prevalence of bacterial vaginosis: 2001–2004 national health and nutrition examination survey data. *Obstet Gynecol.* 2007;109:114–120.

6. American College of Obstetricians and Gynecologists. Vaginitis. *ACOG Practice Bulletin.* Number 72, May 2006. *Obstet Gynecol.* 2006;107:1195–1206.

7. Nygren P, Fu R, Freeman M, et al; U.S. Preventive Services Task Force. Evidence on the benefits and harms of screening and treating pregnant women who are asymptomatic for bacterial vaginosis: an update review for the U.S. Preventive Services Task Force. *Ann Intern Med.* 2008;148:220–233.

8. American College of Obstetricians and Gynecologists. Assessment of risk factors for preterm birth. *ACOG Practice Bulletin.* Number 31, October 2001. *Obstet Gynecol.* 2001;98:709–716.

9. Briggs GG, Freeman RK, Yaffe SJ. *Drugs in Pregnancy and Lactation: A Reference Guide to Fetal and Neonatal Risk.* 8th ed. Philadelphia: Lippincott Williams & Wilkins, 2008.

10. American College of Obstetricians and Gynecologists. Prenatal and perinatal human immunodeficiency virus testing: expanded recommendations. *ACOG Committee Opinion.* Number 304, November 2004. *Obstet Gynecol.* 2004;104:1119–1124.

11. Centers for Disease Control and Prevention. U.S. Public Health Service Task Force recommendations for use of antiretroviral drugs in pregnant HIV-1-infected women for maternal health and interventions to reduce perinatal HIV-1 transmission in the United States. *MMWR Recomm Rep.* 2002;51(RR-18):1–38.

12. Centers for Disease Control and Prevention. General recommendations on immunization: recommendations of the Advisory Committee on Immunization Practices (ACIP). *MMWR Recomm Rep.* 2006;55(RR-15):1–48.

13. American College of Obstetricians and Gynecologists. Immunization during pregnancy. *ACOG Committee Opinion.* Number 282, January 2003. *Obstet Gynecol.* 2003;101:207–212.

14. Larsen B. Vaginal flora in health and disease. *Clin Obstet Gynecol.* 1993;36:107–121.

15. Pearlman MD, Pierson CL, Faix RG. Frequent resistance of clinical group B streptococci isolates to clindamycin and erythromycin. *Obstet Gynecol.* 1998;92:258–261.

16. Stoll BJ, Hansen N, Fanaroff AA, et al. Changes in pathogens causing early-onset sepsis in very-low-birth-weight infants. *N Engl J Med.* 2002;347:240–247.

17. Chow AW, Jewesson PJ. Pharmacokinetics and safety of antimicrobial agents during pregnancy. *Rev Infect Dis.* 1985;7:287–313.

18. Briggs GG, Ambrose P, Nageotte MP. Gentamicin dosing in postpartum women with endometritis. *Am J Obstet Gynecol.* 1989;160:309–313.

19. Patterson TF, Andriole VT. Bacteriuria in pregnancy. *Infect Dis Clin North Am.* 1987;1:807–822.

20. Nicolle LE, Bradley S, Colgan R, et al. Infectious Diseases Society of America guidelines for the diagnosis and treatment of asymptomatic bacteriuria in adults. *Clin Infect Dis.* 2005;40:643–654.

21. Smaill F. Antibiotics for asymptomatic bacteriuria in pregnancy. *Cochrane Database Syst Rev.* 2001;(2):CD000490.

22. Kass EH. Pregnancy, pyelonephritis and prematurity. *Clin Obstet Gynecol.* 1970;13:239–254.

23. Gibbs RS, Sweet RL, Duff P. Maternal and fetal infectious disorders. In Creasy RK, Resnik R, eds. *Maternal-Fetal Medicine: Principles and Practice.* 5th ed. Philadelphia: WB Saunders, 2004:741–801.

24. Towers CV, Kaminskas CM, Garite TJ, et al. Pulmonary injury associated with antepartum pyelonephritis: can patients at risk be identified? *Am J Obstet Gynecol.* 1991;164:974–978.

25. Angel JL, O'Brien WF, Finan MA, et al. Acute pyelonephritis in pregnancy: a prospective study of oral versus intravenous antibiotic therapy. *Obstet Gynecol.* 1990;76:28–32.

26. Millar LK, Wing DA, Paul RH, et al. Outpatient treatment of pyelonephritis in pregnancy: a randomized controlled trial. *Obstet Gynecol.* 1995;86:560–564.

27. Harris RE, Gilstrap LC. Prevention of recurrent pyelonephritis during pregnancy. *Obstet Gynecol.* 1974;44:637–641.

28. Centers for Disease Control and Prevention. Prevention of perinatal group B streptococcal disease: revised guidelines from CDC. *MMWR Recomm Rep.* 2002;51(RR-11):1–22.

29. Baker CJ, Edwards MS. Group B streptococcal infections. In Remington JS, Klein JO, eds. *Infectious Diseases of the Fetus and Newborn Infant.* 4th ed. Philadelphia: WB Saunders, 1995:980.

30. American College of Obstetricians and Gynecologists. Prevention of early-onset group B streptococcal disease in newborns. *ACOG Committee Opinion.* Number 279, December 2002. *Obstet Gynecol.* 2002;100:1405–1412.

31. Savoia MC. Bacterial, fungal, and parasitic disease. In Burrow GN, Duffy TP, Copel JA, eds. *Medical Complications during Pregnancy.* 6th ed. Philadelphia: Elsevier Saunders, 2004:305–345.

32. Edwards RK, Duff P. Single additional dose postpartum therapy for women with chorioamnionitis. *Obstet Gynecol.* 2003;102:957–961.

33. Smaill F, Hofmeyr GJ. Antibiotic prophylaxis for cesarean section. *Cochrane Database Syst Rev.* 2002;(3):CD000933.

34. American College of Obstetricians and Gynecologists. Prophylactic antibiotics in labor and delivery. *ACOG Practice Bulletin.* Number 47, October 2003. *Obstet Gynecol.* 2003;102:875–882.

35. Chelmow D, Ruehli MS, Huang E. Prophylactic use of antibiotics for nonlaboring patients undergoing cesarean delivery with intact membranes: a meta-analysis. *Am J Obstet Gynecol.* 2001;184:656–661.

36. Currier JS, Tosteson TD, Platt R. Cefazolin compared with cefoxitin for cesarean section prophylaxis: the use of a two-stage study design. *J Clin Epidemiol.* 1993;46:625–630.

37. Carlson C, Duff P. Antibiotic prophylaxis for cesarean delivery: is an extended-spectrum agent necessary? *Obstet Gynecol.* 1990;76:343–346.

38. Bloom SL, Cox SM, Bawdon RE, et al. Ampicillin for neonatal group B streptococcal prophylaxis: how rapidly can bactericidal concentration be achieved? *Am J Obstet Gynecol.* 1996;175:974–976.

39. Fiore MT, Pearlman MD, Chapman RL, et al. Maternal and transplacental pharmacokinetics of cefazolin. *Obstet Gynecol.* 2001;98:1075–1079.

40. Sullivan SA, Smith T, Chang E, et al. Administration of cefazolin prior to skin incision is superior to cefazolin at cord clamping in preventing postcesarean infectious morbidity: a randomized, controlled trial. *Am J Obstet Gynecol.* 2007; 196:455.e1–e5.

41. Costantine MM, Rahman M, Ghulmiyah L, et al. Timing of perioperative antibiotics for cesarean delivery: a metaanalysis. *Am J Obstet Gynecol.* 2008;199:301.e1–e6.

42. Spandorfer SD, Graham E, Forouzan I. Postcesarean endometritis: clinical risk factors predictive of positive blood culture. *J Reprod Med.* 1996;41:797–800.

43. French LM, Smaill FM. Antibiotic regiments for endometritis after delivery. *Cochrane Database Syst Rev.* 2004;(4):CD001067.

44. Brown CE, Stettler RW, Twickler D, et al. Puerperal septic pelvic thrombophlebitis: incidence and response to heparin therapy. *Am J Obstet Gynecol.* 1999;181:143–148.

Nausea and Vomiting of Pregnancy

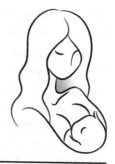

Gerald G. Briggs and Michael P. Nageotte

CHAPTER 24

LEARNING OBJECTIVES

1. Differentiate between nausea and vomiting of pregnancy and hyperemesis gravidarum.

2. Formulate a treatment plan for nausea and vomiting of pregnancy.

3. Formulate a plan to prevent or reduce the severity of nausea and vomiting in a woman with a history of hyperemesis gravidarum in her last pregnancy.

4. Identify the potential toxicity of therapeutic treatment on the embryo/fetus.

I. Introduction

Nausea and vomiting of pregnancy (NVP) is a frequent condition that affects 70%–85% of all pregnant women.[1] Although there are a number of treatment options that can lessen the impact of the condition, many women are undertreated or forego treatment all together, either because of ineffective therapy[1] or fear for the safety of the conceptus.[2] This can result in a significant decrease in the quality of life for the woman or loss when a pregnancy is voluntarily terminated because of unrelenting nausea/vomiting.

The primary goal of therapy is prevention. If NVP does occur, the secondary goal is to mitigate the symptoms so that the condition is tolerable and to prevent progression to more severe nausea/vomiting, such as hyperemesis gravidarum. Complete suppression of the symptoms of NVP is rarely achievable with oral therapy.

Although few women would describe NVP as a benefit, there is substantial evidence that women who experience nausea/vomiting actually have fewer pregnancy losses.[1] The exact cause of NVP has not been determined, but it appears to be associated with higher concentrations of two pregnancy-related hormones, human chorionic gonadotropin (hCG) and estradiol. Higher levels of these hormones have been associated with fewer spontaneous abortions (miscarriages).[1]

A 2000 study of 160 pregnant women with nausea reported the patterns of the symptom.[3] Most women (80%) had nausea lasting all day, whereas only 1.8% had "morning sickness." The mean duration of nausea was about 35 days with relief from the symptoms occurring by gestational week 14 in 50% and by week 22 in 90%.[3]

All clinicians, whether they are physicians, nurses, or pharmacists, who provide care or services to women of reproductive age have a role in the prevention and treatment of NVP. Pharmacists have a vital role because appropriate drug therapy is a critical component of successful prevention and treatment. They are frequently consulted by patients requesting information about the condition and they come in contact with pregnant women when working in clinics or other areas of clinical practice. In these situations, pharmacists can be an important source of information and offer reliable recommendations to prevent and control nausea/vomiting during pregnancy.

II. CASE HISTORY [PART 1]

J.W. is a 20-year-old woman early in her second pregnancy (gravida 2, para 1). Her pregnancy dating, based on the first day of her last menstrual period, is 8 2/7 weeks. She is complaining of intermittent nausea and vomiting that occurs primarily in the evening hours. She also had nausea and vomiting in the first 14 weeks of her first pregnancy that was partially controlled with diet changes and ginger. However, these interventions have not been successful in this pregnancy. She believes the symptoms are much worse than before. Except for motion sickness, her medical history is negative. Her mother had severe NVP that required hospitalization in two of her three pregnancies. She is taking no medications, other than the ginger and prenatal vitamins. She stopped drinking coffee several weeks ago because of the nausea and she does not smoke or drink alcohol, and there is no history of using other abuse substances. Her prepregnancy weight was 86.4 kilograms, but she is now 83.6 kilograms. Her height is 162.6 centimeters, giving her a body mass index of about 32. Electrolytes, urinalysis, and a complete blood count are within normal limits. There is no evidence of a urinary tract infection. Her blood pressure (130/75 mmHg) and pulse (80 beats per minute) are normal.

III. Nausea and Vomiting of Pregnancy

A. Etiology

The causes of NVP and its most severe form, hyperemesis gravidarum, are unknown, but several theories have been advanced.[1,4–8] These include psychological factors, evolutionary adaptation, nutritional deficiencies, thyrotoxicosis, serotonin, upper gastrointestinal dysmotility, liver abnormalities, Helicobacter pylori infection, and hormonal changes.

Although popular in the past, the belief that a psychological disorder, such as an abnormal response to stress or a subconscious attempt to reject an unwanted pregnancy, was responsible for NVP[5–7] has been largely discarded.[1,8] A hypothesis with more credibility is that NVP is an evolutionary adaptation that developed to protect the embryo and fetus from maternal ingestion of potentially toxic substances.[1] However, belief that NVP is a natural consequence of pregnancy can lead to undertreatment and a decrease in the quality of life for the mother.[1]

Although nutritional deficiencies, thyrotoxicosis, serotonin, upper gastrointestinal dysmotility, liver abnormalities, and *H. pylori* infection may have a role in some cases, evidence for a major role in the etiology of NVP is lacking.[4–8]

There is circumstantial evidence from many studies that hCG and estradiol might be responsible for NVP.[1] Peak concentrations of hCG occur at the same time as peak symptoms of nausea/vomiting. Moreover, placental conditions (eg, multiple gestation) that increase the concentration of hCG also increase the risk of severe NVP. Hyperemesis gravidarum also is associated with female fetuses.[9,10] The mechanism is thought to be related to higher concentrations of hCG in maternal blood and placental tissues when the fetus is a female.[10] The concentration of estradiol also is closely associated with the prevalence of nausea/vomiting. It is well known that estrogen in combination oral contraceptives induces nausea/vomiting in a dose-related manner. The frequent observation that women who smoke cigarettes are less likely to experience hyperemesis gravidarum is consistent with the observation that smoking is associated with lower concentrations of hCG and estradiol.[1]

B. Maternal Risk Factors

Several risk factors for NVP, including for the most severe form hyperemesis gravidarum, have been identified. The factors are increased placental mass (eg, multiple gestation), family or personal history of hyperemesis gravidarum, and history of motion sickness or migraine headaches.[1]

C. Effect on the Mother

Although maternal death secondary to NVP is rare, the condition is related to significant morbidity.[1] Wernicke's encephalopathy caused by vitamin B_1 (thiamine) deficiency has been associated with maternal death as well as permanent neurologic disability. Other reported maternal adverse effects are splenic avulsion, esophageal rupture and pneumothorax associated with vomiting, acute tubular necrosis, and marked psychosocial morbidity resulting in pregnancy termination. Depression, somatization, and hypochondriasis also have been associated with NVP.[1]

D. Effect on the Embryo and/or Fetus

Developmental toxicity (growth restriction, structural anomalies, functional/neurobehavioral deficits, or death) is not associated with NVP. In contrast, uncontrolled hyperemesis gravidarum may be associated with an increased risk of a low-birthweight infant (ie, less than the 10th percentile for gestational age). Moreover, uncontrolled hyperemesis may cause the woman to electively terminate her pregnancy. Long-term studies of the health of offspring from mothers with hyperemesis have not been conducted. On the other hand, women with NVP including hyperemesis actually have fewer spontaneous abortions or miscarriages than women who do not experience nausea/vomiting during pregnancy.

E. Differential Diagnosis

The diagnosis of NVP is usually straightforward; an otherwise healthy pregnant woman experiences nausea and vomiting. The onset of the symptoms almost always occurs before 9 weeks of gestation.[1] However, there are many diseases and conditions that mimic this condition and must be excluded, especially if the onset of symptoms occurs after 9 weeks of gestation. Thus, NVP is a diagnosis of exclusion. A 1998 review listed 26 diseases and conditions under six major headings that were involved in the differential diagnosis of NVP.[11] A sampling of these diseases and conditions exemplifies the difficulties that can arise in the diagnosis: gastrointestinal (eg, gastroenteritis, gastroparesis, hepatitis, peptic ulcer disease), genitourinary tract (eg, pyelonephritis, kidney stones, ovarian torsion, uremia), metabolic disease (eg, diabetic ketoacidosis, Addison's disease, hyperthyroidism, porphyria), neurologic disorders (eg, migraine, pseudotumor cerebri, vestibular lesions, central nervous system tumors), miscellaneous (drug toxicity or intolerance, psychological), and pregnancy-related conditions (preeclampsia, acute fatty liver of pregnancy).[1,11] Many of these same diseases and conditions were noted in a 2000 review.[7]

IV. Prevention

A. Diet

Although the benefits are not well documented, obstetricians frequently recommend modifications in a woman's diet to prevent or lessen the effects of NVP.[1] The modifications include avoiding spicy foods, eating frequent small meals, high-protein snacks, and crackers in the morning before arising, and a dry, low-fat, bland diet.[1] "Dry" is defined by some dietitians as no liquids for 30 minutes after a meal. A 1998 study found that a high daily intake of total fat, particularly saturated fat, increased the risk of severe hyperemesis.[12]

B. Multivitamins

Taking multivitamins at the time of conception has been associated with less frequent need for therapy to control vomiting.[1] Women of reproductive potential should be taking multivitamins with folic acid before conception to lessen the chance of neural tube defects in offspring. Decreasing the frequency of medical intervention to control vomiting is an added benefit from the multivitamins.

C. Rest

Although the effect of rest on the symptoms of NVP has not been directly studied, adequate rest is important for overall health, including health during pregnancy. Rest may alleviate the initial symptoms of NVP.[1]

D. Avoidance of Emetogenic Odors

Sensory stimuli, particularly odors, are known to provoke nausea and vomiting.[1] A 1995 publication hypothesized that pregnancy-induced hyperolfaction might be involved in NVP.[13] The range of triggering odors was quite broad and included common background odors in the home such as foods, body odors, cigarette smoke, and perfumed soaps, as well as odors from multiple sources outside of the home. The emetogenic stimuli will vary from patient to patient, but women with NVP should be counseled to avoid or eliminate those odors that trigger symptoms.

E. Avoidance of Iron Tablets

Gastric upset is frequently associated with the ingestion of iron tablets in pregnancy.[1] Even though iron supplementation during gestation is important, women suffering from NVP should be told to stop taking iron until the nausea/vomiting has ceased.

F. Acupuncture and Acupressure

Both acupuncture and acupressure have been studied in the treatment of NVP.[1] Although the majority of studies found a benefit, many have significant methodologic flaws. Two of the largest and best-designed studies showed no benefit other than a large placebo effect.[1] A 2006 study found no difference between acupressure and placebo in terms of the need for antiemetic medications, IV fluids, or the duration of hospital stay.[14]

V. Treatment

A. Intravenous Hydration

Intravenous hydration is a common treatment option for women who have become dehydrated secondary to NVP. Typically, 1–2 liters of isotonic fluids are infused over several hours either in the physician's office or the hospital emergency room. Relief of the patient's symptoms is usually rapid and may last up to a day. However, even if oral antiemetic therapy is initiated, nausea/vomiting frequently returns and repeated courses of IV hydration may be required.

B. Vitamin B$_6$

Pyridoxine (vitamin B$_6$) is the only vitamin known to have an antiemetic effect. The mechanism of the antiemetic action is unknown but, as a B complex vitamin, it acts as an essential coenzyme that is involved in the metabolism of amino acids, carbohydrates, and lipids. The first reported use of pyridoxine for NVP appeared in 1942 and, since then, numerous reports have described successful treatment of NVP.[15] For example, two studies using short courses with oral doses of 10 or 25 mg every 8 hours found significant decreases in nausea and vomiting.[16,17]

The vitamin also was a component, along with doxylamine, of Bendectin, a popular and effective product that was frequently used for NVP.[18] Although Bendectin had been used by more than 30 million pregnant women in the 1960s–1980s, the manufacturer withdrew the product from the market in 1983 because of several large legal awards against the company involving birth defects. However, the large body of scientific evidence indicated that the combination of 10 mg pyridoxine and 10 mg doxylamine was safe and effective.[18] In fact, a similar product, Diclectin, has been available in Canada since 1978, and the individual ingredients (pyridoxine and doxylamine) are available over-the-counter worldwide. In 1999, the FDA added the combination to its published list of "Approved Drug Products with Therapeutic Equivalence Evaluations," commonly known as the "Orange Book." Drugs listed in the Orange Book are considered safe and effective for their stated indications. In this case, the stated indication is the prevention of nausea during pregnancy.

Pyridoxine (Table 1) is a reasonable option for any pregnant woman suffering from NVP. Consideration also should be given to combining pyridoxine with doxylamine if pyridoxine alone does not provide adequate relief (see Doxylamine, in Table 1).

C. Ginger

Ginger has been used in Chinese herbal or folk medicine for the treatment of NVP since ancient times.[19] The mechanism, although uncertain, appears to be a local effect in the gut that inhibits gastrointestinal serotonin, thereby preventing stimulation of the vagus nerve and, subsequently, the vomiting center. Recent studies have shown ginger to be an effective antiemetic without causing adverse pregnancy outcomes.[19] A 2005 review of herbal remedies recommending caution in the use of ginger[20] elicited correspondence that the recommendation was unfounded[21] and a reply.[22] In a randomized, controlled trial, ginger and vitamin B_6 were equally efficacious for reducing nausea, retching, or vomiting.[23]

Either ginger (Table 1) or pyridoxine is a reasonable option for NVP. However, because there are more human data for the vitamin, pyridoxine is the first choice for mild NVP.

Table 1. Prevention and Treatment of Nausea and Vomiting of Pregnancy

Condition	Therapy
Preconception	Multivitamins
Nausea[a]	Avoid spicy foods; frequent small meals; high-protein snacks; dry, low-fat, bland diet; adequate rest; avoid sensory stimuli associated with NV; avoid iron tablets if they cause gastric upset
Mild NV[a]	
No history of HG	Pyridoxine, 25 mg 3–4 times per day
	or
	Ginger powder, 250 mg 4 times per day
	or
	Doxylamine, 12.5 mg *plus*
	Pyridoxine, 25 mg at bedtime
History of HG	Doxylamine, 12.5 mg *plus*
	Pyridoxine, 25 mg twice daily
Moderate NV[a]	Doxylamine, 12.5 mg *plus*
	Pyridoxine, 25 mg 4 times per day
Severe NV[a]	Same as for moderate NV *plus*
(not HG)	IV hydration
	or
	Metoclopramide, 5–10 mg *plus*
	Hydroxyzine, 50 mg 3–4 times per day
	plus IV hydration

HG = hyperemesis gravidarum, History = personal or family history, NV = nausea/vomiting.
[a]According to patient.

D. Pharmacologic Therapy

1. Antihistamines

Although first-generation antihistamines are known to have antiemetic activity, only dimenhydrinate, diphenhydramine, doxylamine, hydroxyzine, meclizine, and tri-methobenzamide have reported use in the treatment of NVP.[24] There are no recent reports describing the use of trimethobenzamide for NVP, and its use for this purpose appears to have been replaced by other antihistamines. The mechanism of antihista-mines probably is related to interruption of signals from the vestibular apparatus in the inner ear to the vomiting center in the medulla oblongata. In addition to their antihis-tamine (H_1 receptor antagonist) activity, they also have anticholinergic and sedative actions. They do not appear to cause embryo or fetal harm.[24] However, their sedating properties might limit their use.

The proprietary combination of doxylamine and pyridoxine (Bendectin) has been used extensively for NVP and is the most studied drug product in human preg-nancy.[15,18] If the patient characterizes her symptoms as moderate to severe, or if she has a history of moderate to severe nausea/vomiting in a previous pregnancy, the extemporaneous combination is the treatment of first choice (Table 1). Patients should be counseled regarding the sedating properties of the antihistamine.

2. Antidopaminergics

The antidopaminergics that have been used for NVP are the butyrophenones, meto-clopramide, and phenothiazines.[24] The primary antiemetic effect appears to be related to inhibition of the dopamine signal from the chemoreceptor trigger zone to the vom-iting center in the medulla oblongata. These agents are usually reserved for women who have not responded to other therapies.

Although two butyrophenones, droperidol and haloperidol, have been used to treat severe NVP, only droperidol is presently used for this purpose. Droperidol is the most potent antiemetic agent, on a weight basis, among the antidopaminergics. Although the data are limited, it does not appear to be associated with embryo-fetal harm.[25] A continuous IV infusion of droperidol has been used for the treatment of hyperemesis gravidarum.[9] The primary adverse effect observed was an extrapyramidal reaction (akathisia). Addition of an antihistamine with anticholinergic activity, such as diphenhydramine significantly reduces the prevalence of akathisia but potentiates sedation.

In 2001, the U.S. Food and Drug Administration (FDA) placed a black box warning for QT prolongation and torsades de pointes on droperidol. However, there have been no published cases of this adverse effect when the drug was used as an antiemetic. The authors have unpublished data in 49 women that continuous infusions of droperidol do not cause a significant change in the QT interval. A 2004 editorial commented that the degree of QT prolongation from antiemetic doses of droperidol had no clinical significance.[26] A study published in 2007 examined all of the cases that the FDA had used for the black box warning.[27] After excluding dupli-cate reports, there were 65 cases of cardiac toxicity possibly caused by droperidol, but only two involved doses used in the United States, one of which involved a patient with preexisting cardiovascular disease. In addition, the FDA used data from

Europe that involved doses 50–100 times higher than those used in the United States. Thus, it did not appear that drugs such as ondansetron were safer than droperidol with regard to QT interval prolongation.[27]

There are numerous reports describing the use of metoclopramide in human pregnancy.[28] The mechanism of action probably is related to its antidopaminergic activity and to increased gastric emptying. It has been used both orally and parenterally for hospitalized and nonhospitalized patients. The drug appears to be safe and effective for the treatment of NVP.[28] However, because it can cause severe adverse reactions, such as dystonia (an extrapyramidal reaction), it is not considered a treatment of first choice (see Table 1 for dose). The addition of a first-generation antihistamine with anticholinergic properties, such as diphenhydramine or hydroxyzine, to prevent dystonia should be considered.

The phenothiazines include the antipsychotics chlorpromazine, perphenazine, and prochlorperazine, and the antihistamine promethazine. The antiemetic effect of the antipsychotics is secondary to the antidopaminergic activity, whereas the effect of promethazine is similar to other antihistamines. Maternal use appears to represent a low risk of embryo-fetal harm.[24] Based on the absence of reports, it appears that perphenazine and chlorpromazine are no longer routinely used in pregnancy as antiemetics. Because the antipsychotic phenothiazines can cause severe dystonia, their primary usefulness has been in hospitalized patients. If they are used, consideration should be given to adding an antihistamine (other than promethazine), such as diphenhydramine, to prevent dystonia. A typical oral dose for prochlorperazine is 5–10 mg four times daily. The rectal dose is a 25-mg suppository twice daily. For promethazine, a common dose is 12.5–25 mg orally, rectally, or intravenously every 4 hours.

3. Selective Serotonin (5-HT$_3$) Receptor Antagonists

Ondansetron is the only agent in this class with published experience in the treatment of NVP.[29] Because serotonin 5-HT$_3$ receptors are located peripherally on vagal nerve terminals and centrally in the chemoreceptor trigger zone, the antiemetic action may be mediated peripherally, centrally, or at both sites.[30] The limited human data do not suggest embryo-fetal risk,[29] but the drug does not appear to represent a significant advancement in the therapy or prevention of NVP. A 1996 randomized, double-blind study comparing IV ondansetron and promethazine found no differences between the drugs in terms of duration of hospitalization, nausea score, number of doses received, treatment failures, and daily weight gain.[31] In three other studies, the IV doses used for NVP were 8–10 mg two to three times daily.[29] A 2007 study concluded that droperidol was as safe and effective as ondansetron.[27] Moreover, selective serotonin (5-HT$_3$) receptor antagonists did not appear to be safer than droperidol with regard to QT prolongation.[27] Although the oral dose for NVP has not been quantified, 4–8 mg three times daily appears to be a reasonable option. However, ondansetron is not a first-line agent for the treatment of NVP but, if it is used, it should be combined with an antihistamine.

4. Corticosteroids

Corticosteroids, such as hydrocortisone and methylprednisolone, have been used for the treatment of hyperemesis gravidarum. However, these agents carry a small risk (1–2 per 1000 live births) for cleft lip and/or palate if used before 10 weeks of gestation.[32]

They should be considered agents of last choice and then only for severe NVP that has not responded to other therapies.[1]

VI. Treatment of Hyperemesis Gravidarum

Hyperemesis gravidarum is the most severe form of NVP. It occurs in approximately 0.5%–2.0% of all pregnancies.[1] Although any definition of hyperemesis is controversial, a good working definition is severe nausea/vomiting that prevents oral intake of food and liquids, and is characterized by at least one of three objective findings: loss of 5% or more from the prepregnancy body weight, hypokalemia, and ketonuria.[9] Hyperemesis is the most common reason for hospital admission in the first part of pregnancy and is second only to preterm labor for hospitalization at any time during pregnancy.[1]

A 2005 study examined the pregnancy outcomes of 2466 hyperemesis cases among a cohort of 520,739 births.[33] Singleton infants from mothers with hyperemesis were smaller (3255 vs 3380 grams, $p < .0001$) and more likely to be small for gestational age (29.2% vs 20.8%, $p < .0001$) than infants whose mothers did not have hyperemesis.

Treatment of hyperemesis involves rest, IV fluids with replacement of electrolytes (potassium, sodium, and magnesium), IV multivitamins (if patient has been unable to take oral multivitamins), diet control, IV drugs, and oral medications upon discharge. Some studies have used only oral drugs, but in such a setting the diagnosis of hyperemesis is questionable. One algorithm for management recommends the following IV drugs (in alphabetical order): dimenhydrinate, 50 mg every 4–6 hours; or metoclopramide, 5–10 mg every 8 hours; or promethazine, 12.5–25 mg every 4 hours.[1,34] If necessary, additional therapy includes the following: oral or IV methylprednisolone, 16 mg every 8 hours for 3 days and then tapered over 2 weeks to the lowest effective dose (maximum duration 6 weeks); or IV ondansetron, 8 mg every 12 hours.[34]

A 1996 study used an IV infusion of droperidol combined with IV diphenhydramine, 50 mg, every 6 hours for about 36 hours (Table 2).[9] After approximately 48

Table 2. Treatment of Hyperemesis Gravidarum

1. Intravenous hydration with isotonic solutions at 250 mL/h for 4 h, then 150 mL/h until discharged from the hospital;
2. Replace electrolytes (potassium, sodium, and magnesium) as needed;
3. Multivitamins plus additional pyridoxine (25 mg/L) in IV fluids;
4. Bland, low-fat, dry, diet with frequent (eg, six) meals per day;
5. Intravenous medications (eg, droperidol[a] or metoclopramide) (see text);
6. Diphenhydramine, 50 mg IV over 30 min every 6 h;
7. Discharge from hospital on oral medications (eg, metoclopramide plus hydroxyzine or doxylamine plus pyridoxine) (see text).

[a]A 12-lead ECG conducted before administering droperidol and continued for 2–3 h after completing treatment is an option but, based on a large amount of data, it appears to be unnecessary. Patients should have normal concentrations of potassium and magnesium and should not receive droperidol if they have a history of QT prolongation (slow heart rate), congestive heart failure, cardiac arrhythmias, or are taking other drugs known to increase the QT interval. Additionally, because there is a genetic component for QT prolongation, women also should be excluded if they have a history of an immediate blood relative (mother, father, or siblings) with QT prolongation or sudden cardiac death secondary to cardiac arrhythmia.
From Nageotte MP et al.[9]

hours of hospitalization, patients were discharged home on oral metoclopramide, 10 mg, and hydroxyzine, 50 mg, both given four times daily (with meals and at bedtime) for approximately 2 weeks. IV fluids included multivitamins and additional pyridoxine. Approximately 15% of the patients required a second hospitalization with the same therapy. Readmission was primarily due to noncompliance with the prescribed diet or, to a lesser extent, stopping the drug therapy prematurely. When compared to a historical cohort of women treated with other medications for hyperemesis gravidarum, this newer protocol was associated with fewer overall hospital days and fewer readmissions for treatment of hyperemesis.[9]

A 2001 Montreal study, using a method similar to that described immediately above, compared droperidol infusions with historical controls for the treatment of hyperemesis gravidarum.[35] The droperidol group had a significantly shorter duration of hospitalization, fewer readmissions, and lower average daily nausea and vomiting scores. No difference between the groups in the number of major defects was observed.[35] In 2003, a second study from Montreal compared two doses (0.5 and 1.0 mg/hour) of droperidol with historical controls and, again, found no differences between the groups in major birth defects.[36]

VII. Effects of Treatment on the Embryo and/or Fetus

With the exception of the corticosteroids, the antiemetics used to prevent or treat NVP appear to be low risk for causing embryo and/or fetal harm.[15,18,19,24,25,29] However, there is inadequate human pregnancy experience for nearly all antiemetics.[24] Combined with the fact that the peak incidence of NVP occurs during organogenesis, antiemetics, with one exception, cannot be considered safe for the embryo-fetus. Only the combination of doxylamine-pyridoxine has sufficient human data to be classified as safe in pregnancy.[15,18]

VIII. CASE HISTORY [PART 2]

Assessment: Relevant information includes her mother's history of hyperemesis, J.W.'s history of NVP and motion sickness, and her current condition. She has not responded to ginger and diet, and she thinks the symptoms are worse than in her first pregnancy. She has lost 3.2% of her prepregnancy weight, her serum potassium is within normal limits, and she does not have ketonuria.

Plan: (1) Discontinue ginger and prenatal vitamins; (2) start doxylamine, 12.5 mg, plus pyridoxine, 25 mg, four times daily (with meals and at bedtime); (3) change diet to six small meals daily that are bland and low fat. Encourage her to drink fluids between meals.

Rationale: The combination of doxylamine-pyridoxine is considered safe and effective. Although the cardinal signs are negative, she is at risk for developing hyperemesis gravidarum. Thus, a higher dose should be started.

Monitoring: The patient should be seen at least weekly for monitoring of her symptoms, hydration, weight gain or loss, and urine ketones (by dipstick). A repeat serum potassium should be considered if her vomiting continues.

Patient Education: Counsel the patient to avoid sensory stimuli, especially odors. Compliance with a low emetogenic diet is critical as is compliance with the drug therapy. Because doxylamine is very sedating, she needs to be cautious with any tasks, such as driving or cooking, that require close attention. She should call the office or clinic if her symptoms worsen.

IX. Summary

Nausea and vomiting of pregnancy is a very common condition. Although it can adversely affect the woman's quality of life and may have direct and indirect effects on the embryo-fetus, it also is associated with fewer spontaneous pregnancy losses. There are several treatment options for NVP and determining which is optimal for a specific patient depends on the gestational age and an understanding of the condition. In addition to the references already cited, two recent reviews offer further information.[37,38]

Clinicians providing services to pregnant women can have a major impact in the treatment of this condition. The provision of factual information regarding NVP to the patient, drug selection based on gestational age and the patient's perception of the severity of her symptoms, appropriate monitoring of the patient's response to therapy, and patient education are vital tasks. Patient education is critical because some women are hesitant to accept treatment because of unfounded fears of risk to their embryo or fetus.[2]

X. References

1. American College of Obstetricians and Gynecologists. Nausea and vomiting of pregnancy. ACOG Technical Bulletin. Number 52, April 2004. *Obstet Gynecol.* 2004;103:803–815.

2. Mazzitta O, Magee LA, Maltepe C, et al. The perception of teratogenic risk by women with nausea and vomiting of pregnancy. *Reprod Toxicol.* 1999;13:313–319.

3. Lacroix R, Eason E, Melzack R. Nausea and vomiting during pregnancy: a prospective study of its frequency, intensity, and patterns of change. *Am J Obstet Gynecol.* 2000;182:931–937.

4. Jarnfelt-Samsioe A. Nausea and vomiting in pregnancy: a review. *Obstet Gynecol Survey.* 1987;41:422–427.

5. Hod M, Orvieto R, Kaplan B, et al. Hyperemesis gravidarum: a review. *J Reprod Med.* 1994;39:605–612.

6. Broussard CN, Richter JE. Nausea and vomiting of pregnancy. *Gastroenterol Clin North Am.* 1998;27:123–151.

7. Eliakim R, Abulafia O, Sherer DM. Hyperemesis gravidarum: a current review. *Am J Perinatol.* 2000;17:207–218.

8. Goodwin TM. Nausea and vomiting of pregnancy: an obstetric syndrome. *Am J Obstet Gynecol*. 2002;186:S184–189.

9. Nageotte MP, Briggs GG, Towers CV, et al. Droperidol and diphenhydramine in the management of hyperemesis gravidarum. *Am J Obstet Gynecol*. 1996;174:1801–1806.

10. Melero-Montes MDM, Jick H. Hyperemesis gravidarum and the sex of the offspring. *Epidemiology*. 2000;12:123–124.

11. Goodwin TM. Hyperemesis gravidarum. *Clin Obstet Gynecol*. 1998;41:597–605.

12. Signorello LB, Harlow BL, Wang S, et al. Saturated fat intake and the risk of severe hyperemesis gravidarum. *Epidemiology*. 1998; 9:636–640.

13. Erick M. Hyperolfaction and hyperemesis gravidarum: what is the relationship? *Nutr Rev*. 1995;289–295.

14. Heazell A, Thorneycroft J, Walton V, et al. Acupressure for the in-patient treatment of nausea and vomiting in early pregnancy: a randomized control trial. *Am J Obstet Gynecol*. 2006;194:815–820.

15. Briggs GG, Freeman RK, Yaffe SJ. Pyridoxine. In *Drugs in Pregnancy and Lactation*. 8th ed. Philadelphia: Lippincott Williams & Wilkins, 2008:1563–1570.

16. Sahakian V, Rouse D, Sipes S, et al. Vitamin B6 is effective therapy for nausea and vomiting of pregnancy: a randomized double-blind placebo-controlled study. *Obstet Gynecol*. 1991;78:33–36.

17. Vutyavanich T, Wongtra-ngan S, Ruangsri R-A. Pyridoxine for nausea and vomiting of pregnancy: a randomized, double-blind, placebo-controlled trial. *Am J Obstet Gynecol*. 1995;173:881–884.

18. Briggs GG, Freeman RK, Yaffe SJ. Doxylamine. In *Drugs in Pregnancy and Lactation*. 8th ed. Philadelphia: Lippincott Williams & Wilkins, 2008:580–586.

19. Briggs GG, Freeman RK, Yaffe SJ. Ginger. In *Drugs in Pregnancy and Lactation*. 8th ed. Philadelphia: Lippincott Williams & Wilkins, 2008:820–822.

20. Marcus DM, Snodgrass WR. Do no harm: avoidance of herbal medicines during pregnancy. *Obstet Gynecol*. 2005;105:1119–1122.

21. Fugh-Berman A, Lione A, Scialli AR. Do no harm: avoidance of herbal medicines during pregnancy (Letter). *Obstet Gynecol*. 2005;106:409–410.

22. Marcus DM, Snodgrass WR. Do no harm: avoidance of herbal medicines during pregnancy (Letter). *Obstet Gynecol*. 2005;106:410–411.

23. Smith C, Crowther C, Willson K, et al. A randomized controlled trial of ginger to treat nausea and vomiting of pregnancy. *Obstet Gynecol*. 2004;103:639–645.

24. Briggs GG, Freeman RK, Yaffe SJ. *Drugs in Pregnancy and Lactation*. 8th ed. Philadelphia: Lippincott Williams & Wilkins, 2008.

25. Briggs GG, Freeman RK, Yaffe SJ. Droperidol. In *Drugs in Pregnancy and Lactation*. 8th ed. Philadelphia: Lippincott Williams & Wilkins, 2008:586–588.

26. White PF. Prevention of postoperative nausea and vomiting—a multimodal solution to a persistent problem. *N Engl J Med*. 2004;350:2511–2512.

27. Jackson CW, Sheehan AH, Reddan JG. Evidence-based review of the black-box warning for droperidol. *Am J Health-Syst Pharm*. 2007;64:1174–1186.

28. Briggs GG, Freeman RK, Yaffe SJ. Metoclopramide. In *Drugs in Pregnancy and Lactation*. 8th ed. Philadelphia: Lippincott Williams & Wilkins, 2008:1197–1201.

29. Briggs GG, Freeman RK, Yaffe SJ. Ondansetron. In *Drugs in Pregnancy and Lactation*. 8th ed. Philadelphia: Lippincott Williams & Wilkins, 2008:1368–1369.

30. Zofran. In *Physicians' Desk Reference*. 62nd ed. Montvale, NJ: Thomson Healthcare; 2008:1649–1652.

31. Sullivan CA, Johnson CA, Roach H, et al. A pilot study of intravenous ondansetron for hyperemesis gravidarum. *Am J Obstet Gynecol.* 1996;174:1565–1568.

32. Briggs GG, Freeman RK, Yaffe SJ. Hydrocortisone. In *Drugs in Pregnancy and Lactation*. 8th ed. Philadelphia: Lippincott Williams & Wilkins, 2008:879–887.

33. Bailit JL. Hyperemesis gravidarum: epidemiologic findings from a large cohort. *Am J Obstet Gynecol.* 2005;193:811–814.

34. Levichek Z, Atanackovic G, Oepkes D, et al. Nausea and vomiting of pregnancy: evidence-based treatment algorithm. *Can Fam Physician.* 2002;48:267–268, 277.

35. Turcotte V, Ferreira E, Duperron L. Utilité du dropéridol et de la diphenhydramine dans l'hyperemesis gravidarum. *J Soc Obstet Gynaecol Can.* 2001;23:133–139.

36. Ferreira E, Bussieres J-F, Turcotte V, et al. Case-control study comparing droperidol plus diphenhydramine with conventional treatment in hyperemesis gravidarum. *J Pharm Technol.* 2003;19:349–354.

37. Mazzotta P, Magee LA. A risk-benefit assessment of pharmacological and non-pharmacological treatments for nausea and vomiting of pregnancy. *Drugs.* 2000;59:781–800.

38. Badell ML, Ramin SM, Smith JA. Treatment options for nausea and vomiting during pregnancy. *Pharmacotherapy.* 2006;26:1273–1287.

QUESTIONS AND ANSWERS

1. The most credible theory on the cause of NVP is:

    a. evolutionary adaptation

    b. serotonin

    c. hCG and estradiol

    d. psychological

2. A woman with hyperemesis gravidarum in a previous pregnancy begins to have mild nausea/vomiting early in her current pregnancy. The best treatment option at this time is:

    a. doxylamine, 12.5 mg, plus pyridoxine, 25 mg, twice daily

    b. pyridoxine, 25 mg QID

    c. intravenous ondansetron, 8 mg every 8 hours

    d. metoclopramide, 10 mg, plus hydroxyzine, 50 mg TID

3. A patient at 14 weeks' gestation has moderately severe nausea/vomiting. She has been treated with pyridoxine, 25 mg QID, and diet but her symptoms have become more severe. At 12 weeks' gestation, she was given IV methylprednisolone, 16 mg, and then started on prednisone, 10 mg daily. What are the risks of the therapy to her developing baby? The best answer is:

    a. There is a small risk of oral clefts from the corticosteroids.

    b. There are no risks of embryo-fetal harm from the therapy.

    c. There is a background risk of birth defects but none from the therapy.

    d. There is a risk of growth retardation from the severe nausea/vomiting as well as from the corticosteroid.

4. A woman at 8 weeks' gestation in her first pregnancy has marked nausea, with little or no vomiting, that lasts throughout the day. Her family history is negative for hyperemesis gravidarum. The best treatment for her at this time is:

    a. lifestyle changes plus ginger powder, 250 mg, four times daily

    b. lifestyle changes plus doxylamine, 12.5 mg, at bedtime

    c. lifestyle changes plus pyridoxine, 25 mg, at bedtime

    d. lifestyle changes such as diet, avoiding stimulating odors, and rest

Answers:

1. c; 2. a; 3. c; 4. d

Autoimmune Diseases in Pregnancy

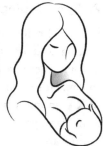

Eliza Chakravarty and Christina Chambers

CHAPTER 25

LEARNING OBJECTIVES

1. Evaluate the effects of pregnancy on underlying autoimmune disease activity using rheumatoid arthritis and systemic lupus erythematosus as examples.

2. Outline the potential adverse effects of underlying autoimmune disease on pregnancy outcome and how these vary by specific type of autoimmune disease.

3. Identify common medication options for treatment of systemic lupus or rheumatoid arthritis and identify those that carry potential teratogenic risks.

I. Introduction

Autoimmune diseases tend to be more common among women and may occur in 1%–2% of females. Although some autoimmune diseases have an average age of onset that is beyond a woman's typical reproductive years, many of these diseases can and do occur in women who have the potential to become pregnant and/or who wish to plan a pregnancy. Changes in the disease course, symptom control, and issues related to appropriate treatment raise important and unique issues during pregnancy. Two examples of autoimmune rheumatologic conditions, rheumatoid arthritis (RA) and systemic lupus erythematosus (SLE) are presented to illustrate the various challenges these diseases and their treatment present in pregnancy.

II. PATIENT CASE (PART 1): RHEUMATOID ARTHRITIS

A 35-year-old woman with long-standing diagnosis of RA found out she was 6 weeks pregnant while being treated with etanercept, prednisone, and nonsteroidal anti-inflammatory drugs (NSAIDs). This was her first pregnancy, and although unplanned, the pregnancy was desired.

A. Epidemiology and Pathophysiology

RA is a chronic systemic autoimmune disease that often leads to chronic joint inflammation and destruction with progressive loss of function. Most patients require chronic therapy with disease-modifying antirheumatic drugs (DMARDs) to control inflammation and prevent or retard progressive damage to the joints. The prevalence of RA among women in the United States is estimated to be approximately 1.4% with a median age of onset of 59 years. Although prevalence estimates among women of childbearing age are not available in the United States, they are approximately 1–2 per 1000 women between ages 16 and 44 years in the United Kingdom.[1] There have been suggestions that underlying RA may reduce fertility, fecundity, or the desire for additional children.[2,3] Recent nationwide estimates suggest that approximately 1000–2000 women with underlying RA become pregnant annually.[2–4] In contrast to SLE, in which flares appear to be common, many patients with underlying RA may expect some degree of amelioration or reduction in symptoms during pregnancy, but most will experience a flare within 4 months postpartum.[2]

The majority of clinical studies of disease activity of RA during pregnancy consistently find that reduction in signs and symptoms occurs in approximately 75% of patients.[2] Improvements are often seen as early as the first trimester of pregnancy and continue through the end of pregnancy.[5] Underlying immunologic mechanisms responsible for this observation remain unknown. While this is encouraging news for women with RA who wish to have children, it still leaves approximately 25% who will not improve and may even worsen during pregnancy. In contrast, one recent prospective study of 30 women with RA using a standardized disease activity index throughout pregnancy found that at least 50% had intermediate to high disease activity during the third trimester.[6] To date, no clinical or standard laboratory variables have been found to be predictive of the course the disease will take during pregnancy. Given that RA is generally a chronic, progressive disease that is not characterized by flares and remissions, achieving disease remission without underlying medical therapy before conception is elusive and usually not feasible.

In past decades, there was not much study of pregnancy outcomes among women with underlying RA. This is largely due to positive data regarding the effects of pregnancy on disease activity. In the absence of the effects of antenatal exposure to potentially teratogenic medications, maternal and fetal outcomes were assumed to be unchanged by maternal RA. It is true that earlier studies did not demonstrate adverse fetal effects.[2] However, more recent studies have begun to show increased rates of adverse pregnancy outcomes among women with RA compared to the general obstetric population. Two studies have found that infants born to mothers with RA have slightly lower birth weight (although generally within the normal range) than those born to healthy mothers,[7,8] and that lower birth weight was associated with increased disease activity of RA during pregnancy.[8] Similarly, studies have shown that underlying RA is associated with an increased risk of prematurity,[9,10] preeclampsia,[4,8] and cesarean delivery.[4,8,10] However, most of these studies do not have sufficient data or are not designed to tease apart the relative effects of underlying disease activity or medication exposure.

Goals for preconception management of RA center on the removal of disease-modifying agents several months before conception and replacement, when necessary, with agents that have a known and acceptable safety profile during pregnancy. There also may be some emerging evidence that increased disease activity during pregnancy may have subtle adverse effects on the fetus.

B. Detection and Screening

It is extremely rare for RA to first present during pregnancy; however, disease onset may begin during the postpartum period. Aside from discontinuation of known teratogenic medications before conception or on discovery of pregnancy, the most critical aspect for monitoring RA during pregnancy is to distinguish underlying activity of RA from normal changes during pregnancy.

In the nonpregnant state, erythrocyte sedimentation rate (ESR) and c-reactive protein (CRP) are two acute-phase proteins that become elevated in association with systemic inflammation, and usually correlate well with increased disease activity of RA. They are key components of different disease activity indices used commonly to quantitate disease activity in the clinic and for research. These parameters have been shown to change by trimester during healthy pregnancies, with more dramatic increases seen with the ESR rather than the CRP.[11] Nonetheless, because of natural changes during pregnancy, increases in either ESR or CRP must be interpreted with caution in the pregnant woman with RA.

In addition to changes in laboratory parameters, some clinical changes during pregnancy may mimic increases in disease activity. As pregnancy progresses, women often experience increased generalized fatigue and mild swelling of the distal extremities. Carpal tunnel syndrome (CTS), often a consequence of inflammatory arthritis of the wrist in those with RA, can occur in otherwise healthy pregnancies. One recent study reported an estimated 2% of pregnant patients, without underlying diabetes mellitus or RA, experienced symptoms of CTS severe enough to lead to referral to an orthopedist.[12] Symptoms generally began during the third trimester of pregnancy and were significantly decreased in the first few weeks after delivery.[12] In pregnant RA patients experiencing CTS, careful examination for evidence of joint swelling and tenderness should be undertaken to help distinguish benign, pregnancy-related CTS from a potential flare of underlying RA.

There are no published data on the prevalence of tender joints or swollen joints that may occur in healthy women as a consequence of pregnancy itself. Similarly, most studies of disease activity during pregnancy report only global measures rather than comparisons of tender and swollen joint counts. Despite the lack of rigorous clinical parameters to assess changes in RA disease activity during pregnancy, the experienced clinician should rely on evaluation for synovitis in the joints most commonly affected by RA in contrast to generalized swelling or puffiness that may extend beyond the joint capsule.

C. Prevention

Prevention is almost exclusively centered on counseling of women with RA before pregnancy. Goals for preconception management of RA include counseling regarding the known risk to the fetus of various medications commonly used by women with RA. However, as can be seen in the section below, Pregnancy Safety for Selected Treatments, only a very small number of these medications have been adequately studied with respect to their teratogenicity, making it very difficult to provide women contemplating pregnancy conclusive information. The best that can be done is to provide a woman with the facts that are available, and to provide her with information that can be used to understand issues relating to the risk/benefit of taking a particular agent during her pregnancy. In addition, it is important to recognize that there may be some emerging evidence that failure to control symptoms (ie, increased disease activity during pregnancy) may have subtle adverse effects on the fetus.

D. Pregnancy Safety of Selected Treatments

1. Corticosteroids

It has long been recognized that a dose-related risk exists for corticosteroids, such as prednisone, and intrauterine growth restriction. In addition, although still controversial, three out of four recent case-control studies and a meta-analysis have concluded that systemic corticosteroids used in the first trimester appear to be associated with a three- to six-fold increased risk for cleft lip with or without cleft palate and possibly cleft palate alone.[13-17] The extent to which this association can be explained by the various underlying maternal diseases involved in these studies or other unmeasured confounders is unknown. However, to put these data into perspective, in that the population risk for oral clefts is approximately 1 per 1000 live births, systemic corticosteroid use would be associated with 3–6 oral clefts for every 1000 pregnancies exposed during the critical period for lip/palatal closure. Based on these data, it is suggested that the risk associated with prenatal exposure to these medications is low.

2. Nonsteroidal Anti-Inflammatory Drugs

Included within the NSAID category are celecoxib, indomethacin, ibuprofen, sulindac, ketoprofen, diclofenac, meloxicam, ketorolac, naproxen, nimesulide, and piroxicam. Based on published studies, it is generally not thought that NSAIDs are serious human teratogens. However, some studies have suggested that NSAIDs may be associated with very low risks for certain specific congenital malformations and possibly for miscarriage. Three case-control studies have examined the association between ibuprofen and gastroschisis, a defect that occurs in approximately 5 per 10,000 live births. One of those studies demonstrated a four-fold increased risk when mothers reported using ibuprofen around the time of conception, while the other two studies showed no such association.[18-20] In addition, one large Swedish cohort study has shown an approximate two-fold increased risk for cardiac defects with any NSAID use in early pregnancy and an approximate three-fold increased risk for oral clefts with early pregnancy of NSAIDs, specifically naproxen.[21] Using the same data source, an approximate two-fold increased risk for cardiac defects in association with early pregnancy use of naproxen was documented in another study.[22] In contrast, in a Danish study of NSAID use in early pregnancy, no increased risk for malformations, preterm delivery, or low birth weight was noted.[23] However, this study, as well as one U.S. study, has shown a two- to seven-fold risk for spontaneous abortion when NSAIDs are used in very early in pregnancy.[23,24] At present these data do not provide sufficient or conclusive evidence that NSAIDs used in early pregnancy cause birth defects or spontaneous abortion, even at a low level of risk.

In contrast, more concern has been raised regarding fetal exposure to NSAIDs late in pregnancy, although the magnitude of the risk is not well documented. Premature closure of the fetal ductus arteriosus with resultant pulmonary hypertension has been noted in association with third-trimester exposure to NSAIDs.[25] Renal dysgenesis leading to oligohydramnios has been reported following late pregnancy exposure to ibuprofen, indomethacin, naproxen, ketoprofen, nimesulide, and piroxicam.[26] Necrotizing enterocolitis and ileal perforation, as well as intraventricular hemorrhage and cystic brain lesions, have been seen in premature infants exposed to indomethacin before delivery.[27,28]

Although in utero ductal constriction seldom occurs with prenatal exposure earlier than 27 weeks' gestation, a significant risk is present at or beyond 32 weeks' gestation. This has led to the recommendation that NSAIDs be discontinued before 32 weeks' gestation.

3. Methotrexate

Both aminopterin and its methyl derivative, methotrexate, have been associated with a specific pattern of malformation in infants born to mothers who took these medications early in pregnancy. The pattern of malformation includes prenatal-onset growth deficiency; severe lack of ossification of the calvarium; hypoplastic supraorbital ridges; small, low-set ears; micrognathia or small jaw; and limb abnormalities. The majority of affected infants have been born to women treated with high-dose methotrexate for psoriasis or neoplastic disease or as an abortifacient.[29]

Pregnancy outcomes in 23 women with RA who had 25 pregnancies in which the fetus was prenatally exposed to methotrexate have been reported.[29–32] The dosage of methotrexate in these pregnancies was low, ranging from 7.5–12.5 mg/wk. Nine of the 25 pregnancies resulted in spontaneous abortion and 14 resulted in normal babies. One woman who received a total methotrexate dose of approximately 100 mg over the first 8 weeks of her pregnancy had a baby with the aminopterin/methotrexate syndrome, and two women electively terminated their pregnancies. In another case series, pregnancy outcome was reported for 28 women, 22 of whom were treated for RA, and for all but one woman, doses were <15 mg/wk during early pregnancy. Five pregnancies ended in elective termination, four in spontaneous abortion, and the remaining 19 resulted in live births. One child presented with mild neonatal abnormalities consisting of bilateral metarsus varus and right eyelid angioma.[33] Based on these cases, it has been suggested that the maternal methotrexate dose necessary to produce the aminopterin/methotrexate syndrome is greater than 10 mg/wk.[29] Furthermore, it has been suggested that the critical period of exposure relative to the risk for the syndrome is between 6 and 8 weeks postconception.[29] However, data are still not sufficient to verify the exact threshold dose, the critical window of exposure, or the magnitude of the risk for the syndrome following first-trimester exposure to methotrexate.

4. Leflunomide

No malformations were reported among the offspring of 10 women who were prescribed leflunomide during pregnancy and whose rheumatologists responded to a questionnaire mailed to them regarding their practices when prescribing DMARDs.[34] An additional three case reports of pregnancy outcome following first-trimester exposure to leflunomide were prospectively reported.[35] Two of these cases ended in elective termination and the third in a normal live birth. An ongoing prospective controlled study of RA medications in pregnancy is being carried out by the North American Organization of Teratology Information Specialists (OTIS). To date, 43 pregnancy outcomes with first-trimester exposure have been presented in abstract.[36] Those 43 leflunomide-exposed pregnant women were compared to 78 women with RA who did not use leflunomide and a second group of 47 women without RA. Based on small numbers, rates of major birth defects were similar between the groups. Infants prenatally exposed to leflunomide were significantly more likely than the nondiseased comparison infants to be born prematurely and were significantly smaller in birth weight. However, lack of large differences on these two measures between the leflunomide-exposed group and the RA comparison group suggest that the underlying disease and/or other medications such as prednisone used to treat RA contribute to these outcomes.

Despite the minimal data in humans, leflunomide has been assigned pregnancy category X by the U.S. Food and Drug Administration (FDA). This is based on its mechanism of action (interference with de novo synthesis of pyrimidines),[37] as well as animal studies in pregnant rats and rabbits that demonstrated an increased risk for congenital malformation in their offspring.[38] However, based on the lack of adequate data in human pregnancy, at present, the teratogenic risk of leflunomide is unknown.

5. Cyclosporine
A meta-analysis of studies evaluating pregnancy outcomes for a combined sample of 410 pregnancies with prenatal exposure to cyclosporine did not produce statistically significantly increased risks for major malformations, prematurity, or low birth weight relative to controls.[39] However, recognized toxicities of cyclosporine include nephrotoxicity and hypertension. Recent animal studies have suggested that prenatal exposure to cyclosporine is associated with long-term systemic and renal effects that may not be noted in the newborn period.[40] At the present time, it is unlikely that there is a substantial risk for malformations following prenatal exposure to cyclosporine. However, long-term effects in humans prenatally exposed to this drug require further evaluation.

6. Cyclophosphamide
Although not commonly used in the treatment of RA, except in patients who have SLE, eight case reports documenting a unique pattern of malformation in infants prenatally exposed to cyclophosphamide have been published.[41] An additional five case reports of cyclophosphamide use to treat lupus have been reported. Two pregnancies with first-trimester exposure ended in spontaneous abortion, two with second-trimester exposure ended in fetal demise, and one with treatment initiated in the second trimester ended with a normal live born infant.[42,43] Although no epidemiologic studies of prenatal exposure to cyclophosphamide have been published, the similar pattern of malformation seen in case reports suggests that cyclophosphamide is a human teratogen, although the magnitude of risk is unknown.

7. Tumor Necrosis Factor Inhibitors: Biologics, Including Etanercept, Infliximab, and Adalimumab
Minimal human pregnancy information is available for any of the tumor necrosis factor (TNF) inhibitors, and the majority of published data consist of isolated case reports, retrospective surveys, and otherwise uncontrolled studies.

No malformations were reported in the offspring of 14 women who were prescribed etanercept during pregnancy and whose rheumatologists responded retrospectively to a mailed survey.[34] Information on pregnancy outcome from 17 pregnant women exposed to etanercept was collected through the British Society of Rheumatology Biologics Register. No birth defects were reported and the rate of spontaneous abortion was comparable to that of the general population. Normal pregnancy outcome was reported in a single case report of a woman with RA and infertility who received chronic therapy with etanercept.[44] Finally, a single case report of a child with the VATER association (a nonrandom co-occurrence of certain defects including vertebral anomalies, anal atresia, tracheoesophageal fistula, esophageal atresia, and renal or radial defects) has been reported in a woman treated with etanercept therapy during pregnancy for psoriatic arthritis.[45]

Three studies involving pregnancy outcome in women receiving infliximab have been published. One involved analysis of 58 spontaneous reports of first-trimester exposed pregnancies either retrospectively or prospectively reported to the drug manufacturer with no comparison group.[46] Of the five live born infants in this series with complications, two were structurally normal but had complicated neonatal courses and three had structural or developmental problems. Of these, one member of a twin pair was developmentally delayed, one child had tetralogy of Fallot, and one had intestinal malrotation. In the second study, based on a retrospective chart review with no comparison group, the offspring of 10 women who received infliximab treatment throughout pregnancy for Crohn's disease were evaluated.[47] All 10 were live born without structural anomalies or intrauterine growth restriction, but three were born prematurely.

With respect to adalimumab, a single case report of a normal full-term infant born to a woman treated with adalimumab throughout pregnancy for Crohn's disease has been published.[48] The British Society of Rheumatology Biologics Register has collected information regarding patients receiving a TNF inhibitor for RA.[49] Information on pregnancy outcome was collected from 17 pregnant women from that Register exposed to etanercept, three exposed to infliximab, and three to adalimumab. No birth defects were reported and the rate of spontaneous abortion was comparable to that of the general population.

An ongoing prospective controlled study of RA medications in pregnancy is being conducted by OTIS.[50] Based on the small number of subjects with known outcome, the data are too preliminary at the present time to draw any conclusions; however, no consistent pattern of abnormalities has been noted among the pregnancies exposed to either etanercept or to adalimumab. Firm conclusions await accumulation of sufficient sample size.

E. Case Resolution

The patient consulted with her rheumatologist and her obstetrician, and decided to discontinue the anti-TNF medication until after delivery, and to continue with prednisone and NSAIDs as needed. Her RA symptoms were virtually nonexistent through the remainder of her uneventful pregnancy. She delivered a healthy 2800-gram infant at 36 weeks' gestation. Breastfeeding was initiated, but shortly after delivery, the mother experienced a flare, and after consulting with her physician, she decided to restart etanercept. Although theoretically of no concern, because little data were available regarding breastfeeding safety, once therapy was initiated, the patient elected to switch the infant to formula feeding.

II. PATIENT CASE (PART 2): SYSTEMIC LUPUS ERYTHEMATOSUS

The patient is a 28-year-old Hispanic woman with an 8-year history of SLE. Her lupus had been complicated in the past by inflammatory arthritis, photosensitivity, malar rash, hemolytic anemia, positive antinuclear antibodies, and antiphospholipid antibody syndrome manifested by a retinal artery occlusion 8 years ago. She has a history of two early pregnancy losses. Her lupus had been clinically quiescent (inactive) for longer than 1 year, and she had discontinued hydroxychloroquine 4 years before any of her pregnancies because of quiescent disease. She denied any history of tobacco, alcohol, or illicit substance abuse. There was no history of lupus nephritis, renal insufficiency, hypertension, or diabetes mellitus. Serologic studies obtained during the first trimester of pregnancy included positive antiphospholipid antibodies, negative anti-SSA/Ro and anti-SSB/La antibodies, persistently low complement levels, and negative anti–double-stranded DNA (dsDNA) antibodies. Medications during pregnancy included low molecular weight heparin, 81 mg daily aspirin, and prenatal vitamins.

A. Epidemiology/Pathophysiology

SLE is a chronic, multisystemic, autoimmune disease that predominantly affects women during the childbearing years. Prevalence estimates of SLE range from 1 to 4 per 1000 women.[51,52] With the exception of premature ovarian failure due to therapy with alkylating agents, fertility rates for women with SLE are normal.[53] In the 1950s, pregnancy among women with SLE was associated with unacceptably high rates of maternal morbidity and mortality; subsequently, women were cautioned against becoming pregnant or carrying pregnancies to term.[54] In more recent decades, pregnancy outcomes for both mother and fetus have become more favorable and many women are able to have successful and healthy pregnancies. This is a function of better understanding of and modification of risk factors associated with adverse pregnancy outcomes as well as better management of disease activity before conception and during pregnancy. Recent studies estimate approximately 3000–4500 pregnancies each year in the United States among women with SLE.[4,55]

Although pregnancy outcomes among women with SLE have improved dramatically over the past 60 years, pregnancy is still associated with increased maternal and fetal morbidity in this population. Estimates vary, but a consensus of studies has demonstrated that approximately 50% of women will have a flare of underlying SLE during pregnancy. The majority of flares will be mild to moderate in nature, with common manifestations in the cutaneous, articular, and hematologic organ systems. Unfortunately, 10%–20% of pregnant women with lupus will have a more severe flare involving the renal or central nervous system that can threaten the health of both mother and fetus.[55]

In addition to risk of flare of underlying disease, pregnancy among women with lupus carries increased risks of other adverse outcomes including preeclampsia, prematurity, growth restriction, and fetal loss.[55] Underlying lupus has been shown to carry increased risks of adverse pregnancy outcomes even after adjustment for other variables including maternal age, ethnicity, and diabetes mellitus.[56] Individual studies have had varying results; however, several risk factors have been identified that are associated with increased risks of lupus flare and other adverse pregnancy outcomes. Many of these risk factors can be minimized by careful planning and timing of pregnancies to coincide with periods of relative disease quiescence.

The risk of developing a lupus flare during pregnancy is increased if the woman has had active lupus during the 6–12 months before conception,[55,57,58] particularly if the woman conceives during times of increased disease activity.[58,59] As expected, based on increased rates of flares following discontinuation of hydroxychloroquine in the non-pregnant lupus population,[60] recent discontinuation of antimalarial therapy preceding pregnancy has been shown to increase risk of flare during pregnancy.[58,61,62] It is important to minimize the occurrence and frequency of lupus flares during pregnancy, not only for the health of the mother, but additionally because a lupus flare is itself a risk factor for other adverse pregnancy outcomes, including preeclampsia, prematurity, intrauterine growth restriction, and fetal loss.[55] Other risk factors for preeclampsia among lupus patients include active disease at conception, thrombocytopenia, hypertension, and a history of renal disease.[55,59] Risk factors for premature delivery and fetal loss include active disease at conception or during pregnancy, hypertension, renal disease, and antiphospholipid antibodies.[55,58,59]

B. Detection and Screening

One of the most critical times for intervention to reduce complications of pregnancy in women with lupus is before conception. Ideally, women should time pregnancies during periods of quiescent or very mild disease activity. This includes monitoring the disease for a period of at least six months after withdrawal of any potentially teratogenic medications or strong immunosuppressive agents. Other parameters that should be addressed before pregnancy include aggressive management of hypertension and underlying renal insufficiency.

In addition to evaluating for signs of overt disease activity or relevant comorbidities (hypertension, renal disease), there are a number of serologic studies that will help to plan appropriate monitoring during pregnancy. Specific autoantibodies can be associated with adverse pregnancy outcomes, whereas others are associated with neonatal lupus syndromes that are characterized by transplacental passage of maternal autoantibodies into the fetal circulation. While the obstetric antiphospholipid antibody syndrome is characterized by late or recurrent early pregnancy loss, preeclampsia, premature delivery, and intrauterine growth restriction, there is less consensus about the role of antiphospholipid antibodies in pregnant women with lupus who do not have a history of clinical events.[63]

Neonatal lupus erythematosus (NLE) syndromes are a series of manifestations that occur within weeks of birth of an affected infant, and generally resolve within 6 months of delivery as maternally derived autoantibodies are eliminated from the fetal circulation. NLE is associated with maternal anti-SSA/Ro or anti-SSB/La antibodies that cross into the fetal circulation beginning in the second trimester of pregnancy. Skin rash and mild transaminitis or cytopenias are the most common manifestations and are transient, having little or no residual effect on the infant. In approximately 2% of infants born to anti-Ro or -La antibody positive mothers, the antibodies will affect the fetal cardiac conduction system and potentially lead to fixed conduction defects with first-, second-, or third-degree heart block that persists and may even progress after birth.[64] Approximately 65% of affected infants will require permanent pacemaker placement.

C. Guidelines

Although no formal guidelines to managing pregnancies exist, and few if any randomized controlled trials have been or will be performed, in women with lupus, general recommendations can be culled from the existing literature.

- All women of childbearing potential with lupus should receive counseling regarding the potential risks of pregnancy to both the mother and fetus. Additionally, preconception evaluation by a specialist in maternal-fetal medicine may provide additional guidance if a women expresses interest in future pregnancies.

- Whenever possible, pregnancy should be delayed until periods of prolonged disease quiescence and potentially teratogenic medications have been discontinued and eliminated from the maternal system.[55]

- Aggressive blood pressure control before and throughout pregnancy in women with underlying lupus, and particularly in women with a history of lupus nephritis.

- Women with underlying SLE should have anti-SSA/Ro and anti-SSA/La antibodies assessed before or shortly after pregnancy is discovered. Those with positive SSA/Ro or SSB/La antibodies should undergo regular monitoring of the PR interval by fetal echocardiography beginning at 16 weeks' gestation to detect early signs of heart block. Clinical trials are currently under way to assess the utility of intervention with antenatal corticosteroids or intravenous immunoglobulin in preventing or limiting heart block in affected fetuses or in women with a history of a child affected by NLE heart block.[64]

- Women should be assessed for a history of thromboses (arterial or venous), prior obstetric manifestations of the antiphospholipid antibody syndrome (late or recurrent early pregnancy losses, premature delivery), and the presence of antiphospholipid antibodies. Women with the antiphospholipid antibody syndrome including a history or thromboses or related obstetric complications should be assessed for treatment with low-dose aspirin, heparin, or a combination of the two. Clinical trials have found that neither corticosteroids nor immunoglobulins have an effect in preventing pregnancy loss in this population.[65]

- Hydroxychloroquine should not be discontinued in women with SLE who become pregnant or are planning a pregnancy. There is less consensus about starting antimalarials during pregnancy.[66]

D. Assessment

Identifying active disease or other potential risk factors before the onset of pregnancy is relatively straightforward, particularly if a woman has been stable off of immunosuppressants for several months. What is much more difficult, however, is assessing lupus disease activity in the context of the physiologic and immunologic changes of pregnancy.

Many normal physiologic changes of pregnancy can mimic active manifestations of underlying lupus. Anemia and thrombocytopenia due to the hemodilutional effects of increased plasma volume are common in normal pregnancies and may be hard to distinguish from the mild cytopenias often seen in lupus. Pregnant women may also develop melasma, a photosensitive hyperpigmentation of the cheeks often occurring in the distribution of a typical malar rash, or generalized palmar and facial erythema. Fatigue, arthralgias, mild edema, and shortness of breath commonly seen in normal pregnancies may be mistaken for lupus flare.[55] Conversely, early signs of a lupus flare may be inadvertently overlooked, as the symptoms may be attributed to the pregnancy alone.

Distinguishing preeclampsia from lupus nephritis is a much more difficult proposition, particularly given the high morbidity associated with both conditions. Not only are lupus patients at increased risk for developing preeclampsia, but those with a history of lupus nephritis are at increased risk for developing severe flares, including active renal disease during pregnancy. Both syndromes will present with nephritic range proteinuria and hypertension. Clinical or laboratory markers to distinguish lupus nephritis from preeclampsia have remained elusive. Serum complement levels will rise during normal pregnancies; however, they may not reach normal levels even in uncomplicated pregnancies in women with lupus. Low complements almost always characterize lupus nephritis in the nongravid state, but normal complement levels do not exclude the diagnosis during pregnancy. An active urinary sediment (pyuria, hematuria, and cellular casts) suggests lupus nephritis, as this is a rare feature of preeclampsia.[55] In the absence of other features of active lupus, and in cases where delivery of the infant carries significant risks, some patients may require renal biopsy to distinguish the underlying disease process. Delivery of the infant and placenta is the definitive treatment for preeclampsia (see Chapter 11, Gestational Hypertension, Preeclampsia, and Eclampsia). In contrast, treatment of lupus nephritis entails combination therapy with corticosteroids and stronger immunosuppressive or cytotoxic agents.

E. Pregnancy Safety for Selected Treatments

Recommendations for the treatment of lupus patients during pregnancy have changed dramatically over past decades. For the most part, these changes surround prophylactic therapy in the absence of active disease.

1. Antimalarials

Antimalarials that contain the 4-aminoquinoline radical, predominantly chloroquine and hydroxychloroquine, are frequently used for the treatment of lupus, and discontinuation of antimalarials has been shown to increase the frequency and severity of flares in the nongravid state.[60] Early reports of chloroquine-induced neonatal ototoxicity and animal models demonstrating retinal deposits lead to recommendations to discontinue antimalarials before pregnancy.[67,68] Hydroxychloroquine crosses the placenta and is present in similar concentrations in cord blood as in maternal serum, and is present in human breast milk at a somewhat reduced concentration.[69]

More recently, the use of hydroxychloroquine during pregnancy has been revisited, due to both concern of morbidity associated with lupus flares during pregnancy and with a growing number of case reports of successful use of hydroxychloroquine during pregnancy without adverse neonatal affects or related congenital malformations. As early as 1988, Parke et al. reported a series of 11 pregnancies in eight women with SLE who took hydroxychloroquine or chloroquine for the duration of pregnancy.[70] Of the six resulting live births, none reported any congenital malformations or oto- or retinal toxicity up to 14 years of age. Since that initial series, a total of 284 live births from 327 pregnancies in lupus patients exposed to hydroxychloroquine have been reported—all without an excess of congenital malformations or of any ocular or auditory damage (Table 1). A randomized,

Table 1. Studies of Hydroxychloroquine during Pregnancy

Study	Exposed	Controls	Length of Follow-Up	Assessment	Live Births (Exposed)	Abnormalities (Live Births)
Parke 1988[70]	8	0	Up to 16 y	G	6	0
Levy 1991[71]	27	0	5.3 y	G	14	0
Parke 1996[72]	9	0	33 mo	G	9	0
Buchanan 1996[73]	36	53	Newborn	G	31	1 Down syndrome
Levy 2001[74]	10	10	1.5–3 y	O	10	0
Klinger 2001[75]	21	0	2.8 y	O		
Motta 2002[76]	35	0	1 y	G,O,D	21	0
Costedoat 2003[77]	133	70	26 mo	G, O	117	4 congenital malformations
Clowse 2006[61]	56	47	Not stated	G	77	No difference in fetal anomalies
					39	2 retinal hemorrhages (not related)
Total	**335**	**180**			**324**	

D = developmental assessment, G = general physical examination, O = ophthalmologic examination.

placebo-controlled trial of hydroxychloroquine compared to placebo in lupus pregnancy was performed with a total of 20 patients.[74] Although the sample size was small, the study found that subjects receiving placebo had increased lupus activity during pregnancy and a 30% incidence of preeclampsia in comparison with mild to quiescent disease and no preeclampsia among subjects receiving hydroxychloroquine. All infants underwent extensive examination including ophthalmologic evaluation at birth, 18 months, and 3 years of age without evidence of teratogenic effects. An observational study of lupus patients who continued or discontinued hydroxychloroquine during pregnancy found similar results.[61] Women who discontinued hydroxychloroquine within 3 months of pregnancy had higher rates of increased lupus activity and required higher doses of corticosteroids during pregnancy than women who continued hydroxychloroquine. Consensus opinion among rheumatologists supports recommendations for the continuation of hydroxychloroquine during pregnancy if a woman has been taking it previously.[78,79] There is little data concerning initiating treatment with hydroxychloroquine during pregnancy, and this practice cannot be recommended at this time.

2. Corticosteroids

During the 1960s and 1970s, it was recommended that all pregnant women with underlying lupus, irrespective of disease activity, receive prednisone to decrease the rate of flares. This practice has largely been abandoned because the risks of side effects to both mother and fetus often outweigh the benefits of treatment, particularly in cases of quiescent disease. The adverse effects of corticosteroids, namely increased blood pressure, glucose intolerance, osteoporosis, and risk of infections are confounded during pregnancy, notably with the increase in insulin resistance during the later stages of pregnancy. Pregnancy-specific concerns with the use of corticosteroids include increased risk of premature rupture of membranes, preterm delivery, and low-birth-weight infants. As noted in the RA section above, controversy still exists regarding the risk of oral clefts with early antenatal exposure to corticosteroids; however, if there is a higher risk for oral clefts, it is estimated to be less than 1%. No other congenital abnormalities have been associated with early antenatal exposure to these agents.[79]

As in the nonpregnant state, systemic corticosteroids remain one of the mainstays of treatment of lupus flares during pregnancy, and are among the most commonly used therapeutics because of the short time to efficacy and the ability to titrate the dose according to disease activity. Approximately 10% of prednisone or prednisolone crosses into the fetal circulation. Given the perinatal morbidity associated with active lupus during pregnancy, judicious use of prednisone or prednisolone to reduce the severity of disease activity during pregnancy is critical. The dose should be carefully titrated to minimize the cumulative exposure to corticosteroids while controlling underlying disease.[55,79] In contrast, fluorinated corticosteroids (betamethasone and dexamethasone) cross into the fetal circulation in much higher concentrations. Use of these agents during pregnancy should be reserved for cases in which treatment is directly targeting the fetus. Examples of this include promoting fetal lung maturity in anticipation of a preterm delivery (see Chapter 9, Fetal Lung Maturity).

3. Immunosuppressives

In some cases, control of underlying lupus requires therapy with stronger immunosuppressive agents, either before conception or for severe flares that occur during an established pregnancy. As with any medication taken during pregnancy, the risks of medication exposure must be balanced by the potential benefits of achieving control of underlying lupus in both the mother and the fetus. The onset of action of many immunosuppressive agents may be weeks to months, so the clinician must be aware of the period of time of exposure without clinical benefit and the effects that exposure may have on the developing fetus. Therefore, immunosuppressive agents should be reserved for situations of moderate to severe disease activity that cannot be managed with other alternatives. For this same reason, caution must also be exercised when interpreting data regarding immunosuppressant use among pregnant women with lupus, as associations of adverse pregnancy outcomes may be confounded by the underlying disease, related comorbid conditions, and concomitant corticosteroid and other medication use.

4. Azathioprine/6-Mercaptopurine

Azathioprine and its metabolite, 6-mercaptopurine, is an immunosuppressant used commonly for the prevention of allograft rejection after solid organ transplantation as well as for management of several autoimmune diseases including lupus. As a purine analog, azathioprine interferes with ribonucleotide synthesis and predominately affects T cells. Most data on gestational use of azathioprine come from small retrospective case series of pregnant women with underlying renal transplantation or autoimmune diseases. A prospective study from Israel compared outcomes of 189 pregnancies exposed to azathioprine for any indication to a control group of 230 women who had no drug exposure or who were exposed to nonteratogenic medications.[80] Women receiving azathioprine tended to be younger and smoked more than controls; however, rates of live births (87%–90%) and congenital malformations (3.0%–3.5%) were comparable between the groups. Notably, pregnancies exposed to azathioprine had shorter gestation periods and were more likely to result in premature delivery.[80] The largest cohort of lupus patients exposed to azathioprine during pregnancy was reported from the Hopkins Lupus Cohort.[81] This study examined outcomes of 31 pregnancies exposed to azathioprine to 227 pregnancies without exposure. There were no differences in miscarriage rates between exposed and nonexposed pregnancies during the first trimester. However, a higher rate of fetal demise was found among pregnancies exposed to azathioprine after 20 weeks' gestation. Even after adjusting for underlying disease activity and presence of antiphospholipid antibody syndrome, azathioprine exposure was associated with a two-fold increased risk of fetal demise.[81]

Recommendations derived from extensive literature review and expert consensus suggest azathioprine may be used at modest doses during pregnancy if indicated by severity of the underlying disease or need for allograft rejection prophylaxis.[79]

5. Other Immunosuppressive Agents

In contrast to recommendations about azathioprine, mycophenolate mofetil and cyclophosphamide should be avoided during pregnancy. Few published reports of pregnancy outcomes with mycophenolate exposure exist, but recent case reports and transplant registry data suggest there may be an increased risk for a specific pattern of malformation consistent with findings in animal studies.[79] The pattern of abnormalities notably includes cleft lip and palate, microtia with atresia of the external auditory canal, micrognathia, and hypertelorism. Cardiac, renal, and diaphragmatic malformations may also be involved.[82]

Based on these animal and human data, the FDA has issued a warning about the fetotoxicity of mycophenolate mofetil and has recommended confirmation of adequate contraception before prescribing to women of childbearing potential.[83]

Cyclophosphamide is an alkylating agent used for the treatment of malignancy, and in lower doses for the treatment of life- or organ-threatening manifestations of lupus and other autoimmune diseases. In lupus, the most common indication for cyclophosphamide is for the treatment of proliferative lupus nephritis. Aside from increasing risks of premature ovarian failure in exposed nonpregnant women of childbearing age, a history of use of cyclophosphamide before the onset of pregnancy does not appear to increase the risk for congenital malformations among offspring.[84,85] The effects of cyclophosphamide use during pregnancy vary by trimester of exposure. It is clear that cyclophosphamide is a potent teratogen with first-trimester antenatal exposure. The "cyclophosphamide embryopathy" described in eight patients with early antenatal exposure is manifest by calvarial abnormalities, microcephaly, cleft palate, limb defects, and developmental delay among surviving infants.[41] Other reports describe isolated cases where there are no apparent congenital malformations following early pregnancy exposure to cyclophosphamide.[81] In contrast, cyclophosphamide, has been used in the second and third trimester of pregnancy for serious maternal disease including malignancy.[87] Few reports are available regarding pregnancy outcomes following second- or third-trimester exposure of cyclophosphamide for the treatment of severe lupus. These have not shown congenital abnormalities, but have varied effects on fetal survival.[42] Cyclophosphamide should only be considered during the later stages of pregnancy in such situations where the benefits to the health of the mother outweigh any potential risks.

F. Case Resolution

The patient had an uncomplicated pregnancy course, with appropriate prenatal care, until gestational week 27, when she developed a pruritic erythematous rash over her anterior chest, neck, and abdomen. In addition to the diffuse erythematous rash, physical examination revealed a faint malar rash and prominent frontal alopecia without other abnormalities. Laboratory studies showed a normal urinalysis and serum creatinine, normal complete blood count, and low serum complement levels. She was given a diagnosis of a moderate mucocutaneous lupus flare and was started on 20 mg prednisone daily with a tapering schedule. The rash on her trunk resolved with moderate prednisone; however, it began to return with a taper of prednisone to 5 mg daily. Her alopecia continued and she developed inflammatory arthritis in the small joints of her hands. Prednisone was increased to 10 mg daily. She delivered a 2630-gram boy at 35 weeks' gestation. The infant had problems with poor feeding and anemia, but otherwise had no skin rash, cardiac, or hepatobiliary abnormalities. Postpartum, the patient continued to have inflammatory arthritis, but was without alopecia or any cutaneous disease. Hydroxychloroquine was started and prednisone was continued at 10 mg daily.

IV. Other Autoimmune Diseases

The above cases illustrate common issues surrounding the management of autoimmune diseases during pregnancy, namely the importance of adequately treating underlying inflammatory disease while minimizing teratogenic risks associated with medication use. In essence, these principles apply for other autoimmune diseases including inflammatory bowel disease and multiple sclerosis. Inflammatory bowel diseases encompass both ulcerative colitis and Crohn's disease, and very commonly affect young women. Similar to RA, inflammatory bowel diseases do not appear to worsen significantly during pregnancy.[88] A meta-analysis of 12 studies encompassing 3907 patients with inflammatory bowel disease found increased risks for preterm birth, low birth weight, and cesarean delivery.[89] Immunomodulating agents commonly used to treat inflammatory bowel disease overlap considerably with therapies for RA and include corticosteroids, methotrexate, azathioprine, cyclosporine, and TNF inhibitors. Similar to inflammatory bowel disease, multiple sclerosis is an autoimmune disease that commonly affects young adults and regarding reproductive issues is paramount to effective counseling and treatment of young women. Like several other autoimmune diseases, multiple sclerosis does not appear to worsen during pregnancy, and may often show clinical improvement before delivery.[90] Recent data are encouraging that rates of adverse pregnancy outcomes among women with multiple sclerosis do not appear significantly increased compared to healthy pregnant women.[91] Aside from common immunosuppressant agents, multiple sclerosis is currently treated with a variety of new biological therapies including interferon β, glatiramer acetate, and anti-integrin therapy.[90] None of these newer agents has sufficient clinical data to adequately assess safety for use during pregnancy.

V. Summary

Most, but not all, women with RA can expect some degree of amelioration of symptoms during pregnancy. In general, the presence of underlying maternal RA does not impart significant risks to the fetus, but emerging data suggest that increased or uncontrolled disease activity during pregnancy may have subtle adverse effects on fetal growth. Several commonly used medications to control disease activity have potential for teratogenicity and ideally should be discontinued and eliminated from the system before pregnancy. In this era of new biological therapies for the treatment of RA, there are insufficient data to draw any conclusions as to pregnancy risks associated with newer medications. Women with RA who are contemplating future pregnancies or those with inadvertent pregnancies should receive careful counseling regarding discontinuation of and potential teratogenic risks of DMARDs.

In general, women with underlying lupus have a greater chance of experiencing a flare of the disease during pregnancy than do women with RA. Careful planning before conception can help to mitigate risks as well as exposure to potentially teratogenic medications. Aside from continuation of hydroxychloroquine, prophylactic immunomodulation during pregnancy is not necessary. Treatment of active disease during pregnancy should be tailored to the severity of active manifestations. Pregnant women with lupus should receive coordinated care with a rheumatologist and maternal-fetal medicine specialists. Special attention should be paid to women with positive antibodies against SSA/Ro, SSB/La, or phospholipids.

VI. References

1. Symons DP. Epidemiology of rheumatoid arthritis: determinants of onset, persistence and outcome. *Best Pract Res Clin Rheumatol.* 2002;16:707–722.

2. Golding A, Haque UJ, Giles JT. Rheumatoid arthritis and reproduction. *Rheum Dis Clin North Am.* 2007;33:319–343.

3. Katz PP. Childbearing decisions and family size among women with rheumatoid arthritis. *Arthritis Rheum.* 2006;55:217–223.

4. Chakravarty EF, Nelson L, Krishnan E. Obstetric hospitalizations in the United States for women with systemic lupus erythematosus and rheumatoid arthritis. *Arthritis Rheum.* 2006;54:899–907.

5. Nelson JL, Hughes KA, Smith AG, et al. Maternal-fetal disparity in HLA class II alloantigens and the pregnancy-induced amelioration of rheumatoid arthritis. *N Engl J Med.* 1993;329:466–471.

6. de Man YA, Hazes JMW, van de Geijn FE, et al. Measuring disease activity and functionality during pregnancy in patients with rheumatoid arthritis. *Arthritis Rheum.* 2007;57:716–722.

7. Bowden AP, Barrett JH, Fallow W, et al. Women with inflammatory polyarthritis have babies of lower birth weight. *J Rheumatol.* 2001;28:355–359.

8. Stomsvoll JF, Ostensen M, Irgens LM, et al. Obstetrical and neonatal outcome in pregnant patients with rheumatic disease. *Scand J Rheumatol Suppl.* 1998;107:109–112.

9. Chambers CD, Johnson DL, Jones KL, et al. Pregnancy outcome in women exposed to anti-TNF-alpha medications: the OTIS rheumatoid arthritis in pregnancy study (abstract). *Dermatology.* 2005;152:205.

10. Reed SD, Vollan TA, Svec MA. Pregnancy outcomes in women with rheumatoid arthritis in Washington State. *Matern Child Health J.* 2006;10:361–366.

11. Ostensen M. The influence of pregnancy on blood parameters in patients with rheumatic disease. *Scand J Rheumatol.* 1984;13:203–208.

12. Finsen V, Zeitlmann H. Carpal tunnel syndrome during pregnancy. *Scand J Plast Reconstr Surg Hand Surg.* 2006;40:41–45.

13. Pradat P, Robert-Gnasia E, Di Tanna GL, et al. Contributors to the MADRE database. First trimester exposure to corticosteroids and oral clefts. *Birth Defects Res A Clin Mol Teratol.* 2003;67:968–970.

14. Czeizel AE, Rockenbauer M. Population-based case-controls study of teratogenic potential of corticosteroids. *Teratology.* 1997;56:335–340.

15. Rodriguez-Pinilla E, Martinez-Frias ML. Corticosteroids during pregnancy and oral clefts: a case-control study. *Teratology.* 1988;58:2–5.

16. Carmichael SL, Shaw GM. Maternal corticosteroid use and risk of selected congenital anomalies. *Am J Med Genet.* 1999;86:242–244.

17. Aselton P, Jick H, Milunsky A, et al. First trimester drug use and congenital disorders. *Obstet Gynecol.* 1985;65:451–455.

18. Torfs CP, Katz EA, Bateson TF, et al. Maternal medications and environmental exposures as risk factors for gastroschisis. *Teratology.* 1996;54:84–92.

19. Werler MM, Mitchell AA, Shapiro S. First trimester maternal medication use in relation to gastroschisis. *Teratology*. 1992;45:361–367.

20. Werler MM, Sheehan JE, Mitchell AA. Maternal medication use and risks of gastroschisis and small intestinal atresia. *Am J Epidemiol*. 2002;155:26–31.

21. Ericson A, Kallen BAJ. Nonsteroidal anti-inflammatory drugs in early pregnancy. *Reprod Toxicol*. 2001;15:371–375.

22. Kallen BAJ, Olausson PO. Maternal drug use in early pregnancy and infant cardiovascular defect. *Reprod Toxicol*. 2003;17:255–261.

23. Nielsen GL, Sorensen HT, Larsen H, et al. Risk of adverse birth outcome and miscarriage in pregnant users of nonsteroidal anti-inflammatory drugs: population based observational study and case-control study. *BMJ*. 2001;322:266–270.

24. Li D-K, Liu L, Odoul R. Exposure to non-steroidal anti-inflammatory drugs during pregnancy and risk of miscarriage: population based cohort study. *BMJ*. 2003;327:368–370.

25. Vermillion ST, Scardo JA, Lashus AG, et al. The effect of indomethacin tocolysis on fetal ductus arteriosus constriction with advancing gestational age. *Am J Obstet Gynecol*. 1997;177:256–259.

26. Kaplan BS, Restaino I, Raval DS, et al. Renal failure in the neonate associated with in utero exposure to non-steroidal anti-inflammatory agents. *Pediatr Nephrol*. 1994;8:700–704.

27. Major CA, Lewis DF, Harding JA. Tocolysis with indomethacin increasing the incidence of necrotizing enterocolitis in the low-birth-weight neonate. *Am J Obstet Gynecol*. 1994;170:102–106.

28. Baerts W, Fetter WP, Hop WC, et al. Cerebral lesions in preterm infants after tocolytic indomethacin. *Dev Med Child Neurol*. 1990;32:910–918.

29. Feldkamp M, Carey JC. Clinical teratology counseling and consultation case report: low dose methotrexate exposure in the early weeks of pregnancy. *Teratology*. 1993;47:533–539.

30. Kozlowski RD, Steinbrunner JW, MacKenzie, et al. Outcome of first-trimester exposure to low-dose methotrexate in eight patients with rheumatic disease. *Am J Med*. 1990;88:589–592.

31. Donnefeld AE, Pastuszak A, Noah JS, et al. Methotrexate exposure prior to and during pregnancy. *Teratology*. 1994;49:79–81.

32. Buckley LM, Bullaboy CA, Leichtman L, et al. Multiple congenital anomalies associated with weekly low-dose methotrexate treatment of the mother. *Arthritis Rheum*. 1997;40:971–973.

33. Lewden B, Vial T, Elefant E, et al. Low dose methotrexate in the first trimester of pregnancy: results of a French collaborative study. *J Rheumatol*. 2004;31:2360–2365.

34. Chakravarty EF, Sanchez-Yamamoto D, Bush TM. The use of disease modifying antirheumatic drugs in women with rheumatoid arthritis of childbearing age: a survey of practice pattern and pregnancy outcomes. *J Rheumatol*. 2003;30:241–246.

35. De Santis M, Straface G, Cavaliere A, et al. Paternal and maternal exposure to leflunomide: pregnancy and neonatal outcome. *Annals Rheum Dis.* 2005;64:1096–1097.

36. Chambers CD, Johnson DL, Macaraeg GR, et al. Pregnancy outcome following early gestational exposure to leflunomide: the OTIS Rheumatoid Arthritis in Pregnancy Study (abstract). *Pharmacoepidemiol Drug Safe.* 2004;13:S252.

37. Prakist A, Jarvis B. Leflunomide. A review of its use in active rheumatoid arthritis. *Drugs.* 1999;58:1137–1164.

38. Brent RL. Teratogen update: reproductive risk of leflunomide (Arava): a pyrimidine synthesis inhibitor: counseling women taking leflunomide before or during pregnancy and men taking leflunomide who are contemplating fathering a child. *Teratology.* 2001;63:106–112.

39. Bar Oz B, Hackman R, Einarson T, et al. Pregnancy outcome after cyclosporine therapy during pregnancy: a meta-analysis. *Transplantation.* 2001;71:1051–1055.

40. Tendron-Franzin A, Gouyon JB, Guignard JP, et al. Long-term effects of *in utero* exposure to cyclosporine A on renal function in the rabbit. *J Am Soc Nephrol.* 2004;15:2687–2693.

41. Vaux KK, Khaole NCO, Jones KL. Cyclophosphamide, methotrexate and cytarabine embryopathy: is apoptosis the common pathway? *Birth Defects Res A Clin Mol Teratol.* 2003;67:403–408.

42. Clowse M, Magder L, Petri M. Cyclophosphamide for lupus during pregnancy. *Lupus.* 2005;14:593–597.

43. Kart Koseoglu H, Yucel A, Kunefeci G, et al. Cyclophosphamide therapy in a serious case of lupus nephritis during pregnancy. *Lupus.* 2001;10:818–820.

44. Sills E, Perloe M, Tucker M, et al. Successful ovulation induction, conception, and normal delivery after chronic therapy with etanercept: a recombinant fusion anticytokine treatment for rheumatoid arthritis. *Am J Reprod Immunol.* 2001;46:366–368.

45. Carter JD, Valeriano J, Vasey FB, et al. Tumor necrosis factor alpha inhibition and VATER association: a causal relationship? *J Rheumatol.* 2006;33:1014–1017.

46. Katz JA, Antoni C, Keenan GF, et al. Outcome of pregnancy in women receiving infliximab for the treatment of Crohn's disease and rheumatoid arthritis. *Am J Gastroenterol.* 2004;99:2385–2392.

47. Mahadevan U, Kane S, Sandborn J, et al. Intentional infliximab use during pregnancy for induction or maintenance of remission in Crohn's disease. *Aliment Pharmacol Ther.* 2005;21:733–738.

48. Vesga L, Terdiman JP, Mahadevan U. Adalimumab use in pregnancy. *Gut.* 2005;54:890–891.

49. Hyrick KL, Symmons DPM, Watson KD, et al. Pregnancy outcome in women who were exposed to anti-tumor necrosis factor agents: results from a national population register. *Arthritis Rheum.* 2006;54:2701–2702.

50. OTIS: arthritis and pregnancy study. Available at http://www.raandpregnancy.org. Accessed May 15, 2008.

51. Uramoto KM, Michet CJ Jr, Thumboo J, et al. Trends in the incidence and mortality of systemic lupus erythematosus, 1950–1992. *Arthritis Rheum.* 1999;42:46–50.

52. Chakravarty EF, Bush TM, Manzi S, et al. Prevalence of adult systemic lupus erythematosus in California and Pennsylvania in 2000: estimates obtained using hospitalization data. *Arthritis Rheum.* 2007;56:2092–2096.

53. Ostensen M. New insights into sexual functioning and fertility in rheumatic diseases. *Best Pract Res Clin Rheumatol.* 2004;18:219–232.

54. Turner SJ, Levine L, Redman A. Lupus erythematosus and pregnancy. *Obstet Gynecol.* 1956;8:601–609.

55. Clowse MEB. Lupus activity in pregnancy. *Rheum Dis Clin North Am.* 2007;33:237–252.

56. Chakravarty EF, Nelson L, Krishnan E. Obstetric hospitalizations in the United States for women with systemic lupus erythematosus and rheumatoid arthritis. *Arthritis Rheum.* 2006;54:899–907.

57. Clowse ME, Magder LS, Witter F, et al. The impact of increased lupus activity on obstetric outcomes. *Arthritis Rheum.* 2005;52:514–521.

58. Cortes-Hernandez J, Ordi-Ros J, Paredes F, et al. Clinical predictors of fetal and maternal outcome in systemic lupus erythematosus: a prospective study of 103 pregnancies. *Rheumatology.* 2002;41:643–650.

59. Chakravarty EF, Colon I, Langen ES, et al. Factors that predict prematurity and preeclampsia in pregnancies that are complicated by systemic lupus erythematosus. *Am J Obstet Gynecol.* 2005;192:1897–1904.

60. The Canadian Hydroxychloroquine Study Group. A randomized study of the effect of withdrawing hydroxychloroquine sulfate in systemic lupus erythematosus. *N Engl J Med.* 1991;324:150–154.

61. Clowse ME, Magder L, Witter F, et al. Hydroxychloroquine in lupus pregnancy. *Arthritis Rheum.* 2006;54:3640–3647.

62. Costedoat-Chalumeau N, Amoura Z, Huong DLT, et al. Safety of hydroxychloroquine in pregnant patients with connective tissue diseases. Review of the literature. *Autoimmun Rev.* 2005;4:111–115.

63. Ruiz-Irastorza G, Khamashta MA. Antiphospholipid syndrome in pregnancy. *Rheum Dis Clin North Am.* 2008;33:287–297.

64. Frankovich J, Sandborg C, Barnes P, et al. Neonatal lupus and related autoimmune disorders of infants. *NeoReviews.* 2008;9:e206–e217.

65. Ruiz-Irastorza G, Khamasta MA. Antiphospholipid syndrome in pregnancy. *Rheum Dis Clin North Am.* 2007;33:287–297.

66. Borden MB, Parke AL. Antimalarial drugs in systemic lupus erythematosus: use in pregnancy. *Drug Safety.* 2001;24:1055–1063.

67. Matz GJ, Naunton RF. Ototoxicity of chloroquine. *Arch Otolaryngol.* 1968;88:370–372.

68. Ullberrg S, Lindquist NG, Sjostrand SE. Accumulation of chorioretinotoxic drugs in the foetal eye. *Nature.* 1970;19:1257–1258.

69. Costedoat-Chalumeau N, Amora Z, Zymard G, et al. Evidence of transplacental passage of hydroxychloroquine in humans. *Arthritis Rheum.* 2002;46:1123–1124.

70. Parke A. Antimalarial drugs and pregnancy. *Am J Med*. 1988;85:30–33.

71. Levy M, Buskila D, Gladmann DD, et al. Pregnancy outcome following first trimester exposure to chloroquine. *Am J Perinatol*. 1991;8:174–178.

72. Parke A, West B. Hydroxychloroquine in pregnant patients with systemic lupus erythematosus. *J Rheumatol*. 1996;23:1715–1718.

73. Buchanan NMM, Toubi E, Khamashta MA, et al. Hydroxychloroquine (HCQ) in lupus pregnancy: review of a series of 36 cases. *Ann Rheum Dis*. 1996;55:486–488.

74. Levy RA, Vilela VS, Cataldo MJ, et al. Hydroxychloroquine (HCQ) in lupus pregnancy: double-blind and placebo-controlled study. *Lupus*. 2001;10:401–404.

75. Klinger G, Morad Y, Westall CA. Ocular toxicity and antenatal exposure to chloroquine or hydroxychloroquine for rheumatic disease. *Lancet*. 2001;358:813–814.

76. Motta M, Tincani A, Faden D, et al. Antimalarial agents in pregnancy. *Lancet*. 2002;359:524–525.

77. Costedoat-Chalumeau N, Amoura Z, Duhaut P, et al. Safety of hydroxychloroquine in pregnant patients with connective tissue diseases: a study of one hundred thirty-three cases compared with a control group. *Arthritis Rheum*. 2003;48:3207–3211.

78. Al-Herz A, Schulzer M, Esdaile JM. Survey of antimalarial use in lupus pregnancy and lactation. *J Rheumatol*. 2002;29:700–706.

79. Ostensen M, Khamashta M, Lockshin M, et al. Anti-inflammatory and immunosuppressive drugs and reproduction. *Arthritis Res Ther*. 2006;8:209–228.

80. Goldstein LH, Dolinsky G, Greenberg, R, et al. Pregnancy outcome of women exposed to azathioprine during pregnancy. *Birth Defects Res A Clin Mol Teratol*. 2007;79:696–701.

81. Clowse MEB, Witter F, Madger LS, Petri M. Azathioprine use in lupus pregnancy. *Arthritis Rheum*. 2005;52 (suppl 9);S386–S387.

82. Perez-Aytes A, Ledo A, Boso V, et al. In utero exposure to mycophenolate mofetil: a characteristic phenotype? *Am J Med Genet A*. 2008;146:1–7.

83. U.S. FDA Medwatch. Available at http://www.fda.gov/medwatch/safety/2007/safety07.htm#Myfortic. Accessed May 15, 2008.

84. Gershenson DM. Menstrual and reproductive function after treatment with combination chemotherapy for malignancy ovarian germ cell tumors. *J Clin Oncol*. 1988;6:270–275.

85. Huong DLT, Amoura Z, Duhaut P, et al. Risk of ovarian failure and fertility after intravenous cyclophosphamide: a study of 84 patients. *J Rheumatol*. 2002;29:2571–2576.

86. Fernandez M, Andrade R, Alarcon GS. Cyclophosphamide use and pregnancy in lupus. *Lupus*. 2006;15:59.

87. Berry DL, Theriault RL, Holmes FA, et al. Management of breast cancer during pregnancy using a standardized protocol. *J Clin Oncol*. 1999;17:855–861.

88. Dubinsky M, Abraham B, Mahadevan U. Management of the pregnant IBD patient. *Inflamm Bowel Dis*. 2008;14:1736–1750.

89. Cornish J, Tan E, Teare J, et al. A meta-analysis on the influence of inflammatory bowel disease on pregnancy. *Gut*. 2007;56:830–837.

90. Houtchens MK. Pregnancy and multiple sclerosis. *Semin Neurol.* 2007;27:434–441.

91. Dahl J, Myhr KM, Daltveit AK, et al. Pregnancy delivery, and birth outcome in women with multiple sclerosis. *Neurology.* 2005;65:1961–1963.

QUESTIONS AND ANSWERS

1. Compare and contrast typical changes in autoimmune disease activity during pregnancy in women with RA versus women with SLE.

2. Describe examples of potential adverse perinatal outcomes that are noted to occur with increased frequency in pregnancies complicated by either RA or SLE.

3. Name two medications used to treat RA and/or SLE that are known to be teratogenic and should be considered carefully with respect to use in pregnancy.

Answers:

1. The majority of women with RA will experience a reduction in symptoms of the disease during pregnancy. More than 50% of pregnant women with SLE will experience a disease flare in pregnancy; 10%–20% will have severe disease flares that involve the central nervous or renal system and may threaten the health of mother and fetus.

2. Pregnancies in mothers with RA are associated with increased risks for preterm delivery and lower birthweight, as well as preeclampsia. Pregnancies complicated by SLE are associated with increased risks for fetal loss, preeclampsia, preterm delivery, fetal growth restriction, and a risk for congenital heart block in infants.

3. Methotrexate for RA and cyclophosphamide for both RA and SLE are known to be teratogenic, depending on timing of exposure and dose.

Thromboembolic Disease in Pregnancy

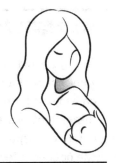

Wendy Abe Fukushima

LEARNING OBJECTIVES

1. Summarize the clinical risk factors for venous thromboembolism in women during pregnancy.

2. Describe the criteria for classification of the antiphospholipid syndrome and which women should be tested.

3. Compare the method(s) of prevention and treatment for acute venous thromboembolism in women preconception, during pregnancy, and postpartum.

4. Identify the risks involved when using oral anticoagulation for prevention or treatment of venous thromboembolism in pregnancy.

5. Identify the situation(s) when vitamin K antagonist therapy is indicated.

I. Introduction

Among the leading causes of obstetric mortality are deep vein thrombosis (DVT) and pulmonary embolism (PE), collectively termed *thromboembolic disease*. During pregnancy, thromboembolism is reported on average with a frequency of approximately one case per thousand pregnancies. Many early studies, when prolonged hospitalization was the norm, suggested a predominance of thromboembolic events during the postpartum period. However, a review of more than 1.4 million pregnancies represented by several studies reported an equal number of DVT and PE events occurred during the antepartum and postpartum periods.[1]

The incidence of a fatal PE can be reduced if a DVT is recognized early and adequately treated. Approximately 30% of isolated episodes of PE have been shown to be associated with a silent DVT. In addition, in patients presenting with DVT symptoms, silent PE frequency ranged as high as 40%–50%.[2] Since the early 1980s the 15% mortality rate in untreated antenatal DVT patients who developed PE improved to 1% with proper anticoagulation treatment.[3] Therefore, to reduce maternal mortality, it is imperative to provide adequate anticoagulant prophylaxis to those who have a high risk for thromboembolic disease and to thoroughly provide proper treatment to any patient with a documented DVT or PE.

II. PATIENT CASE [PART 1]

A 37-year-old primigravid white woman is seen for her first prenatal visit at 10 weeks of gestation. This patient has an unremarkable medical history but has been on bed rest for the last week due to hyperemesis gravidarum. The only medication the patient has been taking for the last several years is an oral contraceptive before conception. Her left calf has had progressive swelling and soreness, which she noticed a few days ago. Currently, she denies shortness of breath, cough, or chest pain and appears at ideal body weight but slightly dehydrated. She does not drink alcohol or participate in recreational drug use and she has no known drug allergies. The patient also reports that her sister had a pulmonary embolism after a knee surgery last year.

III. Pathophysiology

The formation of a thrombus has been thought to occur with possible abnormalities in blood flow, blood vessel integrity, and clotting components. This has been referred to as *Virchow's triad of hypercoagulability*.[4,5] During normal pregnancy, the risk of each triad component to occur is enhanced. Blood flow to the lower extremities can be reduced when an enlarging uterus compresses the pelvic veins and inferior vena cava. A compromised blood flow and birth of the baby may contribute to vessel cell injury. Finally, clotting factor changes during pregnancy are well documented, with marked increases in factors II, VII, VIII, IX, X, and XII and fibrinogen levels during pregnancy.[1,3,6] These all peak at the term of the pregnancy, only returning to normal approximately 8 weeks after birth.[3] Uterine decidual hemorrhage must be avoided during implantation, placentation, and the third stage of labor. Therefore, dramatic changes are necessary in the coagulation, anticoagulant, and fibrinolytic systems to increase the thrombin generating potential. Overall pregnancy is associated with an increased clotting potential, decreased anticoagulant activity, and decreased fibrinolysis, facilitating hemostasis but increasing the risk for venous thromboembolism (VTE) in pregnancy.[6]

Common risk factors for VTE in pregnancy are advanced maternal age, early pregnancy obesity, operative delivery, and a personal or family history of VTE (that could imply an inherited or acquired thrombophilia). Other contributing risk factors have been established (Table 1)[7] that could be important in decisions to consider prophylaxis in this patient population.

Additionally, the incidence of VTE among oral contraceptive users has been reported to be 3.94 per 10,000 exposed woman-years, with risks increasing sharply among obese and older women. Smoking, asthma, and poor health can contribute to a predisposition for VTE among estrogen-containing contraceptive users.[8] There also appears to be a modest increased risk of VTE associated with the use of third- versus second-generation oral contraceptives.[9]

Table 1. Risk Factors for Pregnancy-Associated Venous Thromboembolism (VTE)

Patient factors
  Age older than 35 y
  Obesity (BMI >29 kg/m^2) in early pregnancy
  Thrombophilia
  History of VTE (especially if idiopathic- or thrombophilia-associated)
  Gross varicose veins
  Significant current medical problem (eg, nephritic syndrome)
  Current infection or inflammatory process (eg, active inflammatory bowel disease or urinary
    tract infection)
  Immobility (eg, bed rest or lower limb fracture)
  Paraplegia
  Long-distance travel
  Dehydration
  Intravenous drug abuse
  Ovarian hyperstimulation
Pregnancy/obstetric factors
  Cesarean section, particularly as an emergency in labor
  Operative vaginal delivery
  Major obstetric hemorrhage
  Hyperemesis gravidarum
  Preeclampsia

BMI = body mass index.
From Greer IA, with permission.[7]

IV. Thrombophilias

There are many inhibitory proteins that regulate the coagulation cascade,[1] such as antithrombin III, protein S, protein C, and tissue factor pathway inhibitor.[5] Defects in these protein inhibitors can be either inherited or acquired and are commonly known as thrombophilias.[3] Thrombophilias can lead to hypercoagulability. Some have been linked to recurrent maternal VTE and they are responsible for more than 50% of all thromboembolic events during pregnancy. Typically thrombophilias are detected only after a thromboembolic event has occurred, as most inherited thrombophilias can be clinically insignificant alone. When combined with a precipitating trigger such as surgery, pregnancy, or other contributing risk factor (Table 1),[7] the result is susceptibility to clot formation and possible thrombosis.

Inherited thrombophilia disorders are found only in approximately 15% of the white European population,[10] 3% of African Americans, and virtually absent in African blacks and Asians.[6] Studies suggest that the natural inherited anticoagulation system abnormalities, such as antithrombin (AT) deficiency, activated protein C resistance and protein S or C deficiency, induce varying degrees of increased risk of thrombosis in pregnancy and the puerperium (Table 2).[7,11,12] The most common of the inherited thrombophilias, but the least thrombogenic, are hyperhomocysteinemia/homozygous MTHFR (C677T/A1298C). The rarest, but the most thrombogenic, inherited thrombophilias are AT deficiency, activated protein C resistance or factor V Leiden, and the compound heterozygote of factor V Leiden and prothrombin G20210A mutations.[11,13,14]

Table 2. Thrombophilia and Thromboembolism

Inherited Thrombophilia	General Incidence	VT or VTE	VT/VTE in Pregnancy or Puerperium
Antithrombin deficiency (most thrombogenic)	0.02%–1.17%; 1% in patients with VTE	50% life chance of VTE	50% chance of VTE in pregnancy
APCR or factor V Leiden[a]	3%–7% of white women	Incidence of 20%–30% with VTE	APCR found in 78% with VTE Factor V Leiden in 46% with VTE (predictive value 1:500)

Protein S or C deficiency[b]	0.14%–0.5%	Found in 3.2% with VTE	Protein S 0%–6%
			Protein C 3%–10%
			Postpartum:
			  Protein S 7%–22%
			  Protein C 7%–19%

Factor V Leiden and PGM G20210A	—	—	Predictive value 4.6:100 Prevalence in VTE 9.3% vs 0 in control group
Hyperhomocysteinemia/ homozygous MTHFR (C677T/A1298C)	8%–10% of healthy population	Increased risk	NA

APCR = activated protein C resistance, NA = not available, PGM = prothrombin gene mutation, VT = venous thrombosis, VTE = venous thromboembolism.
[a]Includes causes other than factor V Leiden for resistance to activated protein C.
[b]Protein S levels decrease in pregnancy to below normal standard reference range.
From Duhl AJ, et al, with permission.[11]

An acquired thrombophilia associated with thrombosis, fetal loss, and other clinical manifestations is an autoimmune disease characterized by the presence of antiphospholipid antibodies (APLA), known as the *antiphospholipid syndrome* (APS). These APLA are a heterogeneous group of autoantibodies that act directly against the phospholipids of cell membranes. This results in a complex illness, which most commonly causes thrombosis but can also cause too little coagulation. Antibodies have been shown to be present in up to 20% of individuals with a documented VTE. These APLA pose a major risk factor for VTE with a lifetime prevalence of arterial or VTE of approximately 30% in affected patients with an event rate of 1% per year.[6] The APLA have been reported in up to 10% of healthy individuals, depending on the laboratory assay used, and 30%–50% of patients with systemic lupus erythematosus (SLE).[15] Approximately 70% of individuals with APS are female, many of whom are at a reproductive age.[16] Fifteen to twenty percent of women with the antibodies have been shown to have obstetric complications, such as abruption, severe preeclampsia, fetal growth restriction, and fetal loss. There is also a three- to five-fold increased risk for recurrent fetal loss in those who have lupus anticoagulants and anticardiolipin antibodies, and at least 50% of pregnancy losses with APLA occur after the 10th week of gestation.[6,14,16,17]

Primary APS refers to patients with known APS when there is no other autoimmune disease detected. *Secondary APS* is when individuals meeting criteria for APS have a concurrent autoimmune, rheumatic, or connective tissue disorder, the most common being SLE.[17] Diagnosis of APS is made when a person presents with at least one of the following qualifying clinical criteria and at least one subsequent quantitative laboratory criteria on two or more occasions at least 12 weeks apart.[18]

Clinical criteria[18]:

1. Vascular thrombosis
   a. One or more clinical episodes of arterial, venous, or small-vessel thrombosis in any tissue or organ
   b. Thrombosis must be confirmed by imaging studies or Doppler studies
2. Pregnancy morbidity (when all other causes have been excluded) described as:
   a. >1 unexplained death of a morphologically normal fetus at or beyond the 10th week of gestation,
   b. at least one premature birth of a morphologically normal fetus at or before the 34th week of gestation due to preeclampsia, eclampsia, or placenta insufficiency,
   c. or at least three consecutive spontaneous abortions before the 10th week.

Laboratory criteria[18]:

1. Lupus anticoagulant in serum
2. Anticardiolipin antibody of immunoglobulin (Ig) G and/or IgM isotype in serum or plasma
3. Anti-β_2-glycoprotein I antibody of IgG and/or IgM isotype in serum or plasma

V. Screening

Currently, universal screening for thrombophilia in pregnancy is not supported by any beneficial evidence, nor has it been shown to be cost-effective. Many thrombophilias may not have any clinical implications and, therefore, the need to intervene with positive test results could lead to treatment dilemma. It is also important to be aware that pregnancy can influence the thrombophilia screens; for example, protein S naturally declines in pregnancy and 40% of pregnancies can have activated protein C resistance.[7,16] White patients with a history of thromboembolic events should be tested because there is a high prevalence of the factor V Leiden mutation in this population.[16] Only patients with clotting disorders, pregnancy morbidity (as previously described for APS diagnostic clinical criteria), and a strong family history with vascular thrombosis should be screened for testing at optimal times to produce reliable results. Numerous studies examining the association between inherited thrombophilias and adverse reproductive outcomes have been performed with no clear conclusions drawn. Therefore, patients with a history of unexplained fetal loss at or after 20 weeks' gestation, severe preeclampsia or HELLP (hemolysis, elevated liver enzymes, and low platelets) at or before 34 weeks' gestation, and severe intrauterine growth restriction may also benefit from thrombophilia screening.[11]

VI. Diagnosis

Signs and symptoms commonly consistent with DVT and PE can be nonthrombotic in origin but rather normal physiologic changes in pregnancy. Only one quarter to one third of patients clinically presenting with a DVT actually have it confirmed when reliable objective tests are performed.[1] The clinical signs and symptoms of a DVT include erythema, warmth, muscle pain, edema or swelling, discoloration, tenderness, dilated superficial veins, a palpable deep linear cord, and a positive Homans' sign.[3,5,6] The Homans' sign might be present in only approximately 30% of patients with a DVT, thus making it less reliable as an assessment tool.[5] Venous ultrasonography can be used to assist in making the diagnosis of DVT (see algorithm in Figure 1).[6] The D-dimer assay, which can be used before contrast venography or magnetic resonance imaging, has been excluded. Although a negative D-dimer result can be reassuring, there is a high rate of false positive results for thrombosis in pregnant, puerperal, and postoperative patients, as well as in patients with superficial thrombophlebitis.[6] Proximal DVT is considered important clinically, as it is more commonly associated with serious disease and possibly fatal outcomes. The management of isolated calf-vein thrombosis had been more controversial. However, since most iliofemoral thromboses originate from calf-vein thrombosis, treatment is suggested for symptomatic patients. Furthermore, recurrent VTE data support the need for anticoagulation therapy for all DVT, with the duration of therapy dependent on risk factors and episodes of occurrence.[19] During pregnancy most cases of DVT are predominately in the deep veins of the lower extremity with a propensity to be in the left leg,[1,2] perhaps as a result from compression of the left iliac vein by the right iliac and ovarian arteries, since both cross the vein only on the left side.[20]

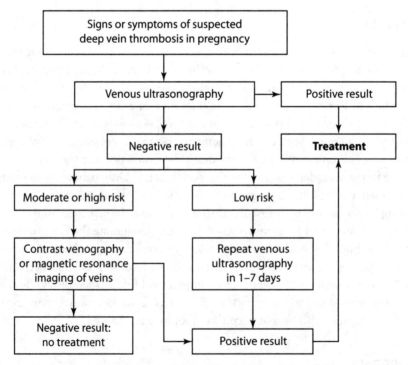

Figure 1. Alternative diagnostic paradigm for the diagnosis of deep vein thrombosis when D-dimer test is unavailable or inappropriate. From Lockwood C, with permission.[6]

The major signs and symptoms of PE are tachypnea (≥20 breaths per minute), dyspnea, pleuritic pain, and apprehension. Small emboli lodged more peripherally can produce infarction accompanied by pleural signs of cough, hemoptysis, tachycardia (heart rate ≥100 beats per minute), temperature, atelectatic rales, pleuritic chest pain with splinting, and a friction rub.[3,6] Symptoms suggestive of a myocardial infarction (such as right-sided heart failure with jugular venous distention, presyncope, syncope, and hypotension) can result from a massive PE, defined as occlusion of at least 50% of the pulmonary arterial circulation.[3] Approximately 90% of acute PE cases arise from lower extremity DVTs and, conversely, among patients with acute PE, 50% will harbor a DVT with only 20% of these patients having no clinical signs or symptoms of the DVT.[21] Therefore, imaging for a DVT is common when a PE is suspected, because a DVT diagnosis in itself will mandate treatment, regardless of pulmonary findings.[6] Specific diagnostic studies indicating the existence of a PE include large mismatched defects in ventilation-perfusion ($\dot{V}/\dot{Q}$) scans, emboli presence in either spiral pulmonary angiographic computed tomography (spiral CT) or magnetic resonance angiography. The spiral CT exposes the fetus to less radiation than $\dot{V}/\dot{Q}$ scanning but more radiation exposure to the breasts. Review of all diagnostic modalities combined that were used in evaluation for VTE resulted in radiation exposure <5 rads, and, thus, they were deemed to pose no known risk of spontaneous abortion, teratogenicity, or perinatal morbidity. Neither administration of gadolinium or of iodinated contrast media has been shown to cause mutagenic or teratogenic effects to the fetus. However, fetal goiter may be of some concern after maternal exposure to radiographic contrast. Therefore, appropriate fetal and neonatal assessments may be warranted for proper thyroid function.[6]

Two potential thrombotic problems occurring postpartum are ovarian vein thrombosis and septic thrombophlebitis, a serious complication of pyogenic pelvic infections. Both are difficult to diagnose because they present as fever, pain, and possibly a mass seen on CT scan. Septic thrombophlebitis should be suspected in patients who have persistent fever despite adequate antibiotic therapy. The addition of heparin can assist with the differential diagnosis of septic thrombophlebitis if fever subsides within 12–36 hours of initiation of therapy. Ovarian vein thrombosis can also be treated with antibiotics and anticoagulation therapy.[3]

VII. Guidelines

During pregnancy, anticoagulant therapy is indicated for the prevention and treatment of VTE, prevention and treatment of systemic embolism in patients with mechanical heart valves, and prevention of pregnancy complications in women with APLAs or other thrombophilia and previous pregnancy complications.

Recommendations about the use of anticoagulants during pregnancy, including duration of therapy and prophylaxis, are based largely on data extrapolated from nonpregnant patients, from case reports, and from case series of pregnant patients. There are no randomized, prospective trials for the treatment of VTE in pregnancy. There are a variety of antithrombotic treatments available for the nonpregnant population, but many have limitations during pregnancy. The management of thromboprophylaxis during pregnancy requires frequent monitoring for weight, renal, and volume of distribution changes. Furthermore, treatment modifications must be used during labor and delivery, and, finally, conversion to oral anticoagulation is needed postpartum.

Evidence-based guidelines and current recommendations for the use of antithrombotic agents during pregnancy were outlined by the American College of Chest Physicians (ACCP) in 2004 and are shown in Figure 2.[22] In 2008, the ACCP reviewed the most recent information concerning VTE in pregnancy, but apparently concluded that the new data did not offer significant improvements over current recommendations because the majority of the 2004 recommendations remained unchanged.[23] Experts from across the United States, organized by Aventis Pharmaceuticals, met to further define recommendations for antithrombotic therapy in pregnancy. Their goal was to provide a concise update, which is outlined in Figure 3.[11] Patients were classified according to their risk of VTE, their risk of an adverse pregnancy outcome (APO), or both. Antithrombotic recommendations were based on an assessment of an individual patient's level of risk. This group also concluded that thromboprophylaxis during cesarean birth is currently not recommended. They also identified more patients who might benefit from thrombophilia screening, particularly those with a history of APO, and further described prophylaxis intensity treatment for various thrombophilias based on the risk for VTE (Figure 3).[11]

VIII. Treatment

Treatment decisions during pregnancy have implications for the health and life of both the mother and fetus. Therefore, careful risk assessments must be performed and individualized for each patient.[23] The combination of mechanical and pharmacologic methods should be used to treat patients with a documented VTE and to provide prophylaxis therapy to those who have a high risk for thromboembolic disease or its recurrence. Mechanical methods increase blood flow to the femoral vessels, reduce venous stasis, and enhance fibrinolysis. Pharmacologic methods are directed at different portions of the clotting cascade to prevent clot formation.[13]

A. Nonpharmacologic

Graduated elastic compression stockings, pneumatic compression devices, the Trendelenburg position, and initial treatment with bed rest are nonpharmacologic interventions aimed at preventing VTE and reducing the occurrence of postphlebitic syndrome after a DVT. Graduated compression stockings must be worn correctly, because improper fit could cause venous stasis or occlusion in blood flow. Intermittent pneumatic compression devices use an inflatable pneumatic sleeve that compresses the calf at regular intervals to help increase blood flow in the femoral vessels, reduce venous stasis, and possibly enhance fibrinolysis.[3,6,13] Gynecologic literature lacks evidence supporting the beneficial use of combining mechanical and pharmacologic methods. However, both the ACCP (in the Seventh Consensus Conference and Eighth Edition) and the American College of Obstetrics and Gynecology (ACOG) support the combined approach in patients at highest risk for VTE.[13,22,23] The Trendelenburg position, elevation of the foot of the bed by approximately 8 inches, and bed

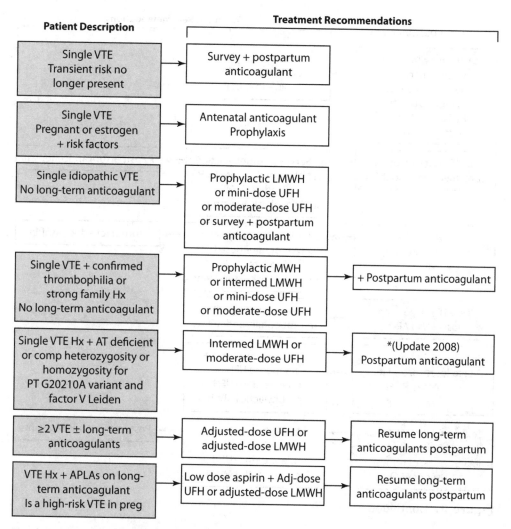

Figure 2. Evidence-Based Guidelines for the Use of Antithrombotic Agents in Pregnancy. APLAs = antiphospholipid antibodies, APO = adverse pregnancy outcome (recurrent preeclampsia, abruptions, unexplained intrauterine death, or intrauterine growth restriction), AT = antithrombin, Comp = compound, Hx = history, Intermed = intermediate, LMWH = low-molecular-weight heparin, Preg = pregnancy, PT = prothrombin, UFH = unfractionated heparin, VTE = venous thromboembolism. Low-dose aspirin = 60–150 mg daily. UFH: mini-dose = 5000 units SC q12h; moderate-dose = SC q12h target anti-Xa (0.1–0.3 U/mL); adjusted-dose = SC q12h target mid-interval activated partial thromboplastin time. LMWH: prophylactic = dalteparin, 5000 units SC q12h or enoxaparin, 40 mg SC q24h; intermediate-dose = SC q12h, weight-adjusted dalteparin, 200 units/kg daily or 100 units/kg q12h, tinzaparin, 175 units/kg daily, or enoxaparin 1 mg/kg q12h (half-life of LMWH is shorter in pregnancy; twice-daily dosing is preferable, at least in the initial treatment phase. Postpartum anticoagulants: warfarin for 4–6 weeks, target international normalized ratio (INR) 2.0–3.0, with initial UFH or LMWH overlap until the INR is ≥2.0. Survey = clinical surveillance is clinical vigilance and aggressive investigation of women with symptoms suspicious of deep venous thrombosis or pulmonary embolism. From Bates SM, et al, with permission.[22,23] (continued)

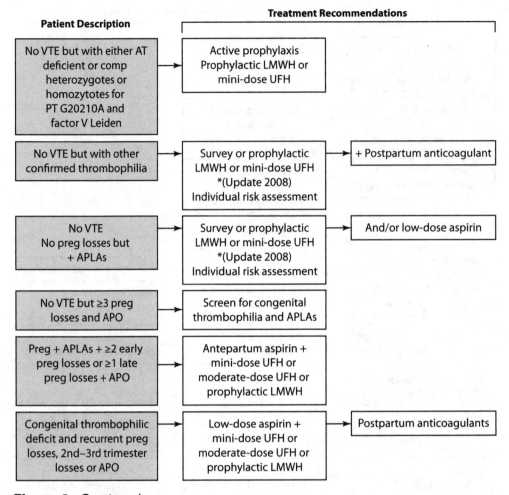

Figure 2. Continued.

rest can promote venous return and decrease edema initially after an extremity DVT event has occurred. As soon as symptoms permit, ambulation should be encouraged for DVT and after 5–7 days for PE to prevent further venous stasis from bed rest. Lastly, oxygen therapy can be very important during pregnancy with suspicious or documented PE for maternal reasons and to assist in preventing fetal damage from a hypoxic mother.[3]

B. Pharmacologic

Thrombosis prophylaxis and treatment use pharmacologic agents that assist clot lysis, hinder platelet adhesion-aggregation, and most importantly, inhibit fibrin formation. Heparin, heparinlike compounds, and coumarin derivatives interfere with fibrin formation and are considered the most important anticoagulants in the treatment of VTE in pregnancy. However, issues of maternal abruption, puerperal hemorrhage, lactation, and fetal teratogenicity or hemorrhage should also be considered.[3]

Standard unfractionated heparin (UFH) is a heterogeneous mixture of glycosaminoglycans of varying molecular weights, which act rapidly as an intravenous or subcutaneous anticoagulant. Its mechanism of action is in its ability to bind to the naturally

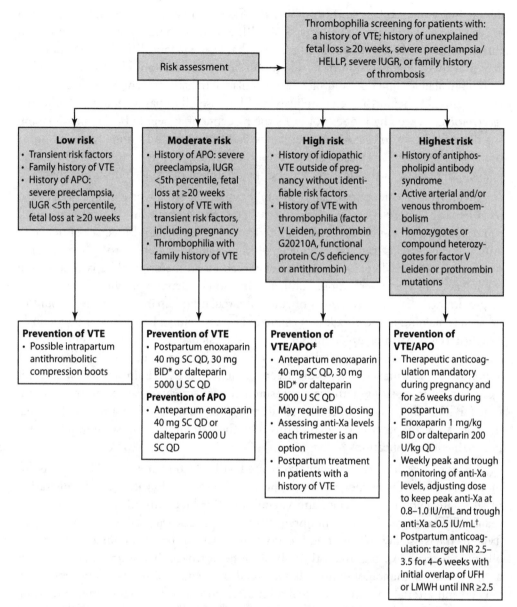

Figure 3. Risk assessment and prevention of venous thromboembolism (VTE) and adverse pregnancy outcomes (APO) in pregnant patients. HELLP = hemolysis, elevated liver enzymes, and low platelets, INR = international normalized ratio, IUGR = intrauterine growth restriction, LMWH = low-molecular$_2$ weight heparin, UFH = unfractimated heparin. *The choice of enoxaparin dose should be tailored according to the individual patient, as these doses have not been compared in this setting. †The dose of enoxaparin may be increased to maintain peak levels at the top of the desired range. ‡Aspirin and heparin are recommended in patients with antiphospholipid antibodies. From Duhl AJ, et al, with permission.[11]

circulating anticoagulant antithrombin III (AT III). The bound complex can then accelerate the anticoagulant effects of AT III, and it becomes a potent inhibitor of thrombin factor IIa affecting clotting factors Xa, IXa, XIa, and XIIa. This overall process prevents the conversion of fibrinogen to fibrin. In addition, UFH has the ability to inhibit platelet function and increase vascular permeability, which could make it a risk for possible hemorrhagic complications.[5] Because UFH has a negative charge and large molecular weight, it does not cross the placenta or appear in breast milk, making it a desirable agent to use during pregnancy and lactation.[3] Additionally, unlike some oral anticoagulants, UFH use during gestation has not been reported to be linked to congenital defects, further leading it to be the treatment of choice during pregnancy.[22]

Hemorrhage, osteoporosis, and thrombocytopenia are adverse effects associated with heparin. There is a 4% incidence of hemorrhage occurring in properly monitored, nonsurgical patients receiving intravenous heparin.[3] Rapid reversal of heparin's anticoagulant effects can be achieved with protamine sulfate. Protamine dosages needed to neutralize heparin can be calculated based on the original heparin dose and the interval since administration. Full neutralization of heparin activity requires 1 mg of protamine sulfate per 100 units of residual circulating heparin, with the amount of heparin remaining in the circulation estimated by assuming a half-life of intravenously administered heparin of 30–60 minutes. Only the calculated dose of protamine should be used, as the excess amount has its own anticoagulant effect.[1] When heparin is administered subcutaneously, reversal can be achieved by administering small infusions of protamine along with serial measurements of activated partial thromboplastin time (aPTT). This may be necessary if UFH has been dosed within 4 hours of vaginal or cesarean birth; otherwise, beyond this time the patient is not at substantial risk for hemorrhagic complications.[6]

Osteoporosis has been strongly correlated with >15,000 units of UFH per day for more than 6 months of therapy, and appears to be reversible with the administration of adequate amounts of calcium and vitamin D.[1,3,6,22] Heparin-induced thrombocytopenia (HIT) can arise in 3% of nonpregnant patients, appearing as two different types. Type I HIT is usually self-limiting, occurs within days of heparin contact, and is usually not associated with a risk of thrombosis or hemorrhage. In contrast, type II HIT is a more rare immunoglobulin-mediated syndrome, inconsistently associated with venous and arterial thrombosis, usually reported to occur 5–14 days after initiation, and requires the termination of heparin therapy.[1,3,5,6,22] Therefore, type II HIT should be suspected when the platelet count falls below 50% of the baseline value or <100 × 10^9/L within the suspected timeframe after heparin exposure.

During pregnancy, VTE treatment is similar to that in nonpregnant patients, using a heparin weight–based dosing nomogram. (Table 3).[24] This is just one method that can be used to achieve a therapeutic aPTT rapidly.[25] IV heparin is initiated via total body pregnancy weight–based dosing with an IV bolus (80 units/kg) followed by a continuous infusion (18 units/kg/h)[26] titrated to achieve full anticoagulation measured by aPTT with a goal of 1.5–2.5 times control (60–80 seconds).[3,5,6] The aPTT response to heparin is often attenuated during pregnancy because of increased levels of factor VIII and fibrinogen.[22] Because the aPTT can be influenced by the coagulation timer and reagents used to perform the test, it is recommended that each laboratory standardize its therapeutic

Table 3. Weight-Based Heparin Dosing Nomogram

Initial dose		80 units/kg bolus, then 18 units/kg/h
aPTT, <35 s	<1.2 × control	80 units/kg bolus, then 4 units/kg/h
aPTT, 35–45 s	1.2–1.5 × control	40 units/kg bolus, then 2 units/kg/h
aPTT, 46–70 s	1.5–2.3 × control	No change
aPTT, 71–90 s	2.3–3 × control	Decrease infusion rate by 2 units/kg/h
aPTT, >90 s	>3 × control	Hold infusion 1 h, then decrease infusion rate by 3 units/kg/h

aPTT = activated partial thromboplastin time.
From Raschke RA, et al, with permission.[24]
The American College of Physicians is not responsible for the accuracy of this translation.

range aPTT to correspond to plasma heparin levels from 0.3 to 0.7 IU/mL anti-Xa activity by the amidolytic assay.[25,26] The aPTT should be measured approximately 6 hours after the bolus dose of heparin, and the continuous IV dose should be adjusted accordingly every 6 hours until goal aPTT steady state has been achieved; then, aPTT monitoring can be reduced to daily. Continuous IV heparin should be administered for at least 3–5 days (before transition to subcutaneous heparin) for active thromboembolic disease or until resolution of symptoms and no evidence of recurrence exists. Treatment for VTE can be transitioned to subcutaneous heparinlike agents for duration of at least 4–6 months to prevent VTE recurrence in pregnancy.[3,6,22] This should be followed by prophylactic doses for the remainder of pregnancy and labor, and stopped just before childbirth, with possible dose adjustments throughout as the blood volume changes in pregnancy.[3] Then postpartum anticoagulation can be transitioned to oral anticoagulant therapy for at least 6–12 weeks postpartum (DVT) or 6 months postpartum (PE).[3]

Subcutaneous UFH administered twice daily has been shown to be as effective and at least as safe as IV UFH for DVT and PE treatment. It is imperative that adequate initial dosing (35,000 units/24 h) is administered and subsequent doses are adjusted to achieve a therapeutic aPTT monitored 6 hours (mid-interval) after administration, and the dose is adjusted to achieve a 1.5 to 2.5 aPTT prolongation.[26] UFH is well absorbed after subcutaneous administration, but should never be administered intramuscularly due to the high incidence of hematoma formation.[3,5] Subcutaneous adjusted dose of UFH can cause a persistent anticoagulant effect at the time of delivery, up to 28 hours after the last injection has been reported.[22]

In prophylactic therapy, much less UFH is required to prevent thrombus formation than to prevent further clotting once a thrombus has formed. Only small amounts of UFH are needed to enhance the action of AT III, the inhibiting factor of Xa, which is essential for thrombus formation.[3] A standard UFH dose of 5000 units every 12 hours has been shown to be effective and safe for the prevention of VTE in high-risk nonpregnant patients.[3,22] However, because this dose does not reliably produce detectable heparin levels, there is concern that this dose could be insufficient in high-risk situations. Therefore, in pregnancy, higher doses of 10,000 units every 12 hours have been used, but no comparative studies have been performed.[22]

Derived from a portion of UFH, low-molecular-weight heparin (LMWH) can inactivate factor Xa by binding more specifically to Xa, but due to its short length (<18 saccharide moieties), it is incapable of forming the heparin–AT III complex necessary to bind factor IIa.[3,5] This property allows LMWHs to retain equivalent antithrombotic effects as standard UFH but have fewer bleeding risks. Multiple well-designed trials comparing LMWH to UFH have shown that LMWHs are a reliable method for thromboprophylaxis and effective treatment for VTE.[13,22] The three LMWHs currently marketed are enoxaparin, tinzaparin, and dalteparin.[3,5] These LMWHs cannot be used interchangeably (unit for unit) with other LMWHs or UFH. Table 4 summarizes the available LMWH preparations, fondaparinux (a synthetic heparin pentasaccharide), and UFH. The advantages of using LMWH over UFH include less HIT,[22] a greater bioavailability after subcutaneous injections, a longer half-life, a closer correlation between body weight and anti-Xa activity, and the reduction or elimination of laboratory monitoring except in patients who are pregnant, morbidly obese, or have renal failure.[6] Because the half-life of LMWH is shorter in pregnancy, it is preferable to use twice-daily dosing, especially during the initial VTE treatment phase.[22] The pharmacokinetics of enoxaparin during early and late phases of pregnancy differs for the same women when not pregnant. The increased renal clearance during pregnancy might reduce the maximum concentration and the plasma activity of enoxaparin.[3] Therefore, anti-Xa activity levels should be used to monitor and adjust enoxaparin therapy with the target peak levels of 0.5–1 IU/mL drawn 4 hours after a dose.[27] A regimen for correcting the enoxaparin dose utilizing anti-Xa levels is outlined in Table 5.[3,27]

LMWHs do not cross the placenta and, as a result, are low risk to the fetus.[1,3,6,22] In 2002, the enoxaparin manufacturer warned of an association of congenital anomalies and increased hemorrhage risks when enoxaparin was used in pregnancy. However, ACOG concluded that these risks were rare, the incidence was not higher than expected, and that no cause-and-effect relationship had been established.[1] The patient should not experience anticoagulation-related problems if vaginal or cesarean birth occurs beyond 12 hours of a prophylactic dose or 24 hours from a therapeutic LMWH dose. Protamine may be necessary to reverse the anticoagulation effects for LMWH, although protamine can only partially (60%) neutralize anti-Xa activity.[11] Regional (spinal and epidural) anesthesia is associated with a 50% decrease in DVT risk when compared with general anesthesia. However, spinal and epidural anesthesia are contraindicated within 18–24 hours of LMWH administration due to the 1997 U.S. Food and Drug Administration (FDA) public health advisory describing 41 patients who developed epidural and spinal hematomas, with resultant long-term neurologic injury, after using enoxaparin and undergoing spinal and epidural anesthesia.[13] Therefore, UFH should be used instead of LMWHs for expectant management at 36–38 weeks of gestation, or earlier if preterm delivery is expected.[3,6]

Sodium warfarin is the most widely employed coumarin derivative used in managing VTE. It is an oral anticoagulant that acts as a vitamin K antagonist, preventing the carboxylation of precursors to produce clotting factors II, VII, IX, and X, and it also depletes the synthesis of protein C and protein S. Its delayed effect is directly related to the diminishing concentrations of each of the warfarin-affected clotting factors.[3,5] Anticoagulation with warfarin is generally contraindicated during pregnancy because it readily crosses the placenta and can cause embryopathy (fetal warfarin syndrome), central nervous system defects, spontaneous abortion, still birth, prematurity, and

Table 4. Low-Molecular-Weight Heparin, Synthetic Heparin, and Unfractionated Heparin

	Enoxaparin	Dalteparin	Tinzaparin	Fondaparinux	Unfractionated Heparin
Trade name	Lovenox®	Fragmin®	Innohep®	Arixtra®	—
Pregnancy category[a]	B	B	B	B	C
Administration	SC	SC	SC	SC	IV or SC
Frequency (BID preferred in pregnancy)	BID or daily	Daily	Daily	Daily	BID or TID
Low-dose prophylaxis in pregnancy	40 mg SC once or twice daily[30]	5000 units SC once or twice daily[30]	—	2.5 mg SC daily[11]	5000–7000 units SC q12h first trimester 7500–10,000 units SC q12h second trimester 10,000 units SC q12h third trimester[30]
Pregnancy-adjusted dose treatment of deep venous thrombosis or pulmonary embolism	30–80 mg q12h or 1 mg/kg q12h[30] SC dose	5000–10,000 units q12h[30] SC dose	175 anti-factor XA IU/kg SC daily[22]	<50 kg 5 mg 50–100 kg 7.5 mg >100 kg 10 mg SC daily[11]	
Monitoring	Anti-Xa peak (4 h after dose) 0.8–1.0 IU/mL and trough (12 h after dose) ≥0.5 IU/mL[11]	—	—	—	Mid-interval aPTT of 1.5–2.5 × control[6]
Breastfeeding[a]	Compatible	Compatible	No human data; probably compatible	No human data; probably compatible	Compatible

aPTT = activated partial thromboplastin time.
[a]Briggs GG, et al.[28]

Table 5. Adjusting Enoxaparin Dosage Based on Anti-Xa Levels

Anti-Xa Level (IU/mL)	Dose	Repeat
<0.35	Increase 25%	24 h to 1 wk
0.35–0.49	Increase 10%	24 h to 1 wk
0.5–1.0	No change	q week to month
1.1–1.5	Decrease 20%	24 h to 1 wk
1.6–2.0	Decrease 30%	24 h to 1 wk
>2.0	None; restart when <0.5, restart at 40% original	24 h

From Laros Jr RK, with permission,[3] and Busby LT, et al, with permission.[27]

hemorrhage.[1,3,28] It is postulated that first-trimester anomalies could be consequential to either a direct teratogenic effect or a vitamin K–deficiency effect, whereas the second- and third-trimester defects may result from fetal hemorrhage. Therefore, women requiring prolonged anticoagulation with coumarin derivatives should be converted to UFH or LMWH before conception, if possible, and counseled on possible negative effects if exposed during the first trimester for longer than the first 14–21 days after conception.[3] Another recommended method is to test frequently for pregnancy and substitute UFH or LMWH for warfarin when pregnancy is achieved.[22] An area of much controversy is anticoagulation for pregnant women with prosthetic heart valves, as oral anticoagulation still appears to be most efficacious at preventing thrombosis in this population. Limited data of UFH or LMWH efficacy in high-risk mechanical valves (eg, older-generation prosthesis valve in mitral position or history of thromboembolism)[23] might possibly be due to inadequate dosing or inappropriate target therapeutic ranges. As a result, definitive recommendations for these patients are difficult, particularly with the fetal concerns.[3,22,23] Despite the apparent contraindication of warfarin therapy during pregnancy, warfarin may have a role in patients unable to master self-administration of heparin, who exhibit heparin allergic reactions, who have a mechanical heart valve prosthesis in situ, or in cases of antithrombin III deficiency.[3] In these very unique cases, warfarin should only be used after 13 weeks of gestation[23] to avoid fetal embryopathy as much as possible, and stopped well in advance of labor (middle of the third trimester). Either UFH or LMWH with aggressively adjusted dosing and appropriate diligent monitoring should be used during the period of warfarin absence.[3,22]

Full doses of UFH or LMWH should be reinstituted 3–6 hours after vaginal birth and 6–8 hours after cesarean surgery. However, the initiation of LMWH therapy after removal of an epidural catheter should be based on bleeding and physical examination, and not begun for at least 10–12 hours.[6] Warfarin should be started as soon as the patient resumes oral intake in most postpartum patients. A warfarin therapeutic dose schedule aims for a smooth reduction in circulating levels of all influenced factors. Large loading doses should be avoided, as they tend only to depress factor VII and produce more bleeding. The usual warfarin dose, 5 mg daily, is initiated until achievement of a therapeutic prolongation of the international normalized ratio (INR). For either prevention or treatment of VTE or for an in situ tissue cardiac valve, the therapeutic INR is 2.0–3.0. A patient with a mechanical cardiac valve should target an INR of 2.5–3.5. The overlap (bridging) with either UFH or LMWH with warfarin therapy should continue until the INR reaches the therapeutic range for two successive days to ensure proper VTE protection.[5,6,22]

Patients with known hypercoagulable conditions, such as protein C or protein S deficiency, should begin warfarin therapy only after adequate heparinization is achieved to avoid an early procoagulant and anticoagulant activity imbalance that can cause skin necrosis as a result of extensive microvascular thrombosis within subcutaneous fat. Although skin necrosis is rare, occurrence is approximately 0.01%–0.1%, it can be serious, requiring temporary cessation of warfarin until symptoms resolve and warfarin at lower doses can be reintroduced.[5] Other adverse effects for warfarin therapy include purple toes syndrome and the most common problem is bleeding.

Other treatment options previously used to improve fetal survival in women with APS include steroids and IV immune globulin to suppress the immune system, heparin and aspirin to prevent thrombosis in the uteroplacental circulation, and low-dose aspirin to improve placental blood flow by decreasing the thromboxane–prostacyclin ratio.[14] Currently, only low-dose aspirin (60–150 mg/d) during the second and third trimesters is recommended.[22,23]

C. Surgical Intervention

Surgical or radiologic intervention with an inferior vena caval filter is reserved for patients in whom anticoagulation therapy is absolutely contraindicated, who develop recurrent acute PE despite adequate anticoagulation therapy, and in whom an acute PE could be fatal.[3] Pregnant patients with type II HIT or severe heparin allergies may also benefit from surgical intervention, but a trial with fondaparinux, a synthetic heparin pentasaccharide, may be a therapeutic option, but should be reserved for those in whom there are no other obvious therapeutic alternatives, as limited experience in pregnancy exists. This agent is considered pregnancy class B by the FDA.[6] There is currently limited experience with direct thrombin inhibitors and thrombolytic agents in pregnancy.[22] The concern is effects on the placenta (eg, premature labor, placental abruption, or fetal demise)[23] and, therefore, these will not be discussed further.

During postpartum hospitalization after cesarean section, thromboprophylaxis with pharmacologic and/or mechanical (graduated compression stockings or intermittent pneumatic compression) prophylaxis is recommended for women considered at risk for VTE. In selected postcesarean patients with very high risk factors for VTE, thromboprophylaxis should be continued after discharge from the hospital for up to 4–6 weeks.[23]

IX. Patient Education

The patient should be counseled:

- to observe for signs/symptoms of clotting problems (calf pain, tenderness, swelling, etc.)
- to recognize bleeding problems (check urine, stools, and gums for blood)
- on the importance of compliance with laboratory tests for monitoring
- on expected progression of pregnancy and need to follow fetal kick counts when at appropriate gestation

- on when to withhold anticoagulation therapy, especially in conjunction with labor or cesarean surgery
- when to notify her physician
- in proper subcutaneous administration technique if using UFH or LMWH, including site of injection into the abdomen and rotation of sites, to minimize bruising by not rubbing the injection site, needle stick prevention, and proper disposal into a sealed sharps container.[29] No special administration techniques are mentioned for pregnancy; therefore, subcutaneous injection into the abdominal fat layer should continue during pregnancy.

If prescribed warfarin, additional patient counseling includes awareness of warfarin drug–drug interactions, possible warfarin teratogenicity effects, special dietary considerations (the need for consistent diet), proper identification of different tablets, the need to inform others about being on this anticoagulant, and how to handle missed dosages.[5]

X. PATIENT CASE [PART 2]

The patient has no personal history of thrombosis or pregnancy loss. However, she does have several risk factors for VTE, which include: age older than 35 years, possible immobility and dehydration due to hyperemesis gravidarum, and positive family history (sister) with a PE. The type of oral contraceptives the patient had been taking should be explored. Although the patient has a first-degree relative with a VTE, her sister's thrombosis occurred after a very thrombogenic stimulus (knee surgery). In addition, she is white, also putting her at risk for a factor V Leiden mutation thrombophilia. The symptoms of left calf swelling and soreness should further heighten the suspicion that the patient is truly experiencing a DVT. The left side propensity for DVT should also be noted.

The patient should be admitted to the hospital for observation, given the risk factors for VTE and the patient's display of symptoms. Because sudden death is not uncommon in pregnant patients,[2] this patient should have objective testing performed expeditiously. Treatment should start once diagnostic venous ultrasonography confirms that a left DVT or high suspicion for a silent DVT continues to be present. Furthermore, thrombophilia testing should be completed before starting treatment. Keep in mind that further testing may be necessary after pregnancy influences are gone. Laboratory tests should include a baseline complete blood count, aPTT, and INR, and graduated compression stockings should be placed on the patient's legs. IV UFH therapy can be initiated after initial blood work has been obtained by using 80 units/kg IV bolus and a continuous infusion of 18 units/kg/h administered simultaneously with the bolus. Monitoring of aPTT should be done 6 hours after the bolus dose and every 6 hours after heparin dose adjustment until a steady state of goal aPTT of 1.5–2 times the control is achieved.

This is followed by daily monitoring of aPTT for at least 5 days for documented DVT, or conversion to subcutaneous UFH or LMWH. Heparin is stopped if a DVT is ruled out and no thrombophilia risk is found. Fetal surveillance, including ultrasound and possibly fetal heart rate monitoring,[11] should be conducted daily along with close observation for bleeding. Platelets should be monitored for possible HIT as recommended by ACOG at baseline, on day 5, and then periodically for the first 2 weeks.[1]

Given that this patient has several risk factors for DVT and a suspicious thrombophilia, prophylactic doses of either UFH or LMWH could be used even if a DVT is ruled out. A recommendation of LMWH over UFH is favored given the advantages of better bioavailability, longer plasma half-life, more predictable pharmacokinetics, and pharmacodynamics, less potential for osteoporosis, a lower incidence of HIT, and less antithrombin activity, which may decrease medical bleeding and wound hematoma formation for LMWH.[11,13] Although the patient is not obese, anti-factor Xa monitoring to target peak levels (0.5–1 IU/mL) 4 hours after the injection for LMWH treatment dosing (or 0.2–0.4 IU/mL for prophylaxis dosing)[11] will be followed during pregnancy because there are many changes, such as weight, renal function, and volume of distribution. Furthermore, pregnancy in itself could mask some thrombophilias. If LMWH is continued throughout her pregnancy, then the patient should be converted to subcutaneous UFH at 36–38 weeks so that regional anesthesia could be used during labor.[3] Subcutaneous UFH, 10,000 units every 12 hours, or dose adjusted by 6-hour mid-interval level of aPTT with target range of 1.5–2.5 times control, can be used. The UFH dose should be stopped 6 hours before labor, if possible. However, if spontaneous labor has occurred, a dose of protamine can be administered to neutralize the estimated active heparin to help avoid bleeding.

Either UFH or LMWH can be resumed in 6 hours after a vaginal birth, 8 hours after a cesarean birth,[6] or 12 hours if an epidural catheter has been removed.[11] Because the patient may be at risk for thrombophilia or APS, therapeutic heparinization should be achieved before initiating warfarin therapy to avoid potential skin necrosis. Warfarin can be initiated with an oral dose of 5 mg, then adjusted daily using the INR to achieve a target INR (2.0–3.0). Overlap of heparin (UFH or LMWH) should continue with warfarin until INR is at target goal for at least 2 days. Then, when the INR remains in target goal and is stable, monitoring can be reduced to weekly intervals. Warfarin therapy should continue for at least 6 weeks postpartum,[1] and possibly longer if thrombophilia testing proves positive and risk factors remain. The total duration of anticoagulation therapy for a pregnant woman with an acute VTE without any risk factors is to continue throughout the remainder of the pregnancy and for a total minimum duration of 6 months, which includes at least 6 weeks of postpartum therapy.[23]

The patient should receive patient education for the low risk of UFH or LMWH to the fetus, on proper administration for subcutaneous dosing, and that both are compatible with breastfeeding.[6] Warfarin has teratogenic effects and, therefore, caution should be taken against conception while on warfarin therapy postpartum. The patient will need a contraception method, but should not take oral contraceptives containing estrogens due to their propensity for possible thrombosis. Warfarin is acceptable with breastfeeding.[1,5]

The patient should be cautioned to observe for bleeding risks while on anticoagulant therapy, possible VTE progression, potential risks for a thrombophilia, and proper fetal monitoring (kick counts when at appropriate gestation). She should be warned about the possible anticoagulant effects of herbal products[6,13] and alcohol's effect on the fetus. Direction on laboratory draws and method for follow-up monitoring should also be established before discharge. Furthermore, the patient should be given hyperemesis gravidarum treatment and education (see Chapter 24, Nausea and Vomiting of Pregnancy).

XI. Summary

Venous thromboembolism continues to be one of the leading causes of morbidity and mortality in women.[6] Thrombophilia and VTE development during pregnancy can have very serious repercussions for both mother and fetus.[11] Therefore, it is imperative to identify those patients at highest risk for VTE development to provide adequate prophylaxis and proper therapeutic treatment to those patients with a documented VTE. There is still a need for clear and concise guidance for pregnant patients at risk for VTE or adverse pregnancy outcomes because most of the current data are still derived from the nonpregnant population.[11] Much of the guideline information presented was developed by consensus groups who are considered experts for VTE, with the goal of further defining treatment and prophylaxis options for the unique needs of the pregnant population.

XII. References

1. Cunningham FG, Leveno KJ, Bloom SL, et al, eds. Thromboembolic disorders. In *Williams Obstetrics*. 22nd ed. New York: McGraw-Hill, 2005:1073–1091.

2. Marik PE, Plante LA. Venous thromboembolic disease and pregnancy. *N Engl J Med*. 2008;359:2025–2033.

3. Laros Jr RK. Thromboembolic disease. In Creasy RK, Resnik R, eds. *Maternal-Fetal Medicine*. 5th ed. Philadelphia: Saunders, 2004:845–857.

4. Brotman DJ, Deitcher SR, Lip GY, et al. Virchow's triad revisited. *Southern Med J*. 2004;97:213–214.

5. Wittkowsky AK. Thrombosis. In Koda-Kimble MA, Young LY, Kradjan WA, et al. *Applied Therapeutics: The Clinical Use of Drugs*.7th ed. Philadelphia: Lippincott Williams & Wilkins, 2001:1–33.

6. Lockwood C. Thrombosis, thrombophilia, and thromboembolism. *Clinical Updates in Women's Health Care*. 2007;6:1–95.

7. Greer IA. Prevention of venous thromboembolism in pregnancy. *Best Pract Res Clin Haematol.* 2003;16:261–278.

8. Geerts WH, Heit JA, Clagett GP, et al. Prevention of venous thromboembolism. *Chest.* 2001;119(suppl 1):132S–175S.

9. Kemmeren JM, Algra A, Grobbee DE. Third generation oral contraceptives and risk of venous thrombosis: meta-analysis. *BMJ.* 2001;323:131.

10. Lockwood CJ. Inherited thrombophilias in pregnant patients: detection and treatment paradigm. *Obstet Gynecol.* 2002;99:333–341.

11. Duhl AJ, Paidas MJ, Ural SH, et al. Antithrombotic therapy and pregnancy. Consensus report and recommendations for prevention and treatment of venous thromboembolism and adverse pregnancy outcomes. *Am J Obstet Gynecol.* 2007;197:457–469.

12. Eldor A. Thrombophilia, thrombosis and pregnancy. *Thromb Haemost.* 2001;86:104–111.

13. American College of Obstetricians and Gynecologists. Prevention of deep vein thrombosis and pulmonary embolism. *ACOG Practice Bulletin.* Number 84. August 2007. *Obstet Gynecol.* 2007;110:429–440.

14. Lockwood CJ, Silver R. Thrombophilias in pregnancy. In Creasy RK, Resnik R, eds. *Maternal-Fetal Medicine.* 5th ed. Philadelphia: Saunders, 2004:1005–1021.

15. Hanly JG. Antiphospholipid syndrome: an overview. *Can Med Assoc J.* 2003; 168:1675–1682.

16. American College of Obstetricians and Gynecologists. Antiphospholipid syndrome. *ACOG Practice Bulletin.* Number 68. November 2005. *Obstet Gynecol.* 2005;106:1113–1125.

17. Lim W, Crowther MA, Eikelboom JW. Management of antiphospholipid antibody syndrome. *JAMA.* 2006;295:1050–1057.

18. Miyakis S, Lockshin MD, Atsumi T, et al. International consensus statement on an update of the classification criteria for definite antiphospholipid syndrome. *J Thromb Haemostat.* 2006;4:295–306.

19. Kearon C, Kahn SR, Agnelli G. Antithrombotic therapy for venous thromboembolic disease. *Chest.* 2008;133(suppl 6):454S–545S.

20. Greer IA. Prevention and management of venous thromboembolism in pregnancy. *Clin Chest Med.* 2003;24:123–137.

21. Fedullo PF, Tapson VF. Clinical practice. The evaluation of suspected pulmonary embolism. *N Engl J Med.* 2003;349:1247–1256.

22. Bates, SM, Greer IA, Hirsch J, et al. Use of antithrombotic agents during pregnancy: the seventh ACCP conference on antithrombotic and thrombolytic therapy. *Chest.* 2004;126(suppl 3):627S–644S.

23. Bates, SM, Greer IA, Pabinger I, et al. Venous thromboembolism, thrombophilia, antithrombotic therapy, and pregnancy: American College of Chest Physicians evidence-based clinical practice guidelines (8th edition). *Chest.* 2008;133(suppl 6):844S–886S.

24. Raschke RA, Reilly BM, Guidry JR, et al. The weight-based heparin dosing nomogram compared with a "standard care" nomogram: a randomized controlled trial. *Ann Intern Med.* 1993;119:874–881.

25. Hirsh J, Raschke R. Heparin and low-molecular-weight heparin. The seventh ACCP conference on antithrombotic and thrombolytic therapy. *Chest.* 2004; 126(suppl 3):188S–203S.

26. Buller HR, Agnelli G, Hull RD, et al. Antithrombotic therapy for venous thromboembolic disease. The seventh ACCP conference on antithrombotic and thrombolytic therapy. *Chest.* 2004;126(suppl 3):401S–428S.

27. Busby LT, Weyman A, Rodgers GM. Excessive anticoagulation in patients with mild renal insufficiency receiving long-term therapeutic enoxaparin. *Am J Hematol.* 2001;67:54–56.

28. Briggs GG, Freeman RK, Yaffe SJ. *Drugs in Pregnancy and Lactation.* 8th ed. Philadelphia: Lippincott Williams & Wilkins, 2008:430–437.

29. Enoxaparin sodium injection. Package Insert, Sanofi-Aventis U.S. LLC; 2006.

QUESTIONS AND ANSWERS

1. Which of the following is not a risk factor for venous thromboembolism in women during pregnancy?

   a. obesity early in pregnancy

   b. family history of venous thromboembolism

   c. maternal age of 33 years

   d. dehydration due to hyperemesis gravidarum

2. Which of the following is not used to diagnose a person with antiphospholipid syndrome?

   a. the presence of lupus anticoagulant in plasma on one laboratory test result

   b. a pregnancy morbidity of at least three consecutive spontaneous abortions before the 10th week of gestation

   c. a confirmed deep venous thrombosis and the presence of anticardiolipin antibody of IgG on two occasions, 14 weeks apart

   d. two unexplained deaths of morphologically normal fetus, both beyond the 10th week of gestation

3. Treatment for a woman on bed rest for preterm labor at 35 weeks' gestation who has a history of an acute VTE should be:

   a. subcutaneous injection of adjusted-dose unfractionated heparin

   b. IV unfractionated heparin (bolus followed by a continuous infusion to maintain aPTT 1.0–1.5 times control)

   c. adjusted-dose low-molecular-weight heparin

   d. only a and c

4. A thin woman with a single episode of a VTE in her history who has a transient risk factor of hyperemesis gravidarum early in this pregnancy (now resolved) should have prevention treatment for a recurrent VTE with:

   a. IV unfractionated heparin

   b. clinical surveillance and postpartum anticoagulation

   c. adjusted-dose low-molecular-weight heparin throughout pregnancy until delivery

   d. subcutaneous injections of unfractionated heparin, 10,000 units, twice daily throughout pregnancy

5. Oral anticoagulation, vitamin K antagonist, might be used in pregnancy during the following:

   a. never in pregnancy

   b. preconception until 4–6 weeks of gestation in a woman with very high risks for VTE

   c. beyond the 13th week gestation through the middle of the third trimester in a woman with a mechanical heart valve

   d. only b and c

Answers:

1. c; 2. a; 3. a; 4. b; 5. d

Thyroid Disease in Pregnancy

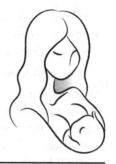

Julie J. Kelsey

LEARNING OBJECTIVES

1. Describe normal maternal and fetal thyroid function throughout pregnancy.

2. Explain the need for more thyroid hormone in hypothyroid pregnant women.

3. Outline a treatment plan for hyperthyroidism in pregnancy.

4. Compare postpartum thyroiditis and Graves' disease.

I. Introduction

The incidence of hypothyroidism and hyperthyroidism in the general population is 4.6% and 1.3%, respectively, according to the Third National Health and Nutrition Examination Survey.[1] The prevalence during pregnancy is approximately 0.3%–0.5% for overt hypothyroidism and 2%–3% for subclinical hypothyroidism. Hyperthyroidism is less common, with only 0.1%–0.4% prevalence for overt disease and 0.4% for subclinical hyperthyroidism.[2] Autoimmune thyroiditis occurs in up to 10% of reproductive age women and can result in either hypothyroidism or hyperthyroidism. Postpartum thyroiditis occurs in approximately 7% following pregnancy.[3]

Similar to other endocrine systems within the female body during pregnancy, the thyroid gland also undergoes new demands. Early in pregnancy, the thyrotrophic activity from production of human chorionic gonadotropin (hCG) causes an elevation of thyroxine (T_4) and a subsequent decrease in thyroid-stimulating hormone (TSH) released from the pituitary.[4] Thyroid binding globulin (TBG) levels are increased secondary to a decrease in hepatic elimination and an increase in synthesis secondary to estrogen stimulation.[4] Free T_4 assays in pregnancy can be altered by increased TBG and decreased albumin levels.[5] This may lead to more women being diagnosed as hypothyroid, especially in the first trimester. Possible ways to obtain a better result include using a free T_4 index or multiplying the total T_4 reference range by 1.5 to obtain a free T_4 reference range.

An increase in dietary iodine is necessary for production of larger amounts of T_4, fetal requirements, as well as increased renal secretion.[6] Consumption of prenatal vitamins helps to boost maternal iodine intake; however, many do not contain the recommended amount of 150 µg as suggested by health experts. The latest U.S. survey concluded that most pregnant women have a sufficient amount of iodine intake.[7]

Metabolism of thyroid hormones is slightly different in pregnancy because the placenta contains two important enzymes.[4] Type II deiodinase converts T_4 to triiodothyronine (T_3), and type III deiodinase, which converts T_4 to reverse T_3 (rT_3) and T_3 to diiodothyronine; both metabolites are inactive. When less T_4 is available, the activity of type II deiodinase increases, thus maintaining adequate levels of T_3 in the placenta. However, deiodinase type III is highly active, restricting the amount of T_3 that is transferred to the fetus.

During the first 10–12 weeks, the mother is responsible for the entire thyroid demands for herself and the embryo. After this time, the fetus has thyroid follicles and can synthesize T_4.[4] The fetus obtains iodine directly from the mother as well as from placental breakdown of T_4 and T_3. This thyroid production is critical for the development of the brain both in utero and in neonatal life. During the first 12 weeks, fluid surrounding the embryo contains T_4 and rT_3 from the mother.[4] By 18–20 weeks, the fetus has developed a pituitary-thyroid axis; however, the feedback system does not completely mature until 35–37 weeks. There is a marked difference between maternal and fetal concentrations of free T_4 and T_3, as these hormones do not cross the placenta in large amounts.[4]

II. PATIENT CASE (PART 1)

U.M. is a 22-year-old primigravida at 8 3/7 weeks' gestation. She states "I can't keep anything down and now haven't eaten in a week," and "my heart keeps racing." Physical examination reveals a moderately distressed patient who is mildly sweating, tachycardic, a little tremulous, and has an enlarged thyroid. She has lost nearly 6% of her weight. Her medical history is unremarkable, including no history of thyroid problems. Her family history is relevant for a sister who had hyperemesis gravidarum during two pregnancies. She is taking no medications and her prenatal vitamins are on hold due to feeling poorly.

Her laboratory values reveal a β-hCG of 38,000, TSH less than 0.1 nmol/L, elevated free T_4 and T_3, TSH receptor antibodies, and her potassium is 2.5 mEq/dL. Urinalysis reveals ketones, but none were found in her blood.

III. Clinical Presentation

Normal thyroid values are shown in Table 1.

Exacerbation of preexisting hypothyroidism can occur due to the increased demands on the thyroid gland during the first trimester; however, it is possible to have de novo development of hypothyroidism during pregnancy. Although many women remain asymptomatic while hypothyroid, clinical features of hypothyroidism include weight gain, hair loss, loss of deep tendon reflexes, cold sensitivity, dry skin, puffiness

Table 1. Normal Thyroid Values

Thyroid Function Test	Normal Range
Thyroid-stimulating hormone	0.5–5 mUnits/L
Total thyroxine (T$_4$)	4–12 µg/dL
Free T$_4$	0.7–2.1 ng/dL
Total triiodothyronine	75–180 ng/dL

From Farwell AP, Ebner SA.[22]

of the hands and face, drowsiness, and constipation.[2,3] Some of these could be misinterpreted as regular complaints of pregnancy.

Hyperthyroidism, especially in early pregnancy, can easily be confused with pregnancy symptoms. These include weight loss, tachycardia, warm moist skin, tremor, wide pulse pressure, and a systolic murmur. Pregnancy, though, usually does not cause a goiter and ophthalmopathy.[3] Distinguishing between gestational hyperthyroidism and true hyperthyroidism can be challenging, but is needed to determine whether the patient will require drug therapy long term, if at all.

IV. Pathophysiology

A. Hypothyroidism

By far, the most common cause of hypothyroidism is Hashimoto's thyroiditis in the United States. Hashimoto's thyroiditis is an autoimmune disorder characterized by a goiter and thyroid antibodies and thyroid antigen–specific T cells circulating throughout the body.[8] In developing countries, and even some areas of Europe, iodine deficiency is the leading cause. In other cases, thyroidectomy or previously being treated for hyperthyroidism with radioactive iodine may be the cause.

Subclinical hypothyroidism is characterized by an elevated TSH with a normal free T$_4$ level. This can represent early Hashimoto's thyroiditis; treatment for this condition is controversial because the T$_4$ level is normal. The chance of subclinical hypothyroidism progressing into full hypothyroidism is dependent on the level of elevation of TSH and antithyroid peroxidase antibodies (TPOAb). The conversion rate is approximately 3%–8% per year in the nonpregnant individual, which most correlates to high TSH levels and the presence of TPOAb.[8]

The presence of TPOAb is commonly associated with Hashimoto's thyroiditis and other autoimmune thyroid diseases. These antibodies prevent the thyroid gland from producing normal amounts of thyroid hormones. It is possible to be not yet hypothyroid and have autoimmune antibodies. These antibodies are of the immunoglobulin (Ig) G type, which can cross the placenta but do not transfer the condition from mother to fetus.[8] There appears to be a connection between presence of these antibodies and recurrent early pregnancy loss in women who are euthyroid.[9]

Maternal complications related to hypothyroidism include decreased fertility, as well as an increased risk for pregnancy loss.[3] Pregnancy complications include anemia, preterm delivery, gestational hypertension and preeclampsia, placental abruption, and postpartum hemorrhage. Adequate treatment with thyroid hormones decreases the risk of these outcomes. Subclinical hypothyroidism may still have an increased risk for these complications, although not all studies show this.[10] Treatment has been shown to improve obstetric outcomes in the subclinical hypothyroid population, but may not alter long-term neurologic development.[3]

Fetal complications can be extensive if overt hypothyroidism goes untreated for a prolonged period of time during the pregnancy. Severe congenital hypothyroidism has been called cretinism for centuries. Although the condition is more commonly associated with iodine deficiency than Hashimoto's thyroiditis, these children are affected by severe mental retardation, cognitive and neurologic impairment, delayed bone maturation, and short stature.[11]

Lesser complications, although still significant, can occur in untreated or under-treated women.[3] Impairment of mental and physical development can occur, as well as low birth weight and premature delivery. An increased risk of congenital anomalies and perinatal morbidity and mortality has been reported in the literature.[2,10] Some authors have suggested that the impaired mental development may be more related to prematurity than the hypothyroid state of the mother.[10,11]

B. Hyperthyroidism

Gestational hyperthyroidism is the term used for the transient hyperthyroidism that can accompany most cases of hyperemesis gravidarum. Elevations of free T_4 and T_3 and suppressed TSH associated with high levels of β-hCG are the hallmarks of the condition. As the pregnancy progresses, gestational hyperthyroidism spontaneously resolves, usually without treatment. Very symptomatic women, especially if they are tachycardic, can be treated with antithyroid agents until the second trimester.[3]

Graves' disease accounts for nearly 85% of hyperthyroid cases.[3,12] Other causes include toxic adenoma, toxic goiter, and thyroiditis. Graves' disease often exacerbates during early pregnancy and again postpartum, as do other autoimmune disorders. Most women with Graves' disease have circulating TPOAb and TSH receptor antibodies (TRAb) that can help distinguish between gestational thyrotoxicosis and hyperthyroidism.[3] If a woman is allergic to antithyroid agents, requires extreme doses of these agents, or is noncompliant, then surgical management may be appropriate.

Thyroid cancer is the second most common malignancy in pregnancy, occurring in approximately 14 of every 100,000 pregnancies that end in a live birth.[13] If diagnosed, a thyroidectomy may be performed during the pregnancy, preferably in the second trimester, or after delivery. Another option is to suppress thyroid function with exogenous T_4 until surgery or radioactive iodine can be accomplished postpartum or postlactation.

Thyroid storm complicates about 1% of pregnancies with hyperthyroidism. It can present with the extreme symptoms of fever, tachycardia, anxiety, confusion, seizures, vomiting, diarrhea, or cardiac arrhythmias, and can cause maternal heart failure and death.[14] There is usually a stressful event that triggers the storm. If the severely hypermetabolic state is left untreated, then shock, stupor, and coma can ensue. Treatment of the underlying cause should also occur along with medical management of thyroid storm.[11,14]

The order of medication administration is also critical in treating a patient experiencing thyroid storm.[14] Because iodine can increase the amount of thyroid hormone released, it is important to give a thionamide as initial therapy. The use of β-blockers is important to control the cardiovascular stimulation of the thyroid hormone. Propranolol is most often used; however, esmolol can be used instead if the patient is in heart failure. Agents for management are listed in Table 2.

Maternal complications related to uncontrolled hyperthyroidism depend on treatment and control. Untreated and inadequately treated women have a higher risk for preterm delivery, preeclampsia, congestive heart failure, and thyroid storm.[3] Thyrotoxicosis complicating pregnancy can be life-threatening if heart failure occurs. The pregnancy outcome is related to the severity of the disease at delivery. Women with thyrotoxicosis who are untreated or insufficiently treated are likely to experience a spontaneous abortion.[3]

Fetal implications of hyperthyroidism include low birth weight, intrauterine growth restriction, and stillbirth. Congenital malformations, such as imperforate anus, anencephaly, and cleft lip have been reported in untreated women.[2] The possibility of neonatal thyroid dysfunction exists with either excessive or insufficient therapy. High TRAb levels often indicate poorly controlled hyperthyroidism either with inadequate or no therapy and can lead to fetal/neonatal hyperthyroidism.[12] Fetal and neonatal hypothyroidism can occur with excessive treatment. Both present with a goiter, although other developments will distinguish between the two. Hyperthyroid fetuses may also have arrhythmias, con-

Table 2. Agents for Thyroid Storm

Drug	Dose	Purpose	Comments
Propylthiouracil	600–800 mg PO initial dose, followed by 150–200 mg q4–6h	Prevent thyroid synthesis, prevent conversion of T_4 to T_3	Only available as 50-mg tablets
Potassium iodide	5 drops PO q6h	Block release of thyroid hormone	Start at least 1 h after propylthiouracil therapy
Propranolol	20–80 mg PO q4–6h	Limit adrenergic effects of thyroid hormone, block T_4 to T_3 conversion	Can use IV at 1–10 mg every 4 h
Dexamethasone	2 mg IV q6h for 24 h	Decrease thyroid hormone release, prevent conversion of T_4 to T_3	Can also use hydrocortisone 100 mg q8h IV
Phenobarbital	30–60 mg PO q4–6h	Reduce agitation and increase metabolism of thyroid hormones	Not included in all thyroid storm regimens
Lithium	300 mg PO q8h	Prevent thyroid synthesis and release from the gland	Used when all other agents are contraindicated
Cholestyramine	4 g PO four times daily	Lower thyroid levels by preventing reabsorption from enterohepatic circulation	Can be used along with antithyroid agents

T_3 = triiodothyronine, T_4 = thyroxine.
From Rashid M, Rashid MH,[11] and Nayak B, Burman K.[14]

gestive heart failure, advanced bone age, craniosynostosis (premature closure of the cranial sutures), and hydrops.[12] Hypothyroidism is more difficult to diagnose, as delayed bone maturation is often the only sign beyond a goiter and thyroid ultrasound findings.

C. Postpartum Thyroiditis

Postpartum thyroiditis occurs in approximately 7% of women within the first year after delivery.[3] The incidence is higher in women with type I diabetes. The presence of TPOAb during the pregnancy seems to be an indicator of postpartum thyroiditis, as up to 60% of these women will develop the condition.[3] Typically, the hyperthyroid phase of thyroiditis occurs within 1–3 months after delivery and persists for a couple of months. This is classically followed by the hypothyroid stage, starting at 3–6 months postpartum, usually lasting 4–6 months. Up to 29% of women will develop permanent hypothyroidism.[15] As many as 70% of women will experience a recurrence with subsequent pregnancies.

The hyperthyroid period of thyroiditis can be confused with an exacerbation or recurrence of Graves' disease. However, women with thyroiditis will not have TRAb concentrations. Symptomatic hyperthyroid women should be treated, typically with β-blocker therapy and not with antithyroid agents. The high amounts of hormones in the system are from increased release, not excessive production, so antithyroid drugs are not indicated.

Treatment of the hypothyroid state is dependent on several factors. Women with a high TSH (>10 mUnits/L) and symptomatic women with elevated TSH values should be treated with levothyroxine.[15] If a woman is anticipating becoming pregnant again soon, she should also be treated, even if she is asymptomatic. Treatment duration is controversial; however, it should continue for approximately 1 year either after therapy initiation or after the woman has completed child-bearing.

V. Screening

At this time, routine screening is not recommended for all pregnant women. However, in women at risk for hypothyroidism, a TSH measurement before pregnancy is justifiable. This would include women with a history of thyroid disease or postpartum thyroiditis, family history of thyroid disease, a goiter, type I diabetes, other autoimmune disorders, or prior radiation to the neck area.[3] Some endocrinologists recommend screening for type II diabetics as well.

Universal screening could become the new standard of care. A recent cost-effectiveness analysis favored screening all asymptomatic women for subclinical hypothyroidism.[16] The model used assumed that treatment would reduce the incidence of mentally impaired offspring, thus lowering the costs of long-term care; whether levothyroxine therapy produces these benefits in this population remains uncertain.

VI. Treatment

The goal of treatment for hypothyroidism is simple, normalization of the TSH. However, it is a little more complicated for hyperthyroidism. There is no reference range for normal total T_4 during the different pregnancy trimesters; therefore, antithyroid agents should be dosed to keep the total T_4 at the upper limit or slightly above the normal value for nonpregnant individuals. Follow-up should continue with vigilance in women with hyperthyroidism, as their disease will likely regress with therapy and the antithyroid agent will need to be tapered back. This will help limit the exposure of the fetus to the agent, minimizing effects on the fetal thyroid.

A. Hypothyroidism

1. Levothyroxine

Levothyroxine is the mainstay of therapy for hypothyroidism. It is the synthetic version of thyroxine. For women with preexisting hypothyroidism, an increase between 30%–50% is often needed during the pregnancy to maintain appropriate levels.[3] This can be achieved by increasing the daily dose or by the addition of 2 extra tablets per week. The dosage increase is dependent on the amount of natural thyroid function remaining. For women with higher TSH values, larger doses of levothyroxine will be needed than in those with only mild TSH elevations. For women with de novo hypothyroidism occurring during pregnancy, the recommendation is to start at 100–150 µg/d or use a body weight titration of 2–2.4 µg/kg/d.[3] Initially, more hormone can be given to rapidly stabilize the amount of thyroid available. Monitoring should occur within a month of dosage changes and every 4–6 weeks thereafter.

2. Liothyronine

Liothyronine, the synthetic version of triiodothyronine, is occasionally used in combination with levothyroxine or as monotherapy. Numerous studies have used the two together and have found higher patient satisfaction, but have not shown more of an improvement in laboratory values. Women with mutations or genetic polymorphisms in type I and II deiodinase genes may need supplementation of liothyronine to maintain normal levels.[17] Also, some individuals with normal thyroid function tests can have a failing sense of well-being. Combination therapy with both hormone supplements may be warranted in these cases. The combination has been shown in some studies to improve psychological function and mood.[17]

Several drugs can interfere with the absorption of thyroid hormone. It is important for the patient not to take her iron or prenatal vitamins within 4 hours of taking her thyroid medication. Adverse reactions associated with thyroid hormones tend to be symptoms of hyperthyroidism indicating overdosing or a hypersensitivity to inert ingredients.

Patient education should include the following counseling points:

- Take your thyroid hormone on an empty stomach with a full glass of water.
- Your dose may change as the pregnancy progresses and you might not return to your prepregnancy dose after you give birth.
- Separate iron tablets, prenatal vitamins, and any calcium-containing products by at least 4 hours from your thyroid pills.
- Do not double up on tablets if a dose is missed.

B. Hyperthyroidism

Agents used in the treatment of hyperthyroidism are shown in Table 3.

1. Propylthiouracil

Propylthiouracil is a thionamide agent and the most widely used antithyroid agent used in pregnancy in the United States. It inhibits thyroid synthesis by blocking thyroid peroxidase–mediated iodination of tyrosine in thyroglobulin.[18] It also prevents the peripheral conversion of T_4 to T_3 via type I deiodinase.[19] Antithyroid agents also seem to play a role in immunosuppression, decreasing important antibodies over time as well as other molecules such as interleukin 2 and 6.[18]

Propylthiouracil is rapidly, although erratically, absorbed by the intestines, peaks in the serum approximately 1 hour later, and then concentrates in the thyroid, despite the fact it is 75%–80% bound to albumin. Dosing should typically be two to three times daily due to the shorter antithyroid effects, despite a relatively long serum half-life. Major side effects of propylthiouracil include leukopenia, agranulocytosis (usually presenting with a fever and sore throat), exfoliative dermatitis, antineutrophil cytoplasmic antibody–positive vasculitis, hepatitis, glomerulonephritis and acute renal failure, interstitial pneumonitis, and a systemic lupus erythematosus (SLE)–like syndrome. Common side effects include edema, fever, vertigo, headache, dizziness, rash, urticaria, pruritus, nausea, vomiting, loss of taste, abdominal pain, constipation, and arthralgias.[20]

Initial doses of propylthiouracil should be 300–450 mg/d in divided doses. Doses of up to 1000 mg can be used for thyroid storm. Propylthiouracil crosses the placenta and can cause fetal hypothyroidism when used in excess of maternal requirements. A widely held belief is that propylthiouracil crosses the placenta to a lesser extent than methimazole. However, this has been disproven with an established placenta model.[21]

The preference for propylthiouracil in pregnancy has stemmed from reports of congenital anomalies associated with methimazole. Aplasia cutis (a congenital anomaly involving skin development, usually on the scalp) has been the most described anomaly; it has also been thought to cause choanal or esophageal atresia.[18] Other studies have not demonstrated a difference in outcomes between propylthiouracil and methimazole.[21] Abnormalities in one study fell within the national average of congenital anomalies (2%–5%) for both agents. Thyroid function in the fetus does not appear to be different

Table 3. Agents for Hyperthyroidism

Drug	Dose	Comments
Propylthiouracil	300–450 mg/d	First-line agent, adjust dose as needed throughout pregnancy to maintain T_4 in high to slightly above normal range
Methimazole	15–30 mg/d	Second-line agent, use only if allergic or not tolerant of propylthiouracil, adjust dose as needed to maintain T_4 in high to slightly above normal range
Iodine	6–40 mg/d	Not recommended, could cause fetal hypothyroidism, can be used for surgery preparation

T_4 = thyroxine.
From Bach-Huynh T-G, Jonklaas J,[6] and Cooper DS.[18]

between the two drugs either. Even though these small studies make it appear that either drug would be acceptable, there are no reports of propylthiouracil causing aplasia cutis, making it the drug of choice in pregnancy. This being said, if the patient is allergic to propylthiouracil, methimazole can be substituted.

Patient education should include:

- Take propylthiouracil spaced as evenly as possible throughout the day.
- It may take several weeks to see results from this medication, be patient.
- Call your health care provider immediately if you have a sore throat with a fever.

2. Methimazole

Methimazole is also a thionamide agent and most widely used antithyroid drug in Europe. Its mechanism of action is the same as propylthiouracil; however, it does not have an effect on peripheral thyroid hormones. Methimazole is rapidly absorbed in the intestines, concentrates in the thyroid, and does not bind to serum proteins. A longer duration of action allows for once-daily dosing of methimazole. Major side effects of methimazole include leukopenia, agranulocytosis, exfoliative dermatitis, hepatitis, nephrotic syndrome, and an SLE-like syndrome. Common side effects include edema, headache, vertigo, drowsiness, rash, urticaria, pruritus, nausea, vomiting, abdominal pain, abnormal taste, constipation, and arthralgias.[20] Side effects from methimazole appear to be related more to dose than the agent itself.

Initial doses of methimazole are 15–30 mg daily. However, doses of up to 60 mg may be required in cases of severe hyperthyroidism. Methimazole may have a faster improvement in normalization of T_4 and T_3,[18] although this difference may be only 1 week in pregnant women.[21] The relative potency between methimazole and propylthiouracil is at least 10:1, making it possible for individuals to be on lower doses of methimazole than the equivalent propylthiouracil dosage.

Patient counseling should include the following points:

- Take the medication with or without food, but try to take it at the same time every day.
- It may take several weeks for this medication to fully work, so keep taking it unless your health care provider says to stop.
- Call your health care provider immediately if you have a sore throat with a fever.

VII. PATIENT CASE [PART 2]

Although U.M. has the classic signs of hyperemesis gravidarum based on her weight loss, ketonuria, and hypokalemia, as well as a significant family history of nausea and vomiting in pregnancy, her symptoms are secondary to her actual diagnosis. U.M. is diagnosed as being overtly hyperthyroid, given her laboratory values of TSH, T_4, T_3, TRAb, and the goiter that was noticed on clinical examination. The patient was started on propylthiouracil at a dose of 150 mg PO every 8 hours, as propylthiouracil is the drug of choice in pregnancy. She is also started on propranolol, 20 mg, three times daily for her symptomatic tachycardia.

She will return to the clinic in 1 month for measurement of her T_4 level and potential adjustment of the propylthiouracil dose. Her propranolol will be discontinued at that time as well. She will be monitored monthly with laboratory values and routine prenatal care.

VIII. Summary

Thyroid disease in pregnancy is not a common occurrence; however, it is essential for fetal and child development that it is appropriately treated. It is also important that the mother is appropriately managed to maintain the pregnancy as well as avoid significant pregnancy complications. Treatment can be accomplished with medications readily available through any pharmacy.

Subclinical hypothyroidism seems to be the most prevalent condition. There is still some debate about whether these women should be treated with thyroid hormones. Pregnancy outcomes in untreated women are slightly better than in women with overt hypothyroidism, but treatment seems to improve overall outcome and may be warranted.

Severe complications can occur with hyperthyroidism during the pregnancy. Thyroid storm and heart failure are the most detrimental to the mother's condition. The chance of fetal and neonatal thyroid disease is significantly higher in this population. Untreated women who are euthyroid but have TSH receptor antibodies still can cause fetal hypothyroidism. However, fetal and neonatal hyperthyroidism is also a possibility. Neonatologists and pediatricians need to be aware of the mother's disease when caring for the newborn.

Overall, thyroid disease can be managed well in most cases by obstetricians, perinatologists, and endocrinologists. Pregnancy outcomes and fetal implications are minimized in women who have optimal treatment throughout their pregnancy.

IX. References

1. Hollowell JG, Staehling NW, Flanders WD, et al. Serum TSH, T(4), and thyroid antibodies in the United States population (1988 to 1994): National Health and Nutrition Examination Survey (NHANES III). *J Clin Endocrinol Metab*. 2002;87:489–499.

2. Roti E, Minelli R, Salvi M. Management of hyperthyroidism and hypothyroidism in the pregnancy woman. *J Clin Endocrinol Metab*. 1996;81:1679–1682.

3. Abalovich M, Amino N, Barbour LA, et al. Management of thyroid dysfunction during pregnancy and postpartum: an endocrine society clinical practice guideline. *J Clin Endocrinol Metab*. 2007;92:S1–S47.

4. Burrow GN, Fisher DA, Larsen PR. Maternal and fetal thyroid function. *N Engl J Med*. 1994;331:1072–1078.

5. Lee RH, Spencer CA, Mestman JH, et al. Free T4 immunoassays are flawed during pregnancy. *Am J Obstet Gynecol*. 2009;200:260.e1–e6.

6. Bach-Huynh T-G, Jonklaas J. Thyroid medications during pregnancy. *Ther Drug Monit*. 2006;28:431–441.

7. Caldwell KL, Miller GA, Wang RY, et al. Iodine status of the U.S. population, national health and nutrition examination survey 2003–2004. *Thyroid.* 2008;18:1207–1214.

8. Brent GA, Larsen PR, Davies TF. Hypothyroidism and thyroiditis. In Kronenberg HM, Melmed S, Polonsky KS, et al, eds. *Williams Textbook of Endocrinology.* 11th ed. Philadelphia: Saunders Elsevier, 2008:333–376.

9. Ambramson J, Stagnaro-Green A. Thyroid antibodies and fetal loss: an evolving story. *Thyroid.* 2001;11:57–63.

10. Idris I, Srinivasan R, Simm A, et al. Maternal hypothyroidism in early and late gestation: effects on neonatal and obstetric outcome. *Clin Endocrinol.* 2005;63:560–565.

11. Rashid M, Rashid MH. Obstetric management of thyroid disease. *Obstet Gynecol Surv.* 2007;62:680–688.

12. Chan GW, Mandel SJ. Therapy insight: management of Graves' disease during pregnancy. *Nature Clin Pract Endocrinol Metab.* 2007;3:470–478.

13. Yasmeen S, Cress R, Romano PS, et al. Thyroid cancer in pregnancy. *Int J Gynecol Obstet.* 2005;91:15–20.

14. Nayak B, Burman K. Thyrotoxicosis and thyroid storm. *Endocrinol Metab Clin.* 2006;35:663–686.

15. Stagnaro-Green A. Postpartum thyroiditis. *Best Pract Res Clin Endocrinol Metab.* 2004;18:303–316.

16. Thung SF, Funai EF, Grobman WA. The cost-effectiveness of universal screening in pregnancy for subclinical hypothyroidism. *Am J Obstet Gynecol.* 2009;200:267.e1–e7.

17. Danzi S, Klein I. Potential uses of T_3 in the treatment of human disease. *Clin Cornerstone.* 2005;7(suppl 2):S9–S15.

18. Cooper DS. Antithyroid drugs. *N Engl J Med.* 2005;352:905–917.

19. Davies TF, Larsen PR. Thyrotoxicosis. In Kronenberg HM, Melmed S, Polonsky KS, et al, eds. *Williams Textbook of Endocrinology.* 11th ed. Philadelphia: Saunders Elsevier, 2008:377–410.

20. Lacy CF, Armstrong LA, Morton MP, et al, eds. *Drug Information Handbook.* 14th ed. Hudson, OH: Lexicomp, 2006:1025–1026, 1343–1344.

21. Chattaway JM, Klepser TB. Propylthiouracil versus methimazole in treatment of Graves' disease during pregnancy. *Ann Pharmacother.* 2007;41:1018–1022.

22. Farwell AP, Ebner SA. Thyroid gland disorders. In Noble J, ed. *Textbook of Primary Care Medicine.* 3rd ed. St. Louis, MO: Harcourt Health Sciences Company, 2001.

QUESTIONS AND ANSWERS

1. Which of the following sentences is not correct when describing maternal and fetal thyroid functioning?

    a. The placenta contains enzymes to metabolize thyroxine and liothyronine.

    b. Iodine insufficiency can cause hypothyroidism in the mother.

c. Large amounts of thyroxine cross the placenta to the fetus.

d. The fetus produces its own thyroid during the third trimester.

2. Pregnant women need more thyroid hormone due to which of the following?

a. An increase in β-hCG causes more thyroid to be metabolized.

b. The demand from the embryo exceeds the normal maternal supply.

c. The fetus needs plenty of thyroxine to be transferred across the placenta.

d. Thyroid-stimulating hormone levels increase, creating less thyroid hormone.

3. The most appropriate treatment for a hyperthyroid pregnant woman includes:

a. propylthiouracil, propranolol, and concentrated iodine

b. methimazole

c. methimazole and propranolol

d. propylthiouracil

4. Adverse outcomes from maternal hypothyroidism include all of the following except:

a. fetal hypothyroidism

b. preterm labor

c. fetal growth restriction

d. gestational hypertension

5. To determine whether a woman has postpartum thyroiditis, which of the following would be most helpful?

a. presence of TSH receptor antibodies (TRAb)

b. presence of antithyroid peroxidase antibodies (TPOAb)

c. history of gestational diabetes mellitus

d. history of Graves' disease

Answers:

1. c; 2. b; 3. d; 4. a; 5. b

Glossary

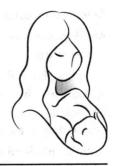

Abruption: synonym for abruptio placenta

Abruptio placentae: clinical condition where placental separation occurs before delivery of the infant, which can cause significant maternal hemorrhage and deprive the fetus

Achondroplasia: a type of dwarfism with short extremities but normal trunk; the head may be enlarged; autosomal dominant inheritance

Acute phase proteins: proteins secreted by inflammatory cells or the liver in response to inflammation; serum concentrations often used as markers of inflammation

Addison's disease: adrenocortical insufficiency

Akathisia: a type of extrapyramidal reaction characterized by an inability to remain in a sitting posture, with motor restlessness and a feeling of muscular quivering; restless legs

Alpha-fetoprotein: a fetal protein that increases in maternal blood during pregnancy and, when detected by amniocentesis, is an important indicator of open neural tube defects in the fetus

Amniocentesis: transabdominal or transcervical procedure for aspiration of amniotic fluid from the uterus

Amnion: fluid-filled sac that encloses the embryo; the extraembryonic membrane that lines the chorion and contains the amniotic fluid and fetus

Amniotic fluid index: four-quadrant evaluation of largest vertical pocket of fluid to assess volume; normal is 6–24 centimeters of amniotic fluid

Amniotomy: artificial rupture of the fetal membranes

Anastomosis: a natural communication, direct or indirect, between two blood vessels or other tubular structures

Anencephaly: congenital defective development of the brain, with absence of the bones of the cranial vault and absent or rudimentary cerebral and cerebellar hemispheres, brain stem, and basal ganglia

Angiotensin: a family of peptides of known and similar sequence, with vasoconstrictive activity, produced by enzymatic action of renin upon angiotensinogen

Anhydramnios: the absence of amniotic fluid; usually from rupture of the membranes

Anotia: congenital absence of one or both auricles of the ears

Antepartum: occurring before childbirth, in reference to the mother

Antidopaminergic: relating to nerve cells or fibers that employ dopamine as their neurotransmitter

Antiphospholipid antibodies: an antibody, usually immunoglobulin (Ig) G but can be IgM or IgA, directed against phospholipid-containing complexes; may paradoxically prolong in vitro phospholipid-dependent tests of coagulation, but are clinically associated with increased risks of arterial or venous thromboses

Antiphospholipid antibody syndrome: a clinical syndrome consisting of the presence of antiphospholipid antibodies in the serum in addition to documented arterial thromboses, venous thromboses, or obstetric complications; obstetric complications include two or more spontaneous pregnancy losses of morphologically normal fetuses after 12 weeks' gestation; three consecutive first-trimester pregnancy losses; prematurity or preeclampsia due to placental insufficiency

Apgar score: an evaluation of a newborn infant's physical status by assigning numeric values (0–2) to each of 5 criteria: heart rate, respiratory effort, muscle tone, response stimulation, and skin color; a score of 8–10 indicates the best possible condition

Aplasia cutis: congenital absence or deficiency of a localized area of skin, with the base of the defect covered by a thin translucent membrane; most often a single area near the vertex of the scalp; occurs spontaneously in approximately 3 infants per 10,000 live births

Apoptosis: single deletion of scattered cells by fragmentation into membrane-bound particles that are phagocytosed by other cells; believed to be due to programmed cell death

Arteriovenous anastomosis: vessels through which blood is shunted from arterioles to venules without passing through the capillaries

Ascites: accumulation of serous fluid in the peritoneal cavity

Atelectasis: in adults, collapse of the lung; at birth, incomplete expansion of the lungs

Biophysical profile: a technique for evaluating fetal status using fetal heart rate monitoring and ultrasound assessment of amniotic fluid volume, fetal movement, and fetal breathing motion

Calvarial hypoplasia: same as hypocalvaria

Cardiomyopathy: disease of the myocardium (heart muscle)

Carpal tunnel syndrome: compression of the medial nerve under the carpal ligament at the wrist leading to a painful entrapment neuropathy in the hand that can radiate into the forearm; common causes of carpal tunnel syndrome include synovitis from rheumatoid and other arthritides, diabetes mellitus, hyperparathyroidism, and pregnancy among others

Cerclage: suture around the cervix to prevent it from opening spontaneously

Chemoreceptor trigger zone: CRTZ; cells in the brain stem that are sensitive to changes in the composition of the blood; stimulation results in a nerve impulse to the vomiting center in the medulla oblongata

Choanal atresia: absence of the opening into the nasopharynx of the nasal cavity on either side

Chorioamnionitis: inflammation or infection of the outer membrane and the fluid-filled sac that encloses the embryo; also referred to as *intraamniotic infection, amnionitis, amniotic fluid infection,* or *intrapartum fever*

Chorion: outermost membrane of the embryo; it develops villi, becomes vascularized, then forms the fetal part of the placenta

Chromaffinoma: a neoplasm composed of chromaffin cells occurring in the medullae of adrenal glands

Complement: a series of enzymatic proteins that interact to mediate the body's immune response to infection or inflammation; can combine with antibodies to form immune complexes that can respond to infection or cause tissue injury; complement components C3 and C4 are often lower than normal in patients with systemic lupus erythematosus and may decrease further during periods of increased disease activity

Conization: cone; surgical removal of precancerous cells from the cervix with a knife

C-reactive protein: CRP; an acute phase protein synthesized and secreted by the liver in response to inflammation

Cushing's disease: adrenal hyperplasia caused by an adrenocorticotropic hormone–secreting basophil adenoma of the pituitary

Cutis laxa: a congenital or acquired condition characterized by deficient elastic fibers of the skin hanging in folds; vascular anomalies may be present

Cytokines: hormonelike low-molecular-weight proteins, secreted by many different cell types, which regulate the intensity and duration of immune responses and are involved in cell-to-cell communication

Decidua basalis: the area of endometrium between the implanted chorionic vesicle and the myometrium, which develops into the maternal part of the placenta

Decidual: mucous membrane that lines the uterus and changes during pregnancy; it is shed at delivery or during menstruation; also called *deciduous membrane*

Deformations: deviation of form from the normal; specifically, an alteration in shape and/or structure of a previously normally formed part; occurs after organogenesis and often involves the musculoskeletal system (eg, clubfoot)

Disease-modifying antirheumatic drugs: DMARDs; medications that have been shown to reduce progression of clinical symptoms or radiographic damage of rheumatoid arthritis, in contrast to medications that simply provide symptom relief

Disseminated intravascular coagulation: DIC; a hemorrhagic syndrome that occurs after the uncontrolled activation of clotting factors and fibrinolytic enzymes throughout small blood vessels; fibrin is deposited, platelets and clotting factors are consumed, and fibrin degradation products inhibit fibrin polymerization, resulting in tissue necrosis and bleeding

Dysphonia: altered voice production

Dyspnea: shortness of breath, a subjective difficulty or distress in breathing, usually associated with disease of the heart or lungs

Dystonia: a type of extrapyramidal reaction characterized by a state of abnormal hypertonicity in the muscles of the face and neck

Ebstein's anomaly: a congenital downward displacement of the tricuspid valve into the right ventricle

Eclampsia: occurrence of one or more convulsions, not attributable to other cerebral conditions such as epilepsy or cerebral hemorrhage, in a patient with preeclampsia

Emetogenic: inducing emesis (vomiting)

Endometritis: inflammation or infection of the endometrium or decidua, with extension into the myometrium and parametrial tissues, occurring more than 24 hours after childbirth

Endometrium: mucous membrane lining the uterus

Epidural analgesia: euphemism for epidural anesthesia; produced by injection of a local anesthetic solution, with or without a narcotic, into the peridural space of the spine

Episiotomy: surgical incision of the perineum and vagina to ease delivery

Erythrocyte sedimentation rate: ESR; rate that red blood cells settle out of suspension in the plasma; ESR is influenced by the amount of proteins present in the plasma and is increased as a result of increased acute phase proteins in the blood; used clinically as a marker of inflammation

Esophageal atresia: congenital failure of the full esophageal lumen to develop

Estradiol: the most potent naturally occurring estrogen in mammals

Exsanguination: removal of blood; making it deprived of blood

Factor V Leiden: participates in the common pathway to coagulation by binding factor Xa to platelet surfaces; deficiency of this factor leads to a rare hemorrhagic tendency; autosomal recessive inheritance

Fern test: the proteins in amniotic fluid crystallize in a certain fashion when allowed to dry and evaluated under a microscope; used to diagnosis premature rupture of membranes (PROM) or preterm PROM

Fetal fibronectin: glycoprotein whose function is to attach the decidua to the membranes

Fibroid: a synonym for fibroleiomyoma; a leiomyoma (a benign neoplasm derived from smooth, nonstriated muscle) containing nonneoplastic collagenous fibrous tissue, which may make the tumor hard; usually arises in the myometrium, and the proportion of fibrous tissue increases with age

Fundus: the bottom or base of an organ

Galactagogue: a drug or other substance that purportedly increases the breastmilk supply

Gastroparesis: a slight degree of gastroparalysis

Gastroschisis: a defect in the abdominal wall resulting from rupture of the amniotic membrane during physiologic gut-loop herniation or, later, due to delayed umbilical ring closure; usually accompanied by protrusion of viscera

Gestational diabetes: onset or first recognition of diabetes during pregnancy

Gestational hypertension: hypertension that occurs after 20 weeks' gestation in women known to be normotensive before pregnancy without any other associated features and resolves in the postpartum period

Goldenhar's syndrome: abnormal tissue development of the eyes, ears, and vertebrae; synonym: oculoauriculovertebral dysplasia

Glomerulonephritis: renal disease characterized by bilateral inflammatory changes in glomeruli that are not the result of infection of the kidneys

Gravid: pregnant

Helicobacter pylori: microaerophilic bacteria that is associated with severe gastroduodenal diseases

Hemorrhagic disease of the newborn: bleeding in the newborn secondary to low levels of vitamin K

Hirschsprung's disease or anomaly: congenital megacolon

Human chorionic gonadotropin: hCG; a hormone produced by the placental trophoblastic cells; in first trimester, stimulates ovarian secretion of estrogen and progesterone required for integrity of embryo; no significant role in the second and third trimesters

Hydrops: abnormal accumulation of serous fluid in the fetal tissues

Hyperbilirubinemia: an abnormally large amount of bilirubin in the circulating blood, resulting in clinically apparent icterus or jaundice when the concentration is sufficient

Hypocalvaria: underdevelopment of the upper domelike portion of the skull

Hypochondriasis: a morbid concern about one's own health and exaggerated attention to any unusual bodily or mental sensations

Hypoglycemia: abnormally small concentrations of glucose in the circulating blood

Hypokalemia: abnormally small concentrations of potassium ions in the circulating blood

Hyponatremia: abnormally small concentrations of sodium ions in the circulating blood

Insulin resistance: the diminished ability of cells to respond to the action of insulin in transporting glucose from the bloodstream into muscle and other tissues

Intrapartum: occurring during childbirth, in reference to the mother

Intrathecal: within either the subarachnoid or the subdural space

Interstitial nephritis: a form of nephritis (inflammation of the kidneys) in which the interstitial connective tissue is chiefly affected

Involution: return of the uterus to the normal size after delivery

Latency period: period from rupture of membranes until labor begins

LEEP: loop electrosurgical excision procedure; preformed on the cervix to remove abnormal precancerous cells

Leukotrienes: products of eicosanoid metabolism (usually, arachidonic acid) with postulated physiologic activity such as mediators of inflammation and roles in allergic reactions

Lochia: vaginal discharge occurring during the first 2 weeks after delivery

Lupus nephritis: a relatively common serious manifestation of systemic lupus erythematosus manifested by immune-complex mediated glomerulonephritis; without treatment will often lead to end-stage renal disease

Mastitis: inflammation of the breast

Meconium: fecal material from the fetus; many times passed in utero, discoloring the amniotic fluid

Medulla oblongata: the caudal subdivision of the brain stem, immediately continuous with the spinal cord

Megaloblastic anemia: any anemia in which there is a predominant number of megaloblastic erythroblasts, and relatively few normoblasts, among the hyperplastic erythroid cells in the bone marrow (as in pernicious anemia)

Meninges: membranous coverings of the brain and spinal cord

Meningomyelocele: protrusion of the spinal cord and its membranes through a defect in the vertebral column

Metalloproteinase: an enzyme with a tightly bound metal ion that catalyzes the hydrolysis of a peptide chain at points well within the chain, not near termini

Methemoglobinemia: the presence of methemoglobin in the circulating blood; methemoglobin is a transformation product of oxyhemoglobin and is useless for respiration

Microphthalmia: abnormal smallness of the eye

Microtia: smallness of the auricle of the ear with a blind or absent external auditory meatus

Milk-to-plasma ratio: the ratio of the concentration of a drug in breastmilk to the concentration in maternal serum

M:P or M/P ratio: abbreviation for the milk-to-plasma ratio

Möbius' syndrome: a developmental bilateral facial paralysis usually associated with oculomotor or other neurologic disorders

Multipara: describes a woman who has given birth at least two times, liveborn or not, weighing 500 g or more, or having an estimated length of gestation of at least 20 weeks

Multiple gestation: a pregnancy with more than one fetus, such as twins

Myometrium: muscular wall of the uterus

Neonate: an infant 28 days of age or less

Nephrosclerosis: induration of the kidney from overgrowth and contraction of the interstitial connective tissue

Newborn: synonym for neonate or neonatal

Neural tube defect: a defect in closure of the neural tube during organogenesis; includes entire spectrum from spina bifida occulta to meningomyelocele

Nitrazine test: a test using pH paper to test for alkaline pH; used to identify amniotic fluid in the vagina suggesting a diagnosis of premature rupture of membranes (PROM) or preterm PROM

Nonstress test: NST; assessment of the fetal heart rate pattern to determine if a fetus is healthy and in a good in utero environment

Nulliparous: describing a woman who has never given birth

Oligohydramnios: the presence of an insufficient amount of amniotic fluid (<300 mL at term); <5 centimeters, see Amniotic fluid index

Oliguria: scanty urine production

Omphalocele: congenital herniation of viscera into the base of the umbilical cord, with a covering membranous sac of peritoneum-amnion; the umbilical cord is inserted into the sac

Organogenesis: the period when organs are formed during pregnancy (34–69 days after the first day of the last menstrual period)

Osteoporosis: reduction in the quantity of bone or atrophy of skeletal tissue

Parametrial: pertaining to the parametrium, the connective tissue of the pelvic floor

Parturition: the process of giving birth; delivery of a baby

Perineum: the area between the thighs extending from the coccyx to the pubis and lying below the pelvic diaphragm; lying between the vulva and the anus in the female

Peripartum: the period immediately before childbirth

Persistent pulmonary hypertension of the newborn: hypertension in the pulmonary circuit

Pheochromocytoma: a functional chromaffinoma, usually benign, derived from adrenal medullary tissue cells and characterized by the secretion of catecholamines, resulting in hypertension, which may be paroxysmal, and associated with attacks of palpitation, headache, nausea, dyspnea, anxiety, pallor, and profuse sweating

Placenta accreta: a condition where chorionic tissue embeds through the decidual lining and into the uterine muscular layer; these placentas cause problems because there is often failure of complete separation and detachment of the placenta from the uterus at delivery, causing massive hemorrhage

Placenta previa (central): a condition in which a complete placenta previa occurs and the central portion of the placenta is directly over the internal cervical os

Placenta previa (complete): a condition in which the lower placental edge completely crosses the internal cervical os

Placenta previa (marginal): a condition in which the lower edge of the placenta is adjacent to the internal cervical os

Placenta previa (partial): a condition in which the lower edge of the placenta partially crosses the internal os from one side

Placenta percreta: a condition in which the chorionic tissue invades through the decidual lining, through the entire muscular layer of the uterus, and reaches the serosal surface or adjacent pelvic organs such as urinary bladder, pelvic vessels, and bowel

Plasmapheresis: removal of whole blood from the body, separation of its cellular elements by centrifugation, and reinfusion of them suspended in saline or some other plasma substitute, thus depleting the body's own plasma without depleting its cells

Pleural effusion: increased amounts of fluid within the pleural cavity, usually due to inflammation

Polycystic kidneys: a progressive disease characterized by formation of multiple cysts of varying size scattered diffusely throughout both kidneys, resulting in compression and destruction of kidney parenchyma, usually with hypertension, gross hematuria, and uremia

Polyhydramnios: too much amniotic fluid (>25 centimeters) (see Amniotic fluid index)

Porphyria: a group of disorders involving heme biosynthesis, characterized by excessive excretion of porphyrins or their precursors

Postpartum: occurring after childbirth, in reference to the mother and usually describing the first 4–6 weeks after parturition

Preeclampsia: development of hypertension with proteinuria or edema or both after the 20th week of pregnancy

Premature rupture of membranes: PROM; rupture of membranes before labor

Preterm premature rupture of membranes: PPROM; rupture of membranes before 37 weeks of gestation

Primigravid: a woman in her first pregnancy

Proteinuria: presence of urinary protein in concentrations greater than 0.3 g in a 24-hour urine collection

Pseudotumor cerebri: a condition of the brain simulating the presence of an intracranial tumor

Pudendal: relating to the external genitals

Puerperal: related to or occurring during childbirth or the period immediately after

Puerperium: the period from the end of labor to the return of uterus to normal size, usually from 3–6 weeks

Pulmonary edema: edema of the lungs

Pulmonary hypoplasia: underdevelopment of the lungs

Pyloric stenosis: stricture or narrowing of the orifice of the pylorus (the muscular tissue surrounding and controlling the outlet of the stomach)

QT prolongation: lengthening of the interval between the start of the Q wave and the end of the T wave in the electrocardiogram

Relative infant dosage: same as weight-adjusted percentage of maternal dosage

Retinopathy: noninflammatory degenerative disease of the retina

Scleroderma: thickening and induration of the skin caused by new collagen formation, with atrophy of pilosebaceous follicles

Scoliosis: abnormal lateral curvature of the vertebral column

Serotonin: a vasoconstrictor, liberated by blood platelets, that inhibits gastric secretion and stimulates smooth muscle

Serotonin syndrome: a constellation of signs and symptoms sometimes observed in newborn infants exposed in utero to selective serotonin reuptake inhibitors and serotonin-norepinephrine reuptake inhibitors; the signs and symptoms resemble those observed with withdrawal

Sjögren's syndrome: keratoconjunctivitis sicca, dryness of mucous membranes, telangiectasias or purpuric spots on the face, and bilateral parotid enlargement

Somatization: the process by which psychological needs are expressed in physical symptoms

Spina bifida: embryologic failure of fusion of one or more vertebral arches

Spina bifida occulta: spina bifida in which there is a spinal defect, but no protrusion of the cord or its membrane, although there is often some abnormality in their development

Spinal analgesia: euphemism for spinal anesthesia; produced by injection of a local anesthetic solution, with or without a narcotic, into the subarachnoid space of the spine

Stippled epiphyses: synonym: dysplasia epiphysialis punctata; abnormal development of a part of a long bone developed from a center of ossification distinct from that of the shaft and separated at first from the latter by a layer of cartilage

Tertiary center: a hospital with personnel to care for high-risk mothers and ill neonates; requires presence of maternal–fetal medicine physicians and neonatologists

Thrombophilia: a disorder of the hemopoietic system in which there is a tendency to the occurrence of thrombosis (blood clots)

Thyrotoxicosis: the state produced by excessive quantities of endogenous or exogenous thyroid hormone

Translabial ultrasound: a form of ultrasound imaging where the covered transducer is placed on the labia to better visualize the cervix and other pelvic organs

Transvaginal ultrasound: a form of ultrasound where a high-frequency ultrasound probe is inserted into the vagina and gently against the cervix to better visualize the cervix and lower uterine segment contents

Thrombin: Factor IIa; an enzyme (proteinase), formed in shed blood, that converts fibrinogen into fibrin by hydrolyzing peptides (and amides and esters) of L-arginine; formed from prothrombin by the action of prothrombinase (factor Xa, another proteinase); causes clotting of blood

Thrombocytopenia: abnormally small number of platelets in the circulating blood

Thrombophilia: a tendency to the occurrence of clot formation

Thymic aplasia: defective development or congenital absence of the thymus gland

Thyroiditis: inflammation of the thyroid gland, often autoimmune mediated, but an infectious process may be involved

Thyrotoxicosis: the state produced by excessive amounts of thyroid hormone

Tocolysis: pharmaceutical intervention to arrest early labor

Tocolytic: any drug used to arrest uterine contractions; often used in an attempt to arrest premature labor contractions

Torsade de pointes: a form of ventricular tachycardia nearly always due to medications and characterized by a long QT interval

Type 2 diabetes: inability to maintain normal glycemic levels due to increases in insulin resistance; also called adult-onset diabetes

Uremia: an excess of urea and other nitrogenous waste in the blood

Vaginitis: inflammation of the vagina

Vaginosis: disease of the vagina, especially one of bacterial infection

Vestibular apparatus: the vestibule of the ear

Weight-adjusted percentage of maternal dosage: the daily dosage of a drug that the infant received in breastmilk divided by the mother's daily dosage, both expressed in mg/kg and multiplied by 100 to create a percentage

Wernicke's encephalopathy: a syndrome secondary to thiamine deficiency that is characterized by disturbances in ocular motility, pupillary alterations, nystagmus, and ataxia with tremors

Index

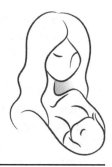

Note: Page numbers followed by t indicate tables; those followed by f indicate figures.